ADVANCES IN
IMMUNOLOGY

CANCER IMMUNOTHERAPY

VOLUME 90

Associate Editors

K. Frank Austen
Division of Rheumatology,
Immunology & Allergy
Harvard Medical School, Boston, Massachusetts, USA

Tasuku Honjo
Graduate School of Medicine and
Faculty of Medicine, Kyoto University
Kyoto, Japan

Fritz Melchers
Department of Cell Biology
University of Basel,
Basel, Switzerland

Jonathan W. Uhr
Department of Microbiology &
Internal Medicine
University of Texas, Dallas, Texas, USA

Emil R. Unanue
Department of Pathology & Immunology
Washington University
St. Louis, Missouri, USA

ADVANCES IN IMMUNOLOGY

CANCER IMMUNOTHERAPY

VOLUME 90

Edited By

James P. Allison
Howard Hughes Medical Institute
Memorial Sloan-Kettering Cancer Center
New York, New York
USA

Glenn Dranoff
Department of Medical Oncology
Dana-Farber Cancer Institute
Boston, Massachusetts
USA

Series Editor

Frederick W. Alt
CBRI Institute for Biomedical Research
Howard Hughes Medical Institute
Children's Hospital Boston
Boston, Massachusetts
USA

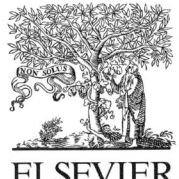

AMSTERDAM • BOSTON • HEIDELBERG • LONDON
NEW YORK • OXFORD • PARIS • SAN DIEGO
SAN FRANCISCO • SINGAPORE • SYDNEY • TOKYO
Academic Press is an imprint of Elsevier

Elsevier Academic Press
525 B Street, Suite 1900, San Diego, California 92101-4495, USA
84 Theobald's Road, London WC1X 8RR, UK

This book is printed on acid-free paper. ∞

Copyright © 2006, Elsevier Ltd. All Rights Reserved.

No part of this publication may be reproduced or transmitted in any form or by any means, electronic or mechanical, including photocopy, recording, or any information storage and retrieval system, without permission in writing from the Publisher.

The appearance of the code at the bottom of the first page of a chapter in this book indicates the Publisher's consent that copies of the chapter may be made for personal or internal use of specific clients. This consent is given on the condition, however, that the copier pay the stated per copy fee through the Copyright Clearance Center, Inc. (www.copyright.com), for copying beyond that permitted by Sections 107 or 108 of the U.S. Copyright Law. This consent does not extend to other kinds of copying, such as copying for general distribution, for advertising or promotional purposes, for creating new collective works, or for resale.
Copy fees for pre-2005 chapters are as shown on the title pages. If no fee code appears on the title page, the copy fee is the same as for current chapters.
0065-2776/2006 $35.00

Permissions may be sought directly from Elsevier's Science & Technology Rights Department in Oxford, UK: phone: (+44) 1865 843830, fax: (+44) 1865 853333, E-mail: permissions@elsevier.co.uk. You may also complete your request on-line via the Elsevier homepage (http://elsevier.com), by selecting "Customer Support" and then "Obtaining Permissions."

For all information on all Academic Press publications
visit our Web site at www.books.elsevier.com

ISBN-13: 978-0-12-022489-0
ISBN-10: 0-12-022489-5

PRINTED IN THE UNITED STATES OF AMERICA
06 07 08 09   9 8 7 6 5 4 3 2 1

**Working together to grow
libraries in developing countries**

www.elsevier.com | www.bookaid.org | www.sabre.org

ELSEVIER   BOOK AID International   Sabre Foundation

Contents

Contributors xi

Preface xv

Cancer Immunosurveillance and Immunoediting: The Roles of Immunity in Suppressing Tumor Development and Shaping Tumor Immunogenicity

Mark J. Smyth, Gavin P. Dunn, and Robert D. Schreiber

1. Introduction 1
2. "Intrinsic" Versus "Extrinsic" Tumor Suppressors 2
3. The Cancer Immunosurveillance Hypothesis: Controversy to Resolution 5
4. Tumor Elimination 7
5. Immunoediting: When Tumor Cells Survive 28
6. Cancer Immunosurveillance/Immunoediting in Humans 32
7. Conclusions 35
   References 36

Mechanisms of Immune Evasion by Tumors

Charles G. Drake, Elizabeth Jaffee, and Drew M. Pardoll

1. Introduction 51
2. Downmodulation of Tumor Antigen Presentation 52
3. Immunologic Barriers Within the Tumor Microenvironment 55
4. Disabled Antigen Presenting Cells 62
5. CD4 T-Cell Tolerance 63
6. Coinhibition 64
7. Regulatory T Cells 66

8. CD8 T-Cell Dysfunction.	68
9. Summary.	69
References	70

Development of Antibodies and Chimeric Molecules for Cancer Immunotherapy

Thomas A. Waldmann and John C. Morris

1. Introduction	84
2. Targets of Monoclonal Antibodies in the Therapy of Cancer	85
3. Monoclonal Antibodies Targeting Host Nonneoplastic Tissues	85
4. Monoclonal Antibodies Targeting Host Immune Cells and Proteins that Act as Inhibitory Checkpoints on the Immune System	87
5. Blockade of CTLA-4 and PD1 Inhibitory Receptors.	88
6. Elimination of $CD4^+$ $CD25^+$ Foxp3 Expressing T Regs (Suppressor T Cells).	89
7. Monoclonal Antibody Targeting of the Inhibitory Cytokine TGF-β.	90
8. Mechanisms of Action of Monoclonal Antibodies	91
9. Engineering Antibodies for Greater Efficacy.	92
10. Genetically Engineered Antibody Fragments for Cancer Immunotherapy	95
11. Unmodified Monoclonal Antibodies Approved by the FDA that Are Directed Toward Neoplastic Cells.	96
12. Antibodies Armed with Cytokines, Chemotherapeutic Agents, Toxins, and Radionuclides Cytokine Armed Monoclonal Antibodies.	107
13. Antibodies Armed with Chemotherapeutic Agents	107
14. Immunotoxins for the Treatment of Cancer	108
15. Systemic Radioimmunotherapy with Monoclonal Antibodies	112
16. Conclusions and Future Prospects.	118
References	121

Induction of Tumor Immunity Following Allogeneic Stem Cell Transplantation

Catherine J. Wu and Jerome Ritz

1. Introduction	134
2. Reconstitution of Donor Hematopoiesis Following Allogeneic HSCT	134

3. Sequence of Immune Reconstitution Following
   Allogeneic HSCT 136
4. The Graft-Versus-Leukemia Effect 138
5. Donor Lymphocyte Infusions Induce GVL Responses After
   Allogeneic HSCT 141
6. The Central Role of Donor T Cells as Mediators of GVL 143
7. Target Antigens of Donor T Cells After Allogeneic HSCT 146
8. Donor Natural Killer Cells as Mediators of GVL 150
9. Donor B Cells as Mediators of GVL 154
10. Future Directions 158
    References 160

Vaccination for Treatment and Prevention of Cancer in Animal Models

Federica Cavallo, Rienk Offringa, Sjoerd H. van der Burg, Guido Forni, and Cornelis J. M. Melief

1. Introduction 176
2. Synthetic Exact MHC Class I Binding Peptide Vaccines for
   Induction of Protective $CD8^+$ Cytotoxic T-Cell Responses
   in Mouse Models 177
3. Therapy of Established Mouse Tumors by Treatment with
   Synthetic Vaccines, in Particular Long Peptides 178
4. Clinical Trials with Synthetic Peptide-Based Cancer Vaccines 181
5. DC Immunotherapy 182
6. Therapeutic Interventions Counteracting Tumor-Induced
   Immunoregulation 183
7. Genetically Modified Mice that Develop Tumors 185
8. Mice Transgenic for Her2 Oncogene 186
9. BALB-*neu*T Mice as a Study Model for Mammary Cancer 188
10. DNA Vaccination Inhibits Her2 Mammary Carcinogenesis 191
11. The Mode of EC-TM Plasmid Delivery is Decisive for
    Vaccine Efficacy 193
12. The Limitations of DNA Vaccination and How They
    Can Be Overcome 196
13. Coordinated Low-Avidity Mechanisms 199
14. Cure Versus Control of Her2 Lesions 204
15. Conclusions 205
    References 206

Unraveling the Complex Relationship Between Cancer Immunity and Autoimmunity: Lessons from Melanoma and Vitiligo

Hiroshi Uchi, Rodica Stan, Mary Jo Turk, Manuel E. Engelhorn, Gabrielle A. Rizzuto, Stacie M. Goldberg, Jedd D. Wolchok, and Alan N. Houghton

1. Introduction 216
2. Immune Ignorance and Tolerance 217
3. Melanoma and Vitiligo 219
4. Active Immunization with Differentiation Antigens as Altered Self.. 222
5. Passive Immunization with Antibodies Against Differentiation Antigens...................................... 226
6. Adoptive Transfer of $CD8^+$ T Cells Specific for Differentiation Antigens in Adoptive Immunotherapy 228
7. Blockade of CTLA-4... 228
8. Overcoming Effects of Suppressor Populations of T Cells 229
9. Dendritic Cells as Adjuvants 230
10. Mouse Model of Spontaneous Melanoma-Associated Vitiligo..... 230
11. Clinical Trials in Melanoma 231
12. Conclusions... 233
    References 234

Immunity to Melanoma Antigens: From Self-Tolerance to Immunotherapy

Craig L. Slingluff, Jr., Kimberly A. Chianese-Bullock, Timothy N. J. Bullock, William W. Grosh, David W. Mullins, Lisa Nichols, Walter Olson, Gina Petroni, Mark Smolkin, and Victor H. Engelhard

1. Introduction 244
2. Molecular Definition of Tumor Antigens Recognized by CD8 T Cells 245
3. Why Study Peptide Vaccines? 246
4. Clinical Studies with Peptide Vaccines....................... 248
5. Vaccination with Single Melanoma Peptide and Nonspecific Helper Peptide in Adjuvant 248
6. Evaluation of Immune Responses in the Sentinel Immunized Node 250

7. Vaccination with Peptides in Adjuvant Is More Immunogenic than a Dendritic Cell Vaccine Using Monocyte Derived Immature DC Pulsed with Peptides 250
8. Low-Dose IL-2 Administered Early with Multipeptide Vaccine Does Not Augment Immunogenicity 251
9. Expanding the Repertoire of Melanoma Reactivity Using Multipeptide Vaccines 252
10. *Ex Vivo* Analyses of T-Cell Responses to Class I MHC Restricted Peptides................................. 259
11. Modulation of Responses by Combination of CD4 and CD8 T-Cell Vaccination, and Modulation of Regulatory Function 260
12. Cancer Vaccine Development Requires Elucidation of Biology of the Host–Tumor Relationship in Human and Murine Systems, *In Vivo* and *In Vitro*.................. 265
13. A Murine Model to Evaluate Immunity to the MDP-Derived Peptide Ag from Tyrosinase........................ 266
14. Nature of Self-Tolerance to $\underline{m}TyR_{369}$ and Its Effect on Tumor Control 267
15. MDP-Specific Immune Responses in Tolerant Mice Enable Control of Tumor Outgrowth 273
16. Peptide-Pulsed Exogenous DC as a Vehicle to Influence the Quality of the Tumor-Specific Immune Response 275
17. Summary of Preclinical and Clinical Studies and Future Directions...................................... 282
References 284

Checkpoint Blockade in Cancer Immunotherapy

Alan J. Korman, Karl S. Peggs, and James P. Allison

1. Introduction 297
2. The Extended CD28:B7 Immunoglobulin Superfamily 300
3. Preclinical Models of Checkpoint Blockade as Tumor Immunotherapy 310
4. Clinical Trials of CTLA-4 Blockade: Overview 317
5. Other Potential Coinhibitory Targets for Checkpoint Blockade ... 323
6. Conclusions... 328
References 329

Combinatorial Cancer Immunotherapy
F. Stephen Hodi and Glenn Dranoff

1. Introduction 341
2. Endogenous Host Responses 342
3. Enhancing Tumor Antigen Presentation 343
4. GM-CSF Secreting Tumor Cell Vaccines 344
5. Targets of Vaccine-Induced Tumor Destruction 347
6. Cytotoxic T Lymphocyte Antigen-4 Antibody Blockade 352
7. Combination Immunotherapy: The Next Paradigm? 358
   References 358

Index.. 369
Contents of Recent Volumes 379

Contributors

Numbers in parenthesis indicated the pages on which the authors' contributions begin.

James P. Allison (297), Howard Hughes Medical Institute, Memorial Sloan-Kettering Cancer Center, New York, New York

Timothy N. J. Bullock (243), Departments of Surgery and Microbiology, Public Health Sciences, Medicine, Pathology, Human Immune Therapy Center, Beirne Carter Center for Immunology Research, University of Virginia, Charlottesville, Virginia

Federica Cavallo (175), Department of Clinical and Biological Sciences, University of Torino, Torino, Italy

Kimberly A. Chianese-Bullock (243), Departments of Surgery and Microbiology, Public Health Sciences, Medicine, Pathology, Human Immune Therapy Center, Beirne Carter Center for Immunology Research, University of Virginia, Charlottesville, Virginia

Charles G. Drake (51), Sidney Kimmel Comprehensive Cancer Center at Johns Hopkins, Baltimore, Maryland

Glenn Dranoff (341), Department of Medical Oncology, Dana-Farber Cancer Institute, Boston, Massachusetts

Gavin P. Dunn (1), Department of Pathology and Immunology, Center for Immunology, Washington University School of Medicine, St. Louis, Missouri

Victor H. Engelhard (243), Departments of Surgery and Microbiology, Public Health Sciences, Medicine, Pathology, Human Immune Therapy Center, Beirne Carter Center for Immunology Research, University of Virginia, Charlottesville, Virginia

Manuel E. Engelhorn (215), Swim Across America Laboratory, Memorial Sloan-Kettering Cancer Center, 1275 York Avenue, New York, New York

Guido Forni (175), Department of Clinical and Biological Sciences, University of Torino, Torino, Italy

Stacie M. Goldberg (215), Swim Across America Laboratory, Memorial Sloan-Kettering Cancer Center, 1275 York Avenue, New York, New York

William W. Grosh (243), Departments of Surgery and Microbiology, Public Health Sciences, Medicine, Pathology, Human Immune Therapy Center, Beirne Carter Center for Immunology Research, University of Virginia, Charlottesville, Virginia

F. Stephen Hodi (341), Department of Medical Oncology, Dana-Farber Cancer Institute, Boston, Massachusetts

Alan N. Houghton (215), Swim Across America Laboratory, Memorial Sloan-Kettering Cancer Center, 1275 York Avenue, New York, New York; Weill Medical and Graduate Schools of Cornell University, 1300 York Avenue, New York, New York

Elizabeth Jaffee (51), Sidney Kimmel Comprehensive Cancer Center at Johns Hopkins, Baltimore, Maryland

Alan J. Korman (297), Medarex Inc., Milpitas, California

Cornelis J. M. Melief (175), Leiden University Medical Center, Leiden, The Netherlands

John C. Morris (83), Metabolism Branch, Center for Cancer Research, National Cancer Institute NIH, Bethesda, Maryland

David W. Mullins (243), Departments of Surgery and Microbiology, Public Health Sciences, Medicine, Pathology, Human Immune Therapy Center, Beirne Carter Center for Immunology Research, University of Virginia, Charlottesville, Virginia

Lisa Nichols (243), Departments of Surgery and Microbiology, Public Health Sciences, Medicine, Pathology, Human Immune Therapy Center, Beirne Carter Center for Immunology Research, University of Virginia, Charlottesville, Virginia

Rienk Offringa (175), Leiden University Medical Center, Leiden, The Netherlands

Walter Olson (243), Departments of Surgery and Microbiology, Public Health Sciences, Medicine, Pathology, Human Immune Therapy Center, Beirne Carter Center for Immunology Research, University of Virginia, Charlottesville, Virginia

Drew M. Pardoll (51), Sidney Kimmel Comprehensive Cancer Center at Johns Hopkins, Baltimore, Maryland

Karl S. Peggs (297), Howard Hughes Medical Institute, Memorial Sloan-Kettering Cancer Center, New York, New York

Gina Petroni (243), Departments of Surgery and Microbiology, Public Health Sciences, Medicine, Pathology, Human Immune Therapy Center, Beirne Carter Center for Immunology Research, University of Virginia, Charlottesville, Virginia

Jerome Ritz (133), Cancer Vaccine Center, Department of Medical Oncology, Dana-Farber Cancer Institute, Boston, Massachusetts

CONTRIBUTORS

Gabrielle A. Rizzuto (215), Swim Across America Laboratory, Memorial Sloan-Kettering Cancer Center, 1275 York Avenue, New York, New York; Weill Medical and Graduate Schools of Cornell University, 1300 York Avenue, New York, New York

Robert D. Schreiber (1), Department of Pathology and Immunology, Center for Immunology, Washington University School of Medicine, St. Louis, Missouri

Craig L. Slingluff, Jr. (243), Departments of Surgery and Microbiology, Public Health Sciences, Medicine, Pathology, Human Immune Therapy Center, Beirne Carter Center for Immunology Research, University of Virginia, Charlottesville, Virginia

Mark Smolkin (243), Departments of Surgery and Microbiology, Public Health Sciences, Medicine, Pathology, Human Immune Therapy Center, Beirne Carter Center for Immunology Research, University of Virginia, Charlottesville, Virginia

Mark J. Smyth (1), Cancer Immunology Program, Peter MacCallum Cancer Centre, East Melbourne, 3002 Victoria, Australia

Rodica Stan (215), Swim Across America Laboratory, Memorial Sloan-Kettering Cancer Center, 1275 York Avenue, New York, New York

Mary Jo Turk (215), Dartmouth-Hitchcock Medical Center, Lebanon, New Hampshire

Hiroshi Uchi (215), Swim Across America Laboratory, Memorial Sloan-Kettering Cancer Center, 1275 York Avenue, New York, New York

Sjoerd H. van der Burg (175), Leiden University Medical Center, Leiden, The Netherlands

Thomas A. Waldmann (83), Metabolism Branch, Center for Cancer Research, National Cancer Institute NIH, Bethesda, Maryland

Jedd D. Wolchok (215), Swim Across America Laboratory, Memorial Sloan-Kettering Cancer Center, 1275 York Avenue, New York, New York; Weill Medical and Graduate Schools of Cornell University, 1300 York Avenue, New York, New York

Catherine J. Wu (133), Cancer Vaccine Center, Department of Medical Oncology, Dana-Farber Cancer Institute, Boston, Massachusetts

Preface

Recent investigations in cancer immunology have yielded important insights into the host–tumor relationship. The development of genetic and biochemical strategies to identify cancer antigens has led to the realization that most tumor-bearing hosts mount innate and adaptive antitumor responses. While these endogenous reactions play a decisive role in shaping the immune characteristics of cancer cells, the formation of clinically evident tumors indicates a failure of host defense. The mechanisms underlying tumor escape have begun to be clarified, however, and this knowledge in turn has created a framework for devising therapeutic schemes that overcome specific immune defects. The clinical activity of human monoclonal antibodies and donor lymphocyte infusions highlights the ability of adaptive immune effector pathways to mediate therapeutic benefits.

In this volume of *Advances in Immunology*, nine groups of investigators working in murine and/or human systems contribute their perspectives on many key problems in cancer immunology. Smyth, Dunn, and Schreiber discuss the impact of endogenous responses on tumor formation, highlighting the ability of host immunity to sculpt the phenotypes of emerging tumor cells. Drake, Jaffee, and Pardoll analyze the pathways of immune escape and illustrate the ways in which unresolved inflammation promotes disease progression. Waldmann and Morris review the therapeutic efficacy of monoclonal antibodies and chimeric proteins in diverse human cancers. Wu and Ritz detail the immune mechanisms involved in the curative effects of allogeneic bone marrow transplantation for hematologic malignancies. Cavallo and colleagues discuss the formulation of prophylactic and therapeutic cancer vaccinations in murine models. Uchi and associates examine the interplay of cancer immunity and autoimmunity using malignant melanoma as a model system. Slingluff and colleagues describe the identification and therapeutic applications of peptides derived from melanoma differentiation antigens. Korman, Peggs, and Allison explore the manipulation of T-cell activation checkpoints as a strategy for cancer immunotherapy. Hodi and Dranoff discuss combinatorial treatments that couple dendritic cell maturation and inhibition of negative immune regulation.

Together, these reviews provide a broad assessment of the current state of research in cancer immunology. We hope that this volume will serve as a useful resource to both students and investigators and help stimulate new efforts aimed at actualizing the considerable potential of cancer immunotherapy.

James Allison
Glenn Dranoff

Cancer Immunosurveillance and Immunoediting: The Roles of Immunity in Suppressing Tumor Development and Shaping Tumor Immunogenicity

Mark J. Smyth,[*] Gavin P. Dunn,[†] and Robert D. Schreiber[†]

[*]Cancer Immunology Program, Peter MacCallum Cancer Centre,
East Melbourne, 3002 Victoria, Australia
[†]Department of Pathology and Immunology, Center for Immunology, Washington University
School of Medicine, St. Louis, Missouri

Abstract.. 1
1. Introduction... 1
2. "Intrinsic" Versus "Extrinsic" Tumor Suppressors 2
3. The Cancer Immunosurveillance Hypothesis: Controversy to Resolution 5
4. Tumor Elimination 7
5. Immunoediting: When Tumor Cells Survive.............................. 28
6. Cancer Immunosurveillance/Immunoediting in Humans.............. 32
7. Conclusions... 35
   References... 36

Abstract

Cellular transformation and tumor development result from an accumulation of mutational and epigenetic changes that alter normal cell growth and survival pathways. For the last 100 years, there has been a vigorous debate as to whether the unmanipulated immune system can detect and eliminate such altered host derived cells despite the fact that cancer cells frequently express either abnormal proteins or abnormal levels of normal cellular proteins that function as tumor antigens. In this review, we discuss the current state of this argument and point out some of the recent key experiments demonstrating that immunity not only protects the host from cancer development (i.e., provides a cancer immunosurveillance function) but also can promote tumor growth, sometimes by generating more aggressive tumors. The terminology "cancer immunoediting" has been used to describe this dual host protective and tumor promoting action of immunity, and herein we summarize the ever-increasing experimental and clinical data that support the validity of this concept.

1. Introduction

After a century of controversy, the notion that the immune system regulates cancer development is experiencing a new resurgence. For the last five decades much of the debate centered on the validity of the cancer immunosurveillance hypothesis originally proposed by Burnet and Thomas (Burnet, 1957; Thomas, 1959) and reflected the inherent difficulties of experimentally revealing whether natural immune defense mechanisms could protect the host against the development of cancers of nonviral origin. Recently, however, an overwhelming amount of definitive experimental data from mouse models together with compelling clinical data from human patients have demonstrated that a cancer immunosurveillance process that functions as an effective extrinsic tumor suppressor mechanism indeed exists. At the same time there has been a growing recognition that tumor elimination represents only one dimension of the complex relationship between the immune system and cancer (Dunn et al., 2002, 2004a,b; Schreiber et al., 2004; Shankaran et al., 2001). When the immune system fails to eliminate all tumor cells, tumors with reduced immunogenicity may emerge that are capable of escaping immune recognition and destruction (Shankaran et al., 2001; Smyth et al., 2000a; Svane et al., 1996; Takeda et al., 2002). This combination of host-protective and tumor-promoting functions of the immune system throughout tumor development has been termed "cancer immunoediting" (Dunn et al., 2002, 2004a,b; Shankaran et al., 2001) and has been envisaged as a dynamic process composed of three phases: elimination, equilibrium, and escape. Elimination embodies the classical concept of cancer immunosurveillance, equilibrium is the period of immune-mediated latency after incomplete tumor destruction, and escape refers to the final outgrowth of tumors that have outstripped immunological restraints of the equilibrium phase. This review represents an extension of our previous review articles (Dunn et al., 2002, 2004a,b; Smyth et al., 2001c) and not only reflects a convergence of thinking by our two laboratories about the process of cancer immunoediting but also our collective optimism that an enhanced understanding of naturally occurring immune system/tumor interactions will lead to the development of more effective immunologically based cancer therapies.

2. "Intrinsic" Versus "Extrinsic" Tumor Suppressors

Cancers arise by an evolutionary process during which somatic cells mutate and escape the restraints that normally rein in their untoward expansion. Suppressing the emergence of such dysregulated autonomously growing cells is an evolutionary necessity of metazoans, particularly in large, long-lived organisms where cells in regenerative tissues retain the potential for neoplastic chaos throughout life. Consequently, multiple cellular mechanisms have arisen to forestall uncontrolled cell division (Fig. 1). A variety of "intrinsic" tumor-suppressive mechanisms exist that trigger apoptosis, repair, or senescence, should proliferation become aberrant. The primary cell death program

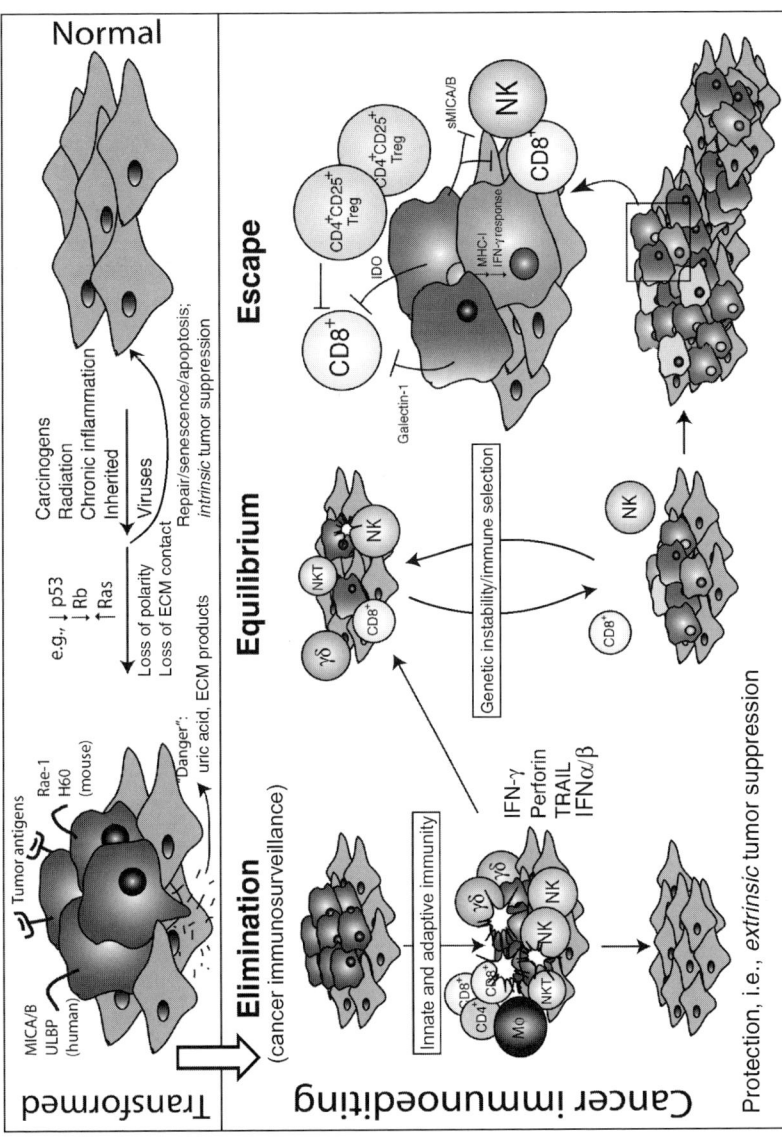

Figure 1 Examples of intrinsic vs. extrinsic tumor suppression. A variety of intrinsic tumor suppressor mechanisms exist to control aberrant cell division. Transformed cells escaping intrinsic control are then subjected to extrinsic tumor suppressor mechanisms. The immune system can function as an extrinsic tumor suppressor: by detecting and eliminating developing tumors long before they become clinically apparent. This function has been termed cancer immunosurveillance and is now known as the elimination phase of a broader process that has been termed cancer immunoediting (Dunn et al., 2002, 2004a,b; Shankaran et al., 2001). Cancer immunoediting takes into account the observation that the immune system not only protects the host against tumor development but also can promote tumor growth. Cancer immunoediting is now envisaged as a process composed of three phases: elimination (i.e., cancer immunosurveillance), equilibrium (a phase of tumor dormancy where tumor cells and immunity enter into a dynamic equilibrium that keeps tumor expansion in check), and escape (where tumor cells emerge that either display reduced immunogenicities or engage immunosuppressive mechanisms to attenuate the antitumor immune responses leading to the appearance of clinically detectable, progressively growing tumors). These phases have been termed the three Es of cancer immunoediting.

integrating the responses to the signals of survival factors, cell stress and injury relies on mitochondria (Cory et al., 2003; Danial and Korsmeyer, 2004; Green and Kroemer, 2004). Mitochondria sequester a variety of proapoptotic effectors that, when released, trigger cellular demise by terminal activation of executioner caspases. The balance between the proapoptotic Bax/Bak proteins and their anti-apoptotic Bcl-2/Bcl$_{XL}$ cousins determines mitochondrial permeability. Transcriptional and posttranscriptional regulation of the Bcl2/BH3-only family members and the expression of death-effector components and a class of caspase inhibitors known as "inhibitors of apoptosis" (IAPs) control the process. In contrast, a second cell-death pathway is activated through ligation of cell-surface "death receptors," such as Fas/CD95, tumor necrosis factor receptor, and tumor necrosis factor apoptosis-inducing ligand (TRAIL) receptor 2 (TRAIL-R2, DR5) (Peter and Krammer, 2003). When ligated by corresponding members of the TNF superfamily, these receptors form the "death-inducing signaling complex" (DISC) that activates the apical caspase-8.

A number of cellular proteins function as sensors for perturbations caused by potentially mutagenic insults and can act directly on the apoptotic-effector machinery, that is, they function as intrinsic tumor suppressors (Lowe et al., 2004). For example, in response to a variety of cellular stresses, such as DNA damage, hypoxia, and nutrient deprivation, the transcription factor p53 engages cellular programs for apoptosis, senescence, and repair (Fridman and Lowe, 2003; Mihara et al., 2003). Oncogenes can also target various components of the cell-death machinery independently of p53. The relative importance of p53-independent versus p53-dependent apoptotic mechanisms in suppressing tumorigenesis varies depending on tumor type and on the nature and sequence of oncogenic mutations within any specific cell undergoing transformation. Activated oncogenes can also trigger cellular senescence, a state characterized by permanent cell-cycle arrest and specific changes in morphology and gene expression that distinguish the process from quiescence (reversible cell-cycle arrest) (Serrano et al., 1997). Escape from oncogene-induced senescence is a prerequisite for the transformation of cells. For maintenance, cancers must acquire cooperating lesions that uncouple mitogenic Ras signaling from senescence. In general terms, both senescence and apoptosis act as potent barriers to the further evolution of any preneoplastic cell.

Alternatively at least three general "extrinsic" mechanisms have been identified by which cells and their adjacent tissues "sense" the presence of cancerous cells. One depends on the obligatory social dependency of cells for specific trophic signals in the microenvironment that quell their innate suicidal tendencies (e.g., epithelial cell—extracellular matrix (ECM) association). In this context, excessive proliferation leads to the disruption of the normal tissue architecture and separation from the ECM, triggering a cell death process called "anoikis." The second appears to involve key links between cell polarity genes that control cellular junctions and cell proliferation (Humbert et al., 2003). The third mechanism involves the detection and elimination and/or cytostasis of transformed cells by leukocytes. These immune system derived effector cells employ extremely diverse mechanisms to kill tumor targets that involve both mitochondrial and cell death receptor pathways. In combination, these diverse intrinsic and extrinsic tumor-suppressing mechanisms are remarkably effective and specific. On average, cancers arise less than once in a human lifetime despite trillions of potential target cells, each harboring hundreds of susceptible cancer-causing genes and all subject to a significant mutation rate.

3. The Cancer Immunosurveillance Hypothesis: Controversy to Resolution

The notion that the immune system protected the host from neoplastic disease was first proposed by Paul Ehrlich (1909). Interestingly, at a similar point in time (1891), William B. Coley made the amazing observation that some cancer patients who developed bacterial infections also experienced tumor regression. Coley subsequently injected cultures of heat-inactivated bacteria or spent bacterial culture supernatants into cancer patients with advanced disease, and some patients experienced marked regression of their tumor and prolonged survival after the treatment. "Coley's toxins" (Coley, 1991) as we now know contained bacterial products with strong immunomodulatory potential. Yet the concept of immune control of cancer was not extensively pursued until some 40 years later (1950s) after Medawar and colleagues clarified the role of cellular components of the immune system in recognizing and mediating allograft rejection (Medawar, 1944). This work cast some doubt on the existence of tumor-specific immunity because it argued that experimental tumors were probably seen simply as foreign grafts. However, soon after, with the development of inbred strains of mice, it was possible to examine whether tumors arising in such animals were immunologically distinguishable from normal tissues in the same strain. The demonstration that syngeneic mice immunized against a tumor rejected a secondary challenge with the same tumor cells but did not react against the corresponding nontransformed cells functionally documented the existence of tumor-specific antigens and thereby showed that tumor-specific immune responses did indeed occur (Klein, 1966; Old and Boyse, 1964). Together this work showed that immune cells could detect the presence of transformed tissue either by recognizing specific structures on the tumor cell surface or by responding to soluble molecules secreted by the tumor itself. On the basis of an emerging understanding of the cellular basis of transplantation and tumor immunity (Klein, 1966; Medawar, 1944;

Old and Boyse, 1964), Burnet and Thomas predicted that lymphocytes were responsible for eliminating continuously arising, nascent-transformed cells and thus formally introduced the cancer immunosurveillance hypothesis (Burnet, 1964, 1970, 1971; Thomas, 1959, 1982).

One logical prediction that stemmed from these initial and subsequent experiments is that hosts with impaired or suppressed immune systems should display higher cancer incidences than their immunocompetent counterparts (Kaplan, 1971; Stutman, 1975). Early on, several groups tried to test this prediction using mice that had undergone neonatal thymectomy to induce immunosuppression but the results were inconsistent (Burstein and Law, 1971; Grant and Miller, 1965; Johnson, 1968; Nomoto and Takeya, 1969; Sanford et al., 1973). Mice rendered immunodeficient in this manner demonstrated an increased susceptibility to virus-induced tumors and spontaneous lymphomas compared with immunocompetent mice. However, the prevailing view was that this result reflected the greater susceptibility of immunocompromised hosts to infections by oncogenic viruses. Furthermore, others explained the greater frequency of lymphomas to the establishment of a state of chronic infection resulting in unresolved antigenic stimulation, increased lymphocyte proliferation, somatic mutation and ultimately to lymphoma formation (Klein, 1973; Stutman, 1975). Perhaps the strongest challenges to the validity of the cancer immunosurveillance hypothesis came from the observations that CBA/H strain nu/nu (nude athymic) mice did not form carcinogen [methylcholanthrene (MCA)]-induced tumors either earlier or more frequently than their immunocompetent littermates (Stutman, 1974) and that incidences of spontaneous, nonviral tumors were similar between nude and wild-type mice (Outzen et al., 1975; Rygaard and Povlsen, 1974a,b; Stutman, 1979). Although these results were used to strongly argue against the cancer immunosurveillance hypothesis, we now appreciate that there were several experimental design problems that the investigators could not have known at the time. Specifically, it is now known that nude mice are not totally immunocompromised [they still have nonthymic-dependent T cell populations and an innate immune system (Hunig and Bevan, 1980; Ikehara et al., 1984; Maleckar and Sherman, 1987)]. Furthermore, since CBA/H strain mice produce a very high specific activity isoform of the aryl hydoxylase enzyme needed to convert MCA into its carcinogenic form these mice are highly sensitive to chemical carcinogen-induced tumor formation (Heidelberger, 1975), and thus immunity to sarcoma may have been overwhelmed in this strain. Finally, the tumor monitoring periods of 3–7 months were too short to detect spontaneous tumor formation. Only recently, with the development of gene targeting and transgenic mouse technologies and the capacity to produce highly specific blocking monoclonal antibodies (mAb) to particular immune components, has the cancer immunosurveillance hypothesis become testable in unequivocal, molecularly defined murine models of immunodeficiency. Over the past 15 years, the use of these improved *in vivo* mouse cancer models and observations in humans have provided strong and convincing data that rekindled interest in the cancer immunosurveillance hypothesis (Dunn *et al.*, 2002, 2004a,b; Smyth *et al.*, 2001c).

However, despite strong evidence supporting the existence of a functional cancer immunosurveillance process, immunocompetent individuals still develop cancers that are refractory to many treatment approaches. This clinical reality may be explained by the failure of the initial host innate and adaptive immune responses to eradicate all the transformed cells. This failure in the face of continued immune pressure favors the outgrowth of tumors with reduced immunogenicity. The term "cancer immunoediting" has been used to emphasize the dual roles of immunity in both eliminating and shaping neoplastic disease during periods of equilibrium and escape (Dunn *et al.*, 2002, 2004a,b; Shankaran *et al.*, 2001). The elimination, equilibrium, and escape phases of this process are described in more detail in the following sections. In particular, we focus on the leukocytes involved, the methods by which leukocytes recognize cellular transformation, and the effector functions used to control, eliminate, and sculpt tumors.

4. Tumor Elimination

4.1. Synopsis of the Tumor Elimination Phase of Cancer Immunoediting

The elimination phase encompasses the original concept of cancer immunosurveillance since it represents the most complete form of the immunoediting process without progression to the two subsequent phases. As an extrinsic tumor suppressor, we envisage that the immune system manifests its effects only after transformed cells have circumvented their intrinsic tumor-suppressor mechanisms (Macleod, 2000). However, in reality, triggers such as infection with potentially oncogenic viruses may stimulate immunity concurrently with the activation of intrinsic tumor suppressor mechanisms. Immunologic rejection of a developing tumor, as in host defense to microbial pathogens, likely requires an integrated response involving both the innate and adaptive arms of the immune system (Fig. 2). We propose that initiation of the antitumor immune response occurs when cells of the innate immune system become alerted to the presence of a growing tumor (Fig. 2A), at least in part owing to the local tissue disruption that occurs as a result of angiogenesis (Carmeliet and

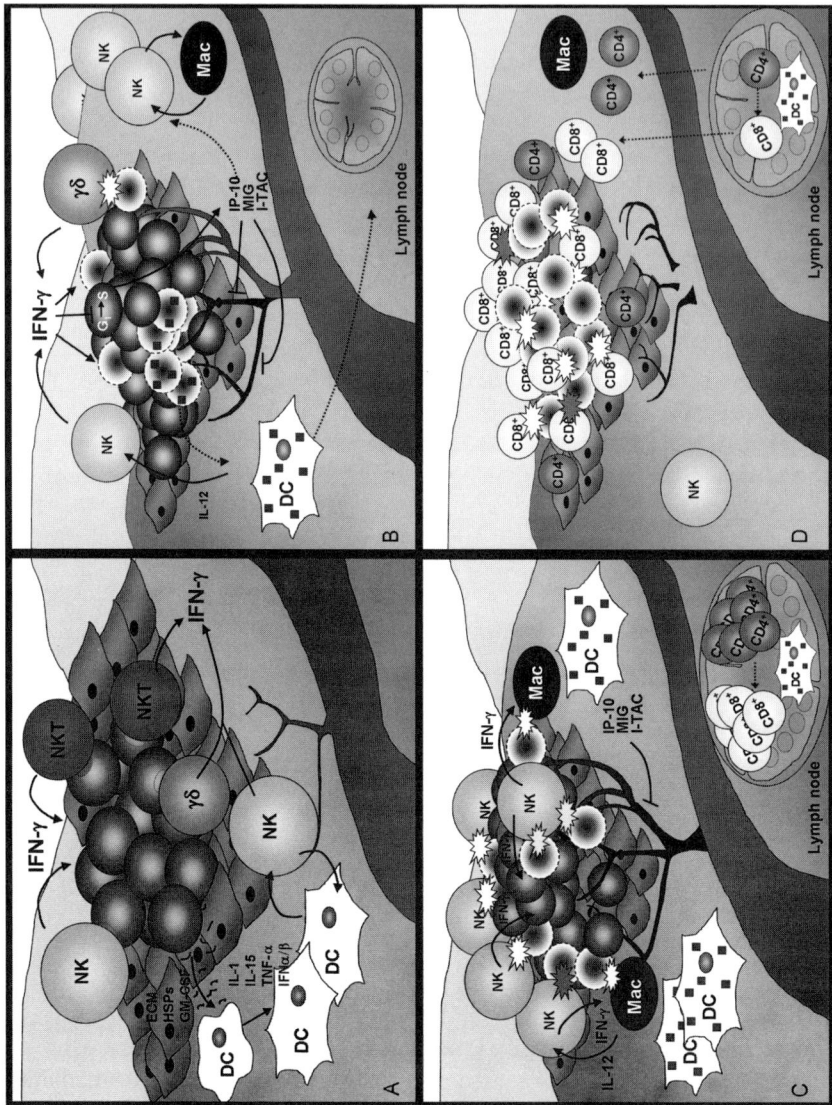

Figure 2 A proposed cellular and molecular model for the elimination phase of cancer immunoediting. The events that are depicted in each panel are described in the text.

Jain, 2000; Hanahan and Folkman, 1996) or tissue-invasive growth (Hanahan and Weinberg, 2000; Sternlicht and Werb, 2001). The stromal remodeling induced during these processes could produce proinflammatory molecules that, together with chemokines that may be produced by the tumor cells themselves (Vicari and Caux, 2002), summon cells of the innate immune system to this new source of local "danger" (Matzinger, 1994). Consistent with the "danger model" (Matzinger, 1994), it is possible that dendritic cells (DCs) act as sentinel cells for monitoring tissue stress, damage and/or transformation, and danger signals can take the form of heat-shock proteins (HSPs) (released as a result of tumor-cell damage or necrosis), extracellular matrix breakdown products or proinflammatory factors (including cytokines released by degenerating tumor cells and reactive host innate cells). Some of these cytokines (e.g., interleukin-1 (IL-1), TNF-α, type I IFN, granulocyte-macrophage colony-stimulating factor (GM-CSF), and IL-15) can promote DC differentiation and activity by multiple mechanisms, including increased cross talk between DCs and NK cells, and later DCs and T cells.

NK cells, macrophages, $\gamma\delta^+$ T cells, and/or NKT cells may be immediately recruited to the "danger" site and recognize molecules, such as the stress ligands for NKG2D, that have been induced on tumor cells either by the incipient inflammation or the cellular transformation process itself (Fig. 2B). In addition, T cells and NKT cells may recognize developing tumors via TCR interaction with either MHC/tumor associated peptide complexes or glycolipid-CD1 complexes expressed on tumor cells, respectively (Smyth et al., 2002). These immune cells may then employ cytotoxic effector mechanisms to eliminate the transformed cell(s) and secrete IFNs that control tumor growth and amplify the immune response by a variety of mechanisms. The initial IFN-γ released at the tumor site could then induce the local production of chemokines that recruit more cells of the innate immune system to the tumor. Products generated during remodeling of the extracellular matrix may induce a feedback loop between tumor-infiltrating macrophages [to produce IL-12 (Hodge-Dufour et al., 1997)] and tumor-infiltrating NK cells (IFN-γ) (Bancroft et al., 1991). Additionally, a number of IFN-γ-dependent processes including anti-proliferative (Bromberg et al., 1996), proapoptotic (Kumar et al., 1997), and angiostatic (Coughlin et al., 1998; Luster and Leder, 1993; Qin and Blankenstein, 2000) effects may also occur that result in the killing of a proportion of the tumor. Macrophages, activated by IFN-γ that express tumoricidal products such as reactive oxygen and reactive nitrogen intermediates (MacMicking et al., 1997; Schreiber et al., 1983) and NK cells activated either by IFN-γ or via engagement of their activating receptors may kill tumor cells via TRAIL-dependent (Smyth et al., 2001a; Takeda et al., 2001) or perforin-dependent (Hayakawa et al., 2002) mechanisms, respectively.

In the next phase, tumor antigens liberated by a variety of cell death pathways and in the context of a milieu of innate immune signals drive the development of tumor-specific adaptive immune responses (Fig. 2C). Immature DCs that have been recruited to the tumor site become activated either by exposure to the cytokine milieu created during the ongoing attack on the tumor by innate immunity or by interacting with tumor-infiltrating NK cells (Gerosa et al., 2002). The activated DCs may then acquire tumor antigens either directly by ingestion of tumor cell apoptotic bodies or via indirect mechanisms involving transfer to DCs of complexes of tumor cell derived heat shock proteins and tumor antigens (Li et al., 2002; Srivastava, 2002). Dendritic cells can then acquire a highly activated mature phenotype and, in response to distinct chemokines and/or cytokines, migrate to the lymph nodes (Sallusto et al., 2000) where they induce the activation of naïve tumor-specific Th1 $CD4^+$ T cells. Th1 cells facilitate the development of tumor-specific $CD8^+$ CTL induced via cross-presentation of antigenic tumor peptides on DC MHC class I molecules (Huang et al., 1994). In some cases, peptides derived from tumor-associated antigens are presented to $CD4^+$ or $CD8^+$ T cells in the context of MHC class-II or class-I molecules, respectively, and the activation of B cells may also occur.

In the last phase, the development of tumor-specific adaptive immunity provides the host with a capacity to completely eliminate the developing tumor (Fig. 2D). Tumor-specific $CD4^+$ and $CD8^+$ T cells home to the tumor site, where they participate in the killing of antigen-positive tumor cells. $CD4^+$ T cells produce IL-2 that, together with host cell production of IL-15, helps to maintain the function and viability of the tumor-specific $CD8^+$ T cells. Tumor-specific $CD8^+$ T cells will efficiently recognize their tumor targets [owing to the enhanced immunogenicity of tumor cells that have been exposed to the IFN-γ produced (Shankaran et al., 2001)] and will induce tumor cell death by both direct and indirect mechanisms. It is likely that these $CD8^+$ T cells directly kill many of the tumor cells in vivo. However, these cells will also produce large amounts of IFN-γ following interaction with their tumor targets and thus might also induce tumor cell cytostasis and killing by the IFN-γ-dependent mechanisms of cell cycle inhibition, apoptosis, angiostasis, and induction of macrophage tumoricidal activity. These two scenarios are not mutually exclusive and most likely occur concomitantly; however, their relative contributions may vary among different tumors. Thus, the elimination phase of cancer immunoediting (i.e., the cancer immunosurveillance phase) is an ever-ongoing process that must be repeated each time antigenically distinct neoplastic cells arise. For this reason, it is particularly noteworthy that cancer is more prevalent in aged populations where immune system functions and therefore, cancer immunosurveillance, begins to decline.

In the next sections, we discuss and summarize the evidence showing that the unmanipulated immune system is indeed capable of recognizing and eliminating tumor cells. We specifically address the following three central mechanistic questions: (1) What cells protect the host from tumor development? (2) How does the immune system distinguish between a transformed cell and its normal progenitor? (3) What are the critical effector mechanisms that the immune system uses to carry out its cancer immunosurveillance function?

4.2. The Roles of Innate and Adaptive Immunity

4.2.1. T Cells

A number of cellular components of both the innate and adaptive immune system have now been implicated in naturally occurring tumor immunity (summarized in Table 1). Although the early studies did not document spontaneous tumor development in nude mice (Stutman, 1975), one very well-controlled study had suggested that germ-free nude mice did develop a low frequency of B cell lymphoma compared with heterozygote littermates (Gershwin *et al.*, 1983). In addition, nude mice stimulated with anti-μ developed an even higher frequency of lymphoma. Mice lacking RAG-2 (or its obligate partner RAG-1) cannot somatically rearrange lymphocyte antigen receptors and therefore are completely devoid of peripheral T cells, B cells, and NKT cells (Shinkai *et al.*, 1992). Unlike other genetic models of immunodeficiency (such as SCID mice), the absence of RAG-2 does not affect DNA damage repair pathways in nonimmune cells undergoing transformation. Recently it was shown that approximately 50% of 129/Sv RAG-2-deficient mice spontaneously developed gastrointestinal malignancies by the age of 18 months (Shankaran *et al.*, 2001). In addition, *Helicobacter*-negative RAG-2$^{-/-}$ 129/Sv mice aged in a specific pathogen-free mouse facility and maintained on broad-spectrum antibiotics administered every other month developed significantly more spontaneous epithelial tumors (gastrointestinal and lung) than did wild-type counterparts (Shankaran *et al.*, 2001). Consistent with these observations, 129/Sv RAG-2-deficient mice that also lack STAT1 showed an earlier onset and broader spectrum of malignancy, including the development of colon and mammary adenocarcinomas (Shankaran *et al.*, 2001). Following subcutaneous injection of the carcinogen methylcholanthrene (MCA), 129/Sv RAG-2$^{-/-}$ mice developed sarcomas at the injection site faster and with greater frequency than strain-matched wild-type controls (Shankaran *et al.*, 2001). Similar findings were obtained in C57BL/6 RAG-1$^{-/-}$ mice (Smyth *et al.*, 2001b) and BALB/c

Table 1 Leukocyte Subsets that Effect/Regulate Tumor Immunity

Mice or treatment	Deficiency	Tumor susceptibility
Nude-LPS/anti-μ	T cells	B cell lymphoma (Gershwin et al., 1983)
RAG-2$^{-/-}$	T, B, and NKT cells	MCA-induced sarcomas
		Spontaneous intestinal neoplasia (Shankaran et al., 2001)
RAG-2$^{-/-}$ × STAT1$^{-/-}$	T, B, and NKT cells IFN-γ and IFN-α/β mediated signaling	MCA-induced sarcomas Spontaneous intestinal and mammary neoplasia (Shankaran et al., 2001)
RAG-1$^{-/-}$	T, B, and NKT cells	MCA-induced sarcomas (Smyth et al., 2001b)
SCID	T, B, and NKT cells	MCA-induced sarcomas (Smyth et al., 2001b)
TCRβ$^{-/-}$	αβ T cells	MCA-induced sarcomas (Girardi et al., 2001)
TCRδ$^{-/-}$	γδ T cells	MCA-induced sarcomas
		DMBA/TPA induced skin tumors (Girardi et al., 2001)
TCRβ$^{-/-}$γ$^{-/-}$	αβ T cells and γδ T cells	DMBA/TPA-induced skin tumors (Girardi et al., 2003)
Jα18$^{-/-}$	Vα14 TCR$^+$ NKT cells	MCA-induced sarcomas (Smyth et al., 2000a)
Anti-asialoGM1	NK cells	MCA-induced sarcomas (Smyth et al., 2001b)
Anti-NK1.1	NK cells	MCA-induced sarcomas (Smyth et al., 2000a)
Anti-Thy1	T cells	MCA-induced sarcomas (Smyth et al., 2000a)
Anti-CD25	CD4$^+$CD25$^+$ Treg cells	Reduced MCA sarcoma susceptibility (Tawara et al., 2002)

RAG-1$^{-/-}$ mice (Smyth, unpublished data) treated with MCA. Thus, lymphocytes protect mice against both chemically induced and spontaneous tumor formation.

4.2.2. NKT Cells and Other Regulatory T Cells

Several T cell subpopulations are known for their ability to regulate immune responses (Godfrey et al., 2000; Sakaguchi, 2004), and in this context such regulatory T cells may also contribute to tumor immunosurveillance (Sakaguchi, 2002; Smyth and Godfrey, 2000; Smyth et al., 2002). NKT cells are CD1d-dependent and MHC-independent and express NK cell receptors in combination with a highly biased TCR repertoire [most TCR-α are Vα14Jα18 and either Vβ8.2, Vβ2, or Vβ7 (Godfrey et al., 2000)]. NKT cells also exist in humans and are commonly defined by coexpression of an invariant TCR-α chain (Vα24JαQ) and TCR Vβ11—TCR homologues of those used by mouse NKT cells. While the CD1d-reactive marine sponge glycolipid, α-galactosylceramide (α-GalCer), has been shown to activate mouse and human NKT cells and promote antitumor function (Hayakawa *et al.*, 2004), the more recently described potential natural ligand for the TCR of NKT cells, isoglobotrihexylceramide (Godfrey *et al.*, 2004; Zhou *et al.*, 2004), has not been examined in this context. The first clear evidence that NKT cells naturally participate in cancer immunosurveillance was obtained in C57BL/6 $J\alpha 18^{-/-}$ mice, lacking Vα14Jα18-expressing invariant NKT cells (Cui *et al.*, 1997). These mice developed MCA-induced sarcomas at two to three times higher frequency than wild-type controls (Smyth *et al.*, 2000a). Subsequently, it was shown that NK cells, CD1d, perforin, and IFN-γ were all necessary in NKT cell-mediated control of the same MCA sarcoma when transplanted into $J\alpha 18^{-/-}$ mice (Crowe *et al.*, 2002). In addition, mice treated with the NKT cell-activating ligand α-GalCer throughout MCA-induced tumorigenesis exhibited a reduced incidence of tumors and displayed a longer latency period to tumor formation than control mice (Hayakawa *et al.*, 2003). It will be important now to examine the broader function of NKT cells in a variety of mouse models of cancer as well as establishing their role in human malignancy. To this end, a study illustrated that human NKT cell dysfunction correlated well with the progression of multiple myeloma (Dhodapkar *et al.*, 2003).

$CD4^+$ $CD25^+$ regulatory T cells (Treg) comprise 5–10% of the total $CD4^+$ T cell population and function largely to maintain immune tolerance (Sakaguchi, 2000, 2004; Shevach, 2002). Treg are critical in host suppression of organ-specific autoimmune diseases, and they promote a dominant state of tolerance during infections and allogeneic transplantation. Treg also suppress immune responses to tumors at both the priming and effector phases (Onizuka *et al.*, 1999; Shimizu *et al.*, 1999; Steitz *et al.*, 2001; Sutmuller *et al.*, 2001; Turk *et al.*, 2004), and depletion of Treg (Onizuka *et al.*, 1999; Turk *et al.*, 2004) improves T cell-based tumor clearance. Cancer patients have increased numbers of peripheral and tumor-infiltrating Treg cells that functionally inhibit tumor-specific T cells and predict poor survival (Curiel *et al.*, 2004; Liyanage *et al.*, 2002; Woo *et al.*, 2001). Although these regulatory T cells are thought to recognize self-antigen peptides in the context of MHC class II, the molecular profiles of the antigens they respond to remain poorly defined. A recent study using TCR $J\alpha 18^{-/-}$ and wild-type mice responding to an MCA-induced sarcoma and immunized with SEREX-defined autoantigens has suggested that $CD8^+$ T and NKT cell antimetastatic activity may be suppressed by $CD4^+CD25^+$ cells (Nishikawa *et al.*, 2003). This study highlights the potential complex immunoregulation of the response to tumor.

4.2.3. NK Cells and $\gamma\delta^+$ T Cells

The role of innate immune cells, such as NK cells and $\gamma\delta TCR^+$ T cells, in immune surveillance of tumors remains controversial. Both NK cells and $\gamma\delta TCR^+$ T cells express perforin (Nakata *et al.*, 1990; Smyth *et al.*, 1990), mediate spontaneous cytotoxicity, and produce many antitumor cytokines, such as IFN-γ, when they recognize target cells via one or more of several cell surface receptors (Cerwenka and Lanier, 2001; Natarajan *et al.*, 2002). NK cells can spontaneously kill MHC class I-deficient tumor cell lines *in vivo* (Smyth *et al.*, 1999, 2000b; van den Broek *et al.*, 1995) and suppress experimental and spontaneous metastasis in mice. Forty years ago Hodgkin's-like B lymphomas spontaneously arising in aging C57L mice (25% incidence at 21 months of age) were first reported, but only recently were these B cell lymphomas shown to express costimulatory molecules and found to be controlled by NK cells in syngeneic mice (Erianne *et al.*, 2000). Another study demonstrated that B cell lymphomas arose with higher frequency in Fas mutant lpr mice that were additionally deficient in $\gamma\delta^+$ T cells or $\alpha\beta^+$ T cells (Peng *et al.*, 1996). Although these experiments were performed on a mixed C57BL/6/MRL background, they nevertheless suggest that $\gamma\delta^+$ T cells could contribute to the suppression of spontaneously arising B cell lymphomas. B cell lymphomas arising in mice deficient in perforin and β2m were shown to be rejected by either NK cells or $\gamma\delta^+$ T cells when transplanted into syngeneic wild-type mice (Street *et al.*, 2004).

In contrast, only a few models have been described thus far where NK cells or $\gamma\delta TCR^+$ T cells prevent primary tumor formation (Girardi *et al.*, 2001; Smyth *et al.*, 2000a, 2001a,b). C57BL/6 mice, depleted of both NK and NKT cells by using the anti-NK1.1 mAb, were two to three times more susceptible to MCA-induced tumorigenesis than wild-type controls (Smyth *et al.*, 2001b). A similar effect was observed in C57BL/6 mice treated with anti-asialo-GM1, which selectively depletes NK cells and activated macrophages, but not NKT cells. Mice lacking $\gamma\delta^+$ T cells (TCR$\delta^{-/-}$ mice) are more susceptible to MCA-induced tumor formation than wild-type mice (on either an FVB or C57BL/6 genetic background) (Gao *et al.*, 2003; Girardi *et al.*, 2001). In addition, using a carcinogenesis model involving initiation with 7,12-dimethylbenz [*a*]anthracene (DMBA) and promotion with 12-*O*-tetradecanoylphorbol 13-acetate (TPA), host protection against tumor formation was found to be more dependent on the action of $\gamma\delta^+$ T cells than $\alpha\beta^+$ T cells (Girardi *et al.*, 2001, 2003). However, TCR$\beta^{-/-}$ × TCR$\delta^{-/-}$ mice were significantly more susceptible to DMBA/TPA carcinogenesis than singly deficient TCR$\delta^{-/-}$ mice (Girardi *et al.*, 2003), revealing a host-protective role for $\alpha\beta$ T cells in the setting of $\gamma\delta^+$ T cell deficiency. Interestingly, in the same study TCRδ$^{-/-}$ mice exhibited the highest ratio of carcinomas to papillomas, suggesting that γδ$^+$ T cells regulate the progression of developing papillomas to more aggressive carcinomas. More recent studies have highlighted the important protective role of IFN-γ secreted by γδ$^+$ T cells (Gao *et al.*, 2003) and CD4$^+$ αβ$^+$ T cells (Girardi *et al.*, 2004) in this model system. While it has not been possible to formally test the importance of these innate lymphocyte subsets in natural human immunity to cancer, several recent studies in patients receiving HLA haplotype mismatch transplants (Ruggeri *et al.*, 2002), monoclonal antibodies to human CD20 and Ep-CAM (Liljefors *et al.*, 2003; O'Hanlon, 2004) or the c-kit tyrosine kinase inhibitor, Gleevec (Borg *et al.*, 2004), indicate an important role for NK cells in the human anticancer response.

4.2.4. Other Leukocytes

Other leukocyte populations may also play important roles in promoting tumor immunity. Very early studies documented that beige mice were susceptible to lymphoma, and while this phenotype was attributed to a lack of NK cell function; these mice have a general defect in the function of many granulocytes (Haliotis *et al.*, 1985). A number of studies have indicated that neutrophils also have a function in tumor immunity (Di Carlo *et al.*, 2001). An important study of breast tumor vaccination in mice revealed that multiple mechanisms involving various innate and adaptive immune components can be important in tumor eradication (Curcio *et al.*, 2003). More recently, a provocative study by Cui *et al.* (2003) provided further evidence that innate immune cells comprise an important arm of the immunosurveillance network. A BALB/c mouse line was found that carries a germline transmissible, aged-related cancer resistance trait controlled by at least two autosomal dominant loci. These "spontaneous regression/complete remission" (SR/CR) mice are able to kill a range of both syngeneic and allogeneic tumor cells derived from multiple tissue sites. Resistance was also observed when the SR/CR trait was bred onto a nude genetic background, suggesting that innate immune cells predominantly mediate the SR/CR phenotype. Characterization of the loci controlling the SR/CR phenotype should provide new insights into innate immune control of tumor growth. It is clear we have a lot more to learn about innate mechanisms of immunity toward tumors, but first we need to generate mice with specific deficiencies in defined leukocyte subsets (e.g., NK cells, DCs, and monocyte subsets) on pure genetic backgrounds. For example, there is very good evidence that, once mobilized, eosinophils can destroy tumor metastases (Mattes *et al.*, 2003) and now that eosinophil-deficient mice have recently been created (Lee *et al.*, 2004); their natural role in tumor immunosurveillance can be studied. In addition, more specific function modifying monoclonal antibodies are needed [such as those that prevent IFN secretion by specific DC subpopulations (Blasius *et al.*, 2004)] in order to rapidly dissect out the antitumor role of innate immune components in wild-type mice. Thus far, there have been no reports of spontaneous tumor formation in mice deficient in one or more of the Toll-like receptor pathways, however, not surprisingly, TLR4 and the MyD88 adapter are crucial for adjuvant-induced induction of antitumor CTL cytotoxicity (Akazawa *et al.*, 2004; Okamoto *et al.*, 2004).

Immunosurveillance is thus a multivariable process requiring the actions of different immune effectors in a manner dependent on the tumor's cell type of origin, mode of transformation, anatomic localization, stromal response, cytokine and chemokine microenvironment, and mechanism of immunologic recognition. Thus, it remains critical to assess the effects of a wide range of immunologic components on tumor development in many different models—both chemically induced and spontaneous—to determine whether the immunosurveillance of all cancer-susceptible tissues of the body is globally similar or locally distinct.

4.3. Recognition of Cancer by Immune Cells

Exactly how do cells of the immunosurveillance network distinguish nascent transformed or established tumor cells from normal cells? We now know a number of recognition systems that immune cells may use to detect transformation (summarized in Table 2). A systematic survey of the humoral and cellular immune responses of patients to their own tumors was initiated in the 1970s using an approach termed autologous typing (Old, 1981). Tumor cell lines were established from a large series of patients with melanoma or other tumor types that could be propagated *in vitro*, and these cells were used as targets for analysis of the humoral or cellular antitumor immune responses of the autologous patient. Fibroblasts and other autologous normal cell types served as control targets to assess the specificity of the antitumor response. Using this system, a small subset of patients was identified who had specific antibody to cell-surface antigens (Carey *et al.*, 1976; Ueda *et al.*, 1979) or who had T cells that recognized the autologous tumor (Knuth *et al.*, 1984). The characterization of the molecular targets recognized by autologous typing was made possible by applying the gene cloning and expression systems developed by Boon and colleagues to identify tumor antigens recognized by $CD8^+$ T cells (Traversari *et al.*, 1992; van der Bruggen *et al.*,

Table 2 Modes of Tumor Recognition

Class	Host	Tumor
Protein Ag	CD8$^+$ T/TCR	MHC class I/peptide
	CD4$^+$ T/TCR	MHC class II/peptide
		Differentiation Ag
		Mutational Ag
		Overexpressed/amplified Ag
		Cancer-testis (CT) Ag
		Viral Ag
	B cell/BCR	As above
Glycolipid Ag	NKT/CD1	Glycolipid
Stress ligand	NKG2D	NKG2D-L
TLR ligands	DC/TLR	HSP, dsRNA
Peptidoglycan Recognition proteins	DC	Peptidoglycans
Danger	DC	Dying cell—Uric acid

1991) and by Pfreundschuh and colleagues for antibody-defined tumor antigens (Sahin et al., 1995). More recently, it has been possible to identify MHC class II restricted tumor antigens recognized by CD4$^+$ T cells (Wang and Rosenberg, 1999).

Since the first human tumor antigen was identified in 1991 (van der Bruggen et al., 1991), many tumor antigens have been cloned and can be segregated into five categories: (1) differentiation antigens (e.g., melanocyte differentiation antigens, Melan-A/MART-1, tyrosinase), and gp-100; (2) mutational antigens (e.g., abnormal forms of p53); (3) overexpressed/amplified antigens (e.g., Her-2/*neu*); (4) cancer-testis (CT) antigens (e.g., MAGE and NY-ESO-1); and (5) viral antigens, (e.g., EBV and HPV) (Boon and van der Bruggen, 1996; Old, 2003; Rosenberg, 1999). Because of their unique characteristics, CT antigens are of particular interest (Scanlan et al., 2002). In adult normal tissues, their expression is limited to germ cells in the testis, whereas in cancer, a variable proportion of a wide range of different tumor types expresses CT antigens. The serological expression cloning technique (SEREX) developed by Pfreundschuh and colleagues (Sahin et al., 1995) to detect the humoral response to human cancer has greatly expanded the list of CT antigens, including NY-ESO-1 (Chen et al., 1997) as well as other categories of tumor antigens, and there are now more than 20 CT antigens or antigen families recognized in human cancer (Scanlan et al., 2002). Using the currently available methodologies, the search for immunogenic human tumor antigens continues (https://www2.licr.org/CancerImmunomeDB/).

In addition to tumor antigens presented on MHC molecules, transformed cells may overexpress other molecular signposts that can function as recognition targets in the immunosurveillance process. The NKG2D-activating receptor, expressed on NK cells, $\gamma\delta^+$ T cells, and $CD8^+$ T cells (Bauer et al., 1999; Raulet, 2003), is one important component that is used by both adaptive and innate immune cells to distinguish cancer cells from normal cells. Functional NKG2D receptor complexes consist of the NKG2D ligand binding polypeptide and either the activating DAP10 or DAP12 signaling polypeptide (Gilfillan et al., 2002). In humans, NKG2D binds to the MHC class I chain-related proteins A and B (MICA/B), as well as the UL16 binding proteins (ULBPs) (Cosman et al., 2001; Pende et al., 2002) and the recently discovered lymphocyte effector cell toxicity-activating ligand (Letal) (Conejo-Garcia et al., 2003) [first reported as RAET1E (Radosavljevic et al., 2002) and also termed ULBP4 (Jan Chalupny et al., 2003)]. The MICA/B proteins are highly polymorphic, nonclassical MHC cell surface glycoproteins that do not associate with β2m or require TAP1 for expression (Groh et al., 1996). While MIC expression in normal tissues has only been documented on the gastrointestinal epithelium of the stomach and large intestines, MICA/B proteins are often expressed in primary carcinomas of the lung, kidney, prostate, ovary, colon (Groh et al., 1996), and liver (Jinushi et al., 2003b), as well as in melanomas (Vetter et al., 2002). In addition, ULBPs (Pende et al., 2002) and Letal (Conejo-Garcia et al., 2003) are also frequently expressed on tumor cells. In mice, NKG2D binds to the retinoic acid early transcript 1 (Rae-1) family proteins Rae-1-, the minor histocompatibility antigen H60 (Cerwenka and Lanier, 2001; Diefenbach et al., 2000), and mouse UL16 binding protein-like transcript (MULT-1) (Carayannopoulos et al., 2002; Diefenbach et al., 2003). NKG2D ligand expression has been observed on a wide range of murine tumors (Diefenbach et al., 2000).

Two data sets link MICA/B recognition to immunosurveillance. First, Groh et al. (1998) demonstrated that MIC-expressing cells were recognized and killed by the Vδ1 γδ T-cell subset, and observed a strong *in vivo* correlation ($p < 0.0001$) between MICA/B expression on tumors and tumor infiltration by Vδ1 γδ T cells (Groh et al., 1999). Second, recent data demonstrated a correlation between downregulation of NKG2D on TILs and the expression of MICA/B in the tumor (Groh et al., 2002). Compared with NKG2D expression in lymphocytes from patients with MIC$^-$ tumors, NKG2D expression was reduced on tumor-infiltrating $CD8^+$ T cells, $\gamma\delta^+$ T cells, and NK cells and also on peripheral blood mononuclear cells (PBMCs) from individuals with MIC$^+$ tumors. Further analysis revealed a correlation between the presence of soluble MIC proteins in the circulation of 7/14 cancer patients and a downregulated expression of NKG2D on lymphocytes. Results of a separate study suggested that shedding of MIC proteins from tumor cell surfaces was the result of the actions of an unknown matrix metalloproteinase (Salih et al., 2002). The finding that soluble MIC proteins may attenuate the expression/function of NKG2D on host immune cells provides one explanation for how a growing tumor could escape cancer immunosurveillance. Sustained or conditional localized expression of Rae-1 in transgenic mice appears to systemically suppress NK cell function rendering these mice more susceptible to carcinogen-induced tumor formation (Oppenheim et al., 2005).

Other work has also established the general importance of NKG2D-dependent tumor recognition in mouse experimental tumor models (Cerwenka et al., 2001; Diefenbach et al., 2001, 2003). Tumor rejection occurred by a combination of NK cell and $CD8^+$ T cell-mediated mechanisms depending on the tumor MHC class I expression, and it appears that the NKG2D receptor functions in vivo primarily by stimulating perforin-mediated cytotoxicity (Hayakawa et al., 2002). A recent study illustrated that cytokines that mediated their antimetastatic activity via perforin were dependent on the NKG2D-NKG2D ligand pathway (Smyth et al., 2004). There still exists some controversy over whether NKG2D-mediated tumor rejection can generate adaptive immunity to NKG2D ligand-negative tumors (Cerwenka et al., 2001; Diefenbach et al., 2001; Westwood et al., 2004). A recent study has illustrated that monoclonal antibody inhibition of NKG2D in mice can increase their sensitivity to MCA-induced fibrosarcoma, directly implicating this pathway in host control of tumor initiation (Smyth et al., 2005).

NKG2D ligands are often described as "stress molecules," but to date no cancer-relevant signaling pathways have been causally linked to their expression. MICA/B gene expression has been induced in several nontransformed human cell lines by heat shock (Groh et al., 1999), infection with virus (Groh et al., 2001), exposure to bacteria (Das et al., 2001; Tieng et al., 2002), or type I interferon (Jinushi et al., 2003a). However, it remains unclear how these conditions overlap the molecular cascades that underlie neoplastic transformation (Hahn and Weinberg, 2002). In mice, Rae-1 is expressed early in development (Raulet, 2003), upregulated by retinoic acid treatment of F9 cells (Nomura et al., 1994) and induced in mouse skin after topical application of DMBA and TPA (Girardi et al., 2001). It has recently been shown that genotoxic stress induces molecules such as the NKG2D ligands (Gasser et al., 2005), a result that directly links the tumorigenesis process to enhanced immune recognition. Further study on the immunology of transformation will be necessary to detail when—and how—in the course of tumorigenesis a cancer cell becomes immunogenic. In the past, it was argued that cellular transformation did not provide a sufficient proinflammatory or "danger" signal to alert the immune system to the presence of a developing tumor (Matzinger,

1994; Pardoll, 2003). However, it is now clear that tumor-stromal interactions may provide the necessary proinflammatory signals. For example: (1) danger signals, such as uric acid (Shi et al., 2003), may arise from the inherent biology of the tumor itself (Seong and Matzinger, 2004) and (2) induction of proinflammatory responses through the generation of potential Toll-like receptor ligands, such as heat shock proteins (Srivastava, 2002), or extracellular matrix derivatives, such as hyaluronic acid (Termeer et al., 2002) or heparin sulfates (Johnson et al., 2002), may share similarities to the events that underlie activation of innate immune responses to microbial pathogens (Janeway, 1989). Similarly, tumor-derived ligands for peptidoglycan recognition receptors or CD1 molecules may also trigger early immune responses to tumors. The function of a large number of innate immune recognition molecules remains to be discovered in mammals. It also remains unknown whether leukocytes like macrophages, neutrophils, and eosinophils can directly recognize tumors. Indeed, even the role that indirect FcR-mediated activation by tumor reactive antibodies plays in natural host immunity to cancer remains a mystery.

4.4. Immune Effector Molecules that Control Cancer

Pivotal studies (Dighe et al., 1994; Kaplan et al., 1998; Shankaran et al., 2001; Smyth et al., 2000a,b; Street et al., 2001, 2002; van den Broek et al., 1996) have shown that deficiencies in key immunologic effector molecules enhanced host susceptibility to both chemically induced and spontaneous tumors, in large part substantiating the cancer immunosurveillance hypothesis (summarized in Table 3). For the purpose of this review, effector mechanisms mediating tumor immunosurveillance have been separated into groups—cytokines and cytotoxic mediators.

4.4.1. Cytokines

Cytokines are most certainly involved in the activation of immune effector mechanisms that limit the growth of the tumor. However, they may also be involved in carcinogenesis and malignant transformation, tumor growth, invasion, and metastasis [See Chapter 9 (Dranoff)]. Cytokines are produced by host stromal and immune cells in response to molecules secreted by the cancer cells or as part of inflammation that frequently accompanies tumor growth. Malignant cells also produce cytokines in the same environment. How a local cytokine network operates in tumors is determined by the array of expressed cytokines, their relative concentrations and cytokine receptor expression patterns. The net cytokine environment likely fluctuates at various stages of tumor development. While a number of cytokines, such as IL-12,

Table 3 Effector Molecules that Mediate Tumor Suppression

Mice or treatment	Deficiency	Tumor susceptibility
IFNGR1$^{-/-}$	IFN-γ receptor 1, IFN-γ sensitivity	MCA-induced sarcomas Wider spectrum in p53$^{-/-}$ background (Kaplan et al., 1998)
IFN-γ$^{-/-}$	IFN-γ production	MCA-induced sarcomas (Street et al., 2001) Spontaneous disseminated lymphomas Spontaneous lung adenocarcinomas in BALB/c background (Street et al., 2002) HLTV1-tax induced T cell lymphoma (Mitra-Kaushik et al., 2004)
IFNAR1$^{-/-}$	IFN-α/β receptor 1	MCA-induced sarcomas (Dunn et al., 2005a)
Anti-IFN-α/β	IFN-α/β	Syngeneic tumors (Gresser et al., 1983)
STAT1$^{-/-}$	IFN-γ and IFN-α/β mediated signal	MCA-induced sarcomas Wider spectrum in p53$^{-/-}$ background (Kaplan et al., 1998) Mammary carcinomas (Shankaran et al., 2001)
GM-CSF$^{-/-}$ × IFN-γ$^{-/-}$	GM-CSF and IFN-γ production	Spontaneous lymphomas Variety of non-lymphoid solid tumors (Enzler et al., 2003)
Perforin$^{-/-}$	Perforin-mediated cytotoxicity	MCA-induced sarcomas (van den Broek et al., 1996) Spontaneous disseminated lymphomas (Smyth et al., 2000b)
Perforin$^{-/-}$ × IFN-γ$^{-/-}$	Perforin-mediated cytotoxicity and IFN-γ production	MCA-induced sarcomas (Street et al., 2001) Spontaneous disseminated lymphomas (Street et al., 2002)
TRAIL$^{-/-}$	TRAIL-mediated cytotoxicity	MCA-induced sarcomas (Cretney et al., 2002)
Anti-TRAIL	TRAIL-mediated cytotoxicity	MCA-induced sarcomas Spontaneous sarcomas, disseminated lymphomas in p53$^{+/-}$ background (Takeda et al., 2002)
IL-12 p40$^{-/-}$	IL-12 p40 subunit, IL-12 and IL-23 production	MCA-induced sarcomas (Smyth et al., 2000a)
LMP2$^{-/-}$	IFN-γ-inducible low molecular mass polypeptide-2 (LMP2) subunit	Spontaneous uterine neoplasias (Hayashi and Faustman, 2002)

IL-18, GM-CSF, Flt3L, and the common γ chain cytokines, may play an important role in tumor immunosurveillance given their therapeutic effects, this section will concentrate on IFNs, whose role in natural tumor immunity has been more thoroughly assessed.

4.4.2. IFN-γ

Endogenously produced IFN-γ has been shown to protect the host against the growth of transplanted tumors and also the formation of primary, chemically induced and spontaneous tumors (Dighe *et al.*, 1994; Kaplan *et al.*, 1998; Shankaran *et al.*, 2001; Street *et al.*, 2001, 2002). Injection of neutralizing mAb for IFN-γ into mice bearing transplanted, established Meth A tumors blocked LPS-induced tumor rejection (Dighe *et al.*, 1994). In addition, transplanted fibrosarcomas grew faster and more efficiently in mice treated with IFN-γ-specific mAbs. Overexpression of a dominant-negative mutant of IFN-γ receptor in these sarcoma cell lines abrogated their sensitivity to IFN-γ, and those tumors with mutant receptors showed reduced immunogenicity in syngeneic mice. Thus, the IFN-γ sensitivity of the developing tumor is critical for its immune recognition and elimination. In models of primary tumor formation, IFN-γ-insensitive 129/Sv mice lacking either the IFNGR1 ligand binding subunit of the IFN-γ receptor or STAT1, the transcription factor that mediates much of IFN-γ's biologic effects on cells (Bach *et al.*, 1997), were found to be 10–20 times more sensitive than wild-type mice to MCA tumor induction (Kaplan *et al.*, 1998). Similar results were obtained in independent experiments that used C57BL/6 mice lacking the gene encoding IFN-γ (Street *et al.*, 2001). These findings were further supported by studies using mice lacking p53 and either the IFN-γ receptor (IFN-γR), STAT1 (Kaplan *et al.*, 1998), or IFN-γ (Street *et al.*, 2001, 2002), which showed that endogenously produced IFN-γ suppressed spontaneous tumor formation in p53 mutant mice. STAT1-deficient mice also display a significant incidence of mammary gland tumor development in both the 129/Sv and C57BL/6 backgrounds (Chan and Schreiber, unpublished observation; Shankaran *et al.*, 2001). It was also shown that a small proportion (<15%) of BALB/c IFN-γ deficient mice developed lung adenocarcinoma but otherwise failed to develop tumors, whereas almost half the IFN-γ-deficient mice on a C57BL/6 background developed a spectrum of various T cell lymphomas (Street *et al.*, 2002). In addition, C57BL/6 mice deficient for both perforin and IFN-γ develop more B cell lymphomas with earlier onset, suggesting in the absence of perforin, IFN-γ can play a role in controlling lymphoma in the C57BL/6 strain of mice. Collectively, the findings suggest that the immune system does regulate some lymphoid and epithelial malignancies through pathways controlled by IFN-γ and the genetic background of mice appears to an important factor in spontaneous tumor development. The overlap between the IFN-γ- and lymphocyte-dependent tumor suppressor pathways was revealed by comparing MCA tumor formation in 129/Sv mice lacking IFN-γ responsiveness (IFNGR1$^{-/-}$ or STAT1$^{-/-}$ mice), lymphocytes (RAG-2$^{-/-}$ mice), or both (RAG-2$^{-/-}$ x STAT1$^{-/-}$) (RkSk mice) (Shankaran et al., 2001). Whereas RkSk mice displayed increased sensitivities to MCA tumor induction compared to wild-type mice, they were no more susceptible than mice lacking IFN-γ responsiveness or lymphocytes only. However, RkSk mice developed spontaneous breast tumors that were not observed in either wild-type or RAG-2$^{-/-}$ mice, therefore demonstrating that the overlap between the two pathways was incomplete.

Recent work using bone marrow chimeric mice suggests that γδ$^+$ T cells are an important source of IFN-γ during the development of protective antitumor responses to MCA-induced sarcomas (Gao et al., 2003). Additional work is required to identify if there are other cellular sources of IFN-γ during tumor development and to determine whether other IFN-γ-producing cells participate in responses to different types of tumors.

More is known about the physiologically relevant targets of IFN-γ's actions. Host and tumor cells are both important targets of IFN-γ during development of protective antitumor immune responses. The data substantiating this conclusion has already been extensively reviewed (Dunn et al., 2002, 2004a,b). Through its capacity to promote the generation of tumor-specific CD4$^+$ Th1 T cells and cytolytic T cells (CTL) and to activate cytocidal activity in macrophages, IFN-γ facilitates development of powerful antitumor effector functions mediated by both adaptive and innate immunity. However, the tumor cells themselves have also been shown to represent critical cellular targets of IFN-γ (Dighe et al., 1994; Kaplan et al., 1998; Shankaran et al., 2001), revealing that IFN-γ's ability to upregulate tumor immunogenicity is sufficient to explain the effects on tumor detection and elimination in immunocompetent hosts. Other potential IFN-γ-dependent effects on developing tumors such as antiproliferative (Bromberg et al., 1996; Chin et al., 1996), proapoptotic (Chin et al., 1997; Xu et al., 1998), and angiostatic (Coughlin et al., 1998; Luster and Leder, 1993) effects may also contribute to the rejection process; however, a physiologic role for these effects in the process must first be established.

Increased tumor formation in LMP2 (the IFN-γ-inducible low-molecular mass polypeptide-2 subunit)-deficient mice (Hayashi and Faustman, 2002) and increased tumor metastasis or tumor formation in mice lacking IL-12 (Noguchi et al., 1996; Smyth et al., 2000a) further demonstrate the diverse role IFN-γ plays in tumor immunity. IL-12 produced by phagocytic cells, B cells, DCs, and possibly other APC acts on T cells and NK cells to generate cytotoxic lymphocytes and facilitate potent production of IFN-γ. Endogenous IL-12 appears also to be important for host resistance to transplantable tumors and to MCA-induced fibrosarcoma (Smyth et al., 2000a). Another study revealed a more indirect immunological action of IFN-γ at the level of the host in preventing tumor development (Enzler et al., 2003). Both GM-CSF/IFN-γ doubly deficient and GM-CSF/IL-3/IFN-γ triple deficient mice were found to be highly susceptible to bacterial infection, displayed acute and chronic inflammation in a variety of different organs, and developed high incidences of spontaneous lymphoma and nonlymphoid solid cancers. The incidences of infection, inflammation, and neoplasia were much reduced in mice lacking GM-CSF alone, IL-3 and GM-CSF only, or IFN-γ alone. Tumor development in the IL-3/GM-CSF/IFN-triple gene-targeted mice was prevented or delayed by maintaining the mice on broad-spectrum antibiotics from birth. These results suggest a role for IFN-γ, in combination with GM-CSF, in controlling chronic infections that can lead to a chronic inflammatory state that ultimately may result in cancer development. Clearly, the relationship between bacterial/microbial immunosurveillance and cancer immunosurveillance warrants further analysis but must await the development of *in vivo* models that can unequivocally differentiate between the two processes.

4.4.3. Type I Interferons (IFN-α/β)

Type I interferons are encoded by a family of structurally related genes, giving rise to more than 13 different proteins that induce overlapping responses in target cells following interaction with a common type I IFN receptor (Pestka et al., 2004). In mice and humans, 14 or 12, respectively distinct IFN-α proteins and the single IFN-β protein represent the major forms of type I IFN. IFN-α has long been known to induce effective antitumor activity against mouse and human malignancies [reviewed in (Belardelli et al., 2002; Gresser and Belardelli, 2002)]. Although type I IFNs can have direct effects on tumor cells (such as inhibiting tumor cell proliferation), it has been postulated that IFN-α/β induces its antitumor effects primarily through host-dependent mechanisms, either by stimulating NK cell proliferation and cytotoxicity, enhancing the production or secretion of other cytokines by NK cells through an autocrine IFN-γ loop, or by influencing $CD8^+$ T-cell and B-cell adaptive-immune responses by upregulating class I and class II MHC expression and increasing antigen presentation. However, the latter hypothesis comes largely from experiments where type I IFN was exogenously administered. Until recently, little was known about the role of type I interferons in promoting natural immunity to tumors, that is in immunosurveillance. Early studies indicated that neutralization of IFN-α/β in mice enhanced the progressive growth of transplanted syngeneic tumors (Affabris et al., 1987; Gresser et al., 1983) or abrogated the rejection of allogeneic or xenogeneic tumors (Gresser et al., 1988). More recent *in vitro* work has pointed to a potential role for IFN-α/β in preventing cellular transformation through mechanisms involving enhanced cellular expression of the p53 tumor suppressor gene in cells exposed to type I IFN (Takaoka et al., 2003). However, this conclusion was based on *in vitro* transformation experiments, and additional work is needed to determine whether this IFN function plays a physiologically important role in preventing tumor development *in vivo*.

Most recently a clear role for type I IFNs has been documented in preventing development of MCA-sarcomas in mice and in promoting rejection of immunogenic transplantable tumors (Dunn et al., 2005a; Smyth, 2005). Mice lacking the IFNAR1 subunit of the type I IFN receptor were more susceptible to MCA carcinogenesis compared to WT mice. In addition, IFNAR1$^{-/-}$ mice were unable to reject highly immunogenic RAG regressor MCA sarcomas, a result that was recapitulated using WT mice pretreated with a blocking IFNAR1 mAb. A search for the functionally relevant targets of type I IFN in these models revealed that tumor cells were not the critical targets of IFN-α/β actions, a result that differentiated IFN-α/β's actions from those of IFN-γ. In contrast, development of a protective antitumor immune response obligatorily required type I sensitivity at the level of host hematopoietic cells. MCA sarcomas derived from IFNAR1$^{-/-}$ mice displayed a highly immunogenic phenotype indicating that they were not edited during their development. Additional work is needed to identify the precise cellular targets of IFN-α/β in the cancer immunosurveillance process and to determine the immunologic pathways that IFN-α/β promotes that lead to cancer immunosurveillance and immunoediting.

4.4.4. Cytotoxic Mediators: Granule Exocytosis

Many cancer vaccine strategies have been based on the premise that specific cytotoxic T cells may eliminate tumor cells. Cytotoxic lymphocytes principally kill tumor cells by two distinct mechanisms, granule exocytosis and death receptor-mediated apoptosis. Perforin (pfp) is the key calcium-dependent pore-forming protein critical for death mediated by lymphocyte granule exocytosis, inserting into the tumor cell plasma membrane and enabling the cytosolic delivery of additional granule proteins including the serine protease granzyme family (Trapani and Smyth, 2002). Importantly, pfp-deficient mice are more permissive to growth of transplantable tumors and develop MCA-induced sarcomas more rapidly and with greater frequency than their wild-type counterparts (Smyth et al., 1999, 2000b; Street et al., 2001; van den Broek et al., 1996). C57BL/6 wild-type and pfp-deficient mice had a similar incidence of Moloney murine sarcoma and leukemia virus-induced sarcomas, but tumors were larger and regression was delayed in pfp-deficient mice. Thus, pfp-dependent cytotoxicity is not only a crucial mechanism of both cytotoxic T lymphocyte- and NK cell-dependent resistance to injected tumor cell lines but also operates during viral and chemical carcinogenesis *in vivo*. In addition, coincident loss of alleles encoding p53 and pfp revealed a specific requirement for pfp in host protection against spontaneous lymphomagenesis (Smyth *et al.*, 2000b). Interestingly, increased susceptibility to all spontaneous tumor formation in p53 mutant mice was observed with IFN-γR or STAT1 deficiencies (Kaplan *et al.*, 1998), whereas only disseminated lymphomas, but not sarcomas, were increased in pfp-deficient mice (Smyth *et al.*, 2000b). Surprisingly, pfp-deficient mice on either a C57BL/6 or BALB/c background develop disseminated B cell lymphomas and plasmacytomas after 15 months of age (Street *et al.*, 2002). These B cell lymphomas express many costimulatory molecules and were avidly rejected by T cells when transplanted into syngeneic WT mice. Mice deficient in pfp and β2m developed even more B cell lymphomas and onset was earlier (Street *et al.*, 2004). Collectively, this evidence implied that pfp was a major immunoregulatory/effector molecule that controls the integrity of the B cell compartment. Exactly how these B cell lymphomas arise and how T cells so effectively recognize and reject these tumors in WT mice remains to be uncovered. The activities of other cytotoxic granule components, such as granzymes and granulysin, depend on pfp activity. Thus far there is no strong evidence that these molecules play a role other than in microbial infection (Smyth *et al.*, 2003a; Stenger *et al.*, 1998; Trapani and Smyth, 2002), although to date experimentation in this area has been limited.

4.4.5. Cytotoxicity: TNF Family Death Ligands

Members of the TNF superfamily that induce tumor cell apoptosis have been shown to contribute to tumor immunity. Tumor necrosis factor apoptosis-inducing ligand (TRAIL) is a member of the TNF superfamily that induces apoptosis through engagement of the TRAIL-R2 (DR5) receptor in mice (Smyth *et al.*, 2003b). TRAIL is expressed constitutively on a subset of liver NK cells and is induced by IFN-γ, IFN-α/β, or TLR signals in monocytes, NK cells, neutrophils, dendritic cells, and T cells (Smyth *et al.*, 2003b). The antimetastatic function of NK cells against TRAIL-sensitive tumor cells in mice was shown to be partly dependent on TRAIL (Smyth *et al.*, 2001a; Takeda *et al.*, 2001). Neutralization of TRAIL promoted tumor development in mice inoculated with MCA and this protective effect of TRAIL was at least partly mediated by NK cells and totally dependent on IFN-γ (Cretney *et al.*, 2002; Takeda *et al.*, 2002). IFN-γ may regulate TRAIL-mediated tumor surveillance, not only by regulating TRAIL expression on effector cells, but also by sensitizing tumor cells to TRAIL-mediated cytotoxicity. A substantial contribution of TRAIL to immune surveillance against spontaneous tumor development caused by p53 mutation was also recently demonstrated (Takeda *et al.*, 2002; Zerafa *et al.*, 2005). Furthermore about 25% of aging C57BL/6 TRAIL-deficient mice were shown to develop spontaneous lymphoma (Zerafa *et al.*, 2005). Considering that the TRAIL-R2 receptor is upregulated by p53 in response to DNA damage (Wu *et al.*, 1997), TRAIL killing may be a critical link between target cell genotoxic distress and immune-mediated destruction. Further study is required to identify the specific innate cell subsets that manifest the TRAIL-dependent antitumor effects, since other cell types such as neutrophils and dendritic cells may also play some role (Ludwig *et al.*, 2004). In addition, a clear role for TRAIL in the T cell-mediated immune defense against tumor growth was formally shown in various grafts versus leukemia models in mice (Schmaltz *et al.*, 2002). Interestingly, a recent study of TRAIL-R-deficient mice bred with $p53^{-/-}$ or adenomatous polyposis coli (APCi) mutant mice did not indicate any significant role for the TRAIL-R pathway in tumor control (Yue *et al.*, 2005). Furthermore, TRAIL-deficient mice bred with Her-2/*neu* transgenic mice did not reveal any critical role for TRAIL in mammary carcinoma progression (Smyth *et al. J. Immunol.* in press, 2005). Collectively, from this work it is clear that complete p53 loss may preclude TRAIL-TRAIL-R function. Although DC vaccines have been shown to protect mice from colon tumors caused by APCi mutation (Iinuma *et al.*, 2004), the role of natural immunity in host protection from colon tumors is not established and the TRAIL/TRAIL-R pathway needs to be assessed in other mouse models of tumor immune surveillance.

Among other members of the TNF superfamily, mice and humans mutant for Fas ligand have also been shown to develop lymphoid malignancies (Davidson *et al.*, 1998; Straus *et al.*, 2001), whereas C57BL/6 mice deficient in TNF do not display an increased incidence of spontaneous tumors compared to syngeneic wild-type controls (Street *et al.*, 2004). TNF is a vital cytokine involved in inflammation, immunity, and cellular organization (Locksley *et al.*, 2001). Although TNF is capable of initiating a tumor apoptotic response, TNF is rarely cytotoxic to tumor cells *in vitro* unless an additional stress (e.g., an RNA or protein synthesis inhibitor) is provided (Wong *et al.*, 1989). Overall, TNF has a dual role in cancer, inducing destruction of blood vessels and cell-mediated killing of certain tumors, as well as acting as a tumor promoter. TNF-deficient mice have provided evidence of both a role in tumor immunosurveillance for TNF (Baxevanis *et al.*, 2000; Smyth *et al.*, 1998) and a role for TNF in tumor development and metastasis (Knight *et al.*, 2000; Moore *et al.*, 1999; Suganuma *et al.*, 1999). Expression studies have confirmed high concentrations of TNF in tumors and associations between single nucleotide polymorphisms (SNPs) in the TNF gene and a variety of cancers exist [reviewed in (Szlosarek and Balkwill, 2003)]. Its role in cancer progression has stimulated interest in the use of TNF antagonists for the prevention and treatment of cancer. Other potential pathways of tumor destruction, such as those mediated by nitric oxide and ROS, do influence tumor development, but have been previously reviewed in depth (Lala and Chakraborty, 2001; Seifried et al., 2003).

5. Immunoediting: When Tumor Cells Survive

Even when the elimination/immunosurveillance phase of cancer immunoediting fails, the relationship between immunity and cancer is far from over. An appreciation of the complexity of the immune system/tumor interaction is based on work that compared the immunogenicities of tumors derived from immunocompromised versus immunocompetent mice. MCA-induced sarcomas formed in an immunodeficient environment ($RAG^{-/-}$, SCID, nude, or NKT cell-deficient mice) are, as a group, more immunogenic than tumors that develop in immunocompetent hosts (Engel et al., 1996; Shankaran et al., 2001; Smyth et al., 2000a; Svane et al., 1996). Moreover, sarcomas from WT mice treated with anti-TRAIL were significantly more TRAIL-sensitive ex vivo than similar sarcomas derived from control Ig treated WT mice (Takeda et al., 2002). Interestingly, lymphomas from $pfp^{-/-}$ mice grew avidly when transplanted into $pfp^{-/-}$ recipients, but most were rejected when transplanted into wild-type mice (Street et al., 2002). Taken together, these results show that tumors are imprinted by the immunologic environment in which they form. By eliminating tumor cells of high intrinsic immunogenicity, this imprinting process may select for tumor cell variants of reduced immunogenicity and therefore favor the generation of tumors that are either poorly recognized by the immune system or that have acquired mechanisms that suppress immune effector functions. We envisage that a tumor that has breached the elimination phase of the immunoediting process may experience two subsequent phases in its interactions with the host's immune system: equilibrium, followed by escape (Dunn et al., 2002, 2004a,b).

5.1. Equilibrium

Although the elimination phase of the cancer immunoediting process can eradicate a significant percentage of transformed cells, there can exist a period of latency extending from the end of the elimination phase to the beginning of the escape phase and the emergence of clinically detectable malignant disease. This potentially protracted period in the course of the immune system/tumor interaction that occurs prior to the detection of clinically apparent tumors constitutes the equilibrium phase. Equilibrium is probably the longest of the three phases and may occur over a period of many years in humans. Indeed, it has been estimated that for many solid human tumors there can be a 20-year interval between initial carcinogen exposure and clinical detection of the tumor (Loeb *et al.*, 2003). The events that occur in the equilibrium phase of cancer immunoediting are likely quite similar to those previously envisaged to occur in a process termed tumor "dormancy" (Uhr *et al.*, 1997; Wheelock *et al.*, 1981). Although many of the original tumor cells are destroyed, new variants arise carrying more mutations that provide them with increased resistance to immune attack. Ultimately, the dynamic interaction between immunity and cancer in the equilibrium phase produces new populations of tumor cells that are better suited for survival in the immunocompetent host. During this period, the heterogeneity and genetic instability of cancer cells that survive the elimination phase are possibly the principal forces that enable tumor cells to eventually resist host immunity. The tumor, which immune cells continuously act on, can contain cancer cells that harbor thousands of mutations (Loeb, 1991; Loeb *et al.*, 2003). It has been proposed that the "mutator phenotype" of tumor cells (Loeb, 1991) may result from the three types of genetic instability observed in cancer: nucleotide-excision repair instability (NIN), microsatellite instability (MIN), and chromosomal instability (CIN) (Lengauer *et al.*, 1998). Of the three, CIN is thought to be the predominant mechanism responsible for destabilizing genomic integrity, and the observation that cancer cell genomes display gains or losses of whole chromosomes (i.e., aneuploidy) associated with an estimated loss of 25–50% of their alleles reflects the degree of genomic upheaval associated with the CIN phenotype (Lengauer *et al.*, 1998). Of the three phases of the cancer immunoediting process, the least is currently known about equilibrium and more work is needed to prove its existence. A complete mechanistic understanding of the equilibrium phase will require the development of new tumor models to better define the cell-intrinsic mechanisms that generate new tumor phenotypes and to identify the tumor-sculpting immune "editors." We envision three possible outcomes for a tumor that has entered the latent period of equilibrium: (1) eventual elimination by the immune system, (2) permanent maintenance in the equilibrium phase by the cellular and molecular controls of immunity, or (3) escape from immune pressure and transit to the final escape phase of the immunoediting process.

5.2. Escape

In the escape phase, some of the tumor cell variants that emerge from the equilibrium phase develop the capacity to grow in an immunologically intact environment. This breach of the host's immune defenses most likely occurs either when genetic and epigenetic changes in the tumor cell confer resistance to immune detection and/or elimination or when the tumor induces a state of immunologic suppression or tolerance in the host allowing the tumors to expand and become clinically detectable. Because both the adaptive and innate compartments of the immune system function in the cancer immunosurveillance network, tumors most likely would have to circumvent either one or both arms of immunity in order to achieve progressive growth. Individual tumor cells may employ multiple immunoevasive strategies to elude the powerful integrated innate and adaptive antitumor immune responses to their immunogenic progenitors. Thus, it is likely that several distinct immunologically driven tumor-sculpting events must occur before the final immunogenic phenotype of a malignant cell is ultimately established. The degree to which the immunogenicity of a tumor is shaped by its interaction with the host immune system may be determined by the identities of the immune editors operative during the equilibrium phase. It is possible that tumor escape from each different tissue site of origin may be mechanistically distinct. It therefore follows that metastatic lesions may experience the most significant immunologic sculpting.

Much work has recently focused on defining the molecular basis of tumor escape although it must be said some of the processes remain more theoretical than proven. It is now recognized that tumor escape mechanisms fall into two basic categories: (1) tumor intrinsic mechanisms associated with tumor cells and tumor-associated antigens and (2) tumor extrinsic mechanisms associated with the host immune system. The former group includes: (a) lack of expression of MHC class II molecules and costimulatory molecules; (b) down regulation or loss of expression of MHC class I molecule proteins (Algarra *et al.*, 2000; Marincola *et al.*, 2000); (c) downregulation or expression of genes associated with antigen presentation (such as transporter associated with antigen processing (TAP), low-molecular-weight protein (LMP) and β2-microglobulin) (Seliger *et al.*, 2000); (d) low level of expression of tumor-associated antigens at early phases of tumor growth (Spiotto *et al.*, 2004); (e) loss of antigenic epitopes; (f) physical barrier preventing effector cells accessing tumors; and (g) loss of response to IFNs (Dunn *et al.*, 2005b; Kaplan *et al.*, 1998; Wong *et al.*, 1997).

Mechanisms associated with the host immune system include: (a) ignorance; (b) tolerance of T cells to tumor-specific antigens resulting from anergy or deletion caused by host APC, myeloid cells, or regulatory T cells; (c) suppression of T cells caused by tumor derived factors [e.g., TGF-β, IL-10, VEGF, FasL, galectin, indoleamine 2,3-dioxygenase (IDO)], immunosuppressive myeloid or regulatory T cells (Gabrilovich *et al.*, 1996; Gorelik and Flavell, 2001, 2002; Hahne *et al.*, 1996; Khong and Restifo, 2002; Loeffler *et al.*, 1992;

Rubinstein *et al.*, 2004; Uyttenhove *et al.*, 2003); (d) secretion of soluble ligands that block lymphocyte activation (e.g., NKG2D-L) (Groh *et al.*, 2002); (e) defects in antigen presentation by professional APC; and (f) impaired APC maturation (Wang *et al.*, 2004). One very recent example showing that tumor-dependent effects on host immunity can indeed lead to tumor escape comes from the analysis of wild-type mice engineered to sporadically express a dormant viral oncogene (SV40 large T antigen, Tag), which develop progressively growing Tag-expressing tumors after a very long latency period (Willimsky and Blankenstein, 2005). This study uses an elegant genetic model to demonstrate a fact that has long been known that certain tumors can induce a state of immune unresponsiveness that allows progressive tumor growth. Thus, the study provides additional support for tumor extrinsic mechanisms that operate within the escape phase of the cancer immunoediting process. Curiously the authors attempt to use the results of this study to argue against the cancer immunosurveillance/immunoediting process. However, this is an invalid argument since tumor development and tumor immunogenicities from immunocompetent versus immunodeficient mice were never compared. Thus, rather than disputing the role of immunity in preventing and shaping tumor development, the results of this study in fact support it. Because the mechanisms that target the immune system to achieve tumor escape are so extensive and have been the subject of recent review articles (Khong and Restifo, 2002; Marincola *et al.*, 2000), they are not specifically discussed further.

Interest has focused on the premise that DC defects are responsible for much of the inability of the immune system to adequately respond to tumor development (Gabrilovich, 2004). There is now sufficient evidence indicating that these defects are caused by the abnormal differentiation of myeloid cells, which results in the decreased production of fully differentiated DCs and the accumulation of immature DCs and myeloid cells (iDCs and iMCs). Both iMCs and iDCs can directly suppress antigen-specific T cell responses. Abnormal myeloid-cell differentiation is caused by several tumor-derived factors. One of the mechanisms driving their effect on myeloid cells is constitutive activation of *STAT3*. This activation of *STAT3* promotes the continuous proliferation and accumulation of iMCs and, together with inhibition of NF-kB (directly or indirectly), prevents the differentiation and activation of DCs. This greatly contributes to the suppression of tumor-specific immune responses and, ultimately, leads to tumor escape from immune-system control (Gabrilovich, 2004; Wang *et al.*, 2004).

An important related question is what attracts myeloid precursor cells to the tumor microenvironment. Some important work in mouse models has shed some light on this question. The development, progression, and metastasis of tumors depend on blood vessels, and a number of recent findings demonstrated that angioblasts, the progenitors for endothelial cells contribute to tumor vascular formation (Asahara et al., 1997; Lyden et al., 2001; Rafii et al., 2002). These progenitor cells were further identified as VEGFR2-positive BM-derived cells. The monocyte/macrophage/DC system is closely related to ECs, and it has recently been shown that Gr^+CD11b^+ myeloid immune suppressor cells, found in large numbers in tumor bearing mice and patients with cancer (Bronte et al., 2000; Gabrilovich et al., 1999; Melani et al., 2003), can differentiate into ECs under certain conditions (Yang and Carbone, 2004). These Gr^+CD11b^+ cells actively contribute to tumor angiogenesis by producing MMP9, and differentiating into ECs. An analogous study has illustrated that tumor-derived β-defensins recruit DC precursors through CCR6 into the tumor, where VEGF-A transforms them into endothelial like cells that engage in vasculogenesis and function as promoters of tumor progression (Conejo-Garcia et al., 2004). Very clearly, this concept requires further validation and in particular the sequence of cross talk between epithelium, stroma, and hematopoietic elements in the microenvironment of the transformed cell mass will be key to model and experimentally dissect. It is intriguing that the immunosuppressive T cell populations, such as IL-13-producing CD1d-restricted T cells (Terabe et al., 2000) or $CD4^+CD25^+$ regulatory T cells (Tregs), may function to suppress tumor immunity following their recruitment and/or interaction with such myeloid suppressor populations (Terabe et al., 2003). Thus, the tumor may take the opportunity of ultimately suppressing subsequent innate and adaptive immune responses in the course of fulfilling its hunger for nutrients.

6. Cancer Immunosurveillance/Immunoediting in Humans

Clearly, immunodeficient humans have a far greater susceptibility to lethal viruses and pathogens than immune compromised mice in pathogen free mouse animal facilities, and therefore the opportunities of observing increased spontaneous tumor formation in people with mutations in specific genes encoding immune effector molecules are rare. Studies in broadly immunodeficient patients have documented a highly elevated incidence of virus-induced malignancies such as non-Hodgkin's lymphoma, Kaposi's sarcoma, and cancers of the anal and urogenital tracts compared with immunocompetent individuals (Boshoff and Weiss, 2002; Penn and Starzl, 1970). In contrast, cancers of nonviral origins may take many years to develop and the variety of viral and bacterial infections to which these immunodeficient/immunosuppressed patients were susceptible may always confound results. Nevertheless, one can draw upon three lines of evidence to suggest that cancer immunosurveillance indeed occurs in humans: (a) immunosuppressed transplant recipients display higher incidences of nonviral cancers than age-matched immunocompetent control populations, (b) cancer patients can develop spontaneous adaptive and innate immune responses to the tumors that they bear, and (c) the presence of lymphocytes within the tumor can be a prognostic indicator of patient's survival.

A variety of studies in immunosuppressed transplant recipients have been extensively reviewed of late (Dunn et al., 2002, 2004b). Suffice it to say that assessment of thousands of transplant patients across the Western world have detected increased relative risk ratios for a broad subset of tumors with no apparent viral origin (e.g., colon, lung, bladder, pancreas, kidney, ureter carcinomas, melanomas, squamous cell carcinoma, and endocrine tumors). Thus, individuals with normal immune systems who undergo immunosuppression display an increased probability of developing a variety of cancers that have not been linked to a viral etiology. This observation may indicate that immunosuppressive intervention predisposed the transplant patients either to *de novo* tumor formation or allowed the outgrowth of occult tumors whose growth was contained by a functioning immune system and were thus held in a state of durable equilibrium. Indeed, a clinical scenario that likely demonstrates the existence of the equilibrium phase in humans is the transmission of cancer from organ transplant donors to recipients. One recent study reported the occurrence of metastatic melanoma 1–2 years posttransplant in two allograft recipients who had each received kidneys from the same donor (MacKie et al., 2003). Upon subsequent investigation, it was found that the donor had been treated for primary melanoma 16 years before her death, but was considered tumor free at the time of organ donation. This study, together with others in the literature (Elder et al., 1997; Penn, 1996; Suranyi et al., 1998), suggests that the pharmacologic suppression of the immune systems of these transplant recipients facilitated the rapid and progressive outgrowth of occult tumors that were maintained in the equilibrium phase by the donor's intact immune system. Overall, these results suggest a protective action of immunity in preventing human tumors.

Natural immune responses to both cancer and normal tissues that share antigens can be detected in patients with autoimmune paraneoplastic neurologic disorders/degenerations (PNDs) (Albert and Darnell, 2004; Darnell and Posner, 2003). Clinically, PNDs may affect any part of the nervous system and are most commonly associated with tumors of the breast, lung, and ovary. In the 1980s, an immunologic link between neuronal degeneration and the presence of cancer was established by the discovery that the serum and cerebrospinal fluid of PND patients harbored high titers of antibodies that reacted with neuronal antigens present in both the affected neuronal population and the associated cancer [antigens are discussed in depth in (Darnell, 1996; Musunuru and Darnell, 2001)]. Furthermore, CTLs have been identified in the peripheral blood (Albert *et al.*, 1998) and cerebrospinal fluid (Albert *et al.*, 2000) of PND patients that can react with peptides from one of these antigens. Data from several clinical studies have noted a positive correlation between the presence of antibody and the extent of disease, response to anticancer therapy, and survival (Darnell and DeAngelis, 1993; Graus *et al.*, 1997). Clearly, these types of studies will increase in impact as emerging technologies provide improved mechanisms to identify the effects of the immune system on developing and established human tumors.

Another line of mounting evidence that a cancer immunosurveillance process exists in humans is the strong correlation between the presence of lymphocytes infiltrating a tumor and patient survival [Table 4 and also reviewed in (Dunn *et al.*, 2002, 2004b)]. These observations of tumor infiltrating T lymphocytes have been validated in large numbers of patients with primary melanoma (Clemente *et al.*, 1996; Mihm *et al.*, 1996), ovarian carcinoma (Zhang *et al.*, 2003), Dukes' colorectal tumors (Naito *et al.*, 1998) and esophageal carcinoma (Schumacher *et al.*, 2001). Other studies have shown similar positive correlations between NK cell infiltration and patient survival for gastric carcinoma (Ishigami *et al.*, 2000), squamous cell lung carcinoma (Villegas *et al.*, 2002), and colorectal cancer (Coca *et al.*, 1997). Regulatory T cells can also be detected in a variety of human cancers (Liyanage *et al.*, 2002; Woo *et al.*, 2001), and a recent study has indicated the specific recruitment of such T cells in ovarian carcinoma (perhaps by tumor and/or macrophage secreted CCL22) enables immune privilege and predicts a reduced patient survival (Curiel *et al.*, 2004). An even more important parameter may prove to be the location of the infiltrating $CD8^+$ cells relative to the location of the cancer versus regulatory cells in the tumor (Odunsi, 2005). It will be important in the future to clarify,

Table 4 TIL and Prognosis in Human Cancer

Cell type	Disease	Prognosis
$CD8^+$ T	Melanoma	Brisk TIL = better (Clemente *et al.*, 1996) (Mihm *et al.*, 1996)
$CD8^+$ T	Ovarian Ca.	TIL = better (Zhang *et al.*, 2003)
$CD8^+$ T	Duke's Colorectal Ca.	TIL = better (Naito *et al.*, 1998)
$CD8^+$ T	Esophageal Ca.	TIL = better (Schumacher *et al.*, 2001)
T cell	Follicular lymphoma	Signature TIL = better (Dave *et al.*, 2004)
NK cell	Gastric Ca.	TIL = better (Ishigami *et al.*, 2000)
NK cell	Squamous cell Ca.	TIL = better (Villegas *et al.*, 2002)
NK cell	Colorectal Ca.	TIL = better (Coca *et al.*, 1997)
Treg	Ovarian Ca.	Poor (Curiel *et al.*, 2004)
NKT	Multiple myeloma	Functional NKT = better (Dhodapkar *et al.*, 2003)

which particular immune cells are prognostic for each distinct type of cancer. The molecular features of tumor infiltrating immune cells and defined immune response signatures have recently been used to predict survival in human follicular lymphoma patients (Dave et al., 2004). Gene expression profiling and proteomics are going to play a key part in defining the major positive and negative immune indicators in human cancer progression.

7. Conclusions

In this review, we have summarized the strong evidence that now supports the existence of an effective cancer immunosurveillance process that prevents cancer development in both mice and humans. We have discussed the various leukocyte subsets, effector molecules, and methods of tumor recognition that contribute to natural host immune suppression of tumors. Moreover, we have presented the rationale for refining the cancer immunosurveillance hypothesis into one that we have termed cancer immunoediting, wherein the malignant cell's immunogenic phenotype is sculpted by its interaction with the host immune system, determining its fitness for continued survival and growth in an immunocompetent environment. We have tried to highlight in this review several of the remaining critical questions as we see them whose answers will ultimately frame a full understanding of host immunity to cancer. An improved understanding of the immunobiology of cancer immunoediting and a molecular definition of how tumors are shaped by this process will undoubtedly bring us closer to a more effective use of immunotherapy to control and/or eradicate neoplastic disease.

Acknowledgments

This review is dedicated to Dr. Lloyd J. Old on the occasion of his retirement as Scientific Director of the Ludwig Institute for Cancer Research. Lloyd Old has been a constant source of inspiration, information, encouragement and support to the field of tumor immunology in general and to the authors of this review in particular. The authors also wish to acknowledge the particularly helpful contributions of science and discussion that Dr. Yoshohiro Hayakawa made to this review. We are grateful to many individuals who have either been members of our laboratories or our close collaborators during the past 5 years who made significant contributions to the field including: Drs. Jack Bui, Ruby Chan, Erika Cretney, Mark Diamond, Hiroaki Ikeda, Catherine Koebel, Joseph Trapani, Jeremy Swann, Vijay Shankaran, Kathleen C.F. Sheehan, and Ravi Uppaluri. Work performed in the MJS laboratory was supported by grants from the National Health and Medical Research Council of Australia, cancer Council of Victoria and the National Cancer Institute, NIH (CA106377). Work in the RDS laboratory was supported by grants from the National Cancer Institute (CA43059 and CA 107527), The Ludwig Institute for Cancer Research, The Cancer Research Institute, and The Susan G. Komen Breast Cancer Foundation.

References

Affabris, E., Romeo, G., Federico, M., Coccia, E., Locardi, C., Belardelli, F., and Rossi, G. B. (1987). Molecular mechanisms of action of interferons in the Friend virus-induced leukemia cell system. *Haematologica* **72**, 76–78.

Akazawa, T., Masuda, H., Saeki, Y., Matsumoto, M., Takeda, K., Tsujimura, K., Kuzushima, K., Takahashi, T., Azuma, I., Akira, S., Toyoshima, K., and Seya, T. (2004). Adjuvant-mediated tumor regression and tumor-specific cytotoxic response are impaired in MyD88-deficient mice. *Cancer Res.* **64**, 757–764.

Albert, M. L., Austin, L. M., and Darnell, R. B. (2000). Detection and treatment of activated T cells in the cerebrospinal fluid of patients with paraneoplastic cerebellar degeneration. *Ann. Neurol.* **47**, 9–17.

Albert, M. L., Darnell, J. C., Bender, A., Francisco, L. M., Bhardwaj, N., and Darnell, R. B. (1998). Tumor-specific killer cells in paraneoplastic cerebellar degeneration. *Nat. Med.* **4**, 1321–1324.

Albert, M. L., and Darnell, R. B. (2004). Paraneoplastic neurological degenerations: Keys to tumour immunity. *Nat. Rev. Cancer* **4**, 36–44.

Algarra, I., Cabrera, T., and Garrido, F. (2000). The HLA crossroad in tumor immunology. *Hum. Immunol.* **61**, 65–73.

Asahara, T., Murohara, T., Sullivan, A., Silver, M., van der Zee, R., Li, T., Witzenbichler, B., Schatteman, G., and Isner, J. M. (1997). Isolation of putative progenitor endothelial cells for angiogenesis. *Science* **275**, 964–967.

Bach, E. A., Aguet, M., and Schreiber, R. D. (1997). The IFN gamma receptor: A paradigm for cytokine receptor signaling. *Annu. Rev. Immunol.* **15**, 563–591.

Bancroft, G. J., Schreiber, R. D., and Unanue, E. R. (1991). Natural immunity: A T-cell-independent pathway of macrophage activation, defined in the scid mouse. *Immunol. Rev.* **124**, 5–24.

Bauer, S., Groh, V., Wu, J., Steinle, A., Phillips, J. H., Lanier, L. L., and Spies, T. (1999). Activation of NK cells and T cells by NKG2D, a receptor for stress-inducible MICA. *Science* **285**, 727–729.

Baxevanis, C. N., Voutsas, I. F., Tsitsilonis, O. E., Tsiatas, M. L., Gritzapis, A. D., and Papamichail, M. (2000). Compromised anti-tumor responses in tumor necrosis factor-alpha knockout mice. *Eur. J. Immunol.* **30**, 1957–1966.

Belardelli, F., Ferrantini, M., Proietti, E., and Kirkwood, J. M. (2002). Interferon-alpha in tumor immunity and immunotherapy. *Cytokine Growth Factor Rev.* **13**, 119–134.

Blasius, A., Vermi, W., Krug, A., Facchetti, F., Cella, M., and Colonna, M. (2004). A cell-surface molecule selectively expressed on murine natural interferon-producing cells that blocks secretion of interferon-alpha. *Blood* **103**, 4201–4206.

Boon, T., and van der Bruggen, P. (1996). Human tumor antigens recognized by T lymphocytes. *J. Exp. Med.* **183**, 725–729.

Borg, C., Terme, M., Taieb, J., Menard, C., Flament, C., Robert, C., Maruyama, K., Wakasugi, H., Angevin, E., Thielemans, K., Le Cesne, A., Chung-Scott, V., et al. (2004). Novel mode of action of c-kit tyrosine kinase inhibitors leading to NK cell-dependent antitumor effects. *J. Clin. Invest.* **114**, 379–388.

Boshoff, C., and Weiss, R. (2002). AIDS-related malignancies. *Nat. Rev. Cancer* **2**, 373–382.

Bromberg, J. F., Horvath, C. M., Wen, Z., Schreiber, R. D., and Darnell, J. E., Jr. (1996). Transcriptionally active Stat1 is required for the antiproliferative effects of both interferon alpha and interferon gamma. *Proc. Natl. Acad. Sci. USA* **93**, 7673–7678.

Bronte, V., Apolloni, E., Cabrelle, A., Ronca, R., Serafini, P., Zamboni, P., Restifo, N. P., and Zanovello, P. (2000). Identification of a CD11b(+)/Gr-1(+)/CD31(+) myeloid progenitor capable of activating or suppressing CD8(+) T cells. *Blood* **96**, 3838–3846.

Burnet, F. M. (1964). Immunological factors in the process of carcinogenesis. *Br. Med. Bull.* **20**, 154–158.
Burnet, F. M. (1970). The concept of immunological surveillance. *Prog. Exp. Tumor Res.* **13**, 1–27.
Burnet, F. M. (1971). Immunological surveillance in neoplasia. *Transplant Rev.* **7**, 3–25.
Burnet, M. (1957). Cancer: A biological approach. III. Viruses associated with neoplastic conditions. IV. Practical applications. *Br. Med. J.* **1**, 841–847.
Burstein, N. A., and Law, L. W. (1971). Neonatal thymectomy and non-viral mammary tumours in mice. *Nature* **231**, 450–452.
Carayannopoulos, L. N., Naidenko, O. V., Fremont, D. H., and Yokoyama, W. M. (2002). Cutting edge: Murine UL16-binding protein-like transcript 1: A newly described transcript encoding a high-affinity ligand for murine NKG2D. *J. Immunol.* **169**, 4079–4083.
Carey, T. E., Takahashi, T., Resnick, L. A., Oettgen, H. F., and Old, L. J. (1976). Cell surface antigens of human malignant melanoma: Mixed hemadsorption assays for humoral immunity to cultured autologous melanoma cells. *Proc. Natl. Acad. Sci. USA* **73**, 3278–3282.
Carmeliet, P., and Jain, R. K. (2000). Angiogenesis in cancer and other diseases. *Nature* **407**, 249–257.
Cerwenka, A., Baron, J. L., and Lanier, L. L. (2001). Ectopic expression of retinoic acid early inducible-1 gene (RAE-1) permits natural killer cell-mediated rejection of a MHC class I-bearing tumor *in vivo*. *Proc. Natl. Acad. Sci. USA* **98**, 11521–11526.
Cerwenka, A., and Lanier, L. L. (2001). Ligands for natural killer cell receptors: Redundancy or specificity. *Immunol. Rev.* **181**, 158–169.
Chen, Y. T., Scanlan, M. J., Sahin, U., Tureci, O., Gure, A. O., Tsang, S., Williamson, B., Stockert, E., Pfreundschuh, M., and Old, L. J. (1997). A testicular antigen aberrantly expressed in human cancers detected by autologous antibody screening. *Proc. Natl. Acad. Sci. USA* **94**, 1914–1918.
Chin, Y. E., Kitagawa, M., Kuida, K., Flavell, R. A., and Fu, X. Y. (1997). Activation of the STAT signaling pathway can cause expression of caspase 1 and apoptosis. *Mol. Cell. Biol.* **17**, 5328–5337.
Chin, Y. E., Kitagawa, M., Su, W. C., You, Z. H., Iwamoto, Y., and Fu, X. Y. (1996). Cell growth arrest and induction of cyclin-dependent kinase inhibitor p21 WAF1/CIP1 mediated by STAT1. *Science* **272**, 719–722.
Clemente, C. G., Mihm, M. C., Jr., Bufalino, R., Zurrida, S., Collini, P., and Cascinelli, N. (1996). Prognostic value of tumor infiltrating lymphocytes in the vertical growth phase of primary cutaneous melanoma. *Cancer* **77**, 1303–1310.
Coca, S., Perez-Piqueras, J., Martinez, D., Colmenarejo, A., Saez, M. A., Vallejo, C., Martos, J. A., and Moreno, M. (1997). The prognostic significance of intratumoral natural killer cells in patients with colorectal carcinoma. *Cancer* **79**, 2320–2328.
Coley, W. B. (1991). The treatment of malignant tumors by repeated inoculations of erysipelas. With a report of ten original cases 1893. *Clin. Orthop.* **262**, 3–11.
Conejo-Garcia, J. R., Benencia, F., Courreges, M. C., Kang, E., Mohamed-Hadley, A., Buckanovich, R. J., Holtz, D. O., Jenkins, A., Na, H., Zhang, L., Wagner, D. S., Katsaros, D., *et al.* (2004). Tumor-infiltrating dendritic cell precursors recruited by a beta-defensin contribute to vasculogenesis under the influence of Vegf-A. *Nat. Med.* **10**, 950–958.
Conejo-Garcia, J. R., Benencia, F., Courreges, M. C., Khang, E., Zhang, L., Mohamed-Hadley, A., Vinocur, J. M., Buckanovich, R. J., Thompson, C. B., Levine, B., and Coukos, G. (2003). Letal, A tumor-associated NKG2D immunoreceptor ligand, induces activation and expansion of effector immune cells. *Cancer Biol. Ther.* **2**, 446–451.
Cory, S., Huang, D. C., and Adams, J. M. (2003). The Bcl-2 family: Roles in cell survival and oncogenesis. *Oncogene* **22**, 8590–8607.
Cosman, D., Mullberg, J., Sutherland, C. L., Chin, W., Armitage, R., Fanslow, W., Kubin, M., and Chalupny, N. J. (2001). ULBPs, novel MHC class I-related molecules, bind to CMV

glycoprotein UL16 and stimulate NK cytotoxicity through the NKG2D receptor. *Immunity* **14**, 123–133.

Coughlin, C. M., Salhany, K. E., Gee, M. S., LaTemple, D. C., Kotenko, S., Ma, X., Gri, G., Wysocka, M., Kim, J. E., Liu, L., Liao, F., Farber, J. M., *et al.* (1998). Tumor cell responses to IFNgamma affect tumorigenicity and response to IL-12 therapy and antiangiogenesis. *Immunity* **9**, 25–34.

Cretney, E., Takeda, K., Yagita, H., Glaccum, M., Peschon, J. J., and Smyth, M. J. (2002). Increased susceptibility to tumor initiation and metastasis in TNF-related apoptosis-inducing ligand-deficient mice. *J. Immunol.* **168**, 1356–1361.

Crowe, N. Y., Smyth, M. J., and Godfrey, D. I. (2002). A critical role for natural killer T cells in immunosurveillance of methylcholanthrene-induced sarcomas. *J. Exp. Med.* **196**, 119–127.

Cui, J., Shin, T., Kawano, T., Sato, H., Kondo, E., Toura, I., Kaneko, Y., Koseki, H., Kanno, M., and Taniguchi, M. (1997). Requirement for Valpha14 NKT cells in IL-12-mediated rejection of tumors. *Science* **278**, 1623–1626.

Cui, Z., Willingham, M. C., Hicks, A. M., Alexander-Miller, M. A., Howard, T. D., Hawkins, G. A., Miller, M. S., Weir, H. M., Du, W., and DeLong, C. J. (2003). Spontaneous regression of advanced cancer: Identification of a unique genetically determined, age-dependent trait in mice. *Proc. Natl. Acad. Sci. USA* **100**, 6682–6687.

Curcio, C., Di Carlo, E., Clynes, R., Smyth, M. J., Boggio, K., Quaglino, E., Spadaro, M., Colombo, M. P., Amici, A., Lollini, P. L., Musiani, P., and Forni, G. (2003). Nonredundant roles of antibody, cytokines, and perforin in the eradication of established Her-2/neu carcinomas. *J. Clin. Invest.* **111**, 1161–1170.

Curiel, T. J., Coukos, G., Zou, L., Alvarez, X., Cheng, P., Mottram, P., Evdemon-Hogan, M., Conejo-Garcia, J. R., Zhang, L., Burow, M., Zhu, Y., Wei, S., *et al.* (2004). Specific recruitment of regulatory T cells in ovarian carcinoma fosters immune privilege and predicts reduced survival. *Nat. Med.* **10**, 942–949.

Danial, N. N., and Korsmeyer, S. J. (2004). Cell death: Critical control points. *Cell* **116**, 205–219.

Darnell, R. B. (1996). Onconeural antigens and the paraneoplastic neurologic disorders: At the intersection of cancer, immunity, and the brain. *Proc. Natl. Acad. Sci. USA* **93**, 4529–4536.

Darnell, R. B., and DeAngelis, L. M. (1993). Regression of small-cell lung carcinoma in patients with paraneoplastic neuronal antibodies. *Lancet* **341**, 21–22.

Darnell, R. B., and Posner, J. B. (2003). Observing the invisible: Successful tumor immunity in humans. *Nat. Immunol.* **4**, 201.

Das, H., Groh, V., Kuijl, C., Sugita, M., Morita, C. T., Spies, T., and Bukowski, J. F. (2001). MICA engagement by human Vgamma2Vdelta2 T cells enhances their antigen-dependent effector function. *Immunity* **15**, 83–93.

Dave, S. S., Wright, G., Tan, B., Rosenwald, A., Gascoyne, R. D., Chan, W. C., Fisher, R. I., Braziel, R. M., Rimsza, L. M., Grogan, T. M., Miller, T. P., LeBlanc, M., *et al.* (2004). Prediction of survival in follicular lymphoma based on molecular features of tumor-infiltrating immune cells. *N. Engl. J. Med.* **351**, 2159–2169.

Davidson, W. F., Giese, T., and Fredrickson, T. N. (1998). Spontaneous development of plasmacytoid tumors in mice with defective Fas-Fas ligand interactions. *J. Exp. Med.* **187**, 1825–1838.

Dhodapkar, M. V., Geller, M. D., Chang, D. H., Shimizu, K., Fujii, S., Dhodapkar, K. M., and Krasovsky, J. (2003). A reversible defect in natural killer T cell function characterizes the progression of premalignant to malignant multiple myeloma. *J. Exp. Med.* **197**, 1667–1676.

Di Carlo, E., Forni, G., Lollini, P., Colombo, M. P., Modesti, A., and Musiani, P. (2001). The intriguing role of polymorphonuclear neutrophils in antitumor reactions. *Blood* **97**, 339–345.

Diefenbach, A., Hsia, J. K., Hsiung, M. Y., and Raulet, D. H. (2003). A novel ligand for the NKG2D receptor activates NK cells and macrophages and induces tumor immunity. *Eur. J. Immunol.* **33**, 381–391.
Diefenbach, A., Jamieson, A. M., Liu, S. D., Shastri, N., and Raulet, D. H. (2000). Ligands for the murine NKG2D receptor: Expression by tumor cells and activation of NK cells and macrophages. *Nat. Immunol.* **1**, 119–126.
Diefenbach, A., Jensen, E. R., Jamieson, A. M., and Raulet, D. H. (2001). Rae1 and H60 ligands of the NKG2D receptor stimulate tumour immunity. *Nature* **413**, 165–171.
Dighe, A. S., Richards, E., Old, L. J., and Schreiber, R. D. (1994). Enhanced *in vivo* growth and resistance to rejection of tumor cells expressing dominant negative IFN gamma receptors. *Immunity* **1**, 447–456.
Dunn, G. P., Bruce, A. T., Ikeda, H., Old, L. J., and Schreiber, R. D. (2002). Cancer immunoediting: From immunosurveillance to tumor escape. *Nat. Immunol.* **3**, 991–998.
Dunn, G. P., Bruce, A. T., Sheehan, K. C., Shankaran, V., Uppaluri, R., Bui, J. D., Diamond, M. S., Koebel, C. M., Arthur, C., White, J. M., and Schreiber, R. D. (2005a). A critical function for type I interferons in cancer immunoediting. *Nat. Immunol.* **6**, 722–729.
Dunn, G. P., Old, L. J., and Schreiber, R. D. (2004a). The immunobiology of cancer immunosurveillance and immunoediting. *Immunity* **21**, 137–148.
Dunn, G. P., Old, L. J., and Schreiber, R. D. (2004b). The three Es of cancer immunoediting. *Annu. Rev. Immunol.* **22**, 329–360.
Dunn, G. P., Sheehan, K. C., Old, L. J., and Schreiber, R. D. (2005b). IFN unresponsiveness in LNCaP cells due to the lack of JAK1 gene expression. *Cancer Res.* **65**, 3447–3453.
Ehrlich, P. (1909). Uber den jetzigen Stand der Karzinomforschung. *Ned. Tijdschr. Genees.* **5**, 273–290.
Elder, G. J., Hersey, P., and Branley, P. (1997). Remission of transplanted melanoma—clinical course and tumour cell characterisation. *Clin. Transplant.* **11**, 565–568.
Engel, A. M., Svane, I. M., Mouritsen, S., Rygaard, J., Clausen, J., and Werdelin, O. (1996). Methylcholanthrene-induced sarcomas in nude mice have short induction times and relatively low levels of surface MHC class I expression. *Apmis* **104**, 629–639.
Enzler, T., Gillessen, S., Manis, J. P., Ferguson, D., Fleming, J., Alt, F. W., Mihm, M., and Dranoff, G. (2003). Deficiencies of GM-CSF and interferon gamma link inflammation and cancer. *J. Exp. Med.* **197**, 1213–1219.
Erianne, G. S., Wajchman, J., Yauch, R., Tsiagbe, V. K., Kim, B. S., and Ponzio, N. M. (2000). B cell lymphomas of C57L/J mice; the role of natural killer cells and T helper cells in lymphoma development and growth. *Leuk. Res.* **24**, 705–718.
Fridman, J. S., and Lowe, S. W. (2003). Control of apoptosis by p53. *Oncogene* **22**, 9030–9040.
Gabrilovich, D. (2004). Mechanisms and functional significance of tumour-induced dendritic-cell defects. *Nat. Rev. Immunol.* **4**, 941–952.
Gabrilovich, D. I., Chen, H. L., Girgis, K. R., Cunningham, H. T., Meny, G. M., Nadaf, S., Kavanaugh, D., and Carbone, D. P. (1996). Production of vascular endothelial growth factor by human tumors inhibits the functional maturation of dendritic cells. *Nat. Med.* **2**, 1096–1103.
Gabrilovich, D. I., Ishida, T., Nadaf, S., Ohm, J. E., and Carbone, D. P. (1999). Antibodies to vascular endothelial growth factor enhance the efficacy of cancer immunotherapy by improving endogenous dendritic cell function. *Clin. Cancer Res.* **5**, 2963–2970.
Gao, Y., Yang, W., Pan, M., Scully, E., Girardi, M., Augenlicht, L. H., Craft, J., and Yin, Z. (2003). Gamma delta T cells provide an early source of interferon gamma in tumor immunity. *J. Exp. Med.* **198**, 433–442.
Gasser, S., Orsulic, S., Brown, E. J., and Raulet, D. H. (2005). The DNA damage pathway regulates innate immune system ligands of the NKG2D receptor. *Nature* **436**, 1186–1190.

Gerosa, F., Baldani-Guerra, B., Nisii, C., Marchesini, V., Carra, G., and Trinchieri, G. (2002). Reciprocal activating interaction between natural killer cells and dendritic cells. *J. Exp. Med.* **195**, 327–333.

Gershwin, M. E., Ohsugi, Y., Castles, J. J., Ikeda, R. M., and Ruebner, B. (1983). Anti-mu induces lymphoma in germfree congenitally athymic (nude) but not in heterozygous (nu/+) mice. *J. Immunol.* **131**, 2069–2073.

Gilfillan, S., Ho, E. L., Cella, M., Yokoyama, W. M., and Colonna, M. (2002). NKG2D recruits two distinct adapters to trigger NK cell activation and costimulation. *Nat. Immunol.* **3**, 1150–1155.

Girardi, M., Glusac, E., Filler, R. B., Roberts, S. J., Propperova, I., Lewis, J., Tigelaar, R. E., and Hayday, A. C. (2003). The distinct contributions of murine T cell receptor (TCR)gammadelta+ and TCRalphabeta+ T cells to different stages of chemically induced skin cancer. *J. Exp. Med.* **198**, 747–755.

Girardi, M., Oppenheim, D., Glusac, E. J., Filler, R., Balmain, A., Tigelaar, R. E., and Hayday, A. C. (2004). Characterizing the protective component of the alphabeta T cell response to transplantable squamous cell carcinoma. *J. Invest. Dermatol.* **122**, 699–706.

Girardi, M., Oppenheim, D. E., Steele, C. R., Lewis, J. M., Glusac, E., Filler, R., Hobby, P., Sutton, B., Tigelaar, R. E., and Hayday, A. C. (2001). Regulation of cutaneous malignancy by gammadelta T cells. *Science* **294**, 605–609.

Godfrey, D. I., Hammond, K. J., Poulton, L. D., Smyth, M. J., and Baxter, A. G. (2000). NKT cells: Facts, functions and fallacies. *Immunol. Today* **21**, 573–583.

Godfrey, D. I., Pellicci, D. G., and Smyth, M. J. (2004). Immunology. The elusive NKT cell antigen—is the search over? *Science* **306**, 1687–1689.

Gorelik, L., and Flavell, R. A. (2001). Immune-mediated eradication of tumors through the blockade of transforming growth factor-beta signaling in T cells. *Nat. Med.* **7**, 1118–1122.

Gorelik, L., and Flavell, R. A. (2002). Transforming growth factor-beta in T-cell biology. *Nat. Rev. Immunol.* **2**, 46–53.

Grant, G. A., and Miller, J. F. (1965). Effect of neonatal thymectomy on the induction of sarcomata in C57 BL mice. *Nature* **205**, 1124–1125.

Graus, F., Dalmou, J., Rene, R., Tora, M., Malats, N., Verschuuren, J. J., Cardenal, F., Vinolas, N., Garcia del Muro, J., Vadell, C., Mason, W. P., Rosell, R., *et al.* (1997). Anti-Hu antibodies in patients with small-cell lung cancer: Association with complete response to therapy and improved survival. *J. Clin. Oncol.* **15**, 2866–2872.

Green, D. R., and Kroemer, G. (2004). The pathophysiology of mitochondrial cell death. *Science* **305**, 626–629.

Gresser, I., and Belardelli, F. (2002). Endogenous type I interferons as a defense against tumors. *Cytokine Growth Factor Rev.* **13**, 111–118.

Gresser, I., Belardelli, F., Maury, C., Maunoury, M. T., and Tovey, M. G. (1983). Injection of mice with antibody to interferon enhances the growth of transplantable murine tumors. *J. Exp. Med.* **158**, 2095–2107.

Gresser, I., Maury, C., Vignaux, F., Haller, O., Belardelli, F., and Tovey, M. G. (1988). Antibody to mouse interferon alpha/beta abrogates resistance to the multiplication of Friend erythroleukemia cells in the livers of allogeneic mice. *J. Exp. Med.* **168**, 1271–1291.

Groh, V., Bahram, S., Bauer, S., Herman, A., Beauchamp, M., and Spies, T. (1996). Cell stress-regulated human major histocompatibility complex class I gene expressed in gastrointestinal epithelium. *Proc. Natl. Acad. Sci. USA* **93**, 12445–12450.

Groh, V., Rhinehart, R., Randolph-Habecker, J., Topp, M. S., Riddell, S. R., and Spies, T. (2001). Costimulation of CD8alphabeta T cells by NKG2D via engagement by MIC induced on virus-infected cells. *Nat. Immunol.* **2**, 255–260.

Groh, V., Rhinehart, R., Secrist, H., Bauer, S., Grabstein, K. H., and Spies, T. (1999). Broad tumor-associated expression and recognition by tumor-derived gamma delta T cells of MICA and MICB. *Proc. Natl. Acad. Sci. USA* **96,** 6879–6884.

Groh, V., Steinle, A., Bauer, S., and Spies, T. (1998). Recognition of stress-induced MHC molecules by intestinal epithelial gammadelta T cells. *Science* **279,** 1737–1740.

Groh, V., Wu, J., Yee, C., and Spies, T. (2002). Tumour-derived soluble MIC ligands impair expression of NKG2D and T-cell activation. *Nature* **419,** 734–738.

Hahn, W. C., and Weinberg, R. A. (2002). Modelling the molecular circuitry of cancer. *Nat. Rev. Cancer* **2,** 331–441.

Hahne, M., Rimoldi, D., Schroter, M., Romero, P., Schreier, M., French, L. E., Schneider, P., Bornand, T., Fontana, A., Lienard, D., Cerottini, J., and Tschopp, J. (1996). Melanoma cell expression of Fas(Apo-1/CD95) ligand: Implications for tumor immune escape. *Science* **274,** 1363–1366.

Haliotis, T., Ball, J. K., Dexter, D., and Roder, J. C. (1985). Spontaneous and induced primary oncogenesis in natural killer (NK)-cell-deficient beige mutant mice. *Int. J. Cancer* **35,** 505–513.

Hanahan, D., and Folkman, J. (1996). Patterns and emerging mechanisms of the angiogenic switch during tumorigenesis. *Cell* **86,** 353–364.

Hanahan, D., and Weinberg, R. A. (2000). The hallmarks of cancer. *Cell* **100,** 57–70.

Hayakawa, Y., Godfrey, D. I., and Smyth, M. J. (2004). Alpha-galactosylceramide: Potential immunomodulatory activity and future application. *Curr. Med. Chem.* **11,** 241–252.

Hayakawa, Y., Kelly, J. M., Westwood, J. A., Darcy, P. K., Diefenbach, A., Raulet, D., and Smyth, M. J. (2002). Cutting edge: Tumor rejection mediated by NKG2D receptor-ligand interaction is dependent upon perforin. *J. Immunol.* **169,** 5377–5381.

Hayakawa, Y., Rovero, S., Forni, G., and Smyth, M. J. (2003). Alpha-galactosylceramide (KRN7000) suppression of chemical- and oncogene-dependent carcinogenesis. *Proc. Natl. Acad. Sci. USA* **100,** 9464–9469.

Hayashi, T., and Faustman, D. L. (2002). Development of spontaneous uterine tumors in low molecular mass polypeptide-2 knockout mice. *Cancer Res.* **62,** 24–27.

Heidelberger, C. (1975). Chemical carcinogenesis. *Annu. Rev. Biochem.* **44,** 79–121.

Hodge-Dufour, J., Noble, P. W., Horton, M. R., Bao, C., Wysoka, M., Burdick, M. D., Strieter, R. M., Trinchieri, G., and Pure, E. (1997). Induction of IL-12 and chemokines by hyaluronan requires adhesion-dependent priming of resident but not elicited macrophages. *J. Immunol.* **159,** 2492–2500.

Huang, A. Y., Golumbek, P., Ahmadzadeh, M., Jaffee, E., Pardoll, D., and Levitsky, H. (1994). Role of bone marrow-derived cells in presenting MHC class I-restricted tumor antigens. *Science* **264,** 961–965.

Humbert, P., Russell, S., and Richardson, H. (2003). Dlg, Scribble and Lgl in cell polarity, cell proliferation and cancer. *Bioessays* **25,** 542–553.

Hunig, T., and Bevan, M. J. (1980). Specificity of cytotoxic T cells from athymic mice. *J. Exp. Med.* **152,** 688–702.

Iinuma, T., Homma, S., Noda, T., Kufe, D., Ohno, T., and Toda, G. (2004). Prevention of gastrointestinal tumors based on adenomatous polyposis coli gene mutation by dendritic cell vaccine. *J. Clin. Invest.* **113,** 1307–1317.

Ikehara, S., Pahwa, R. N., Fernandes, G., Hansen, C. T., and Good, R. A. (1984). Functional T cells in athymic nude mice. *Proc. Natl. Acad. Sci. USA* **81,** 886–888.

Ishigami, S., Natsugoe, S., Tokuda, K., Nakajo, A., Che, X., Iwashige, H., Aridome, K., Hokita, S., and Aikou, T. (2000). Prognostic value of intratumoral natural killer cells in gastric carcinoma. *Cancer* **88,** 577–583.

Jan Chalupny, N., Sutherland, C. L., Lawrence, W. A., Rein-Weston, A., and Cosman, D. (2003). ULBP4 is a novel ligand for human NKG2D. *Biochem. Biophys. Res. Commun.* **305,** 129–135.

Janeway, C. A., Jr. (1989). Approaching the asymptote? Evolution and revolution in immunology. *Cold Spring Harb. Symp. Quant. Biol.* **54**(Pt. 1), 1–13.

Jinushi, M., Takehara, T., Kanto, T., Tatsumi, T., Groh, V., Spies, T., Miyagi, T., Suzuki, T., Sasaki, Y., and Hayashi, N. (2003a). Critical role of MHC class I-related chain A and B expression on IFN-alpha-stimulated dendritic cells in NK cell activation: Impairment in chronic hepatitis C virus infection. *J. Immunol.* **170,** 1249–1256.

Jinushi, M., Takehara, T., Tatsumi, T., Kanto, T., Groh, V., Spies, T., Kimura, R., Miyagi, T., Mochizuki, K., Sasaki, Y., and Hayashi, N. (2003b). Expression and role of MICA and MICB in human hepatocellular carcinomas and their regulation by retinoic acid. *Int. J. Cancer* **104,** 354–361.

Johnson, G. B., Brunn, G. J., Kodaira, Y., and Platt, J. L. (2002). Receptor-mediated monitoring of tissue well-being via detection of soluble heparan sulfate by Toll-like receptor 4. *J. Immunol.* **168,** 5233–5239.

Johnson, S. (1968). Effect of thymectomy on the induction of skin tumours by dibenzanthracene, and of breast tumours by dimethylbenzanthracene, in mice of the IF strain. *Br. J. Cancer* **22,** 755–761.

Kaplan, D. H., Shankaran, V., Dighe, A. S., Stockert, E., Aguet, M., Old, L. J., and Schreiber, R. D. (1998). Demonstration of an interferon gamma-dependent tumor surveillance system in immunocompetent mice. *Proc. Natl. Acad. Sci. USA* **95,** 7556–7561.

Kaplan, H. S. (1971). Role of immunologic disturbance in human oncogenesis: Some facts and fancies. *Br. J. Cancer* **25,** 620–634.

Khong, H. T., and Restifo, N. P. (2002). Natural selection of tumor variants in the generation of "tumor escape" phenotypes. *Nat. Immunol.* **3,** 999–1005.

Klein, G. (1966). Tumor antigens. *Annu. Rev. Microbiol.* **20,** 223–252.

Klein, G. (1973). Immunological surveillance against neoplasia. *Harvey Lect.* **69,** 71–102.

Knight, B., Yeoh, G. C., Husk, K. L., Ly, T., Abraham, L. J., Yu, C., Rhim, J. A., and Fausto, N. (2000). Impaired preneoplastic changes and liver tumor formation in tumor necrosis factor receptor type 1 knockout mice. *J. Exp. Med.* **192,** 1809–1818.

Knuth, A., Danowski, B., Oettgen, H. F., and Old, L. J. (1984). T-cell-mediated cytotoxicity against autologous malignant melanoma: Analysis with interleukin 2-dependent T-cell cultures. *Proc. Natl. Acad. Sci. USA* **81,** 3511–3515.

Kumar, A., Commane, M., Flickinger, T. W., Horvath, C. M., and Stark, G. R. (1997). Defective TNF-alpha-induced apoptosis in STAT1-null cells due to low constitutive levels of caspases. *Science* **278,** 1630–1632.

Lala, P. K., and Chakraborty, C. (2001). Role of nitric oxide in carcinogenesis and tumour progression. *Lancet Oncol.* **2,** 149–156.

Lee, J. J., Dimina, D., Macias, M. P., Ochkur, S. I., McGarry, M. P., O'Neill, K. R., Protheroe, C., Pero, R., Nguyen, T., Cormier, S. A., Lenkiewicz, E., Colbert, D., *et al.* (2004). Defining a link with asthma in mice congenitally deficient in eosinophils. *Science* **305,** 1773–1776.

Lengauer, C., Kinzler, K. W., and Vogelstein, B. (1998). Genetic instabilities in human cancers. *Nature* **396,** 643–649.

Li, Z., Menoret, A., and Srivastava, P. (2002). Roles of heat-shock proteins in antigen presentation and cross-presentation. *Curr. Opin. Immunol.* **14,** 45–51.

Liljefors, M., Nilsson, B., Hjelm Skog, A. L., Ragnhammar, P., Mellstedt, H., and Frodin, J. E. (2003). Natural killer (NK) cell function is a strong prognostic factor in colorectal carcinoma patients treated with the monoclonal antibody 17-1A. *Int. J. Cancer* **105,** 717–723.

Liyanage, U. K., Moore, T. T., Joo, H. G., Tanaka, Y., Herrmann, V., Doherty, G., Drebin, J. A., Strasberg, S. M., Eberlein, T. J., Goedegebuure, P. S., and Linehan, D. C. (2002). Prevalence of regulatory T cells is increased in peripheral blood and tumor microenvironment of patients with pancreas or breast adenocarcinoma. *J. Immunol.* **169**, 2756–2761.

Locksley, R. M., Killeen, N., and Lenardo, M. J. (2001). The TNF and TNF receptor superfamilies: Integrating mammalian biology. *Cell* **104**, 487–501.

Loeb, L. A. (1991). Mutator phenotype may be required for multistage carcinogenesis. *Cancer Res.* **51**, 3075–3079.

Loeb, L. A., Loeb, K. R., and Anderson, J. P. (2003). Multiple mutations and cancer. *Proc. Natl. Acad. Sci. USA* **100**, 776–781.

Loeffler, C. M., Smyth, M. J., Longo, D. L., Kopp, W. C., Harvey, L. K., Tribble, H. R., Tase, J. E., Urba, W. J., Leonard, A. S., Young, H. A., *et al.* (1992). Immunoregulation in cancer-bearing hosts. Down-regulation of gene expression and cytotoxic function in CD8+ T cells. *J. Immunol.* **149**, 949–956.

Lowe, S. W., Cepero, E., and Evan, G. (2004). Intrinsic tumour suppression. *Nature* **432**, 307–315.

Ludwig, A. T., Moore, J. M., Luo, Y., Chen, X., Saltsgaver, N. A., O'Donnell, M. A., and Griffith, T. S. (2004). Tumor necrosis factor-related apoptosis-inducing ligand: A novel mechanism for Bacillus Calmette-Guerin-induced antitumor activity. *Cancer Res.* **64**, 3386–3390.

Luster, A. D., and Leder, P. (1993). IP-10, a -C-X-C- chemokine, elicits a potent thymus-dependent antitumor response *in vivo. J. Exp. Med.* **178**, 1057–1065.

Lyden, D., Hattori, K., Dias, S., Costa, C., Blaikie, P., Butros, L., Chadburn, A., Heissig, B., Marks, W., Witte, L., Wu, Y., Hicklin, D., *et al.* (2001). Impaired recruitment of bone-marrow-derived endothelial and hematopoietic precursor cells blocks tumor angiogenesis and growth. *Nat. Med.* **7**, 1194–1201.

MacKie, R. M., Reid, R., and Junor, B. (2003). Fatal melanoma transferred in a donated kidney 16 years after melanoma surgery. *N. Engl. J. Med.* **348**, 567–568.

Macleod, K. (2000). Tumor suppressor genes. *Curr. Opin. Genet. Dev.* **10**, 81–93.

MacMicking, J., Xie, Q. W., and Nathan, C. (1997). Nitric oxide and macrophage function. *Annu. Rev. Immunol.* **15**, 323–350.

Maleckar, J. R., and Sherman, L. A. (1987). The composition of the T cell receptor repertoire in nude mice. *J. Immunol.* **138**, 3873–3876.

Marincola, F. M., Jaffee, E. M., Hicklin, D. J., and Ferrone, S. (2000). Escape of human solid tumors from T-cell recognition: Molecular mechanisms and functional significance. *Adv. Immunol.* **74**, 181–273.

Mattes, J., Hulett, M., Xie, W., Hogan, S., Rothenberg, M. E., Foster, P., and Parish, C. (2003). Immunotherapy of cytotoxic T cell-resistant tumors by T helper 2 cells: An eotaxin and STAT6-dependent process. *J. Exp. Med.* **197**, 387–393.

Matzinger, P. (1994). Tolerance, danger, and the extended family. *Annu. Rev. Immunol.* **12**, 991–1045.

Medawar, P. (1944). The behaviour and fate of skin autografts and skin homografts in rabbits. *J. Anat.* **78**, 176–199.

Melani, C., Chiodoni, C., Forni, G., and Colombo, M. P. (2003). Myeloid cell expansion elicited by the progression of spontaneous mammary carcinomas in c-erbB-2 transgenic BALB/c mice suppresses immune reactivity. *Blood* **102**, 2138–2145.

Mihara, M., Erster, S., Zaika, A., Petrenko, O., Chittenden, T., Pancoska, P., and Moll, U. M. (2003). p53 has a direct apoptogenic role at the mitochondria. *Mol. Cell* **11**, 577–590.

Mihm, M. C., Jr., Clemente, C. G., and Cascinelli, N. (1996). Tumor infiltrating lymphocytes in lymph node melanoma metastases: A histopathologic prognostic indicator and an expression of local immune response. *Lab. Invest.* **74**, 43–47.

Mitra-Kaushik, S., Harding, J., Hess, J., Schreiber, R., and Ratner, L. (2004). Enhanced tumorigenesis in HTLV-1 tax-transgenic mice deficient in interferon-gamma. *Blood* **104**, 3305–3311.
Moore, R. J., Owens, D. M., Stamp, G., Arnott, C., Burke, F., East, N., Holdsworth, H., Turner, L., Rollins, B., Pasparakis, M., Kollias, G., and Balkwill, F. (1999). Mice deficient in tumor necrosis factor-alpha are resistant to skin carcinogenesis. *Nat. Med.* **5**, 828–831.
Musunuru, K., and Darnell, R. B. (2001). Paraneoplastic neurologic disease antigens: RNA-binding proteins and signaling proteins in neuronal degeneration. *Annu. Rev. Neurosci.* **24**, 239–262.
Naito, Y., Saito, K., Shiiba, K., Ohuchi, A., Saigenji, K., Nagura, H., and Ohtani, H. (1998). CD8+ T cells infiltrated within cancer cell nests as a prognostic factor in human colorectal cancer. *Cancer Res.* **58**, 3491–3494.
Nakata, M., Smyth, M. J., Norihisa, Y., Kawasaki, A., Shinkai, Y., Okumura, K., and Yagita, H. (1990). Constitutive expression of pore-forming protein in peripheral blood gamma/delta T cells: Implication for their cytotoxic role *in vivo*. *J. Exp. Med.* **172**, 1877–1880.
Natarajan, K., Dimasi, N., Wang, J., Margulies, D. H., and Mariuzza, R. A. (2002). MHC class I recognition by Ly49 natural killer cell receptors. *Mol. Immunol.* **38**, 1023–1027.
Nishikawa, H., Kato, T., Tanida, K., Hiasa, A., Tawara, I., Ikeda, H., Ikarashi, Y., Wakasugi, H., Kronenberg, M., Nakayama, T., Taniguchi, M., Kuribayashi, K., *et al.* (2003). CD4+ CD25+ T cells responding to serologically defined autoantigens suppress antitumor immune responses. *Proc. Natl. Acad. Sci. USA* **100**, 10902–10906.
Noguchi, Y., Jungbluth, A., Richards, E. C., and Old, L. J. (1996). Effect of interleukin 12 on tumor induction by 3-methylcholanthrene. *Proc. Natl. Acad. Sci. USA* **93**, 11798–11801.
Nomoto, K., and Takeya, K. (1969). Immunologic properties of methylcholanthrene-induced sarcomas of neonatally thymectomized mice. *J. Natl. Cancer Inst.* **42**, 445–453.
Nomura, M., Takihara, Y., and Shimada, K. (1994). Isolation and characterization of retinoic acid-inducible cDNA clones in F9 cells: One of the early inducible clones encodes a novel protein sharing several highly homologous regions with a *Drosophila* polyhomeotic protein. *Differentiation* **57**, 39–50.
O'Hanlon, L. H. (2004). Natural born killers: NK cells drafted into the cancer fight. *J. Natl. Cancer Inst.* **96**, 651–653.
Odunsi, K. (2005). Lessons from a pilot clinical trial of vaccine therapy with an NY-ESO-1 peptide of dual MHC class I and II specificites in ovarian cancer. *Cancer Immun.* **5**, S22.
Okamoto, M., Ahmed, S. U., Oshikawa, T., Tano, T., and Sato, M. (2004). [Anti-tumor effect of intratumoral administration of dendritic cells in combination with TS-1 and OK-432]. *Gan To Kagaku Ryoho* **31**, 1627–1630.
Old, L. J. (1981). Cancer immunology: The search for specificity—G. H. A. Clowes Memorial lecture. *Cancer Res.* **41**, 361–375.
Old, L. J. (2003). Cancer vaccines 2003: Opening address. *Cancer Immun.* **3**(Suppl. 2), 1.
Old, L. J., and Boyse, E. A. (1964). Immunology of experimental tumors. *Annu. Rev. Med.* **15**, 167–186.
Onizuka, S., Tawara, I., Shimizu, J., Sakaguchi, S., Fujita, T., and Nakayama, E. (1999). Tumor rejection by *in vivo* administration of anti-CD25 (interleukin-2 receptor alpha) monoclonal antibody. *Cancer Res.* **59**, 3128–3133.
Oppenheim, D. E., Roberts, S. J., Clarke, S. L., Filler, R., Lewis, J. M., Tigelaar, R. E., Girardi, M., and Hayday, A. C. (2005). Sustained localized expression of ligand for the activating NKG2D receptor impairs natural cytotoxicity *in vivo* and reduces tumor immunosurveillance. *Nat. Immunol.* **6**, 928–937.
Outzen, H. C., Custer, R. P., Eaton, G. J., and Prehn, R. T. (1975). Spontaneous and induced tumor incidence in germfree "nude" mice. *J. Reticuloendothel. Soc.* **17**, 1–9.

Pardoll, D. (2003). Does the immune system see tumors as foreign or self? *Annu. Rev. Immunol.* **21**, 807–839.

Pende, D., Rivera, P., Marcenaro, S., Chang, C. C., Biassoni, R., Conte, R., Kubin, M., Cosman, D., Ferrone, S., Moretta, L., and Moretta, A. (2002). Major histocompatibility complex class I-related chain A and UL16-binding protein expression on tumor cell lines of different histotypes: Analysis of tumor susceptibility to NKG2D-dependent natural killer cell cytotoxicity. *Cancer Res.* **62**, 6178–6186.

Peng, S. L., Robert, M. E., Hayday, A. C., and Craft, J. (1996). A tumor-suppressor function for Fas (CD95) revealed in T cell-deficient mice. *J. Exp. Med.* **184**, 1149–1154.

Penn, I. (1996). Malignant melanoma in organ allograft recipients. *Transplantation* **61**, 274–278.

Penn, I., and Starzl, T. E. (1970). Malignant lymphomas in transplantation patients: A review of the world experience. *Int. Z. Klin. Pharmakol. Ther. Toxikol.* **3**, 49–54.

Pestka, S., Krause, C. D., and Walter, M. R. (2004). Interferons, interferon-like cytokines, and their receptors. *Immunol. Rev.* **202**, 8–32.

Peter, M. E., and Krammer, P. H. (2003). The CD95(APO-1/Fas) DISC and beyond. *Cell Death Differ.* **10**, 26–35.

Qin, Z., and Blankenstein, T. (2000). CD4+ T cell-mediated tumor rejection involves inhibition of angiogenesis that is dependent on IFN gamma receptor expression by nonhematopoietic cells. *Immunity* **12**, 677–686.

Radosavljevic, M., Cuillerier, B., Wilson, M. J., Clement, O., Wicker, S., Gilfillan, S., Beck, S., Trowsdale, J., and Bahram, S. (2002). A cluster of ten novel MHC class I related genes on human chromosome 6q24.2–q25.3. *Genomics* **79**, 114–123.

Rafii, S., Lyden, D., Benezra, R., Hattori, K., and Heissig, B. (2002). Vascular and haematopoietic stem cells: Novel targets for anti-angiogenesis therapy? *Nat. Rev. Cancer* **2**, 826–835.

Raulet, D. H. (2003). Roles of the NKG2D immunoreceptor and its ligands. *Nat. Rev. Immunol.* **3**, 781–790.

Rosenberg, S. A. (1999). A new era for cancer immunotherapy based on the genes that encode cancer antigens. *Immunity* **10**, 281–287.

Rubinstein, N., Alvarez, M., Zwirner, N. W., Toscano, M. A., Ilarregui, J. M., Bravo, A., Mordoh, J., Fainboim, L., Podhajcer, O. L., and Rabinovich, G. A. (2004). Targeted inhibition of galectin-1 gene expression in tumor cells results in heightened T cell-mediated rejection; A potential mechanism of tumor-immune privilege. *Cancer Cell* **5**, 241–251.

Ruggeri, L., Capanni, M., Urbani, E., Perruccio, K., Shlomchik, W. D., Tosti, A., Posati, S., Rogaia, D., Frassoni, F., Aversa, F., Martelli, M. F., and Velardi, A. (2002). Effectiveness of donor natural killer cell alloreactivity in mismatched hematopoietic transplants. *Science* **295**, 2097–2100.

Rygaard, J., and Povlsen, C. O. (1974a). Is immunological surveillance not a cell-mediated immune function? *Transplantation* **17**, 135–136.

Rygaard, J., and Povlsen, C. O. (1974b). The mouse mutant nude does not develop spontaneous tumours. An argument against immunological surveillance. *Acta Pathol. Microbiol. Scand. [B] Microbiol. Immunol.* **82**, 99–106.

Sahin, U., Tureci, O., Schmitt, H., Cochlovius, B., Johannes, T., Schmits, R., Stenner, F., Luo, G., Schobert, I., and Pfreundschuh, M. (1995). Human neoplasms elicit multiple specific immune responses in the autologous host. *Proc. Natl. Acad. Sci. USA* **92**, 11810–11813.

Sakaguchi, S. (2000). Regulatory T cells: Key controllers of immunologic self-tolerance. *Cell* **101**, 455–458.

Sakaguchi, S. (2002). Immunologic tolerance maintained by regulatory T cells: Implications for autoimmunity, tumor immunity and transplantation tolerance. *Vox Sang.* **83**(Suppl. 1), 151–153.

Sakaguchi, S. (2004). Naturally arising CD4+ regulatory t cells for immunologic self-tolerance and negative control of immune responses. *Annu. Rev. Immunol.* **22**, 531–562.

Salih, H. R., Rammensee, H. G., and Steinle, A. (2002). Cutting edge: Down-regulation of MICA on human tumors by proteolytic shedding. *J. Immunol.* **169,** 4098–4102.

Sallusto, F., Mackay, C. R., and Lanzavecchia, A. (2000). The role of chemokine receptors in primary, effector, and memory immune responses. *Annu. Rev. Immunol.* **18,** 593–620.

Sanford, B. H., Kohn, H. I., Daly, J. J., and Soo, S. F. (1973). Long-term spontaneous tumor incidence in neonatally thymectomized mice. *J. Immunol.* **110,** 1437–1439.

Scanlan, M. J., Gure, A. O., Jungbluth, A. A., Old, L. J., and Chen, Y. T. (2002). Cancer/testis antigens: An expanding family of targets for cancer immunotherapy. *Immunol. Rev.* **188,** 22–32.

Schmaltz, C., Alpdogan, O., Kappel, B. J., Muriglan, S. J., Rotolo, J. A., Ongchin, J., Willis, L. M., Greenberg, A. S., Eng, J. M., Crawford, J. M., Murphy, G. F., Yagita, H., *et al.* (2002). T cells require TRAIL for optimal graft-versus-tumor activity. *Nat. Med.* **8,** 1433–1437.

Schreiber, R. D., Old, L. J., Hayday, A. C., and Smyth, M. J. (2004). Response to "A cancer immunosurveillance controversy." *Nat. Immunol.* **5,** 4–5.

Schreiber, R. D., Pace, J. L., Russell, S. W., Altman, A., and Katz, D. H. (1983). Macrophage-activating factor produced by a T cell hybridoma: Physiochemical and biosynthetic resemblance to gamma-interferon. *J. Immunol.* **131,** 826–832.

Schumacher, K., Haensch, W., Roefzaad, C., and Schlag, P. M. (2001). Prognostic significance of activated CD8(+) T cell infiltrations within esophageal carcinomas. *Cancer Res.* **61,** 3932–3936.

Seifried, H. E., McDonald, S. S., Anderson, D. E., Greenwald, P., and Milner, J. A. (2003). The antioxidant conundrum in cancer. *Cancer Res.* **63,** 4295–4298.

Seliger, B., Maeurer, M. J., and Ferrone, S. (2000). Antigen-processing machinery breakdown and tumor growth. *Immunol. Today* **21,** 455–464.

Seong, S. Y., and Matzinger, P. (2004). Hydrophobicity: An ancient damage-associated molecular pattern that initiates innate immune responses. *Nat. Rev. Immunol.* **4,** 469–478.

Serrano, M., Lin, A. W., McCurrach, M. E., Beach, D., and Lowe, S. W. (1997). Oncogenic ras provokes premature cell senescence associated with accumulation of p53 and p16INK4a. *Cell* **88,** 593–602.

Shankaran, V., Ikeda, H., Bruce, A. T., White, J. M., Swanson, P. E., Old, L. J., and Schreiber, R. D. (2001). IFNgamma and lymphocytes prevent primary tumour development and shape tumour immunogenicity. *Nature* **410,** 1107–1111.

Shevach, E. M. (2002). CD4+ CD25+ suppressor T cells: More questions than answers. *Nat. Rev. Immunol.* **2,** 389–400.

Shi, Y., Evans, J. E., and Rock, K. L. (2003). Molecular identification of a danger signal that alerts the immune system to dying cells. *Nature* **425,** 516–521.

Shimizu, J., Yamazaki, S., and Sakaguchi, S. (1999). Induction of tumor immunity by removing CD25+CD4+ T cells: A common basis between tumor immunity and autoimmunity. *J. Immunol.* **163,** 5211–5218.

Shinkai, Y., Rathbun, G., Lam, K. P., Oltz, E. M., Stewart, V., Mendelsohn, M., Charron, J., Datta, M., Young, F., Stall, A. M., *et al.* (1992). RAG-2-deficient mice lack mature lymphocytes owing to inability to initiate V(D)J rearrangement. *Cell* **68,** 855–867.

Smyth, M. J. (2005). Type I interferon and cancer immunoediting. *Nat. Immunol.* **6,** 646–648.

Smyth, M. J., Cretney, E., Takeda, K., Wiltrout, R. H., Sedger, L. M., Kayagaki, N., Yagita, H., and Okumura, K. (2001a). Tumor necrosis factor-related apoptosis-inducing ligand (TRAIL) contributes to interferon gamma-dependent natural killer cell protection from tumor metastasis. *J. Exp. Med.* **193,** 661–670.

Smyth, M. J., Crowe, N. Y., and Godfrey, D. I. (2001b). NK cells and NKT cells collaborate in host protection from methylcholanthrene-induced fibrosarcoma. *Int. Immunol.* **13,** 459–463.

Smyth, M. J., Crowe, N. Y., Hayakawa, Y., Takeda, K., Yagita, H., and Godfrey, D. I. (2002). NKT cells—conductors of tumor immunity? *Curr. Opin. Immunol.* **14,** 165–171.

Smyth, M. J., and Godfrey, D. I. (2000). NKT cells and tumor immunity—a double-edged sword. *Nat. Immunol.* **1,** 459–460.

Smyth, M. J., Godfrey, D. I., and Trapani, J. A. (2001c). A fresh look at tumor immunosurveillance and immunotherapy. *Nat. Immunol.* **2,** 293–299.

Smyth, M. J., Kelly, J. M., Baxter, A. G., Korner, H., and Sedgwick, J. D. (1998). An essential role for tumor necrosis factor in natural killer cell-mediated tumor rejection in the peritoneum. *J. Exp. Med.* **188,** 1611–1619.

Smyth, M. J., Ortaldo, J. R., Shinkai, Y., Yagita, H., Nakata, M., Okumura, K., and Young, H. A. (1990). Interleukin 2 induction of pore-forming protein gene expression in human peripheral blood CD8+ T cells. *J. Exp. Med.* **171,** 1269–1281.

Smyth, M. J., Street, S. E., and Trapani, J. A. (2003a). Cutting edge: Granzymes A and B are not essential for perforin-mediated tumor rejection. *J. Immunol.* **171,** 515–518.

Smyth, M. J., Swann, J., Cretney, E., Zerafa, N., Yokoyama, W. M., and Hayakawa, Y. (2005). NKG2D function protects the host from tumor initiation. *J. Exp. Med.* **200,** 1325–1335.

Smyth, M. J., Swann, J., Kelly, J. M., Cretney, E., Yokoyama, W. M., Diefenbach, A., Sayers, T. J., and Hayakawa, Y. (2004). NKG2D recognition and perforin effector function mediate effective cytokine immunotherapy of cancer. *J. Exp. Med.* **200,** 1325–1335.

Smyth, M. J., Takeda, K., Hayakawa, Y., Peschon, J. J., van den Brink, M. R., and Yagita, H. (2003b). Nature's TRAIL—on a path to cancer immunotherapy. *Immunity* **18,** 1–6.

Smyth, M. J., Thia, K. Y., Cretney, E., Kelly, J. M., Snook, M. B., Forbes, C. A., and Scalzo, A. A. (1999). Perforin is a major contributor to NK cell control of tumor metastasis. *J. Immunol.* **162,** 6658–6662.

Smyth, M. J., Thia, K. Y., Street, S. E., Cretney, E., Trapani, J. A., Taniguchi, M., Kawano, T., Pelikan, S. B., Crowe, N. Y., and Godfrey, D. I. (2000a). Differential tumor surveillance by natural killer (NK) and NKT cells. *J. Exp. Med.* **191,** 661–668.

Smyth, M. J., Thia, K. Y., Street, S. E., MacGregor, D., Godfrey, D. I., and Trapani, J. A. (2000b). Perforin-mediated cytotoxicity is critical for surveillance of spontaneous lymphoma. *J. Exp. Med.* **192,** 755–760.

Spiotto, M. T., Rowley, D. A., and Schreiber, H. (2004). Bystander elimination of antigen loss variants in established tumors. *Nat. Med.* **10,** 294–298.

Srivastava, P. (2002). Interaction of heat shock proteins with peptides and antigen presenting cells: Chaperoning of the innate and adaptive immune responses. *Annu. Rev. Immunol.* **20,** 395–425.

Steitz, J., Bruck, J., Lenz, J., Knop, J., and Tuting, T. (2001). Depletion of CD25(+) CD4(+) T cells and treatment with tyrosinase-related protein 2-transduced dendritic cells enhance the interferon alpha-induced, CD8(+) T-cell-dependent immune defense of B16 melanoma. *Cancer Res.* **61,** 8643–8646.

Stenger, S., Hanson, D. A., Teitelbaum, R., Dewan, P., Niazi, K. R., Froelich, C. J., Ganz, T., Thoma-Uszynski, S., Melian, A., Bogdan, C., Porcelli, S. A., Bloom, B. R., et al. (1998). An antimicrobial activity of cytolytic T cells mediated by granulysin. *Science* **282,** 121–125.

Sternlicht, M. D., and Werb, Z. (2001). How matrix metalloproteinases regulate cell behavior. *Annu. Rev. Cell Dev. Biol.* **17,** 463–516.

Straus, S. E., Jaffe, E. S., Puck, J. M., Dale, J. K., Elkon, K. B., Rosen-Wolff, A., Peters, A. M., Sneller, M. C., Hallahan, C. W., Wang, J., Fischer, R. E., Jackson, C. M., et al. (2001). The development of lymphomas in families with autoimmune lymphoproliferative syndrome with germline Fas mutations and defective lymphocyte apoptosis. *Blood* **98,** 194–200.

Street, S. E., Cretney, E., and Smyth, M. J. (2001). Perforin and interferon-gamma activities independently control tumor initiation, growth, and metastasis. *Blood* **97,** 192–197.

Street, S. E., Hayakawa, Y., Zhan, Y., Lew, A. M., MacGregor, D., Jamieson, A. M., Diefenbach, A., Yagita, H., Godfrey, D. I., and Smyth, M. J. (2004). Innate immune surveillance of spontaneous B cell lymphomas by natural killer cells and gammadelta T cells. *J. Exp. Med.* **199**, 879–884.

Street, S. E., Trapani, J. A., MacGregor, D., and Smyth, M. J. (2002). Suppression of lymphoma and epithelial malignancies effected by interferon gamma. *J. Exp. Med.* **196**, 129–134.

Stutman, O. (1974). Tumor development after 3-methylcholanthrene in immunologically deficient athymic-nude mice. *Science* **183**, 534–536.

Stutman, O. (1975). Immunodepression and malignancy. *Adv. Cancer Res.* **22**, 261–422.

Stutman, O. (1979). Chemical carcinogenesis in nude mice: Comparison between nude mice from homozygous matings and heterozygous matings and effect of age and carcinogen dose. *J. Natl. Cancer Inst.* **62**, 353–358.

Suganuma, M., Okabe, S., Marino, M. W., Sakai, A., Sueoka, E., and Fujiki, H. (1999). Essential role of tumor necrosis factor alpha (TNF-alpha) in tumor promotion as revealed by TNF-alpha-deficient mice. *Cancer Res.* **59**, 4516–4518.

Suranyi, M. G., Hogan, P. G., Falk, M. C., Axelsen, R. A., Rigby, R., Hawley, C., and Petrie, J. (1998). Advanced donor-origin melanoma in a renal transplant recipient: Immunotherapy, cure, and retransplantation. *Transplantation* **66**, 655–661.

Sutmuller, R. P., van Duivenvoorde, L. M., van Elsas, A., Schumacher, T. N., Wildenberg, M. E., Allison, J. P., Toes, R. E., Offringa, R., and Melief, C. J. (2001). Synergism of cytotoxic T lymphocyte-associated antigen 4 blockade and depletion of CD25(+) regulatory T cells in antitumor therapy reveals alternative pathways for suppression of autoreactive cytotoxic T lymphocyte responses. *J. Exp. Med.* **194**, 823–832.

Svane, I. M., Engel, A. M., Nielsen, M. B., Ljunggren, H. G., Rygaard, J., and Werdelin, O. (1996). Chemically induced sarcomas from nude mice are more immunogenic than similar sarcomas from congenic normal mice. *Eur. J. Immunol.* **26**, 1844–1850.

Szlosarek, P. W., and Balkwill, F. R. (2003). Tumour necrosis factor alpha: A potential target for the therapy of solid tumours. *Lancet Oncol.* **4**, 565–573.

Takaoka, A., Hayakawa, S., Yanai, H., Stoiber, D., Negishi, H., Kikuchi, H., Sasaki, S., Imai, K., Shibue, T., Honda, K., and Taniguchi, T. (2003). Integration of interferon-alpha/beta signalling to p53 responses in tumour suppression and antiviral defence. *Nature* **424**, 516–523.

Takeda, K., Hayakawa, Y., Smyth, M. J., Kayagaki, N., Yamaguchi, N., Kakuta, S., Iwakura, Y., Yagita, H., and Okumura, K. (2001). Involvement of tumor necrosis factor-related apoptosis-inducing ligand in surveillance of tumor metastasis by liver natural killer cells. *Nat. Med.* **7**, 94–100.

Takeda, K., Smyth, M. J., Cretney, E., Hayakawa, Y., Kayagaki, N., Yagita, H., and Okumura, K. (2002). Critical role for tumor necrosis factor-related apoptosis-inducing ligand in immune surveillance against tumor development. *J. Exp. Med.* **195**, 161–169.

Tawara, I., Take, Y., Uenaka, A., Noguchi, Y., and Nakayama, E. (2002). Sequential involvement of two distinct CD4+ regulatory T cells during the course of transplantable tumor growth and protection from 3-methylcholanthrene-induced tumorigenesis by CD25-depletion. *Jpn. J. Cancer Res.* **93**, 911–916.

Terabe, M., Matsui, S., Noben-Trauth, N., Chen, H., Watson, C., Donaldson, D. D., Carbone, D. P., Paul, W. E., and Berzofsky, J. A. (2000). NKT cell-mediated repression of tumor immunosurveillance by IL-13 and the IL-4R-STAT6 pathway. *Nat. Immunol.* **1**, 515–520.

Terabe, M., Matsui, S., Park, J. M., Mamura, M., Noben-Trauth, N., Donaldson, D. D., Chen, W., Wahl, S. M., Ledbetter, S., Pratt, B., Letterio, J. J., Paul, W. E., *et al.* (2003). Transforming growth factor-beta production and myeloid cells are an effector mechanism through which CD1d-restricted T cells block cytotoxic T lymphocyte-mediated tumor immunosurveillance: Abrogation prevents tumor recurrence. *J. Exp. Med.* **198**, 1741–1752.

Termeer, C., Benedix, F., Sleeman, J., Fieber, C., Voith, U., Ahrens, T., Miyake, K., Freudenberg, M., Galanos, C., and Simon, J. C. (2002). Oligosaccharides of Hyaluronan activate dendritic cells via toll-like receptor 4. *J. Exp. Med.* **195**, 99–111.

Thomas, L. (1959). Discussion. *In* "Cellular and Humoral Aspects of the Hypersensitive States" (H. S. Lawrence, Ed.), pp. 529–532. Hoeber-Harper, New York.

Thomas, L. (1982). On immunosurveillance in human cancer. *Yale J. Biol. Med.* **55**, 329–333.

Tieng, V., Le Bouguenec, C., du Merle, L., Bertheau, P., Desreumaux, P., Janin, A., Charron, D., and Toubert, A. (2002). Binding of *Escherichia coli* adhesin AfaE to CD55 triggers cell-surface expression of the MHC class I-related molecule MICA. *Proc. Natl. Acad. Sci. USA* **99**, 2977–2982.

Trapani, J. A., and Smyth, M. J. (2002). Functional significance of the perforin/granzyme cell death pathway. *Nat. Rev. Immunol.* **2**, 735–747.

Traversari, C., van der Bruggen, P., Van den Eynde, B., Hainaut, P., Lemoine, C., Ohta, N., Old, L., and Boon, T. (1992). Transfection and expression of a gene coding for a human melanoma antigen recognized by autologous cytolytic T lymphocytes. *Immunogenetics* **35**, 145–152.

Turk, M. J., Guevara-Patino, J. A., Rizzuto, G. A., Engelhorn, M. E., and Houghton, A. N. (2004). Concomitant tumor immunity to a poorly immunogenic melanoma is prevented by regulatory T cells. *J. Exp. Med.* **200**, 771–782.

Ueda, R., Shiku, H., Pfreundschuh, M., Takahashi, T., Li, L. T., Whitmore, W. F., Oettgen, H. F., and Old, L. J. (1979). Cell surface antigens of human renal cancer defined by autologous typing. *J. Exp. Med.* **150**, 564–579.

Uhr, J. W., Scheuermann, R. H., Street, N. E., and Vitetta, E. S. (1997). Cancer dormancy: Opportunities for new therapeutic approaches. *Nat. Med.* **3**, 505–509.

Uyttenhove, C., Pilotte, L., Theate, I., Stroobant, V., Colau, D., Parmentier, N., Boon, T., and Van den Eynde, B. J. (2003). Evidence for a tumoral immune resistance mechanism based on tryptophan degradation by indoleamine 2,3-dioxygenase. *Nat. Med.* **9**, 1269–1274.

van den Broek, M. E., Kagi, D., Ossendorp, F., Toes, R., Vamvakas, S., Lutz, W. K., Melief, C. J., Zinkernagel, R. M., and Hengartner, H. (1996). Decreased tumor surveillance in perforin-deficient mice. *J. Exp. Med.* **184**, 1781–1790.

van den Broek, M. F., Kagi, D., Zinkernagel, R. M., and Hengartner, H. (1995). Perforin dependence of natural killer cell-mediated tumor control *in vivo. Eur. J. Immunol.* **25**, 3514–3516.

van der Bruggen, P., Traversari, C., Chomez, P., Lurquin, C., De Plaen, E., Van den Eynde, B., Knuth, A., and Boon, T. (1991). A gene encoding an antigen recognized by cytolytic T lymphocytes on a human melanoma. *Science* **254**, 1643–1647.

Vetter, C. S., Groh, V., thor Straten, P., Spies, T., Brocker, E. B., and Becker, J. C. (2002). Expression of stress-induced MHC class I related chain molecules on human melanoma. *J. Invest. Dermatol.* **118**, 600–605.

Vicari, A. P., and Caux, C. (2002). Chemokines in cancer. *Cytokine Growth Factor Rev.* **13**, 143–154.

Villegas, F. R., Coca, S., Villarrubia, V. G., Jimenez, R., Chillon, M. J., Jareno, J., Zuil, M., and Callol, L. (2002). Prognostic significance of tumor infiltrating natural killer cells subset CD57 in patients with squamous cell lung cancer. *Lung Cancer* **35**, 23–28.

Wang, R. F., and Rosenberg, S. A. (1999). Human tumor antigens for cancer vaccine development. *Immunol. Rev.* **170**, 85–100.

Wang, T., Niu, G., Kortylewski, M., Burdelya, L., Shain, K., Zhang, S., Bhattacharya, R., Gabrilovich, D., Heller, R., Coppola, D., Dalton, W., Jove, R., *et al.* (2004). Regulation of the innate and adaptive immune responses by Stat-3 signaling in tumor cells. *Nat. Med.* **10**, 48–54.

Westwood, J. A., Kelly, J. M., Tanner, J. E., Kershaw, M. H., Smyth, M. J., and Hayakawa, Y. (2004). Cutting edge: Novel priming of tumor-specific immunity by NKG2D-triggered NK cell-mediated tumor rejection and Th1-independent CD4+ T cell pathway. *J. Immunol.* **172,** 757–761.

Wheelock, E. F., Weinhold, K. J., and Levich, J. (1981). The tumor dormant state. *Adv. Cancer Res.* **34,** 107–140.

Willimsky, G., and Blankenstein, T. (2005). Sporadic immunogenic tumours avoid destruction by inducing T-cell tolerance. *Nature* **437,** 141–146.

Wong, G. H., Elwell, J. H., Oberley, L. W., and Goeddel, D. V. (1989). Manganous superoxide dismutase is essential for cellular resistance to cytotoxicity of tumor necrosis factor. *Cell* **58,** 923–931.

Wong, L. H., Krauer, K. G., Hatzinisiriou, I., Estcourt, M. J., Hersey, P., Tam, N. D., Edmondson, S., Devenish, R. J., and Ralph, S. J. (1997). Interferon-resistant human melanoma cells are deficient in ISGF3 components, STAT1, STAT2, and p48-ISGF3gamma. *J. Biol. Chem.* **272,** 28779–28785.

Woo, E. Y., Chu, C. S., Goletz, T. J., Schlienger, K., Yeh, H., Coukos, G., Rubin, S. C., Kaiser, L. R., and June, C. H. (2001). Regulatory CD4(+)CD25(+) T cells in tumors from patients with early-stage non-small cell lung cancer and late-stage ovarian cancer. *Cancer Res.* **61,** 4766–4772.

Wu, G. S., Burns, T. F., McDonald, E. R., 3rd, Jiang, W., Meng, R., Krantz, I. D., Kao, G., Gan, D. D., Zhou, J. Y., Muschel, R., Hamilton, S. R., Spinner, N. B., et al. (1997). KILLER/DR5 is a DNA damage-inducible p53-regulated death receptor gene. *Nat. Genet.* **17,** 141–143.

Xu, X., Fu, X. Y., Plate, J., and Chong, A. S. (1998). IFN-gamma induces cell growth inhibition by Fas-mediated apoptosis: Requirement of STAT1 protein for up-regulation of Fas and FasL expression. *Cancer Res.* **58,** 2832–2837.

Yang, L., and Carbone, D. P. (2004). Tumor-host immune interactions and dendritic cell dysfunction. *Adv. Cancer Res.* **92,** 13–27.

Yue, H. H., Diehl, G. E., and Winoto, A. (2005). Loss of TRAIL-R does not affect thymic or intestinal tumor development in p53 and adenomatous polyposis coli mutant mice. *Cell Death Differ.* **12,** 94–97.

Zerafa, N., Westwood, J. A.., Cretney, E., Mitchell, S., Waring, P., Iezzi, M., and Smyth, M. J. (2005). Cutting edge: TRAIL deficiency accelerates hematological malignancies. *J. Immunol.* **175,** 5586–5590.

Zhang, L., Conejo-Garcia, J. R., Katsaros, D., Gimotty, P. A., Massobrio, M., Regnani, G., Makrigiannakis, A., Gray, H., Schlienger, K., Liebman, M. N., Rubin, S. C., and Coukos, G. (2003). Intratumoral T cells, recurrence, and survival in epithelial ovarian cancer. *N. Engl. J. Med.* **348,** 203–213.

Zhou, D., Mattner, J., Cantu, C., 3rd, Schrantz, N., Yin, N., Gao, Y., Sagiv, Y., Hudspeth, K., Wu, Y. P., Yamashita, T., Teneberg, S., Wang, D., et al. (2004). Lysosomal glycosphingolipid recognition by NKT cells. *Science* **306,** 1786–1789.

Mechanisms of Immune Evasion by Tumors

Charles G. Drake, Elizabeth Jaffee, and Drew M. Pardoll

Sidney Kimmel Comprehensive Cancer Center at Johns Hopkins, Baltimore, Maryland

Abstract 51
1. Introduction 51
2. Downmodulation of Tumor Antigen Presentation 52
3. Immunologic Barriers Within the Tumor Microenvironment 55
4. Disabled Antigen Presenting Cells 62
5. CD4 T-Cell Tolerance 63
6. Coinhibition 64
7. Regulatory T Cells 66
8. CD8 T-Cell Dysfunction 68
9. Summary 69
    References 70

Abstract

In the past decade, basic studies in animal models have begun to elucidate the physiological barriers which impede a successful antitumor immune response. These barriers operate at a number of levels, and involve the tumor, the tumor microenvironment and various components of the innate and adaptive immune systems. In this review, we discuss the multiple mechanisms by which tumors evade an immune response, with an emphasis on clinically relevant strategies to overcome these inhibitory checkpoints.

1. Introduction

While there has been recent focus on regulatory and organizational barriers to the development of successful antitumor immunotherapy (Pardoll and Allison, 2004), we must not lose sight of the multitude of physiological barriers to generation of successful antitumor immune responses that must be overcome before cancer immunotherapy strategies can hope to be highly efficacious in humans. In the past decade, basic studies in animal models have begun to elucidate these immunologic barriers and to suggest potential compensatory interventions. These barriers operate at a number of different levels along the pathway from induction to successful execution of antitumor immune responses, and multiple checkpoints may be in place simultaneously. In a general sense, one can divide immune evasion by tumors into two general categories: (1) tolerance induction by the developing tumor and (2) resistance to killing by activated immune effector cells. Each of these general categories can be subdivided into multiple mechanisms, some of which are becoming elucidated at the molecular level. For example, tumor-induced tolerance could occur because the tumor is "ignored" by the immune system or because the tumor somehow actively induces anergy among tumor-specific T cells, reduces regulatory T cells or mediates deletion of tumor-specific T cells. If tumor tolerance were predominantly due to ignorance, therapeutic tumor vaccination by itself would likely be much more effective clinically than experience has demonstrated. With occasional exceptions, the majority of murine tumor studies indicate that a more active form of tumor-induced tolerance appears to be operative. While deletion of tumor reactive T cells may indeed be occurring, there is ample evidence that significant repertoires of tumor-specific T cells remain, albeit in an anergic or suppressed state. A critical issue relevant to prospects for immunotherapy is the reversibility of this anergic/inactive state achievable through specific interventions.

This review provides an overview of the recently described checkpoints to antitumor immunity that represent biologic barriers to successful immunotherapy, with an emphasis on those that operate at the T cell level.

2. Downmodulation of Tumor Antigen Presentation

Immune recognition of tumors as distinct from their normal tissue counterparts fundamentally depends on T cell recognition of tumor-specific or tumor-associated antigens. It is now well established that tumors differ from their normal cell counterparts in antigenic composition. The molecular hallmark of carcinogenesis is genetic instability (Fearon and Vogelstein, 1990). Genetic instability in cancers is a consequence of deletion and/or mutational inactivation of genome guardians such as p53 (Lu and Lane, 1993). New antigens are constantly being generated in tumors as a consequence of genetic instability as the carcinogenic process develops and progresses. This does not occur in normal, nontransformed tissues, which maintain a very stable antigenic profile. In addition to the thousands of mutational events that occur during tumorigenesis, epigenetic changes as a consequence of hyper- and hypo-methylation alter expression levels of hundreds of genes (Jones and Baylin, 2002). While these epigenetic changes do not formally create tumor-specific neoantigens, they raise the concentration of encoded proteins many orders of magnitude, thereby dramatically affecting antigenicity.

The first mechanism of tumor immune evasion to be recognized and studied involved the inhibition of tumor antigen presentation (Fig. 1). Downregulation of the antigen processing machinery—particularly the MHC class I pathway—has been documented extensively in a large variety of tumors. In the human, downregulation of the MHC class I molecules has been observed in a diversity

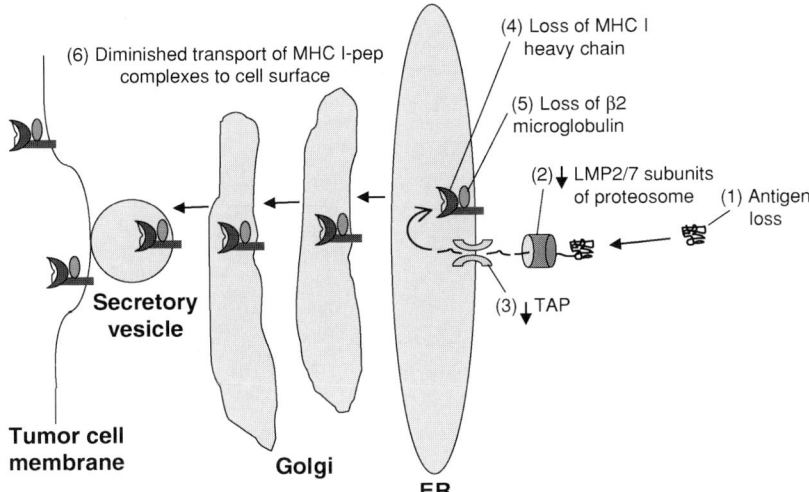

Figure 1 Tumors can downmodulate multiple components of the MHC I processing pathway in order to avoid recognition by tumor specific CTL. In addition to antigen loss, downmodulation of proteosome subunits, transporter associated with antigen presentation (TAP), β2 microglobulin, and MHC I heavy chain can diminish presentation of MHC-peptide complexes on the tumor surface as a means of evasion of CTL recognition. In addition, transport of MHC-peptide complexes from endoplasmic reticulum (ER) through the Golgi to the cell membrane can be diminished. While mutation or deletion has been documented in some tumors, most examples of downregulation of MHC I processing and presentation components are epigenetic and reversible with interferon treatment. (**See Plate 1 in color insert at the end of the book.**)

of tumor types, such as breast cancer, prostate cancer, and lung cancer (Cabrera et al., 1996, 1998; Esteban et al., 1989, 1990, 1996; Ferrone and Marincola, 1995; Marincola et al., 2000; Natali et al., 1983, 1984, 1985, 1989; Perez et al., 1986; Ruiz-Cabello et al., 1989, 1991; van den Ingh et al., 1987; van Driel et al., 1996; Whitwell et al., 1984; Zuk, 1987). In many cases, individual HLA alleles are selectively lost and this has been suggested to represent downmodulation of presentation of immunodominant tumor antigens; however, this notion has never been directly proven. Global MHC class I loss or downmodulation has also been observed in tumors. The most common mechanism for global MHC class I loss is mutations + deletion of β2-microglobulin genes (Benitez et al., 1998; D'Urso et al., 1991; Wang et al., 1993). Loss of heterozygosity at the β2-microglobulin locus with mutation of the remaining allele is the typical scenario. Downmodulation of MHC class I genes can result from multiple mechanisms affecting transcription (Blanchet et al., 1992; Doyle et al., 1985). Downregulation of TAP genes as well as components of the immunoproteosome, such as LMP-2 and LMP-7, have likewise been documented in a number of tumor types (Alpan *et al.*, 1996; Hilders *et al.*, 1994; Restifo *et al.*, 1996; Rowe *et al.*, 1995; Sanda *et al.*, 1995; Seliger *et al.*, 1996). In the majority of cases where the MHC class I processing machinery is downmodulated, it is usually rapidly upregulated by γ-IFN, suggesting that the diminished expression is epigenetic in origin and reversible. Not infrequently, tumors express higher levels of MHC class I molecules and processing machinery than their normal tissue of origin. For example, virtually all renal cancers express quite high levels of MHC class I, whereas normal renal epithelium expresses barely detectable levels of surface MHC class I and very low levels of TAP until exposed to stimuli such as γ-IFN.

Attempts to correlate levels of MHC expression with clinical prognosis in humans or tumor growth rates in the mouse have generated inconsistent outcomes, depending on the tumor type or system. Some human studies suggest that expression of MHC molecules by the tumor is a poor prognostic indicator. Other studies have suggested that high expression of HLA molecules correlates with a favorable prognosis. An example of human cancer in which MHC class I level is consistently downmodulated by multiple mechanisms in the progression from premalignant lesions to malignancy is cervical cancer (Clarke and Chetty, 2002; Koopman *et al.*, 2000). This may be due to the viral (HPV) etiology and the fact that most premalignant HPV lesions are naturally eliminated in immunocompetent but not immunocompromised individuals (Moretta *et al.*, 1997).

Needless to say, since NK cells demonstrate enhanced recognition and killing of cells with low MHC class I levels (Hui *et al.*, 1984; Lanier and Phillips, 1996), downmodulation of the MHC class I processing machinery would not necessarily represent an effective strategy by the tumor to cloak itself from recognition by the immune system. Indeed, while some reports suggested that increasing the level of MHC expression resulted in diminished *in vivo* tumor growth of some murine tumors (Haywood and McKhann, 1971; Ljunggren and Karre, 1985; Wallich *et al.*, 1985), other tumors demonstrate exactly the opposite outcome—namely, diminished growth with lower levels of MHC expression consequent to enhanced NK cell recognition (Karre *et al.*, 1986; Urban *et al.*, 1982). In conclusion, while the modulation of MHC levels and antigen processing machinery is often observed during the progression of cancer, it is yet unclear whether this is a true consequence of development of immune resistance in response to a robust immune surveillance system.

Arguments about loss of tumor-associated antigens (TAA) as an escape mechanism from immune surveillance are equally inconclusive. Heterogeneity of TAA expression and attempts to correlate TAA loss are well documented in murine tumor models with transplantation of immunogenic tumors or after vaccination (Lethe *et al.*, 1992; Urban *et al.*, 1986; Uyttenhove *et al.*, 1983; Ward *et al.*, 1989; Wortzel *et al.*, 1983; Yee *et al.*, 2002). Likewise, Yee *et al.* demonstrated specific loss of cognate melanoma antigens in relapsing tumors from patients treated with adoptive transfer of melanoma antigen-specific CD8$^+$ T cells (Jager *et al.*, 1997). Similarly, there are anecdotal reports of specific antigen loss after treatment of melanoma patients with peptide vaccines (de Vries *et al.*, 1998; Ohnmacht *et al.*, 2001). Together, these reports support the concept of TAA loss as a robust mechanism to escape immunotherapeutically induced antitumor responses. However, despite attempts to document TAA loss with natural tumor progression in humans (particularly in melanoma) (Cormier *et al.*, 1998, 1999; Riker *et al.*, 1999; Scheibenbogen *et al.*, 1996; Schmid *et al.*, 1995), there is no clear evidence that TAA loss is a tumor escape response to immune surveillance in the unmanipulated host.

3. Immunologic Barriers Within the Tumor Microenvironment

While uncontrolled growth is certainly a common biological feature of all tumors, the major pathophysiologic characteristics of malignant cancer responsible for morbidity and mortality are the ability to invade across natural tissue barriers and to metastasize. Both of these characteristics, which are never seen with normal tissues or benign tumors, are associated with dramatic disruption of tissue architecture. One of the important consequences of tissue disruption, even when caused by noninfectious mechanisms, is the elaboration of proinflammatory signals. These signals, generally in the form of cytokines and chemokines, are central initiators of both innate and adaptive immune responses. Thus, unlike normal tissues, cancers are constantly confronted with potential inflammatory responses as they invade tissues and metastasize through the body. How they handle and modulate these responses dictates the interplay with the host immune system. Despite the potential inflammatory and immunogenic consequences of tissue disruption associated with tissue invasion by tumors, the immune system is generally tolerant to established cancers.

In fact, chronic inflammatory responses in the tumor microenvironment not only typically fail to result in tumor elimination, but rather, can also enhance the transformation and growth of tumors. NFκB signaling in hematopoietic cells has been reported to play a critical procarcinogenic role. Selective IKK-β knockout in macrophages and neutrophils resulted in decreases in both number and growth rate of carcinogen-induced tumors in a carcinogen-induced colon cancer model. The general hypothesis to explain these results is that NFκB activation within infiltrating hematopoietic elements is thought to result in production of various proinflammatory cytokines and chemokines, a number of which enhance proliferative responses among IECs as well as providing an antiapoptotic effect (Greten *et al.*, 2004; Karin and Greten, 2005). In particular, these include cytokines, such as TNF, IL-1, IL-6, and CSF-1, type I interferons and multiple chemokines (e.g., IL-8). These proinflammatory cytokines/chemokines have been proposed to promote carcinogenesis in a number of ways, though specific mechanistic details remain to be worked out. Cytokines, such as TNF, can induce an NFκB cascade in adjacent epithelial cells (Lind et al., 2004). IL-6 and CSF-1 can act as growth factors in some cases (Klein et al., 1995; Lin et al., 2002). In addition, NFκB-dependent activation of certain hematopoietic elements, such as macrophages, will induce production of reactive nitrogen species (i.e., NO) through induction of iNOS. Activation of the cytochrome oxidase and NADPH oxidase pathway in neutrophils can result in production of reactive oxygen species (ROS). In some cases, the combination of reactive oxygen and nitrogen species can result in the production of peroxynitrites. These are all highly chemically reactive molecules that can cause oxidative stress in adjacent tumor cells (Bakkenist and Kastan, 2004). The result of ROS and RNS production can be tumoricidal in certain cases but can also promote carcinogenesis through induction of DNA damage under circumstances where the DNA damage response has been disabled, as is commonly the case in cancers.

Together, the accumulating body of information demonstrates that inflammation within the tumor microenvironment, as defined by infiltrating hematopoietically derived cells, can either be bad for the tumor or promote its development and growth. In striking contrast to the inflammatory response associated with infection, the inflammatory response within a tumor does not appear to result in activation of adaptive antitumor immunity. As described later, experiments employing TCR transgenic mice have provided strong evidence for the capacity of tumor cells to induce tolerance to their antigens. Tolerance appears to be operative predominately at the level of T cells; B-cell tolerance to tumors is less certain since there is ample evidence for the induction of antibody responses in animals bearing tumors as well as human patients with tumors. Numerous adoptive transfer studies have demonstrated the potent capacity of T cells to kill growing tumors, either directly through CTL activity or indirectly through multiple CD4-dependent effector mechanisms. It is thus likely that from the tumor's standpoint, induction of antigen-specific tolerance among T cells is of paramount importance for survival.

Mounting evidence supports the idea that tumors actively inhibit the release and sensing of danger signals in order to invade tissues and metastasize without evoking antitumor immune responses that would inhibit their growth, thereby converting inflammatory responses to those that could instead potentiate tumor growth (Fig. 2). Studies have in fact demonstrated that oncogenic signaling pathways not only promote tumor growth and survival in a cell-intrinsic fashion but also actively modulate their immunologic microenvironment. The

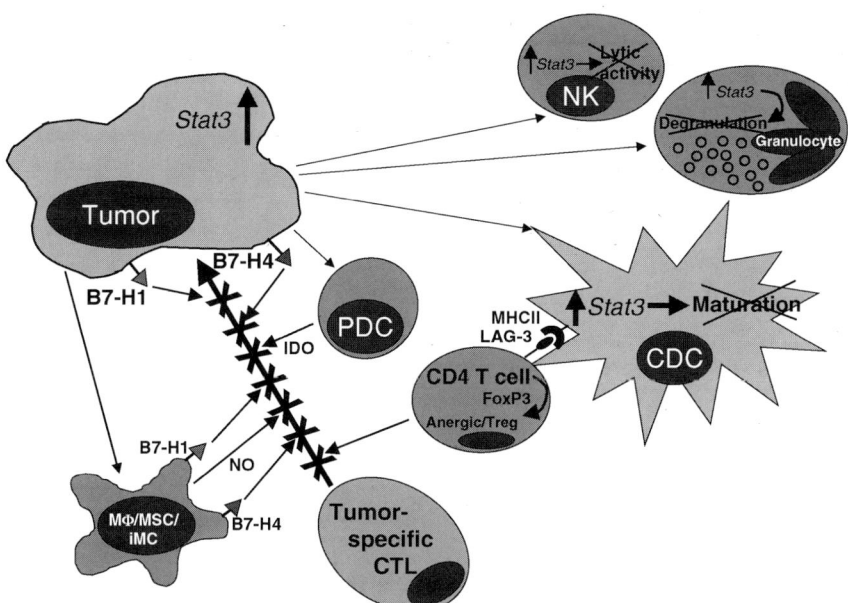

Figure 2 Multiple immunologic checkpoints in the tumor microenvironment. Tumors release factors that induce inhibition of both innate and adaptive antitumor immunity. Stat3 activation in tumors, as well as Braf activation, can induce release of factors such as IL10 that induce Stat3 signaling in NK cells, granulocytes, inhibiting their tumoricidal activity. Stat3 is also activated within conventional dendritic cells (CDC) in the tumor, converting them to toleragenic DC, which can induce T cell anergy and possibly regulatory T cells (Treg). Plasmacytoid DC (PDC) or PDC-related cells in the tumor microenvironment upregulate indoleamine 2,3-dioxygenase (IDO), an enzyme that metabolizes tryptophan. T cells are very sensitive to tryptophan depletion. Tumors can express coinhibitory B7 family members, such as B7-H1 and B7-H4, which downregulate T cell activation and/or cytolytic activity. They can also induce B7-H1 and B7-H4 expression on tumor associated macrophages (TAM). Related immature myeloid cells or myeloid suppressor cells can further inhibit antitumor T cells via production of NO by the enzyme arginase. (**See Plate 2 in color insert at the end of the book.**)

best-studied oncogenic signaling pathway to downmodulate antitumor immune responses is the *Stat3* pathway. *Stat3* is commonly constitutively activated in diverse cancers of both hematopoietic and epithelial origin. Constitutively activated *Stat3* enhances tumor cell proliferation and prevents apoptosis. Indeed, it was found that constitutive *Stat3* activity in tumors negatively regulates inflammation, DC activity and T-cell immunity. Constitutive activation of *Stat3* in tumor cells has been shown to upregulate cell cycle regulatory, proangiogenic and antiapoptotic genes critical to the transformation process (Bowman *et al.*, 2001; Bromberg *et al.*, 1999; Niu *et al.*, 2002; Turkson *et al.*,

1998). As described previously, successful development of invasive, metastatic cancer would require the modulation of genes in a manner that inhibits activation of both innate and adaptive elements of the immune surveillance system. The *Stat3* signaling pathway in tumor cells appears to accomplish this both by inhibiting the production of proinflammatory danger signals and by inducing expression of factors that inhibit functional maturation of dendritic cells (DCs) and other tumor infiltrating hematopoietically derived cells responsible for innate immunity. Blockade of constitutive *Stat3* signaling in tumor cells resulted in the dramatic upregulation of proinflammatory cytokine genes, such as *TNF-α* and *IFN-β*. Proinflammatory chemokine genes, such as *IP-10* and *RANTES*, were also upregulated. These cytokines begin to be produced without any exogenous inductive stimuli when *Stat3* was inhibited, indicating that *Stat3* signaling restrains a natural propensity of tumors to produce these molecules (Wang *et al.*, 2004). Conversely, induction of *Stat3* signaling in 3T3 cells inhibited their production of proinflammatory cytokines and chemokines in response of TLR agonists such as LPS.

It has also been shown that elements of the tumor microenvironment can promote immune tolerance, at least in part, by bone marrow-derived DCs (Hawiger *et al.*, 2001). Indeed, DCs are immature and functionally impaired in both cancer patients and tumor-bearing animals (Almand *et al.*, 2000; Vicari *et al.*, 2002). Dysfunction of DCs in tumor-bearing hosts may be due to the lack of "danger" signals necessary for DC activation together with factors in the tumor milieu inhibiting functional maturation of DCs. *Stat3* activity additionally was found to promote the production of multiple factors, among them VEGF and IL-10, that activate *Stat3* signaling and inhibiting functional DC maturation in culture (Wang *et al.*, 2004). Inhibition of *Stat3* activity in DC cell progenitors has also been shown to reduce accumulation of immature DCs in the tumor microenvironment (Nefedova *et al.*, 2004). Tumors do not invent their own physiology but rather, dysregulate normal physiologic mechanisms to suit their own purposes. The *Stat3* pathway in tumors may represent a dysregulated wound healing response. It is well established that wounding, which causes disruption of cell–cell interactions and tissue architecture, induces release of proinflammatory cytokines. In fact, *Stat3* activation has been shown to be critical to wound healing (Sano *et al.*, 1999). Furthermore, defective wound healing in mice with selective disruption of *Stat3* in keratinocytes was associated with increased inflammatory infiltrates at wound sites. Thus, as with other aspects of cancer biology, the ability of *Stat3* activation to evade the immune system likely reflects a natural function for *Stat3* in normal physiology.

In addition to its role in tumor cells, *Stat3* activation in tumor infiltrating hematopoietic elements appears to be a major checkpoint for innate and adaptive antitumor responses (Kortylewski et al., 2005). The role of hematopoietic *Stat3* signaling was investigated by staining for phospho-*Stat3* in tumor infiltrating cells as well as inducible hematopoietic knockout of *Stat3*. Analysis of phospho-*Stat3* by flow cytometry reveals that *Stat3* is also constitutively activated in tumor-infiltrating NK cells and neutrophils. Induction of *Stat3* deletion considerably increased the number of splenic granulocytic lineage cells and reduced *Stat3* signaling in neutrophils and enhanced their cytolytic activity against target tumor cells. Furthermore, tumor-infiltrating NK cells from hematopoietically *Stat3* ablated mice demonstrated strongly enhanced cytolytic activity compared to those derived from tumor-free control mice. Many tumor-associated factors, including IL-10, VEGF, and IL-6, are activators of *Stat3*, and IL-10 is abundantly produced by tumor-associated macrophages in many different tumors (Halak et al., 1999). The findings of increased function of purified $Stat3^{-/-}$ NK cells and neutrophils from tumor-bearing mice together with an increase in *Stat3* activity directly within these populations in tumor indicates that the role of *Stat3* signaling in downregulating function of these cell types is at least in part, cell intrinsic.

The inhibition of innate responses and DC maturation mediated by *Stat3* pathway activation in hematopoietic cells infiltrating tumors further contributes to the failure to prime tumor-specific T cells. Thus, T cells from hematopoietically *Stat3* ablated mice were able to mount stronger responses against tumor antigens than their $Stat3^{+/+}$ counterparts. This is associated with a considerably higher infiltration by T lymphocytes into tumor tissues from the hematopoietically *Stat3* ablated mice as well as decreases in the number of tumor infiltrating regulatory T cells (see later). These broad ranging inhibitory effects of *Stat3* signaling on innate and adaptive immune responses translate into *in vivo* antitumor responses. Ablating the *Stat3* alleles in hematopoietic cells before tumor challenge significantly inhibited growth of a number of tumor types whereas hematopoietic ablation of *Stat3* after tumor establishment resulted in either slowed growth or outright regression of tumors.

The central role of *Stat3* signaling in both tumors and hematopoietic cells as an immunologic checkpoint defines it as an interesting target for antagonism to enhance antitumor immunity. Recently, a small molecule *Stat3* inhibitor, CPA-7, was identified. CPA-7 disrupts *Stat3* DNA-binding activity, which is followed, within hours, by a reduction of phospho-*Stat3* protein in the treated cells *in vitro* (Turkson et al., 2005). Tumor-infiltrating DCs from mice receiving CPA-7 displayed considerably reduced phospho-*Stat3* compared to vehicle-treated mice. CPA-7 treatment *in vivo* also led to a significant growth inhibition of established tumors that was both T cell and NK cell dependent.

Similar results were observed using a Jak2/*Stat3* inhibitor, JSI-124 (Nefedova *et al.*, 2005).

In addition to its role in inhibiting the activation and effector function of DC, granulocytes, and NK cells in the tumor microenvironment, *Stat3* signaling has also been reported to play a role in guiding immature myeloid cells (iMC) to differentiate into myeloid suppressor cells (MSC) rather than DC with APC activity. Immature myeloid cells (Kusmartsev and Gabrilovich, 2005; Young *et al.*, 2001) and MSC (Bronte *et al.*, 2000, 2003; Mazzoni *et al.*, 2002; Zea *et al.*, 2005) represent a cadre of myeloid cell types, including tumor-associated macrophages (TAM), that share the common feature of inhibiting both the priming and effector function of tumor-reactive T cells. It is still not clear whether these myeloid cell types represent distinct lineages or different states of the same general immune inhibitory cell subset. In mice, iMC and MSC are characterized by coexpression of CD11b (considered a macrophage marker) and Gr1 (considered a granulocyte marker) while expressing low or no MHC class II or the CD86 costimulatory molecule. In humans, they are defined as $CD33^+$ but lacking markers of mature macrophages, DCs or granulocytes and are DR^-. A number of molecular species reported to be produced by tumors tend to drive iMC/MSC accumulation. These include IL-6, CSF-1, IL-10, and gangliosides. IL-6 and IL-10 are potent inducers of *Stat3* signaling. Another cytokine reported to induce iMC/MSC accumulation is GM-CSF (Serafini *et al.*, 2004). This finding is somewhat paradoxical, since GM-CSF is a critical inducer of DC differentiation and GM-CSF transduced tumor vaccines enhance antitumor T-cell immunity via accumulation of DCs at the vaccine site followed by increased DC numbers in vaccine draining LN. It appears that the paradox is solved based on levels of GM-CSF. High-local levels drive DC differentiation at the vaccine site whereas chronic production of low levels of GM-CSF can promote iMC/MSC accumulation. GM-CSF transduced vaccines that produce extremely high GM-CSF levels can induce iMC/MSC accumulation at distant sites (i.e., spleen and LNs) because they release enough GM-CSF systemically to drive iMC/MSC accumulation.

A number of mechanisms have been proposed to explain how iMC/MSC inhibit T-cell responses. Most include the production of ROS and/or RNS. NO production by iMC/MSC as a result of arginase activity, which is high in these cells, has been well documented and inhibition of this pathway with a number of drugs can mitigate the inhibitory effects of iMC/MSC. ROS, including H_2O_2, have been reported to block T-cell function associated with the down-modulation of the ζ chain of the TCR signaling complex (Schmielau and Finn, 2001); a phenomenon well recognized in T cells from cancer patients and associated with generalized T-cell unresponsiveness.

Another mediator of T-cell unresponsiveness associated with cancer is the production of indolamine 2,3-dioxygenase (IDO) (Munn et al., 2002). IDO appears to be produced by DCs either within tumors or in tumor draining LN. Interestingly, IDO in DCs has been reported to be induced via backward signaling by B7-1/2 upon ligation with CTLA-4 (Baban et al., 2005; Mellor et al., 2004). Apparently, the major IDO producing DC subset is either a plasmacytoid DC (PDC) or a PDC-related cell that is $B220^+$ (Munn et al., 2004). IDO appears to inhibit T-cell responses through catabolism of tryptophan. Activated T cells are highly dependent on tryptophan and are therefore sensitive to tryptophan depletion. Thus, Munn and Mellor have proposed a bystander mechanism, whereby DCs in the local environment deplete tryptophan via IDO upregulation, thereby inducing metabolic apoptosis in locally activated T cells.

Another inhibitory molecule produced by many cell types that has been implicated in blunting antitumor immune responses is transforming growth factor beta (TGF-β), which is produced by a variety of cell types, including tumor cells, and which has pleiotropic physiological effects. For most normal epithelial cells, TGF-β is a potent inhibitor of cell proliferation, causing cell cycle arrest in the G1 stage (Blobe et al., 2000). In many cancer cells, however, mutations in the TGF-β pathway confer resistance to cell cycle inhibition, allowing uncontrolled proliferation. Additionally, in cancer cells, the production of TGF-β is increased, and may contribute to invasion by promoting the activity of matrix metaloproteinases. *In vivo*, TGF-β directly stimulates angiogenesis; this stimulation can be blocked by anti-TGF-β antibodies (Pepper, 1997). A bimodal role of TGF-β in cancer has been verified in a transgenic animal model using a keratinocyte-targeted overexpression (Cui et al., 1996). Initially, these animals are resistant to the development of early-stage or benign skin tumors. However, once tumors form, they progress rapidly to a more aggressive spindle-cell phenotype. While this clear bimodal pattern of activity is more difficult to identify in a clinical setting—it should be noted that elevated serum TGF-β levels are associated with poor prognosis in a number of malignancies, including prostate cancer (Shariat et al., 2001), lung cancer (Hasegawa et al., 2001), gastric cancer (Saito et al., 1999) and bladder cancer (Shariat et al., 2001).

From an immunological perspective, TGF-β possesses broadly immunosuppressive properties and TGF-β knockout mice develop widespread inflammatory pathology and corresponding accelerated mortality (Letterio and Roberts, 1998). Interestingly, a majority of these effects seem to be T-cell mediated, as targeted disruption of T cell TGF-β signaling also results a similar autoimmune phenotype (Gorelik and Flavell, 2000). Recent experiments by Chen et al. (2005) rather convincingly demonstrated a role for TGF-β in Treg mediated suppression of CD8 T cell antitumor responses. In these experiments, adoptive transfer of $CD4^+ CD25^+$ regulatory T cells inhibited an antitumor CD8 T-cell effector response, and that this inhibition was ameliorated when the CD8 T cells came from animals with a dominant negative TGF-β1 receptor. In an analogous manner, Zhang *et al.* (2005) performed *ex vivo* transduction of CD8 T cells with a dominant negative TGF-β receptor and then adoptively transferred these cells back into mice with progressive, endogenous prostate tumors. Treated animals showed tumor regression and enhanced survival, demonstrating that TGF-β mediated attenuation of endogenous CD8 T-cell function might be important in tumor progression. Recent data from Ahmadzadeh *et al.* extend these findings to an *in vitro* examination of CD8 T cells from patients who received a gp100 targeted vaccine for melanoma (Ahmadzadeh and Rosenberg, 2005). These cells showed impaired effector function when TGF-β was present in the initial antigen activation cultures, and this attenuation was also noted in melanoma specific T-cell clones. Taken together, these data suggest that either antibody mediated (Lucas *et al.*, 1990), or pharmacological (Callahan *et al.*, 2002; Laping *et al.*, 2002) blockade of TGF-β may prove to be an important component of combinatorial immunotherapy strategies.

4. Disabled Antigen Presenting Cells

One of the unresolved issues in the study of tumor immune evasion relates to the mechanisms by which tumors induce antigen-specific T-cell tolerance. While the many mechanisms described earlier, including *Stat3* signaling dependent mechanisms, IDO, ROS, RNS, TGF-β, etc., clearly inhibit priming of T-cell responses and/or tumor killing by activated effector T cells, it remains to be definitively determined which processes actively induce antigen-specific T-cell tolerance that has been documented in transgenic models. Self-tolerance induction for peripheral tissue antigens is now thought to involve specific presentation of tissue-specific antigens to mature T cells in the absence of appropriate costimulatory signals. Similar mechanisms are likely operative in the case of tumor-induced tolerance. Originally, the relevant costimulatory signals were envisioned to be provided by B7 family costimulatory molecules expressed by DCs (Schwartz, 1992). It is now becoming clear that additional proinflammatory cytokines, such as interferons, IL-12, TNF, etc., are critical in the distinction between effector T-cell induction and tolerance induction.

An emerging concept is that immature or not fully matured DCs are critical in presenting self-antigens to induce T-cell tolerance in the absence of TLR-mediated danger signals associated with infection (Bonifaz *et al.*, 2002; Hawiger *et al.*, 2001; Steinman *et al.*, 2003). Unquestionably, DCs found within the tumor microenvironment have a relatively immature, inactivated phenotype characterized by low levels of proinflammatory cytokine production, CD86, and surface MHC class II expression. As described earlier, a major inhibitory signaling pathway induced in tumor infiltrating DC is the *Stat3* pathway which, when activated, strongly antagonizes TLR and CD40-mediated DC activation. As mentioned, tumor-derived factors, such as IL-10, IL-6, and VEGF (in part induced by *Stat3* signaling in the tumor cell), can induce *Stat3* activation in DCs. Activated *Stat3* in DCs may directly inhibit NFκB signaling either at the level of IKK or further downstream within the nucleus. Additional oncogenic signaling in tumors may contribute to inhibition of activation of DCs in the tumor microenvironment. Recently, constitutive BRAF signaling in melanoma cells (due to an activating mutation found in over 60% of melanomas) has been shown to induce release of factors that inhibit DC activation (Sumimoto *et al.*, 2006). These immature "activation-inhibited" DCs clearly represent a prime candidate for the induction of tumor-specific T-cell tolerance.

It remains an open question as to whether iMC/MSC represent a distinct intertumoral cell subset capable of presenting antigens to T cells in a toleragenic fashion (Kusmartsev *et al.*, 2004). A recent report indeed suggested that iMC loaded with antigen and adoptively transferred into mice can induce antigen-specific T-cell tolerance. Finally, it has been suggested that IDO-expressing DC can induce antigen-specific T-cell tolerance because IDO-mediated tryptophan selectively kills or inhibits proliferation of activated T cells (Munn *et al.*, 2005). According to this model, IDO-expressing DCs would present antigen to T cells inducing activation followed by activation-associated cell death mediated by depletion of local tryptophan stores by the IDO in the presenting DCs. As described later, regulatory T cells play an additional important role in induction or maintenance of tumor antigen-specific T-cell tolerance. Whether Treg cells mediate T-cell tolerance independently from immature or tolerogenic APCs or whether the two mechanisms are completely interrelated (i.e., tolerogenic DCs inducing a Treg phenotype among antigen-specific T cells and antigen-specific Treg cells acting upon DCs to enhance their tolerogenic capacity) remains to be definitely determined.

5. CD4 T-Cell Tolerance

The immune system has evolved multiple mechanisms to avoid a CD4-mediated autoimmune response (Schwartz, 1999). Perhaps the most well studied of these is the deletion of autoreactive T cells at the CD4/CD8 double positive stage in the thymus (Blackman *et al.*, 1992; Hugo *et al.*, 1991; Kappler *et al.*, 1987; MacDonald *et al.*, 1988; Surh and Sprent, 1994). In an animal model, Bogen *et al.* have provided convincing evidence that such events may occur in the progression of myeloma (Bogen *et al.*, 2000; Lauritzsen *et al.*, 1998). In an elegant system, mice were engineered to express a T-cell receptor specific for a myeloma protein. These TCR transgenic mice are quite adept at responding to and rejecting small implanted tumors (Bogen *et al.*, 1995). However, when the primary implant becomes larger than 0.5 cm, the tumors become increasingly progressive. Analysis of thymic T cells in these mice revealed deletion at the double positive stage of ontogeny, strongly resembling that seen in classical thymic deletion models (Lauritzsen *et al.*, 1998). A second, perhaps more subtle, tolerance mechanism involves anergy, a state of antigen-specific unresponsiveness, which occurs when the T-cell receptor engages the MHC antigen-peptide complex in the absence of appropriate costimulatory signals (Bretschen, 1970; Quill and Schwartz, 1987; Schwartz *et al.*, 1989). Anergy as a mechanism for T-cell tolerance to tumors has been demonstrated in several model systems (Mizoguchi *et al.*, 1992; Staveley-O'Carroll *et al.*, 1998). In one such system, A20 lymphoma cells were stably transfected with the influenza hemagglutinin peptide (HA) to provide a unique tumor antigen. When HA-specific T cells are adoptively transferred to mice bearing progressive A20 (HA) lymphomas, the result was not the vigorous immune rejection one might have predicted (and hoped for). In fact, the transferred-specific T cells were rapidly rendered anergic, incapable of proliferating *in vitro* to specific antigen. Perhaps more importantly, A20 (HA) tumors progressed at an identical rate whether the mice received specific adoptively transferred T cells.

Antigen-specific T priming of T cells can be either direct (i.e., via Class I-antigen complexes expressed on the target cell type) or indirect (i.e., via complexes presented on bone marrow-derived professional antigen presenting cells) (Adler *et al.*, 1998). For most tumor types, direct presentation appears to be minimal whereas cross-presentation represents the dominant presentation pathway (Huang *et al.*, 1994). However, a number of groups have noted that this cross priming pathway is not especially efficient, leading to circumstances in which small, evolving tumors are mostly "ignored" by the host immune system (Ochsenbein *et al.*, 1999). Tolerance would, therefore, remain intact until tumors become metastatic to draining lymph nodes, at which time the host could potentially mount an antitumor response (Ochsenbein *et al.*, 2005).

6. Coinhibition

While the Bretscher and Cohn two signal model of T-cell activation has gained wide acceptance and is backed by copious experimental data, recent studies have suggested that this model may be inadequate under certain circumstances, and that T-cell activation and effector function may ultimately be controlled by a balance between costimulatory molecules (such as CD28) and coinhibitory molecules (Chen et al., 2004). The canonical coinhibitory pathway is that mediated by the interaction between CTLA-4 (on T cells) and its ligands (B7-1 and B7-2) on antigen presenting cells. CTLA-4 is not robustly expressed on naïve T cells, but is rapidly induced after T-cell activation, and, as is the case for TGF-β, CTLA-4 knockout mice develop lymphoproliferative autoimmunity, indicating a tonic role for CTLA-4—B7-1/B7-2 interactions in the prevention of autoimmunity (Waterhouse et al., 1995). Based on these data, CTLA-4 blockade would be expected to function mostly during T cell priming events, facilitating or enhancing an immune response. In a number of murine systems, CTLA-4 blockade exerts a pronounced antitumor effect (Chambers et al., 2001), generating enthusiasm for translating these observations to the clinic. Clinical trials to date have primarily evaluated a single agent approach, using a human anti-CTLA-4 monoclonal blocking antibody (MDX010, Medarex, Inc.). While some clinical efficacy has been demonstrated at higher antibody doses (Phan et al., 2003), a number of autoimmune side effects have been observed, including inflammatory bowel pathology. Interestingly, this pathology bears a remarkable resemblance to that seen in the CTLA-4 knockout mice, highlighting the utility of preclinical models in the study of immunotherapy.

A second coinhibitory molecule on T cells is PD1 (programmed death 1), a T cell surface molecule originally discovered in a T-cell hybridoma undergoing apoptosis (Ishida et al., 1992). Further studies of PD1 identified expression on activated, but not naïve T and B cells, in addition to potential overexpression in anergized CD4 T cells (Hatachi et al., 2003; Lechner et al., 2001). Recent data show that PD1 is also expressed on the surface of certain CD8 T cells, where it serves as a marker for T cells that have been "exhausted" by exposure to persistent viral antigen in vivo (R. Ahmed, unpublished observations). As is the case for CTLA-4 and TGF-β, PD1 knockout mice develop strain-dependent autoimmune disease (Nishimura et al., 1999, 2001). In murine models of experimental autoimmune encephalomyelitis (EAE) and diabetes, anti-PD1 antagonist antibodies enhance disease progression (Ansari et al., 2003; Salama et al., 2003). There are currently two known ligands for PD1, B7-H1 (also known as PD-L1) and B7-DC (also known as PD-L2). These ligands have very different tissue distribution patterns, wit B7-DC expression is primarily confined to DCs and macrophages (Tseng et al., 2001). B7-H1 mRNA is widely expressed, but cell surface protein is not detectable in normal tissues other than a subset of macrophages (Dong et al., 1999). Interestingly, B7-H1 expression can be detected in a number of tumor types (Dong et al., 2002), and engagement of PD1 by tumor associated B7-H1 promotes CD8 T-cell apoptosis. Clinically, it has been reported that B7-H1 expression is correlated with poor prognosis in renal cell carcinoma (Thompson et al., 2004). Thus, it seems that PD1/B7-H1 interactions mediate a potent and specific immunoregulatory effect, preventing activated and trafficking CD8 T cells from lysing their targets *in vivo*. In recent data, this observation has been confirmed in murine tumor models, where blockade of either PD1 or of the PD1 ligand B7-H1 potentiates an antitumor immune response (Hirano *et al.*, 2005). In contrast, the molecular role of B7-DC ligation in an immune response is complex (Chen *et al.*, 2004), and under some circumstances ligation of B7-DC on antigen presenting cells appears to potentiate a costimulatory interaction with T cells (Nguyen *et al.*, 2002a,b; Shin *et al.*, 2003). Clearly, further research is required to determine the relative roles of these two PD1 ligands in human tumor immunology. However, all of the currently available data do strongly support a role for PD1 blockade in the potentiation of an antitumor immune response.

Murphy and colleagues, have recently described a new member of the coinhibitor group of molecules, which they coined BTLA (B and T lymphocyte attenuator) (Watanabe *et al.*, 2003). The BTLA is expressed on activated T cells as well as B cells and DCs. Interestingly, like PD1, BTLA also appears to be relatively upregulated on anergic CD4 T cells (Hurchla *et al.*, 2005). While CTLA-4 and PD1 bind to B7 family members, the ligand for BTLA has been identified as HVEM (herpesvirus entry mediator) (Sedy *et al.*, 2005), which is a member of the TNFR superfamily (Croft *et al.*, 2005). This interaction is interesting and represents a unique mechanism for potential crosstalk between the CD28-B7 family and the TNFR-TNF family. Dissecting the overall immune outcome mediated by interactions between BTLA and HVEM is complicated by the fact that HVEM also binds to two additional ligands (LIGHT and secreted lymphotoxin) (Croft *et al.*, 2005). Based on this complexity, a number of signaling models are possible, all of which await further experimental confirmation.

7. Regulatory T Cells

Aside from the burgeoning families of coinhibitory and costimulatory molecules, a great deal of interest in both tumor immunity and infectious immunity has focused on regulatory T cells (Treg) (von Boehmer, 2005). This interest dates back to the observations of Sakaguchi *et al.*, who created a renaissance in T-cell suppression by demonstrating that CD4 T cells that were $CD25^+$ could prevent the development of autoimmunity mediated by neonatal thymectomy (Sakaguchi *et al.*, 1995). The regulatory potential of thymic $CD4^+CD25^+$ T cells was subsequently confirmed in a number of autoimmunity, infection, and tumor models (Shevach, 2004) (Fig. 3). Perhaps the most convincing data concerning a role for $CD4^+CD25^+$ regulatory T cells in human cancer come from the recent work of Curiel *et al.*, who showed that the presence of such regulatory T cells in ascites fluid from women with advanced ovarian cancer

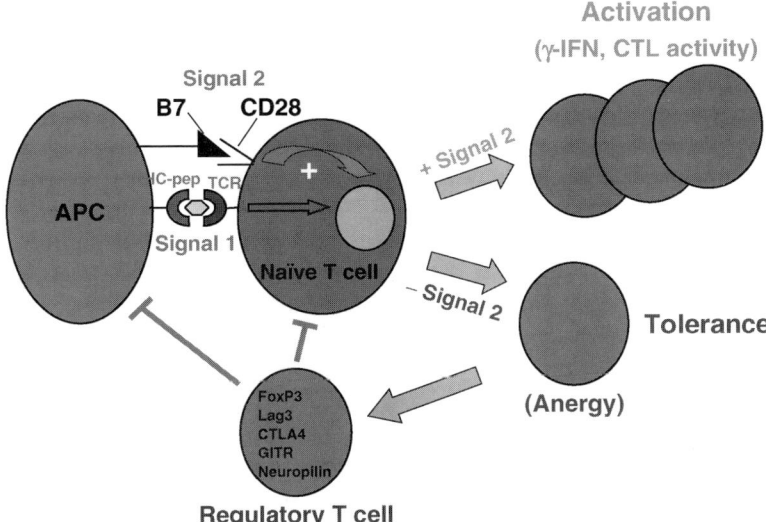

Figure 3 Regulatory T cells are an important inhibitor of antitumor immunity. T cell activation in the absence of appropriate costimulatory signals leads to T cell anergy and generation of induced regulatory T cells (Treg). Treg, characterized by the FoxP3 transcription factor, upregulate a number of cell membrane molecules, including Lag3, CTLA4, GITR, and neuropilin. Treg can inhibit effector T cell activation and function via T-T inhibition or inhibition of antigen presenting cells. **(See Plate 3 in color insert at the end of the book.)**

was associated with decreased survival (Curiel et al., 2004). In addition, these cells were shown to exhibit regulatory function in ex vivo Treg assays. Subsequently, tumor-associated Treg have been identified in lung, pancreatic, ovarian, and breast cancer specimens (Liyanage et al., 2002).

There is presently no single cell surface marker that uniquely identifies Treg. As has been described, CD25 (the IL-2 receptor alpha chain) marks activated as well as regulatory T cells, and thus CD4 CD25 T cells contain a mixture of activated as well as regulatory T cells. Other potential Treg markers include the glucocorticoid-induced TNF receptor (GITR) (McHugh et al., 2002), neuropilin (Bruder et al., 2004), and lymphocyte activation gene-3 (Lag-3) (Huang et al., 2004). This lack of a clear cell surface marker not only complicates the study of Treg in model systems but also makes it difficult to envision Treg specific intervention strategies. Nonetheless, absolute specificity may not be completely necessary; in many systems, systemic depletion of CD4 CD25 T cells by monoclonal antibodies (PC-61 in the mouse) or by a CD25 targeted toxin (Ontac) clearly augments a specific immune response (Terabe and Berzofsky, 2004). Another interesting methodology for functionally targeting Treg stems from seminal observations made by Robert North in the late 1970s, who showed that low doses of the common chemotherapy agent cyclophosphamide appeared to selectively deplete cells with regulatory activity (North, 1982). This observation has been widely confirmed in the clinical setting (Berd *et al.*, 1982, 1986), and recent studies using murine models of prostate and breast cancer have helped to define the mechanism of this effect (Machiels *et al.*, 2001; Nigam *et al.*, 1998). Perhaps the most intriguing data regarding the effect of cyclophosphamide in a tumor model come from Ercolini *et al.*, who showed that immunoregulatory doses of cyclophosphamide seemed to selectively unmask a high affinity population of tumor-specific CD8 T cells (Ercolini *et al.*, 2005). Based on the relatively low toxicity of these regimens (no lymphopenia is induced), there seems little reason not to consider the addition of low-dose cyclophosphamide to antitumor immunotherapy approaches.

8. CD8 T-Cell Dysfunction

Because tumors have likely been present for years before they are clinically detectable, endogenous tumor-specific CD8 T cells have been exposed to tumor antigens for protracted time periods. This situation of persistent antigen has been investigated using a number of chronic viral models (Zajac *et al.*, 1998). Data from such systems are consistent in showing impaired CD8 T-cell function under these conditions. Interestingly, antigen-specific CD8 T cells do not appear to be specifically deleted, but rather enter a state where they cannot transition between an effector memory ($CD62L^{low}$) and central memory ($CD62L^{high}$) phenotype. This phenomenon has been termed "exhaustion" and may play a role in impaired CD8 T-cell response to persistent tumor antigens as well. In a way, the phenomenon of CD8 T-cell exhaustion is actually encouraging from the perspective of immunotherapy, suggesting that tumor-specific CD8 T cells may be present and partially primed, even in the tumor-bearing host. The removal of persistent antigen can have profound effects under such conditions—den Boer *et al.* recently showed that CD8 T cells isolated from tumor bearing hosts could regain function in tumor free animals; functionally mediating protection from tumor challenge (den Boer *et al.*, 2004). These findings echo seminal experiments performed by Ramsdell and Fowlkes, who, over two decades ago showed that elimination of persistent antigen could restore T-cell function *in vivo* (Ramsdell and Fowlkes, 1992). Translating these observations to the clinical setting is not straightforward but suggests that immunotherapy approaches may prove most efficacious in the setting of minimal residual disease (Finn, 2003). For certain tumor types, i.e. chemosensitive small cell lung cancer (SCLC) or hormone responsive prostate cancer, a minimal residual disease state is routinely encountered following standard therapy, representing an attractive patient population for clinical trials.

Animal models of insulinoma have shed some light on the response of tumor-specific CD8 T cells *in vivo* (Lyman *et al.*, 2004; Nguyen *et al.*, 2002a,b). In one such model, Nguyen *et al.* showed that adoptively transferred tumor-specific CD8 T cells differentiated into an effector phenotype, and mediated a modicum of protection *in vivo* (Nguyen *et al.*, 2002a,b). Using a different CD8 T-cell transgenic donor, Lyman *et al.* reported similar findings, that adoptively transferred CD8 T cells proliferated and acquired cytolytic activity *in vivo* (Lyman *et al.*, 2004). Together these data suggest that CD8 T-cell tolerance to tumors may not be as profound as that of CD4 T cells, and that provision of adequate CD4 T-cell help to low affinity tumor-specific T cells may be sufficient to overcome a relative of *in vivo* cytolytic efficacy (Lyman *et al.*, 2004).

When CD8 T cells are activated by antigen presenting cells in a manner that facilitates the acquisition of full effector function, they lyse target cells by a combination of granzyme and perforin-mediated mechanisms. The antigen presenting cells themselves appear to be far less susceptible to CD8 T-cell mediated lysis. One of the mechanisms for this protection has recently been elucidated and stems from the observation that activated antigen presentation cells express a serine protease inhibitor (SPI)-6, a member of the serpin family that specifically inactivates granzyme B and blocks CTL-induced apoptosis (Medema *et al.*, 2001). Surprisingly, recent data show that several colon carcinoma cell lines resistant to CTL-mediated killing express SPI-6 in addition to an additional required serpin known as SPI-CI (serine protease inhibitor involved in cytotoxicity inhibition) (Bots *et al.*, 2005). These data are relatively recent, but they suggest yet another pathway by which tumors may resist killing by activated CD8 T cells. Future studies examining the relative expression of serpins in various tumor types should elucidate the magnitude to which this mechanism inhibits an antitumor immune response in the clinical setting.

9. Summary

While immunologic checkpoints that potentially block antitumor immune responses are becoming well defined at the molecular level, the relative importance of circumventing any individual checkpoint *in vivo* remains to be determined. There has been a tendency to focus upon model systems in which a single intervention renders a previously ineffective immunotherapy approach markedly efficacious. Over the next several years, it will be of primary importance to begin to develop a sense of which checkpoint intervention approaches are of most crucial, both in laboratory models as well as in the clinical situation. It is particularly challenging to clinically develop combinatorial strategies in which blockade of multiple checkpoints is evaluated. For example, if CTLA-4 is blocked, does inhibition of Treg with low-dose cyclophosphamide still have an effect? Or, if TGF-β is neutralized with a blocking antibody or pharmacological inhibitor, would Treg depletion with an anti-CD25 targeted monoclonal antibody be redundant? As Phase II clinical trials to evaluate combination immunotherapy approaches are difficult to design and costly to implement, strong preclinical data from multiple model systems would go a long way toward guiding clinical development. Regardless of the eventual therapeutic development pathway involved, the plethora of barriers present in the tumor-bearing host makes it unlikely that single interventions (i.e., vaccination alone) or blockade of a single checkpoint would achieve a meaningful survival or quality of life benefit in patients with advanced metastatic cancer. Rather, in a manner analogous to combination chemotherapy, it seems that rational combinations targeting multiple nonoverlapping checkpoints will be required. For example, multiple datasets concur that immunological approaches are most successful in the setting of minimal residual disease, or perhaps even in the adjuvant setting, where radiologically detectable tumor may not be present. Thus, the first part of a combination strategy might be to minimize tumor antigen load using hormonal therapy, surgery, radiation, or conventional chemotherapy. Next, checkpoints that affect the processing and presentation of tumor antigen—such as *Stat3* or TGF-β might be blocked. Following this, specific immunization might be employed, using one of several immunization approaches currently under Phase III evaluation. As T cells respond to vaccination, checkpoints like CTLA-4, which affect the priming phase of a T-cell response, might be blocked. Finally, those checkpoints that affect CD8 T-cell function in the tumor environment, such as B7-H1, might be targeted. While such a sequential, combinatorial approach may seem hopelessly complex to a laboratory-based immunologist, far more involved clinical regimens, employing multiple highly toxic chemotherapy regimens in sequence, are utilized every day in the treatment of human cancer. Immunologic strategies may need to approach this level of complexity in order to succeed.

References

Adler, A. J., Marsh, D. W., Yochum, G. S., Guzzo, J. L., Nigam, A., Nelson, W. G., and Pardoll, D. M. (1998). CD4+ T cell tolerance to parenchymal self-antigens requires presentation by bone marrow-derived antigen-presenting cells. *J. Exp. Med.* **187**(10), 1555–1564.

Ahmadzadeh, M., and Rosenberg, S. A. (2005). TGF-beta 1 attenuates the acquisition and expression of effector function by tumor antigen-specific human memory CD8 T cells. *J. Immunol.* **174**(9), 5215–5223.

Almand, B., Resser, J. R., Lindman, B., Nadaf, S., Clark, J. I., Kwon, E. D., Carbone, D. P., and Gabrilovich, D. I. (2000). Clinical significance of defective dendritic cell differentiation in cancer. *Clin. Cancer Res.* **6**(5), 1755–1766.

Alpan, R. S., Zhang, M., and Pardee, A. B. (1996). Cell cycle-dependent expression of TAP1, TAP2, and HLA-B27 messenger RNAs in a human breast cancer cell line. *Cancer Res.* **56**(19), 4358–4361.

Ansari, M. J., Salama, A. D., Chitnis, T., Smith, R. N., Yagita, H., Akiba, H., Yamazaki, T., Azuma, M., Iwai, H., Khoury, S. J., Auchincloss, H., Jr., and Sayegh, M. H. (2003). The programmed death-1 (PD-1) pathway regulates autoimmune diabetes in nonobese diabetic (NOD) mice. *J. Exp. Med.* **198**(1), 63–69.

Baban, B., Hansen, A. M., Chandler, P. R., Manlapat, A., Bingaman, A., Kahler, D. J., Munn, D. H., and Mellor, A. L. (2005). A minor population of splenic dendritic cells expressing CD19 mediates IDO-dependent T cell suppression via type I IFN signaling following B7 ligation. *Int. Immunol.* **17**(7), 909–919.

Bakkenist, C. J., and Kastan, M. B. (2004). Initiating cellular stress responses. *Cell* **118**(1), 9–17.

Benitez, R., Godelaine, D., Lopez-Nevot, M. A., Brasseur, F., Jimenez, P., Marchand, M., Oliva, M. R., van Baren, N., Cabrera, T., Andry, G., Landry, C., Ruiz-Cabello, F., *et al.* (1998). Mutations of the beta2-microglobulin gene result in a lack of HLA class I molecules on melanoma cells of two patients immunized with MAGE peptides. *Tissue Antigens* **52**(6), 520–529.

Berd, D., Mastrangelo, M. J., Engstrom, P. F., Paul, A., and Maguire, H. (1982). Augmentation of the human immune response by cyclophosphamide. *Cancer Res.* **42**(11), 4862–4866.

Berd, D., Maguire, H. C., Jr., and Mastrangelo, M. J. (1986). Induction of cell-mediated immunity to autologous melanoma cells and regression of metastases after treatment with a melanoma cell vaccine preceded by cyclophosphamide. *Cancer Res.* **46**(5), 2572–2577.

Blackman, M. A., Lund, F. E., Surman, S., Corley, R. B., and Woodland, D. L. (1992). Major histocompatibility complex-restricted recognition of retroviral superantigens by V beta 17+ T cells. *J. Exp. Med.* **176**(1), 275–280.

Blanchet, O., Bourge, J. F., Zinszner, H., Israel, A., Kourilsky, P., Dausset, J., Degos, L., and Paul, P. (1992). Altered binding of regulatory factors to HLA class I enhancer sequence in human tumor cell lines lacking class I antigen expression. *Proc. Natl. Acad. Sci. USA* **89**(8), 3488–3492.

Blobe, G. C., Schiemann, W. P., and Lodish, H. F. (2000). Role of transforming growth factor beta in human disease. *N. Engl. J. Med.* **342**(18), 1350–1358.

Bogen, B., Munthe, L., Sollien, A., Hofgaard, P., Omholt, H., Dagnaes, F., Dembic, Z., and Lauritzsen, G. F. (1995). Naive CD4+ T cells confer idiotype-specific tumor resistance in the absence of antibodies. *Eur. J. Immunol.* **25**(11), 3079–3086.

Bogen, B., Schenck, K., Munthe, L. A., and Dembic, Z. (2000). Deletion of idiotype (Id)-specific T cells in multiple myeloma. *Acta Oncol.* **39**(7), 783–788.

Bonifaz, L., Bonnyay, D., Mahnke, K., Rivera, M., Nussenzweig, M. C., and Steinman, R. M. (2002). Efficient targeting of protein antigen to the dendritic cell receptor DEC-205 in the steady state leads to antigen presentation on major histocompatibility complex class I products and peripheral CD8+ T cell tolerance. *J. Exp. Med.* **196**(12), 1627–1638.

Bots, M., Kolfschoten, I. G., Bres, S. A., Rademaker, M. T., de Roo, G. M., Kruse, M., Franken, K. L., Hahne, M., Froelich, C. J., Melief, C. J., Offringa, R., and Medema, J. P. (2005). SPI-CI and SPI-6 cooperate in the protection from effector cell-mediated cytotoxicity. *Blood* **105**(3), 1153–1161.

Bowman, T., Broome, M. A., Sinibaldi, D., Wharton, W., Pledger, W. J., Sedivy, J. M., Irby, R., Yeatman, T., Courtneidge, S. A., and Jove, R. (2001). Stat3-mediated Myc expression is required for Src transformation and PDGF-induced mitogenesis. *Proc. Natl. Acad. Sci. USA* **98**(13), 7319–7324.

Bretschen, P., and Cohn, M. (1970). A theory of self-nonself discrimination. *Science* **169**, 1042–1049.

Bromberg, J. F., Wrzeszczynska, M. H., Devgan, G., Zhao, Y., Pestell, R. G., Albanese, C., and Darnell, Bronte, J. E., Jr. (1999). Stat3 as an oncogene. *Cell* **98**(3), 295–303.

Bronte, V., Apolloni, E., Cabrelle, A., Ronca, R., Serafini, P., Zamboni, P., Restifo, N. P., and Zanovello, P. (2000). Identification of a CD11b(+)/Gr-1(+)/CD31(+) myeloid progenitor capable of activating or suppressing CD8(+) T cells. *Blood* **96**(12), 3838–3846.

Bronte, V., Serafini, P., De Santo, C., Marigo, I., Tosello, V., Mazzoni, A., Segal, D. M., Staib, C., Lowel, M., Sutter, G., Colombo, M. P., and Zanovello, P. (2003). IL-4-induced arginase 1 suppresses alloreactive T cells in tumor-bearing mice. *J. Immunol.* **170**(1), 270–278.

Bruder, D., Probst-Kepper, M., Westendorf, A. M., Geffers, R., Beissert, S., Loser, K., von Boehmer, H., Buer, J., and Hansen, W. (2004). Neuropilin-1: A surface marker of regulatory T cells. *Eur. J. Immunol.* **34**(3), 623–630.

Cabrera, T., Angustias, F. M., Sierra, A., Garrido, A., Herruzo, A., Escobedo, A., Fabra, A., and Garrido, F. (1996). High frequency of altered HLA class I phenotypes in invasive breast carcinomas. *Hum. Immunol.* **50**(2), 127–134.

Cabrera, T., Collado, A., Fernandez, M. A., Ferron, A., Sancho, J., Ruiz-Cabello, F., and Garrido, F. (1998). High frequency of altered HLA class I phenotypes in invasive colorectal carcinomas. *Tissue Antigens* **52**(2), 114–123.

Callahan, J. F., Burgess, J. L., Fornwald, J. A., Gaster, L. M., Harling, J. D., Harrington, F. P., Heer, J., Kwon, C., Lehr, R., Mathur, A., Olson, B. A., Weinstock, J., *et al.* (2002). Identification of novel inhibitors of the transforming growth factor beta1 (TGF-beta1) type 1 receptor (ALK5). *J. Med. Chem.* **45**(5), 999–1001.

Chambers, C. A., Kuhns, M. S., Egen, J. G., and Allison, J. P. (2001). CTLA-4-mediated inhibition in regulation of T cell responses: Mechanisms and manipulation in tumor immunotherapy. *Annu. Rev. Immunol.* **19**, 565–594.

Chen, L. (2004). Co-inhibitory molecules of the B7-CD28 family in the control of T-cell immunity. *Nat. Rev. Immunol.* **4**(5), 336–347.

Chen, M. L., Pittet, M. J., Gorelik, L., Flavell, R. A., Weissleder, R., von Boehmer, H., and Khazaie, K. (2005). Regulatory T cells suppress tumor-specific CD8 T cell cytotoxicity through TGF-beta signals *in vivo*. *Proc. Natl. Acad. Sci. USA* **102**(2), 419–424.

Clarke, B., and Chetty, R. (2002). Postmodern cancer: The role of human immunodeficiency virus in uterine cervical cancer. *Mol. Pathol.* **55**(1), 19–24.

Cormier, J. N., Abati, A., Fetsch, P., Hijazi, Y. M., Rosenberg, S. A., Marincola, F. M., and Topalian, S. L. (1998). Comparative analysis of the *in vivo* expression of tyrosinase, MART-1/Melan-A, and gp100 in metastatic melanoma lesions: Implications for immunotherapy. *J. Immunother.* **21**(1), 27–31.

Cormier, J. N., Panelli, M. C., Hackett, J. A., Bettinotti, M. P., Mixon, A., Wunderlich, J., Parker, L. L., Restifo, N. P., Ferrone, S., and Marincola, F. M. (1999). Natural variation of the expression of HLA and endogenous antigen modulates CTL recognition in an *in vitro* melanoma model. *Int. J. Cancer* **80**(5), 781–790.

Croft, M. (2005). The evolving crosstalk between co-stimulatory and co-inhibitory receptors: HVEM-BTLA. *Trends Immunol.* **26**(6), 292–294.

Cui, W., Fowlis, D. J., Bryson, S., Duffie, E., Ireland, H., Balmain, A., and Akhurst, R. J. (1996). TGFbeta1 inhibits the formation of benign skin tumors, but enhances progression to invasive spindle carcinomas in transgenic mice. *Cell* **86**(4), 531–542.

Curiel, T. J., Coukos, G., Zou, L., Alvarez, X., Cheng, P., Mottram, P., Evdemon-Hogan, M., Conejo-Garcia, J. R., Zhang, L., Burow, M., Zhu, Y., Wei, S., *et al.* (2004). Specific recruitment of regulatory T cells in ovarian carcinoma fosters immune privilege and predicts reduced survival. *Nat. Med.* **10**(9), 942–949.

de Vries, T. J., Trancikova, D., Ruiter, D. J., and van Muijen, G. N. (1998). High expression of immunotherapy candidate proteins gp100, MART-1, tyrosinase and TRP-1 in uveal melanoma. *Br. J. Cancer* **78**(9), 1156–1161.

den Boer, A. T., van Mierlo, G. J., Fransen, M. F., Melief, C. J., Offringa, R., and Toes, R. E. (2004). The tumoricidal activity of memory CD8+ T cells is hampered by persistent systemic antigen, but full functional capacity is regained in an antigen-free environment. *J. Immunol.* **172**(10), 6074–6079.

Dong, H., Zhu, G., Tamada, K., and Chen, L. (1999). B7-H1, a third member of the B7 family, co-stimulates T-cell proliferation and interleukin-10 secretion. *Nat. Med.* **5**(12), 1365–1369.

Dong, H., Strome, S. E., Salomao, D. R., Tamura, H., Hirano, F., Flies, D. B., Roche, P. C., Lu, J., Zhu, G., Tamada, K., Lennon, V. A., Celis, E., et al. (2002). Tumor-associated B7-H1 promotes T-cell apoptosis: A potential mechanism of immune evasion. *Nat. Med.* **8**(8), 793–800.

Doyle, A., Martin, W. J., Funa, K., Gazdar, A., Carney, D., Martin, S. E., Linnoila, I., Cuttitta, F., Mulshine, J., Bunn, P., and Minna, J. (1985). Markedly decreased expression of class I histocompatibility antigens, protein, and mRNA in human small-cell lung cancer. *J. Exp. Med.* **161**(5), 1135–1151.

D'Urso, C. M., Wang, Z. G., Cao, Y., Tatake, R., Zeff, R. A., and Ferrone, S. (1991). Lack of HLA class I antigen expression by cultured melanoma cells FO-1 due to a defect in B2m gene expression. *J. Clin. Invest.* **87**(1), 284–292.

Ercolini, A. M., Ladle, B. H., Manning, E. A., Pfannenstiel, L. W., Armstrong, T. D., Machiels, J. P., Bieler, J. G., Emens, L. A., Reilly, R. T., and Jaffee, E. M. (2005). Recruitment of latent pools of high-avidity CD8(+) T cells to the antitumor immune response. *J. Exp. Med.* **201**(10), 1591–1602.

Esteban, F., Concha, A., Huelin, C., Perez-Ayala, M., Pedrinaci, S., Ruiz-Cabello, F., and Garrido, F. (1989). Histocompatibility antigens in primary and metastatic squamous cell carcinoma of the larynx. *Int. J. Cancer* **43**(3), 436–442.

Esteban, F., Concha, A., Delgado, M., Perez-Ayala, M., Ruiz-Cabello, F., and Garrido, F. (1990). Lack of MHC class I antigens and tumour aggressiveness of the squamous cell carcinoma of the larynx. *Br. J. Cancer* **62**(6), 1047–1051.

Esteban, F., Redondo, M., Delgado, M., Garrido, F., and Ruiz-Cabello, F. (1996). MHC class I antigens and tumour-infiltrating leucocytes in laryngeal cancer: Long-term follow-up. *Br. J. Cancer* **74**(11), 1801–1804.

Fearon, E. R., and Vogelstein, B. (1990). A genetic model for colorectal tumorigenesis. *Cell* **61**(5), 759–767.

Ferrone, S., and Marincola, F. M. (1995). Loss of HLA class I antigens by melanoma cells: Molecular mechanisms, functional significance and clinical relevance. *Immunol. Today* **16**(10), 487–494.

Finn, O. J. (2003). Cancer vaccines: Between the idea and the reality. *Nat. Rev. Immunol.* **3**(8), 630–641.

Gorelik, L., and Flavell, R. A. (2000). Abrogation of TGFbeta signaling in T cells leads to spontaneous T cell differentiation and autoimmune disease. *Immunity* **12**(2), 171–181.

Greten, F. R., Eckmann, L., Greten, T. F., Park, J. M., Li, Z. W., Egan, L. J., Kagnoff, M. F., and Karin, M. (2004). IKKbeta links inflammation and tumorigenesis in a mouse model of colitis-associated cancer. *Cell* **118**(3), 285–296.

Halak, B. K., Maguire, H. C., Jr., and Lattime, E. C. (1999). Tumor-induced interleukin-10 inhibits type 1 immune responses directed at a tumor antigen as well as a non-tumor antigen present at the tumor site. *Cancer Res.* **59**, 911–917.

Hasegawa, Y., Takanashi, S., Kanehira, Y., Tsushima, T., Imai, T., and Okumura, K. (2001). Transforming growth factor-beta1 level correlates with angiogenesis, tumor progression, and prognosis in patients with nonsmall cell lung carcinoma. *Cancer* **91**(5), 964–971.

Hatachi, S., Iwai, Y., Kawano, S., Morinobu, S., Kobayashi, M., Koshiba, M., Saura, R., Kurosaka, M., Honjo, T., and Kumagai, S. (2003). CD4+ PD-1+ T cells accumulate as unique anergic cells in rheumatoid arthritis synovial fluid. *J. Rheumatol.* **30**(7), 1410–1419.

Hawiger, D., Inaba, K., Dorsett, Y., Guo, M., Mahnke, K., Rivera, M., Ravetch, J. V., Steinman, R. M., and Nussenzweig, M. C. (2001). Dendritic cells induce peripheral T cell unresponsiveness under steady state conditions *in vivo*. *J. Exp. Med.* **194**(6), 769–779.

Haywood, G. R., and McKhann, C. F. (1971). Antigenic specificities on murine sarcoma cells. Reciprocal relationship between normal transplantation antigens (H-2) and tumor-specific immunogenicity. *J. Exp. Med.* **133**(6), 1171–1187.

Hilders, C. G., Houbiers, J. G., Krul, E. J., and Fleuren, G. J. (1994). The expression of histocompatibility-related leukocyte antigens in the pathway to cervical carcinoma. *Am. J. Clin. Pathol.* **101**(1), 5–12.

Hirano, F., Kaneko, K., Tamura, H., Dong, H., Wang, S., Ichikawa, M., Rietz, C., Flies, D. B., Lau, J. S., Zhu, G., Tamada, K., and Chen, L. (2005). Blockade of B7-H1 and PD-1 by monoclonal antibodies potentiates cancer therapeutic immunity. *Cancer Res.* **65**(3), 1089–1096.

Huang, A. Y., Golumbek, P., Ahmadzadeh, M., Jaffee, E., Pardoll, D., and Levitsky, H. (1994). Role of bone marrow-derived cells in presenting MHC class I-restricted tumor antigens. *Science* **264**(5161), 961–965.

Huang, C. T., Workman, C. J., Flies, D., Pan, X., Marson, A. L., Zhou, G., Hipkiss, E. L., Ravi, S., Kowalski, J., Levitsky, H. I., Powell, J. D., Pardoll, D. M., *et al.* (2004). Role of LAG-3 in regulatory T cells. *Immunity* **21**(4), 503–513.

Hugo, P., Boyd, R. L., Waanders, G. A., Petrie, H. T., and Scollay, R. (1991). Timing of deletion of autoreactive V beta 6+ cells and down-modulation of either CD4 or CD8 on phenotypically distinct CD4+8+ subsets of thymocytes expressing intermediate or high levels of T cell receptor. *Int. Immunol.* **3**(3), 265–272.

Hui, K., Grosveld, F., and Festenstein, H. (1984). Rejection of transplantable AKR leukaemia cells following MHC DNA-mediated cell transformation. *Nature* **311**(5988), 750–752.

Hurchla, M. A., Sedy, J. R., Gavrieli, M., Drake, C. G., Murphy, T. L., and Murphy, K. M. (2005). B and T lymphocyte attenuator exhibits structural and expression polymorphisms and is highly induced in anergic CD4+ T cells. *J. Immunol.* **174**(6), 3377–3385.

Ishida, Y., Agata, Y., Shibahara, K., and Honjo, T. (1992). Induced expression of PD-1, a novel member of the immunoglobulin gene superfamily, upon programmed cell death. *EMBO J.* **11**(11), 3887–3895.

Jager, E., Ringhoffer, M., Altmannsberger, M., Arand, M., Karbach, J., Jager, D., Oesch, F., and Knuth, A. (1997). Immunoselection *in vivo*: Independent loss of MHC class I and melanocyte differentiation antigen expression in metastatic melanoma. *Int. J. Cancer* **71**(2), 142–147.

Jones, P. A., and Baylin, S. B. (2002). The fundamental role of epigenetic events in cancer. *Nat. Rev. Genet.* **3**(6), 415–428.

Kappler, J. W., Roehm, N., and Marrack, P. (1987). T cell tolerance by clonal elimination in the thymus. *Cell* **49**(2), 273–280.

Karin, M., and Greten, F. R. (2005). NF-kappaB: Linking inflammation and immunity to cancer development and progression. *Nat. Rev. Immunol.* **5**(10), 749–759.

Karre, K., Ljunggren, H. G., Piontek, G., and Kiessling, R. (1986). Selective rejection of H-2-deficient lymphoma variants suggests alternative immune defence strategy. *Nature* **319**(6055), 675–678.

Klein, S. C., Ljunggren, H. G., Piontek, G., and Kiessling, R. (1995). IL6 and IL6 receptor expression in Burkitt's lymphoma and lymphoblastoid cell lines: Promotion of IL6 receptor expression by EBV. *Hematol. Oncol.* **13**(3), 121–130.

Koopman, L. A., Corver, W. E., van der Slik, A. R., Giphart, M. J., and Fleuren, G. J. (2000). Multiple genetic alterations cause frequent and heterogeneous human histocompatibility leukocyte antigen class I loss in cervical cancer. *J. Exp. Med.* **191**(6), 961–976.

Kortylewski, M., Kujawski, M., Wang, T., Wei, S., Zhang, S., Pilon-Thomas, S., Niu, G., Kay, H., Mule, J., Kerr, W. G., Jove, R., Pardoll, D., *et al.* (2005). Inhibiting *Stat3* signalling in the hematopoietic system elicits multicomponent antitumor immunity. *Nature Med.* **11**, 1314–1321.

Kusmartsev, S., and Gabrilovich, D. I. (2006). Role of immature myeloid cells in mechanisms of immune evasion in cancer. *Cancer Immunol. Immunother.* **55**, 1–9.

Kusmartsev, S., Nefedova, Y., Yoder, D., and Gabrilovich, D. I. (2004). Antigen-specific inhibition of CD8+ T cell response by immature myeloid cells in cancer is mediated by reactive oxygen species. *J. Immunol.* **172**(2), 989–999.

Lanier, L. L., and Phillips, J. H. (1996). Inhibitory MHC class I receptors on NK cells and T cells. *Immunol. Today* **17**(2), 86–91.

Laping, N. J., Grygielko, E., Mathur, A., Butter, S., Bomberger, J., Tweed, C., Martin, W., Fornwald, J., Lehr, R., Harling, J., Gaster, L., Callahan, J. F., et al. (2002). Inhibition of transforming growth factor (TGF)-beta1-induced extracellular matrix with a novel inhibitor of the TGF-beta type I receptor kinase activity: SB-431542. *Mol. Pharmacol.* **62**(1), 58–64.

Lauritzsen, G. F., Hofgaard, P. O., Schenck, K., and Bogen, B. (1998). Clonal deletion of thymocytes as a tumor escape mechanism. *Int. J. Cancer* **78**(2), 216–222.

Lechner, O., Lauber, J., Franzke, A., Sarukhan, A., von Boehmer, H., and Buer, J. (2001). Fingerprints of anergic T cells. *Curr. Biol.* **11**(8), 587–595.

Lethe, B., van den, E. B., Van Pel, A., Corradin, G., and Boon, T. (1992). Mouse tumor rejection antigens P815A and P815B: Two epitopes carried by a single peptide. *Eur. J. Immunol.* **22**(9), 2283–2288.

Letterio, J. J., and Roberts, A. B. (1998). Regulation of immune responses by TGF-beta. *Annu. Rev. Immunol.* **16**, 137–161.

Lin, E. Y., Gouon-Evans, V., Nguyen, A. V., and Pollard, J. W. (2002). The macrophage growth factor CSF-1 in mammary gland development and tumor progression. *J. Mammary Gland Biol. Neoplasia* **7**(2), 147–162.

Lind, M. H., Rozell, B., Wallin, R. P., van Hogerlinden, M., Ljunggren, H. G., Toftgard, R., and Sur, I. (2004). Tumor necrosis factor receptor 1-mediated signaling is required for skin cancer development induced by NF-kappaB inhibition. *Proc. Natl. Acad. Sci. USA* **101**(14), 4972–4977.

Liyanage, U. K., Moore, T. T., Joo, H. G., Tanaka, Y., Herrmann, V., Doherty, G., Drebin, J. A., Strasberg, S. M., Eberlein, T. J., Goedegebuure, P. S., and Linehan, D. C. (2002). Prevalence of regulatory T cells is increased in peripheral blood and tumor microenvironment of patients with pancreas or breast adenocarcinoma. *J. Immunol.* **169**(5), 2756–2761.

Ljunggren, H. G., and Karre, K. (1985). Host resistance directed selectively against H-2-deficient lymphoma variants. Analysis of the mechanism. *J. Exp. Med.* **162**(6), 1745–1759.

Lu, X., and Lane, D. P. (1993). Differential induction of transcriptionally active p53 following UV or ionizing radiation: Defects in chromosome instability syndromes? *Cell* **75**(4), 765–778.

Lucas, C., Bald, L. N., Fendly, B. M., Mora-Worms, M., Figari, I. S., Patzer, E. J., and Palladino, M. A. (1990). The autocrine production of transforming growth factor-beta 1 during lymphocyte activation. A study with a monoclonal antibody-based ELISA. *J. Immunol.* **145**(5), 1415–1422.

Lyman, M. A., Aung, S., Biggs, J. A., and Sherman, L. A. (2004). A spontaneously arising pancreatic tumor does not promote the differentiation of naive CD8+ T lymphocytes into effector CTL. *J. Immunol.* **172**(11), 6558–6567.

MacDonald, H. R., Schneider, R., Lees, R. K., Howe, R. C., Acha-Orbea, H., Festenstein, H., Zinkernagel, R. M., and Hengartner, H. (1988). T-cell receptor V beta use predicts reactivity and tolerance to Mlsa-encoded antigens. *Nature* **332**(6159), 40–45.

Machiels, J. P., Reilly, R. T., Emens, L. A., Ercolini, A. M., Lei, R. Y., Weintraub, D., Okoye, F. I., and Jaffee, E. M. (2001). Cyclophosphamide, doxorubicin, and paclitaxel enhance the antitumor immune response of granulocyte/macrophage-colony stimulating factor-secreting whole-cell vaccines in HER-2/neu tolerized mice. *Cancer Res.* **61**(9), 3689–3697.

Marincola, F. M., Jaffee, E. M., Hicklin, D. J., and Ferrone, S. (2000). Escape of human solid tumors from T-cell recognition: Molecular mechanisms and functional significance. *Adv. Immunol.* **74**, 181–273.

Mazzoni, A., Bronte, V., Visintin, A., Spitzer, J. H., Apolloni, E., Serafini, P., Zanovello, P., and Segal, D. M. (2002). Myeloid suppressor lines inhibit T cell responses by an NO-dependent mechanism. *J. Immunol.* **168**(2), 689–695.

McHugh, R. S., Whitters, M. J., Piccirillo, C. A., Young, D. A., Shevach, E. M., Collins, M., and Byrne, M. C. (2002). CD4(+)CD25(+) immunoregulatory T cells: Gene expression analysis reveals a functional role for the glucocorticoid-induced TNF receptor. *Immunity* **16**(2), 311–323.

Medema, J. P., Schuurhuis, D. H., Rea, D., van Tongeren, J., de Jong, J., Bres, S. A., Laban, S., Toes, R. E., Toebes, M., Schumacher, T. N., Bladergroen, B. A., Ossendorp, F., *et al.* (2001). Expression of the serpin serine protease inhibitor 6 protects dendritic cells from cytotoxic T lymphocyte-induced apoptosis: Differential modulation by T helper type 1 and type 2 cells. *J. Exp. Med.* **194**(5), 657–667.

Mellor, A. L., Chandler, P., Baban, B., Hansen, A. M., Marshall, B., Pihkala, J., Waldmann, H., Cobbold, S., Adams, E., and Munn, D. H. (2004). Specific subsets of murine dendritic cells acquire potent T cell regulatory functions following CTLA4-mediated induction of indoleamine 2,3 dioxygenase. *Int. Immunol.* **16**(10), 1391–1401.

Mizoguchi, H., O'Shea, J. J., Longo, D. L., Loeffler, C. M., McVicar, D. W., and Ochoa, A. C. (1992). Alterations in signal transduction molecules in T lymphocytes from tumor-bearing mice. *Science* **258**(5089), 1795–1798.

Moretta, A., Biassoni, R., Bottino, C., Pende, D., Vitale, M., Poggi, A., Mingari, M. C., and Moretta, L. (1997). Major histocompatibility complex class I-specific receptors on human natural killer and T lymphocytes. *Immunol. Rev.* **155**, 105–117.

Munn, D. H., Sharma, M. D., Lee, J. R., Jhaver, K. G., Johnson, T. S., Keskin, D. B., Marshall, B., Chandler, P., Antonia, S. J., Burgess, R., Slingluff, C. L., Jr., and Mellor, A. L. (2002). Potential regulatory function of human dendritic cells expressing indoleamine 2,3-dioxygenase. *Science* **297**(5588), 1867–1870.

Munn, D. H., Sharma, M. D., Hou, D., Baban, B., Lee, J. R., Antonia, S. J., Messina, J. L., Chandler, P., Koni, P. A., and Mellor, A. L. (2004). Expression of indoleamine 2,3-dioxygenase by plasmacytoid dendritic cells in tumor-draining lymph nodes. *J. Clin. Invest.* **114**(2), 280–290.

Munn, D. H., Sharma, M. D., Baban, B., Harding, H. P., Zhang, Y., Ron, D., and Mellor, A. L. (2005). GCN2 kinase in T cells mediates proliferative arrest and anergy induction in response to indoleamine 2,3-dioxygenase. *Immunity* **22**(5), 633–642.

Natali, P., Bigotti, A., Cavaliere, R., Liao, S. K., Taniguchi, M., Matsui, M., and Ferrone, S. (1985). Heterogeneous expression of melanoma-associated antigens and HLA antigens by primary and multiple metastatic lesions removed from patients with melanoma. *Cancer Res.* **45**(6), 2883–2889.

Natali, P. G., Viora, M., Nicotra, M. R., Giacomini, P., Bigotti, A., and Ferrone, S. (1983). Antigenic heterogeneity of skin tumors of nonmelanocyte origin: Analysis with monoclonal antibodies to tumor-associated antigens and to histocompatibility antigens. *J. Natl. Cancer Inst.* **71**, 439–447.

Natali, P. G., Bigotti, A., Nicotra, M. R., Viora, M., Manfredi, D., and Ferrone, S. (1984). Distribution of human Class I (HLA-A,B,C) histocompatibility antigens in normal and malignant tissues of nonlymphoid origin. *Cancer Res.* **44**(10), 4679–4687.

Natali, P. G., Nicotra, M. R., Bigotti, A., Venturo, I., Marcenaro, L., Giacomini, P., and Russo, C. (1989). Selective changes in expression of HLA class I polymorphic determinants in human solid tumors. *Proc. Natl. Acad. Sci. USA* **86**(17), 6719–6723.

Nefedova, Y., Huang, M., Kusmartsev, S., Bhattacharya, R., Cheng, P., Salup, R., Jove, R., and Gabrilovich, D. (2004). Hyperactivation of Stat3 is involved in abnormal differentiation of dendritic cells in cancer. *J. Immunol.* **172**(1), 464–474.

Nefedova, Y., Nagaraj, S., Rosenbauer, A., Muro-Cacho, C., Sebti, S. M., and Gabrilovich, D. I. (2005). Regulation of dendritic cell differentiation and antitumor immune response in cancer by pharmacologic-selective inhibition of the janus-activated kinase 2/signal transducers and activators of transcription 3 pathway. *Cancer Res.* **65**(20), 9525–9535.

Nguyen, L. T., Radhakrishnan, S., Ciric, B., Tamada, K., Shin, T., Pardoll, D. M., Chen, L., Rodriguez, M., and Pease, L. R. (2002a). Cross-linking the B7 family molecule B7-DC directly activates immune functions of dendritic cells. *J. Exp. Med.* **196**(10), 1393–1398.

Nguyen, L. T., Elford, A. R., Murakami, K., Garza, K. M., Schoenberger, S. P., Odermatt, B., Speiser, D. E., and Ohashi, P. S. (2002b). Tumor growth enhances cross-presentation leading to limited T cell activation without tolerance. *J. Exp. Med.* **195**(4), 423–435.

Nigam, A., Yacavone, R. F., Zahurak, M. L., Johns, C. M. S., Pardoll, D. M., Piantadosi, S., Levitsky, H. I., and Nelson, W. G. (1998). Immunomodulatory properties of antineoplastic drugs administered in conjunction with GM-CSF-secreting cancer cell vaccines. *Int. J. Oncol.* **12**(1), 161–170.

Nishimura, H., Nose, M., Hiai, H., Minato, N., and Honjo, T. (1999). Development of lupus-like autoimmune diseases by disruption of the PD-1 gene encoding an ITIM motif-carrying immunoreceptor. *Immunity* **11**(2), 141–151.

Nishimura, H., Okazaki, T., Tanaka, Y., Nakatani, K., Hara, M., Matsumori, A., Sasayama, S., Mizoguchi, A., Hiai, H., Minato, N., and Honjo, T. (2001). Autoimmune dilated cardiomyopathy in PD-1 receptor-deficient mice. *Science* **291**(5502), 319–322.

Niu, G., Wright, K. L., Huang, M., Song, L., Haura, E., Turkson, J., Zhang, S., Wang, T., Sinibaldi, D., Coppola, D., Heller, R., Ellis, L. M., *et al.* (2002). Constitutive Stat3 activity up-regulates VEGF expression and tumor angiogenesis. *Oncogene* **21**(13), 2000–2008.

North, R. J. (1982). Cyclophosphamide-facilitated adoptive immunotherapy of an established tumor depends on elimination of tumor-induced suppressor T cells. *J. Exp. Med.* **155**(4), 1063–1074.

Ochsenbein, A. F. (2005). Immunological ignorance of solid tumors. *Springer Semin Immunopathol.* **27**, 19–35.

Ochsenbein, A. F., Klenerman, P., Karrer, U., Ludewig, B., Pericin, M., Hengartner, H., and Zinkernagel, R. M. (1999). Immune surveillance against a solid tumor fails because of immunological ignorance. *Proc. Natl. Acad. Sci. USA* **96**(5), 2233–2238.

Ohnmacht, G. A., Wang, E., Mocellin, S., Abati, A., Filie, A., Fetsch, P., Riker, A. I., Kammula, U. S., Rosenberg, S. A., and Marincola, F. M. (2001). Short-term kinetics of tumor antigen expression in response to vaccination. *J. Immunol.* **167**(3), 1809–1820.

Pardoll, D., and Allison, J. (2004). Cancer immunotherapy: Breaking the barriers to harvest the crop. *Nat. Med.* **10**(9), 887–892.

Pepper, M. S. (1997). Transforming growth factor-beta: Vasculogenesis, angiogenesis, and vessel wall integrity. *Cytokine Growth Factor Rev.* **8**(1), 21–43.

Perez, M., Cabrera, T., Lopez Nevot, M. A., Gomez, M., Peran, F., Ruiz-Cabello, F., and Garrido, F. (1986). Heterogeneity of the expression of class I and II HLA antigens in human breast carcinoma. *J. Immunogenet.* **13**(2–3), 247–253.

Phan, G. Q., Yang, J. C., Sherry, R. M., Hwu, P., Topalian, S. L., Schwartzentruber, D. J., Restifo, N. P., Haworth, L. R., Seipp, C. A., Freezer, L. J., Morton, K. E., Mavroukakis, S. A., *et al.* (2003). Cancer regression and autoimmunity induced by cytotoxic T lymphocyte-associated antigen 4 blockade in patients with metastatic melanoma. *Proc. Natl. Acad. Sci. USA* **100**(14), 8372–8377.

Quill, H., and Schwartz, R. H. (1987). Stimulation of normal inducer T cell clones with antigen presented by purified Ia molecules in planar lipid membranes: Specific induction of a long-lived state of proliferative nonresponsiveness. *J. Immunol.* **138**(11), 3704–3712.

Ramsdell, F., and Fowlkes, B. J. (1992). Maintenance of *in vivo* tolerance by persistence of antigen. *Science* **257**(5073), 1130–1134.

Restifo, N. P., Marincola, F. M., Kawakami, Y., Taubenberger, J., Yannelli, J. R., and Rosenberg, S. A. (1996). Loss of functional beta 2-microglobulin in metastatic melanomas from five patients receiving immunotherapy. *J. Natl. Cancer Inst.* **88**(2), 100–108.

Riker, A., Cormier, J., Panelli, M., Kammula, U., Wang, E., Abati, A., Fetsch, P., Lee, K. H., Steinberg, S., Rosenberg, S., and Marincola, F. (1999). Immune selection after antigen-specific immunotherapy of melanoma. *Surgery* **126**(2), 112–120.

Rowe, M., Khanna, R., Jacob, C. A., Argaet, V., Kelly, A., Powis, S., Belich, M., Croom-Carter, D., Lee, S., Burrows, S. R., Trowsdale, J., Moss, D. J., *et al.* (1995). Restoration of endogenous antigen processing in Burkitt's lymphoma cells by Epstein-Barr virus latent membrane protein-1: Coordinate up-regulation of peptide transporters and HLA-class I antigen expression. *Eur. J. Immunol.* **25**(5), 1374–1384.

Ruiz-Cabello, F., Lopez Nevot, M. A., Gutierrez, J., Oliva, M. R., Romero, C., Ferron, A., Esteban, F., Huelin, C., Piris, M. A., and Rivas, C. (1989). Phenotypic expression of histocompatibility antigens in human primary tumours and metastases. *Clin. Exp. Metastasis* **7**(2), 213–226.

Ruiz-Cabello, F., Perez-Ayala, M., Gomez, O., Redondo, M., Concha, A., Cabrera, T., and Garrido, F. (1991). Molecular analysis of MHC-class-I alterations in human tumor cell lines. *Int. J. Cancer Suppl.* **6**, 123–130.

Saito, H., Tsujitani, S., Oka, S., Kondo, A., Ikeguchi, M., Maeta, M., and Kaibara, N. (1999). The expression of transforming growth factor-beta1 is significantly correlated with the expression of vascular endothelial growth factor and poor prognosis of patients with advanced gastric carcinoma. *Cancer* **86**(8), 1455–1462.

Sakaguchi, S., Sakaguchi, N., Asano, M., Itoh, M., and Toda, M. (1995). Immunologic self-tolerance maintained by activated T cells expressing IL-2 receptor alpha-chains (CD25). Breakdown of a single mechanism of self-tolerance causes various autoimmune diseases. *J. Immunol.* **155**(3), 1151–1164.

Salama, A. D., Chitnis, T., Imitola, J., Ansari, M. J., Akiba, H., Tushima, F., Azuma, M., Yagita, H., Sayegh, M. H., and Khoury, S. J. (2003). Critical role of the programmed death-1 (PD-1) pathway in regulation of experimental autoimmune encephalomyelitis. *J. Exp. Med.* **198**(1), 71–78.

Sanda, M. G., Restifo, N. P., Walsh, J. C., Kawakami, Y., Nelson, W. G., Pardoll, D. M., and Simons, J. W. (1995). Molecular characterization of defective antigen processing in human prostate cancer. *J. Natl. Cancer Inst.* **87**(4), 280–285.

Sano, S., Itami, S., Takeda, K., Tarutani, M., Yamaguchi, Y., Miura, H., Yoshikawa, K., Akira, S., and Takeda, J. (1999). Keratinocyte-specific ablation of *Stat3* exhibits impaired skin remodeling, but does not affect skin morphogenesis. *EMBO J.* **18**(17), 4657–4668.

Scheibenbogen, C., Weyers, I., Ruiter, D., Willhauck, M., Bittinger, A., and Keilholz, U. (1996). Expression of gp100 in melanoma metastases resected before or after treatment with IFN alpha and IL-2. *J. Immunother. Emphasis Tumor Immunol.* **19**(5), 375–380.

Schmid, P., Itin, P., and Rufli, T. (1995). *In situ* analysis of transforming growth factor-beta s (TGF-beta 1, TGF-beta 2, TGF-beta 3), and TGF-beta type II receptor expression in malignant melanoma. *Carcinogenesis* **16**(7), 1499–1503.

Schmielau, J., and Finn, O. J. (2001). Activated granulocytes and granulocyte-derived hydrogen peroxide are the underlying mechanism of suppression of T-cell function in advanced cancer patients. *Cancer Res.* **61**(12), 4756–4760.

Schwartz, R. H. (1992). Costimulation of T lymphocytes: The role of CD28, CTLA-4, and B7/BB1 in interleukin-2 production and immunotherapy. *Cell* **71**(7), 1065–1068.

Schwartz, R. H. (1999). Immunological tolerance. *In* "Fundamental Immunology" (W. E. Paul, Ed.), pp. 701–740. Lippincott-Raven, Philadelphia.

Schwartz, R. H., *et al.* (1989). T-cell clonal anergy. *Cold Spring Harb. Symp. Quant. Biol.* **54**(Pt. 2), 605–610.

Sedy, J. R., Gavrieli, M., Potter, K. G., Hurchla, M. A., Lindsley, R. C., Hildner, K., Scheu, S., Pfeffer, K., Ware, C. F., Murphy, T. L., and Murphy, K. M. (2005). B and T lymphocyte attenuator regulates T cell activation through interaction with herpesvirus entry mediator. *Nat. Immunol.* **6**(1), 90–98.

Seliger, B., Hohne, A., Knuth, A., Bernhard, H., Ehring, B., Tampe, R., and Huber, C. (1996). Reduced membrane major histocompatibility complex class I density and stability in a subset of human renal cell carcinomas with low TAP and LMP expression. *Clin. Cancer Res.* **2**(8), 1427–1433.

Serafini, P., Carbley, R., Noonan, K. A., Tan, G., Bronte, V., and Borrello, I. (2004). High-dose granulocyte-macrophage colony-stimulating factor-producing vaccines impair the immune response through the recruitment of myeloid suppressor cells. *Cancer Res.* **64**(17), 6337–6343.

Shariat, S. F., Kim, J. H., Andrews, B., Kattan, M. W., Wheeler, T. M., Kim, I. Y., Lerner, S. P., and Slawin, K. M. (2001). Preoperative plasma levels of transforming growth factor beta(1) strongly predict clinical outcome in patients with bladder carcinoma. *Cancer* **92**(12), 2985–2992.

Shariat, S. F., Shalev, M., Menesses-Diaz, A., Kim, I. Y., Kattan, M. W., Wheeler, T. M., and Slawin, K. M. (2001). Preoperative plasma levels of transforming growth factor beta(1) (TGF-beta(1)) strongly predict progression in patients undergoing radical prostatectomy. *J. Clin. Oncol.* **19**(11), 2856–2864.

Shevach, E. M. (2004). Regulatory/suppressor T cells in health and disease. *Arthritis Rheum.* **50**(9), 2721–2724.

Shin, T., Kennedy, G., Gorski, K., Tsuchiya, H., Koseki, H., Azuma, M., Yagita, H., Chen, L., Powell, J., Pardoll, D., and Housseau, F. (2003). Cooperative B7-1/2 (CD80/CD86) and B7-DC costimulation of CD4+ T cells independent of the PD-1 receptor. *J. Exp. Med.* **198**(1), 31–38.

Staveley-O'Carroll, K., Sotomayor, E., Montgomery, J., Borrello, I., Hwang, L., Fein, S., Pardoll, D., and Levitsky, H. (1998). Induction of antigen-specific T cell anergy: An early event in the course of tumor progression. *Proc. Natl. Acad. Sci. USA* **95**(3), 1178–1183.

Steinman, R. M., Hawiger, D., and Nussenzweig, M. C. (2003). Tolerogenic dendritic cells. *Annu. Rev. Immunol.* **21**, 685–711.

Sumimoto, H., Hirata, K., Yamagata, S., Miyoshi, M., Miyagishi, M., Taira, K., and Kawakami, Y. (2006). Effective inhibition of cell growth and invasion of melanoma by combined suppression of BRAF (V599E) and Skp2 with lentiviral RNAi. *Int. J. Cancer* **118**, 472–476.

Surh, C. D., and Sprent, J. (1994). T-cell apoptosis detected *in situ* during positive and negative selection in the thymus. *Nature* **372**(6501), 100–103.

Terabe, M., and Berzofsky, J. A. (2004). Immunoregulatory T cells in tumor immunity. *Curr. Opin. Immunol.* **16**(2), 157–162.

Thompson, R. H., Gillett, M. D., Cheville, J. C., Lohse, C. M., Dong, H., Webster, W. S., Krejci, K. G., Lobo, J. R., Sengupta, S., Chen, L., Zincke, H., Blute, M. L., *et al.* (2004). Costimulatory B7-H1 in renal cell carcinoma patients: Indicator of tumor aggressiveness and potential therapeutic target. *Proc. Natl. Acad. Sci. USA* **101**(49), 17174–17179.

Tseng, S. Y., Otsuji, M., Gorski, K., Huang, X., Slansky, J. E., Pai, S. I., Shalabi, A., Shin, T., Pardoll, D. M., and Tsuchiya, H. (2001). B7-DC, a new dendritic cell molecule with potent costimulatory properties for T cells. *J. Exp. Med.* **193**(7), 839–846.

Turkson, J., Bowman, T., Garcia, R., Caldenhoven, E., De Groot, R. P., and Jove, R. (1998). Stat3 activation by Src induces specific gene regulation and is required for cell transformation. *Mol. Cell. Biol.* **18**(5), 2545–2552.

Turkson, J., Zhang, S., Mora, L. B., Burns, A., Sebti, S., and Jove, R. (2005). A novel platinum compound inhibits constitutive Stat3 signaling and induces cell cycle arrest and apoptosis of malignant cells. *J. Biol. Chem.* **280**(38), 32979–32988.

Urban, J. L., Burton, R. C., Holland, J. M., Kripke, M. L., and Schreiber, H. (1982). Mechanisms of syngeneic tumor rejection. Susceptibility of host-selected progressor variants to various immunological effector cells. *J. Exp. Med.* **155**(2), 557–573.

Urban, J. L., Kripke, M. L., and Schreiber, H. (1986). Stepwise immunologic selection of antigenic variants during tumor growth. *J. Immunol.* **137**(9), 3036–3041.

Uyttenhove, C., Maryanski, J., and Boon, T. (1983). Escape of mouse mastocytoma P815 after nearly complete rejection is due to antigen-loss variants rather than immunosuppression. *J. Exp. Med.* **157**(3), 1040–1052.

van den Ingh, H. F., Ruiter, D. J., Griffioen, G., van Muijen, G. N., and Ferrone, S. (1987). HLA antigens in colorectal tumours–low expression of HLA class I antigens in mucinous colorectal carcinomas. *Br. J. Cancer* **55**(2), 125–130.

van Driel, W. J., Tjiong, M. Y., Hilders, C. G., Trimbos, B. J., and Fleuren, G. J. (1996). Association of allele-specific HLA expression and histopathologic progression of cervical carcinoma. *Gynecol. Oncol.* **62**(1), 33–41.

Vicari, A. P., Caux, C., and Trinchieri, G. (2002). Tumour escape from immune surveillance through dendritic cell inactivation. *Semin. Cancer Biol.* **12**(1), 33–42.

von Boehmer, H. (2005). Mechanisms of suppression by suppressor T cells. *Nat. Immunol.* **6**(4), 338–344.

Wallich, R., Bulbuc, N., Hammerling, G. J., Katzav, S., Segal, S., and Feldman, M. (1985). Abrogation of metastatic properties of tumour cells by de novo expression of H-2K antigens following H-2 gene transfection. *Nature* **315**(6017), 301–305.

Wang, T., Niu, G., Kortylewski, M., Burdelya, L., Shain, K., Zhang, S., Bhattacharya, R., Gabrilovich, D., Heller, R., Coppola, D., Dalton, W., Jove, R., *et al.* (2004). Regulation of the innate and adaptive immune responses by Stat-3 signaling in tumor cells. *Nat. Med.* **10**(1), 48–54.

Wang, Z., Cao, Y., Albino, A. P., Zeff, R. A., Houghton, A., and Ferrone, S. (1993). Lack of HLA class I antigen expression by melanoma cells SK-MEL-33 caused by a reading frameshift in beta 2-microglobulin messenger RNA. *J. Clin. Invest.* **91**(2), 684–692.

Ward, P. L., Koeppen, H., Hurteau, T., and Schreiber, H. (1989). Tumor antigens defined by cloned immunological probes are highly polymorphic and are not detected on autologous normal cells. *J. Exp. Med.* **170**(1), 217–232.

Watanabe, N., Gavrieli, M., Sedy, J. R., Yang, J., Fallarino, F., Loftin, S. K., Hurchla, M. A., Zimmerman, N., Sim, J., Zang, X., Murphy, T. L., Russell, J. H., *et al.* (2003). BTLA is a lymphocyte inhibitory receptor with similarities to CTLA-4 and PD-1. *Nat. Immunol.* **4**(7), 670–679.

Waterhouse, P., Penninger, J. M., Timms, E., Wakeham, A., Shahinian, A., Lee, K. P., Thompson, C. B., Griesser, H., and Mak, T. W. (1995). Lymphoproliferative disorders with early lethality in mice deficient in Ctla-4. *Science* **270**(5238), 985–988.

Whitwell, H. L., Hughes, H. P., Moore, M., and Ahmed, A. (1984). Expression of major histocompatibility antigens and leucocyte infiltration in benign and malignant human breast disease. *Br. J. Cancer* **49**(2), 161–172.

Wortzel, R. D., Philipps, C., and Schreiber, H. (1983). Multiple tumour-specific antigens expressed on a single tumour cell. *Nature* **304**(5922), 165–167.

Yee, C., Thompson, J. A., Byrd, D., Riddell, S. R., Roche, P., Celis, E., and Greenberg, P. D. (2002). Adoptive T cell therapy using antigen-specific CD8+ T cell clones for the treatment of patients with metastatic melanoma: In vivo persistence, migration, and antitumor effect of transferred T cells. *Proc. Natl. Acad. Sci. USA* **99**(25), 16168–16173.

Young, M. R., Petruzzelli, G. J., Kolesiak, K., Achille, N., Lathers, D. M., and Gabrilovich, D. I. (2001). Human squamous cell carcinomas of the head and neck chemoattract immune suppressive CD34(+) progenitor cells. *Hum. Immunol.* **62**(4), 332–341.

Zajac, A. J., Blattman, J. N., Murali-Krishna, K., Sourdive, D. J., Suresh, M., Altman, J. D., and Ahmed, R. (1998). Viral immune evasion due to persistence of activated T cells without effector function. *J. Exp. Med.* **188**(12), 2205–2213.

Zea, A. H., Rodriguez, P. C., Atkins, M. B., Hernandez, C., Signoretti, S., Zabaleta, J., McDermott, D., Quiceno, D., Youmans, A., O'Neill, A., Mier, J., and Ochoa, A. C. (2005). Arginase-producing myeloid suppressor cells in renal cell carcinoma patients: A mechanism of tumor evasion. *Cancer Res.* **65**(8), 3044–3048.

Zhang, Q., Yang, X., Pins, M., Javonovic, B., Kuzel, T., Kim, S. J., Parijs, L. V., Greenberg, N. M., Liu, V., Guo, Y., and Lee, C. (2005). Adoptive transfer of tumor-reactive transforming growth factor-beta-insensitive CD8+ T cells: Eradication of autologous mouse prostate cancer. *Cancer Res.* **65**(5), 1761–1769.

Zuk, J. A., and Walker, R. A. (1987). Immunohistochemical analysis of HLA antigens and mononuclear infiltrates of benign and malignant breast. *J. Pathol.* **152,** 275–275.

Development of Antibodies and Chimeric Molecules for Cancer Immunotherapy

Thomas A. Waldmann and John C. Morris

Metabolism Branch, Center for Cancer Research, National Cancer Institute NIH, Bethesda, Maryland

Abstract 83
1. Introduction 84
2. Targets of Monoclonal Antibodies in the Therapy of Cancer 85
3. Monoclonal Antibodies Targeting Host Nonneoplastic Tissues 85
4. Monoclonal Antibodies Targeting Host Immune Cells and Proteins that Act as Inhibitory Checkpoints on the Immune System 87
5. Blockade of CTLA-4 and PD1 Inhibitory Receptors 88
6. Elimination of $CD4^+$ $CD25^+$ Foxp3 Expressing T Regs (Suppressor T Cells) 89
7. Monoclonal Antibody Targeting of the Inhibitory Cytokine TGF-β 90
8. Mechanisms of Action of Monoclonal Antibodies 91
9. Engineering Antibodies for Greater Efficacy 92
10. Genetically Engineered Antibody Fragments for Cancer Immunotherapy 95
11. Unmodified Monoclonal Antibodies Approved by the FDA that Are Directed Toward Neoplastic Cells 96
12. Antibodies Armed with Cytokines, Chemotherapeutic Agents, Toxins, and Radionuclides Cytokine Armed Monoclonal Antibodies 107
13. Antibodies Armed with Chemotherapeutic Agents 107
14. Immunotoxins for the Treatment of Cancer 108
15. Systemic Radioimmunotherapy with Monoclonal Antibodies 112
16. Conclusions and Future Prospects 118
    References 121

Abstract

Monoclonal antibodies are among the most rapidly expanding class of therapeutics for cancer treatment. Monoclonal antibodies targeting non-Hodgkin's lymphoma (NHL), Her-2/neu highly expressing metastatic breast cancer, colorectal cancer, acute myelogenous leukemia, and B-cell chronic lymphocytic leukemia (CLL) have received FDA approval. Promising new targets for antibody therapy include cellular growth factor receptors, mediators of tumor-driven neo-angiogenesis, as well as host negative immunoregulatory checkpoints that impede an effective immune response to neoplasia. Antibody efficacy has been increased by genetic engineering to humanize the antibodies and to increase their effector functions including antibody dependent cellular cytotoxicity. Furthermore, antibodies have been armed with cytokines, chemotherapeutic agents, toxins, and radionuclides to augment their efficacy as tumor cytotoxic agents. As a consequence of these advances, 30 years after their first development, monoclonal antibodies have become an important standard approach for the therapy of neoplasia with 19 therapeutic monoclonal antibodies now approved by the FDA including 8 for the treatment of cancer.

1. Introduction

In 1888, Emil Rux and Alexandre Yerson isolated the toxin from the diphtheria bacteria. This provided the scientific basis for the work of Emil von Behring and Shibasaburo Kitasato (1890) who injected small doses of diphtheria toxin into animals to yield sera containing antibodies (antitoxins), which on administration to patients provided passive immunity to treat diphtheria. Hericourt and Richet (1895) administered an antiserum derived from dogs to patients with advanced cancer. Some patients improved although significant immunogenicity problems occurred and given the fact that the antisera lacked specificity and purity, the approach did not yield cures. In the same era Paul Ehrlich (see 1956 for collected papers) proposed to the Royal Society of London in his Croonian lecture "On immunity with special reference to cell life" that "immunizations such as these which are of great theoretic interest may come to be available for clinical application attacking epithelium new formations particularly carcinoma by means of specific anti-epithelial sera." However, this dream of the "magic bullet" of antibody therapy proved elusive until the development of monoclonal antibodies 30 years ago by Köhler and Milestein (1975) captured the imagination of the medical community. Despite the early enthusiasm concerning monoclonal antibodies, clinical results were discouraging and failed to fulfill the great promise for immunotherapy inherent in the specificity of monoclonal antibodies, which permits their selective binding to tumor cells.

For a long time only a single monoclonal antibody, muromonab-CD3 (Orthoclone, OKT-3™) was licensed by the FDA (Goldstein, 1986). A number of factors underlied the low-therapeutic efficacy observed. The unmodified murine monoclonal antibodies had a short *in vivo* survival in humans and induced an immune response that neutralized their therapeutic effect. Furthermore, the therapeutic responses induced by murine antibodies were limited because the agents only weakly recruited human effector elements including those that act through antibody dependent cellular toxicity (ADCC) and were relatively ineffective as cytocidal agents. Furthermore, these early antibodies were not directed against a vital cell surface target, such as a receptor for a growth factor that was required for tumor cell survival and proliferation. To circumvent these problems humanized as well as human antibodies were developed. Furthermore, the cytotoxic activity of monoclonal antibodies was augmented by arming them with cytokines, chemotherapeutic agents, toxins, or radionuclides.

2. Targets of Monoclonal Antibodies in the Therapy of Cancer

Antigenic targets especially immunoglobulin idiotypes, cytokines, growth factor, and death-signal receptors on the tumor cells or epitopes on host cells that include tumor neovasculature as well as an array of host negative immunoregulatory cells (checkpoints) provided more effective targets for monoclonal antibody action (Carter, 2001; Gura, 2002; Miller et al., 1982; Stacy, 2005; von Mehren et al., 2003; Waldmann, 1991, 2003b). Seven monoclonal antibodies directed against diverse antigenic targets on the tumor cells themselves have received FDA approval for cancer therapy (see description of individual antibodies discussed later and in Table 1). In addition, basiliximab (Simulect™) a chimeric antibody as well as the first humanized antibody, daclizumab (anti-Tac, Zenapax™) were approved by the FDA. Both of these later antibodies are directed toward the interleukin (IL)-2R alpha receptor subunit CD25 and interfere with the interaction of IL-2 with its receptor. Although daclizumab was approved by the FDA for use in organ-allograft protocols, it also provided effective therapy for select patients with CD25 (IL-2R alpha) expressing T-cell malignancies (Morris and Waldmann, 2000; Waldmann et al., 1993).

The following seven antibodies directed toward tumor antigens have been approved for cancer therapy by the FDA: rituximab (CD20), ^{131}I-tositumomab (CD20), ^{90}Y-ibritumomab tiuxetan (CD20), gemtuzumab ozogamicin (CD33), alemtuzumab (CD52), cetuximab [epidermal growth factor receptor (EGFR)], and trastuzumab (Her-2/neu).

3. Monoclonal Antibodies Targeting Host Nonneoplastic Tissues

In addition to targeting tumor cells themselves, monoclonal antibodies have been utilized in an alternate strategy to target host tissues or proteins that support tumor growth and expression. For example, a potent inhibitor of neo-vascularization bevacizumab (Avastin™), a humanized antibody directed toward vascular endothelial growth factor (VEGF) in combination with chemotherapy was approved for the therapy of patients with metastatic colon cancer (Presta et al., 1997). In addition to this monoclonal antibody, a receptor Ig fusion protein the VEGF-TRAP has been used to target VEGF in the therapy of tumor xenograft models and in patients with renal cell carcinoma (Dupont et al., 2005). The VEGF-TRAP is composed of the extracellular

Table 1 Monoclonal Antibodies Approved for Therapy of Cancer

Year approved	Brand name	Generic name	Type of mAb	Target	Indication
1997	Rituxan	Rituximab	Chimeric	CD20	NHL
1998	Herceptin	Trastuzumab	Humanized	HER2	Her-2/neu positive breast cancer
2000	Mylotarg	Gemtuzumab ozogamicin	Humanized	CD33	Acute myelogenous leukemia
2001	Campath-I	Alemtuzumab	Humanized	CD52	B-cell CLL
2002	Zevalin	Ibritumomab tiuxetan conjugated to ^{111}In or ^{90}Y	Murine	CD20	NHL
2003	Bexxar	^{131}I-tositumomab	Murine radiolabeled	CD20	NHL
2004	Avastin™	Bevacizumab	Humanized	VEGF	Colorectal cancer
2004	Erbitux	Cetuximab	Chimeric	EGFR (HER-1)	Colorectal cancer

VEGF—vascular endothelial growth factor; EGFR—epidermal growth factor receptor.

domains of the human VEGF receptors VEGFRI (FLT-I) and VEGFR2 (KDR) fused to the Fc portion of human IgG (Dupont et al., 2005).

4. Monoclonal Antibodies Targeting Host Immune Cells and Proteins that Act as Inhibitory Checkpoints on the Immune System

In a novel anticancer strategy, monoclonal antibodies are being employed that are directed toward the host immune cells or proteins that act as inhibitory checkpoints or brakes on the immune system (Table 2). Such host cells may both prevent an effective immune response by patients to their neoplasm and inhibit the actions of administered anticancer vaccines. Agents to remove inhibitory checkpoints that will be considered include antibodies to cytotoxic T-lymphocytic antigen-4 (CTLA-4) and programmed cell death-1 (PD1), proteins that mediate negative T-cell signaling pathways, as well as agents directed toward $CD4^+$ $CD25^+$ (IL-2R alpha) expressing T regs (suppressor T cells) (Hodi et al., 2003; Hurwitz et al., 2000; Kwon et al., 1999; Leach et al., 1996;

Table 2 Monoclonal Antibody Mediated Blockade of Immunoregulatory Negative Checkpoints that Impede Immunotherapy

Host negative immunoregulatory mechanism	Monoclonal antibody mediated intervention to release checkpoint on the immune response
Signals mediated by negative T cell costimulatory molecule CTLA-4 after interaction with CD80, 86 family members on APCs deliver signals that terminate T-cell activation	Antibody-mediated blockade of CTLA-4 enhances antitumor immunity
PD1 interaction with PDL1 or PDL2 inhibits TCR—mediated proliferation and activation of $CD4^+$ T cells	Anti-PDL1 antibody
$CD4^+$ $CD25^+$ negative regulatory Tregs (suppressor T cells) inhibit antitumor immune responses	IL-2 diphtheria toxin denileukin difitox (ONTAK), anti-IL-2Rα *Pseudomonas* toxin (LMB-2), or CD25-directed antibody (PC61) therapy to deplete Tregs
$CD4^+$ NKT cell generation of IL-13 that indirectly (through the action of TGFβ) inhibits $CD8^+$ cell-mediated antitumor responses. TGFβ is also synthesized directly by tumor cells or by host cells via other mechanisms	IL-13Rα2 IgFc or anti-TGFβ monoclonal antibody

APCs—antigen-presenting cells; PD1—programmed cell death-1; PDL1—PD1 Ligand 1; NKT—natural killer T cell; TGF—transforming growth factor; CTLA-4—cytotoxic T-lymphocytic antigen-4.

Phan et al., 2003; Sakaguchi, 2004; Shevach, 2000; Shimizu et al., 1999; Sutmuller et al., 2001; Thornton and Shevach, 2000). Furthermore, additional receptor IgFc fusion protein or monoclonal antibody mediated approaches are being used to target the immuno-inhibitory systems that involve, IL-13 or transforming growth factor-beta (TGF-β), cytokines that impede effective immune responses to tumors (Flavell and Gorelik 2002; Gorelik and Flavell 2001; Terabe et al., 2000).

5. Blockade of CTLA-4 and PD1 Inhibitory Receptors

A strategy for pharmacological immunomodulation using monoclonal antibodies is to remove one or more of the host negative immunoregulatory mechanisms that are normally dedicated toward preventing self-directed destructive immune responses that could lead to autoimmune diseases (Dong et al., 2002; Dranoff, 2005; Freeman et al., 2000; Hodi et al., 2003; Hurwitz et al., 2000; Iwai et al., 2002; Kwon et al., 1999; Leach et al., 1996; Phan et al., 2003). The elimination of immunological checkpoints may permit a robust immune response to a tumor, although this strategy carries with it the risk of developing autoimmunity. Such a strategy directed toward the removal of immunological checkpoints would not be effective unless there were a simultaneous immune response to the tumor. Such an antitumor immune response may be naturally occurring as is observed in some patients with malignant melanoma, renal cell tumors or B-cell malignancies. Alternatively, it may have to be induced by the administration of an antitumor vaccine in association with administration of agents directed toward eliminating the immunological checkpoints. Among the best studied of these checkpoints on the immune system is the cytotoxic T-lymphocyte antigen-4 (CTLA-4, CD152), a negative costimulatory molecule (Dranoff, 2004, 2005; Hodi et al., 2003; Hurwitz et al., 2000; Leach et al., 1996; Phan et al., 2003). The initial interaction of B7 family members with the CD28 receptor provides a pivotal positive costimulatory signal that is required to initiate an effective T-cell immune response, in addition to signaling that occurs through the T-cell receptor (TCR) for antigen. However, the subsequent expression of CTLA-4, a second receptor that has a much higher affinity for B7 than does CD28, is induced after T-cell activation. This receptor ligand interaction inhibits T-cell activation and IL-2 production. Phan et al. (2003) demonstrated that blockade of the B7-CTLA-4 interaction enhanced the antitumor immunity provided by a granulocyte-macrophage colony stimulating factor (GM-CSF) transduced vaccine. This coordinate strategy led to the regression of established syngeneic mouse tumors. Translation of this approach to the clinic in patients with malignant melanoma was associated with clinical remissions in some cases. Dranoff (2004, 2005) observed efficacy with MDX-CTLA-4 when used in patients who had previously been vaccinated with GM-CSF secreting tumor cells. Schwartzentruber et al. (2003) administered a human monoclonal antibody against CTLA-4 (MDX-010) together with melanoma antigen derived peptide vaccines to 14 patients with metastatic melanoma (Schwartzentruber et al., 2003). Three patients developed tumor responses (two complete and one partial). However, six patients also developed serious autoimmune disorders including enterocolitis, hypophysitis, and hepatitis (Schwartzentruber et al., 2003).

Another checkpoint system being targeted for immunomodulation cancer therapy involves the membrane molecule PD-1 (Dong et al., 2002; Freeman et al., 2000; Iwai et al., 2002). Like CTLA-4, PD-1 is an immunoinhibitory molecule that is expressed after T-cell activation. As with CTLA-4 knockout mice, mice deficient in PD-1 manifest autoimmune diseases. Programmed cell death-1 is a receptor for two additional B7 homologs B7-H1/PD1-Ligand-1 (PDL-1) and B7/DC/PDL-2 (Dong et al., 2002; Freeman et al., 2000; Iwai et al., 2002). The interaction of PD-1 with PDL-1 or PDL-2 inhibited TCR mediated proliferation and cytokine secretion by $CD4^+$ T cells. Transgenic expression of PDL-1 in ph-15 tumor cells rendered them less susceptible to specific T-cell antigen receptor mediated lysis by cytotoxic T cells *in vitro*, and enhanced their tumogenesis and invasiveness in *vivo* in syngeneic hosts compared with the parental tumor cells. These effects could be reversed by the administration of an anti-PDL-1 antibody. The growth of melanoma cells expressing PDL-1 in normal syngeneic mice was inhibited significantly, albeit transiently, by the administration of anti-PDL-1 antibodies *in vivo*. Furthermore, tumor growth was absent in syngeneic PDL-1 deficient mice. These results suggest that the expression of the PDL molecules on tumor cells can serve as a mechanism for an otherwise immunogenic tumor to escape from host immune responses. Thus, targeting of the interaction of PD-1 with its PDL ligands using monoclonal antibodies may represent a promising strategy to remove this immunological checkpoint and thereby augment specific tumor immunity.

6. Elimination of $CD4^+$ $CD25^+$ Foxp3 Expressing T Regs (Suppressor T Cells)

Another major immunological checkpoint that can compromise effective immune responses to tumor antigens is mediated by $CD4^+$ $CD25^+$ Foxp3 expressing T-regulatory cells (suppressor T cells) (Sakaguchi, 2004; Shevach, 2000; Shimizu et al., 1999; Sutmuller et al., 2001). As is true of the other checkpoints, $CD4^+CD25^+$ T regs are engaged in the control of self-reactive T cells and thereby contribute to the maintenance of immunological self-tolerance. The marked depletion of these cells leads to the development of autoimmune disease in animals. $CD4^+$ $CD25^+$ expression does not uniquely characterize T regs since activated effector-T cells also manifest this phenotype. Other markers associated with T regs include CTLA-4 and the glucocorticoid-induced TNF related receptor gene (*GITR*). The most specific marker of T regs is Scurfin, the transcription factor Foxp3. The administration to mice of a CD25 (IL-2R alpha) specific monoclonal antibody PC61 led to the depletion of T regs that in turn was associated with an augmented immune response to certain syngeneic tumors. In particular, the administration of PC61 was associated with the induction of CTL and natural killer (NK) cell mediated cytotoxicity that was associated with tumor rejection. CD25 is expressed not only by T regs but also by activated effector-T cells. Therefore, CD25 directed therapy to remove T regs must be performed before but not after the administration of an antitumor vaccine that would induce CD25 expressing effector-T cells. Depletion of $CD4^+CD25^+$ T regs mediated by the administration of the PC61 antibody was synergistic with anti-CTLA-4 therapy in a murine B16 melanoma model. Therefore, simultaneous intervention that is directed toward the elimination of both negative regulatory mechanisms was a useful immunomodulation strategy for the induction of therapeutic antitumor immunity. In humans, the monoclonal antibody daclizumab that blocks the interaction of IL-2 with IL-2R alpha (CD25) was not depletive and was not effective in the removal of T regs. However, T regs could be reduced transiently prior to vaccine administration by the administration of a fusion protein IL-2 diphtheria toxin (denileukin diftitox, Ontak™) (Olsen *et al.*, 2001).

7. Monoclonal Antibody Targeting of the Inhibitory Cytokine TGF-β

A number of biologically active agents either synthesized directly by tumor cells or secreted by host cells in association with tumor growth exert suppressive effects on the immune system. For example, inhibition of cancer immune surveillance is mediated by the $CD4^+$ NKT-cell production of IL-13, which in turn induces the expression of TGF-β, a cytokine that inhibits the antitumor cytotoxicity mediated by $CD8^+$ CTLs (Terabe *et al.*, 2000). Blockade of this negative immune regulatory pathway, by inhibiting IL-13 action using an IL-13 receptor immunoglobulin fusion protein augmented antitumor responses and potentiated the efficacy of vaccines.

One of the most prominent inhibitory cytokines, TGF-β, is not only produced in association with the CD1 NKT-cell IL-13 system but also in association with the action of T regs, natural killer cells, macrophages, epithelial cells, stromal cells, and a wide array of tumor cells (Flavell and Gorelik, 2002; Gorelik and Flavell, 2001). TGF-β is a pleiotropic cytokine that inhibits T-cell proliferation and T-cell differentiation into cytotoxic and helper T cells. Therefore, TGF-β production can have an important role in the suppression of effective antitumor immune responses. Gorelik and Flavell (2001) utilized CD8 T cells genetically altered so that they could not respond to TGF-β to demonstrate that preventing TGF-β signaling in T cells facilitates the generation of tumor-specific T-cell responses that are able to eradicate tumors in mice with thymoma or melanoma tumors. In the future the use of monoclonal antibodies or TGF-βR2 receptor mediated blockade of TGF-β suppression of T-cell signaling could be translated clinically to improve T-cell mediated antitumor immunity.

8. Mechanisms of Action of Monoclonal Antibodies

The mechanisms of action of monoclonal antibodies directed toward the tumor cells themselves include activation of death pathways in the tumor cells, blockade of necessary growth factors/growth factor receptor interaction, induction of ADCC complement dependent cytotoxicity, as well as antibody mediated delivery of cytotoxic agents to the tumor cells. In terms of a direct cytotoxic action on the tumor cells mediated by the monoclonal antibody, Mir *et al.* (2000) proposed that anti-CD30 monoclonal antibodies favored the constitutive tumor necrosis factor 2 (TNF2) mediated death signaling pathways in the tumor rather than the alternative cell proliferation pathway thereby leading to the death of CD30 expressing anaplastic large cell lymphoma cells.

A second mechanism of monoclonal antibody action is mediated by ADCC—a process that involves the redirection of host cytotoxic cells to the tumor. Clynes *et al.* (2000) and Ravetch and Lanier (2000) demonstrated that a mechanism involved in the tumor-cell effector function of monoclonal antibodies in murine xenogenic models of human malignancy involves the engagement by the antibodies of receptors FcRI, III, and IV that utilize the FcRγ subunit (Nimmerjahn *et al.*, 2005). Using FcRγ$^{-/-}$ deficient mice that did not express FcγRIII, the stimulatory Fc receptor, they demonstrated greatly diminished efficacy of antibodies directed toward malignant melanoma cells. Similarly, the effector action mediated by trastuzumab, rituximab, and daclizumab in mouse xenograft models was facilitated by the engagement of the antibody with the FcγRIII receptor (Clynes *et al.*, 2000). In contrast, the HeFi-1 monoclonal antibody directed to CD30 that led to direct tumor cell cytotoxicity in a murine model was equally effective in wild-type and FcRγ$^{-/-}$ deficient mice indicating that a non-ADCC mechanism was involved (Zhang *et al.*, 2004). In contrast to the situation with FcγRIII deficient mice, disruption of the gene that encodes the inhibitory FcγRII B receptor substantially enhanced antitumor activity of the monoclonal antibodies studied.

Clinical trials correlating the rituximab responses in patients with non-Hodgkin's lymphoma (NHL), with polymorphisms in Fc receptors FcγRIIIa or FcγRIIa on immune effector cells support a role for Fc receptor binding and ADCC in the efficacy of monoclonal antibody antitumor action (Cartron et al., 2002; Weng and Levy, 2003). Mutations in the FcγIII give rise to FcγRIII receptor forms with either Valine (V) or phenylalanine (F) at position 158. Cells homozygous for the Valine 158 form (FcγRIII-158VV) have higher affinity for the IgG-1 Fc region than do similar cells homozygous for the phenylalanine form FcγRIII-158FF. The FcγRIII 155VV homozygous patients who had follicular NHL had rituximab response rates that were higher than those expressing the 158VF or 158FF genotypes. A second polymorphism involving the histidine/histidine homozygous genotype in FcγRII at amino acid 131was independently associated with a higher response rate and freedom from progression. These studies provide the scientific basis for the genetic engineering of monoclonal antibodies to augment their binding to the FcγRIII stimulatory receptor while reducing binding to the FcγRII inhibitory Fc receptor.

Complement-dependent cytotoxicity is an additional cytolytic mechanism of monoclonal antibody action. Rituximab was effective in eliminating EL-4 cells that had been stably transduced to express human CD20. However, the protective activity of rituximab was completely abolished in syngeneic knock-out animals lacking C1q the first component of the classical pathway of complement (C1qa$^{-/-}$) (Di Gaetano et al., 2003).

9. Engineering Antibodies for Greater Efficacy

The initial monoclonal antibodies used in clinical therapeutic efforts were murine antibodies. They had advantages over previous efforts with polyclonal antisera in that they were homogeneous agents that could manifest great specificity, distinguishing tumor cell targets from normal cells (Carter, 2001; Carter and McDonagh, 2005; Chester et al., 2004; Hudson and Souriau, 2003) (Fig. 1). They were bivalent and thus could have a high affinity for their target cells. Nevertheless, there were major limitations in the use of murine antibodies. Only one unmodified mouse antibody muromonab-CD3 (Orthoclone OKT-3) used to prevent transplanted organ rejection was approved by the FDA (Goldstein, 1986). The limitations of murine antibodies include the fact that they are foreign proteins and are immunogenic in humans precluding their chronic use. Furthermore, they have a short *in vivo* survival that prevents their use when long-term saturation of a receptor is required for therapeutic efficacy. In addition, they are often ineffective as cytocidal agents in that they

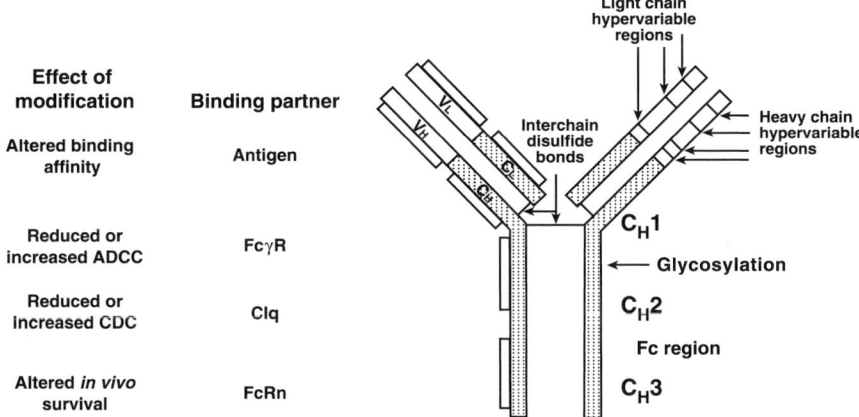

Figure 1 Genetic engineering has been employed to increase the efficacy of monoclonal antibodies. Complementary determining region amino acid sequences have been altered to increase the affinity of the antibody for its target. The Fc element of the monoclonal antibody can be altered to augment binding to FcγRIII agonist receptors and to reduce binding to the FcRγII inhibitory Fc receptor to augment antibody dependent cellular cytotoxic killing of tumor cells. Antibody dependent cellular toxicity has also been enhanced by altering Fc gycosylation with the reduction of fucose. Additional approaches are directed toward reducing or enhancing CDC by modifying the Fc element of the IgG structure. The Fc region of the monoclonal antibody has also been modified to alter its binding to the FcRn receptor thereby altering the pharmacokinetics of the antibody.

often do not fix human complement or function in ADCC with human mononuclear cells. In an effort to reduce immunogenicity, improve pharmacokinetics, and increase effector action, progressive efforts have been taken to make antibodies more human (Hudson and Souriau, 2003; Riechmann et al., 1988; Winter and Milstein, 1991). Initially scientists fused the mouse variable regions (Vh and Vl) to human immunoglobulin constant domains (Fig. 1). These molecules were approximately two-thirds human and one-third murine. Such antibodies termed chimeric antibodies reduced human-anti-mouse antibody (HAMA) responses. Chimeric antibodies include abciximab (Reopro™) directed toward the glycoprotein IIb/IIIa rituximab (anti-CD20 Rituxan™) and infliximab (anti-TNFα, Remicade™), basiliximab (anti-CD25) and cetuximab (anti-EGFR). These chimeric antibodies substantially reduced the HAMA responses, but there were associated serious allergic reactions in some cases. The field was dramatically advanced by the work from Greg Winter's laboratory that produced humanized antibodies that retained from the mouse only the complementarity determining hypervariable regions on the three antibody loops that were involved in antigen binding with the remainder of the molecule being that of a human IgG (Winter and Milstein, 1991). This technique was refined following the recognition that a small number of amino acids not directly involved in the complementarity determining regions from the mouse were still required to maintain the structure of the antigen-binding site and high-affinity binding to targets (Queen et al., 1989). The first approved humanized monoclonal antibody daclizumab (Zenapax^{TM}) directed toward IL-2R alpha blocks the interaction of IL-2 with its receptor (Queen et al., 1989). Daclizumab was approved by the FDA for use in organ-allograft protocols (Vincenti et al., 1998). It also provided effective therapy for patients with CD25 (IL-2Rα) expressing T-cell malignancies and patients with T-cell mediated uveitis and multiple sclerosis (Bielekova et al., 2004; Morris and Waldmann, 2000; Nussenblatt et al., 1999). The majority of the antibodies subsequently receiving FDA approval have been comparable humanized antibodies.

In a further effort to evade the human immune response to the infused monoclonal antibodies, alternative approaches have been utilized to generate fully human antibodies. In one approach the native antibody genes of the mouse have been replaced with their human counterparts MDX-0I0, an anti-CTLA-4 monoclonal antibody is produced with such humanized mouse technology. An alternative approach to produce a human monoclonal antibody employs phage display. Adalimumab (Humira^{TM}), the first fully human monoclonal antibody approved by the FDA targets TNFα and is approved for treatment of rheumatoid arthritis (Weinblatt et al., 2003).

In addition to its use in humanization, genetic engineering has been employed to increase the efficacy of monoclonal antibodies (Fig. 1). Focusing on the complementarity-determining region, amino acid sequences can be altered to increase the affinity of the antibody for its target. In other efforts, the Fc element of the monoclonal antibody can be altered to augment binding to the FcγRIII agonist receptor while reducing binding to the FcRγII inhibitory Fc receptor to augment antibody dependent cellular cytotoxic killing of tumor cells (Shields et al., 2001). Other strategies to enhance ADCC include alteration of Fc gycosylation with reduction of fucose. Lack of fucose on human IgG N-linked oligosaccharides was reported to improve binding to human FcγRIII and ADCC (Shinkawa et al., 2003). Additional approaches are directed toward augmenting antibody dependent phagocytosis. The Fc element of the IgG structure has also been modified to reduce or enhance complement dependent cytolysis (CDC) (Carter and McDonagh, 2005).

An additional focus is on altering the Fc region of the monoclonal antibody to alter binding to the FcRn receptor and thereby alter the pharmacokinetics of the antibody (Junghans and Anderson, 1996). The neonatal Fc receptor (FcRn) is a heterodynamic FcRnα, -β2 microglobulin major histocompatibility (MHC) Class 1 related heterodimeric receptor (Hinton et al., 2004). It interacts with the IgG Fc in a saturable, highly pH dependent manner. The receptor is expressed in microvessel endothelial cells, dendritic cells, monocytes, and neonatal intestinal cells of the rat and mouse, as well as the human placenta. It is involved in the transfer of maternal IgG to the fetus in humans and the neonate in mice and rats. Its receptor is involved in the concentration-catabolism effect that regulates IgG survival (Waldmann and Strober, 1969). IgG on binding in a saturable fashion to the receptor enters endothelial vesicles and remains bound to the receptor and then is recycled back to the vascular lumen. At low concentrations high proportions of this IgG molecule are protected from catabolism and continue to survive in the circulation. At low concentrations of IgG in the serum, as seen in patients with hypogammaglobulinemia, IgG survival is prolonged with a terminal T½ in the serum of up to 40 days as compared to the normal 24 days observed in humans and prolonged to 8–10 days in hypogammaglobulinemic mice as compared to a 3–4 day T½ for normal animals. As the IgG concentration rises by IgG infusion or by endogenous synthesis as in IgG multiple myeloma the proportion of the IgG entering vesicles that is protected reduces and the terminal serum survival T½ is reduced to an asymptotic level of approximately 10 days in humans and 1.5 days in mice.

Several IgG mutants at Fc positions 250 and 428 with increased binding affinity to human FcRn at pH 6.0 were identified. These mutants do not bind to human FcRn at pH 7.5. A pharmacokinetic study of two of these mutant IgG antibodies with increased FcRn binding affinity demonstrated that they had serum half-lives in rhesus monkeys that were approximately twofold longer than wild-type antibody (Hinton et al., 2004). These studies demonstrate the feasibility of Fc engineering to extend the serum survival of antibody therapeutics that might lead to less frequent administration and reduced treatment costs.

10. Genetically Engineered Antibody Fragments for Cancer Immunotherapy

The majority of monoclonal antibodies used clinically are intact bivalent molecules. However, such molecules are quite large and have the limitation that they penetrate tissues, especially solid tumors, very poorly (Jain, 2001). This represents a major limitation when the antibody is used to transport a short-lived cytotoxic agent such as an α-emitting radionuclide to the tumor cell. Furthermore, the long survival of a radiolabeled intact monoclonal antibody in the circulation exposes radiosensitive tissues such as the bone marrow to prolonged irradiation. A series of alternative antibody fragments have been generated with the genetically engineered single chain Fv (scFv) that is one of the most favored (Adams and Weiner, 2005; Adams et al., 1998; Hudson and Souriau, 2003; Olafsen et al., 2004). Such small antibody fragments manifest better pharmacokinetics for tissue penetration but are monovalent and often exhibit fast off rates and poor retention time on the target. Therefore, dimeric, trimetric, or tetrameric conjugates have been engineered to increase their affinity.

Another engineering strategy is used to generate bispecific antibodies that contain two different binding specificities fused together. Antibodies with two distinct binding activities have been generated to deliver radionuclides, toxins, cytotoxic drugs, or host-cytotoxic cells to tumor cell targets (Carter, 2001; Segal et al., 2001; Staerz et al., 1985; Waldmann, 1991). Bispecific antibodies have been prepared by chemical-cross linking, disulfide exchange, or by the production of hybrid-hydridomas (quadromas). Bispecific antibodies have been utilized to retarget cytotoxic cells to tumor cells. To be effective the bispecific antibody must retarget the cytotoxic cells from their natural ligands to the tumor target identified by the monoclonal antibody. Furthermore, the antibody must activate the cytotoxic cells into functional effectors. The most efficient bispecific monoclonal antibodies have targeted the CD3 antigen on cytotoxic T cells or the CD16 (FcγRIII) receptor on natural killer cells as their nonantigen specificity (Waldmann, 1991). Problems that need to be resolved include the immunogenicity of bispecific antibodies and those associated with their manufacture. Additional strategies that are discussed later include genetic engineering to link cytokines and cytocidal agents including toxins to monoclonal antibodies to increase effector action.

11. Unmodified Monoclonal Antibodies Approved by the FDA that Are Directed Toward Neoplastic Cells

11.1. Rituximab (Rituxan™, MabThera™)

Rituximab is a human–mouse chimeric monoclonal antibody that targets the CD20 antigen expressed on the surface of B cells. In 1997, rituximab became the first monoclonal antibody licensed for the treatment of cancer. Its development has revolutionized the treatment of B-cell malignancies. It is approved for the treatment of low-grade or follicular lymphoma, relapsed or refractory, CD20-positive NHL as a single agent. Rituximab (C2B8) was generated from the murine anti-CD20 monoclonal antibody 2B8 by cloning the light and heavy-chain complementary-determining regions (CDR) on to a human IgG1 heavy and kappa light-chain constant region (Reff et al., 1994). The resulting chimeric antibody exhibits powerful B-cell depleting properties.

A pan-B cell marker, CD20, is a 31–37 kDa nonglycosylated cell surface phosphoprotein that is highly expressed on almost all normal B cells and B-cell malignancies (Stashenko et al., 1981). CD20 is nonmodulating and is not shed from the surface of cells making it an ideal target. The mechanism of rituximab action is complex and includes the induction of apoptosis, inhibition of cell growth, complement-mediated cell lysis, sensitization of cells to chemotherapy and radiation, and induction of ADCC (Smith, 2003). Rituximab enhances sensitivity to chemotherapy by downregulating expression of the prosurvival protein BCL-2. Mechanisms of resistance to rituximab are unclear, but may involve alterations in CD20 expression, decreased penetration of tumor masses by the antibody, increased expression of cellular complement inhibitors, enhanced prosurvival pathways, and inhibition of ADCC effector activity. Clynes et al. (2000) demonstrated that full cytotoxic activity could only be achieved in mice expressing the stimulatory γ-chain of the FcγRIII receptor suggesting that this was an important mechanism. A genetic dimorphism in the gene that encodes the human FcγRIIIa has been found to correlate with response to rituximab in patients with follicular NHL (Cartron et al., 2002). The homozygous valine FcγRIIIa-158V polymorphism exhibits a higher affinity for human IgG1 binding and demonstrated enhanced NK cell ADCC in vitro relative to cells from patients expressing the homozygous phenylalanine FcγRIIIa-158F polymorphism or heterozygotes (Cartron et al., 2002; Koene et al., 1997).

Phase I trials identified no maximum tolerated dose of rituximab and established rituximab 375 mg/m^2 intravenously weekly for 4 weeks as the standard treatment (Maloney et al., 1994, 1997) Pharmacokinetic studies showed that rituximab has a plasma half-life of 76.3 h with the first infusion that increases to 205.8 h after the fourth infusion, and it can be detected in the blood for 6 months after completion of therapy (Berinstein et al., 1998). Extending treatment to 8 weekly doses increased the overall response rate, complete response rate, and disease-free survival (Piro et al., 1999). The 8-week course has been subsequently approved for the treatment of bulky (>10 cm) or refractory disease, or patients undergoing re-treatment with rituximab. The efficacy of rituximab was established in a pivotal phase II trial that accrued 166 patients with relapsed NHL (Working Formulation grades A–C) in which a response rate of 48% with 6% complete responses (CR) and a median response duration of 13 months was observed (McLaughlin et al., 1998). Forty-five patients in this group were classified as resistant to their most recent prior chemotherapy treatment. Seventy-six percent experienced at least a 20% reduction in tumor mass.

A peculiar observation has been made concerning the high response rate seen in patients undergoing re-treatment with rituximab after relapse, after prior rituximab treatment. Davis et al. (2000) reported second responses in 38% of patients, including 10 CR. The median duration of response on re-treatment improved from 9.8 months to >15 months. This observation has been confirmed in other studies and may be the result of lower tumor burden present in patients at the time of relapse after initial treatment. Due to its nonoverlapping toxicity with chemotherapy, rituximab in combination with cyclophosphamide, doxorubicin, vincristine and prednisone (CHOP) chemotherapy was compared to CHOP alone for the treatment of high-grade diffuse large B-cell lymphoma in previously untreated patients over the age of 60 (Coiffier et al., 2002). The combination of rituximab with CHOP was found to significantly improve overall response and survival compared to CHOP chemotherapy alone. It is now common to use rituximab in combination with chemotherapy for the treatment of many types of B-cell NHL.

The most common toxicities seen with rituximab include acute infusional reactions including fever, chills, nausea, vomiting, bronchospasm, and hypotension occurring most often with the initial infusion. Other serious adverse events include the "cytokine release syndrome," which is associated with acute increases in the serum levels of IL-6 and TNFα. This is seen most often in patients with high circulating B-cell counts. A "rapid tumor clearance syndrome" associated with fever, chills, hypoxia, hypotension, acute lymphopenia, thrombocytopenia, elevated coagulation parameters, rising serum LDH, and uric acid levels, as well as classical acute tumor lysis syndrome may also be seen. B cell numbers nadir 24–72 h after rituximab infusion and begin to return to normal values at an average of 9 months after therapy. Little change in serum immunoglobulin levels can be documented in patients receiving rituximab and the risk of serious infection is only marginally increased in the months following rituximab treatment.

11.2. Trastuzumab (Herceptin™)

Trastuzumab is a recombinant humanized IgG1 monoclonal antibody directed against the extracellular domain of the human Her-2/*neu* (Her2) protein. Trastuzumab was FDA approved in 1998 as single-agent therapy for patients with metastatic breast cancer whose tumors overexpress the Her2 protein and who have received one or more chemotherapy regimens for metastatic disease. It is also approved for use in combination with paclitaxel for treatment of patients with metastatic breast cancer whose tumors overexpress the Her2 protein and who have not received chemotherapy for their metastatic disease. The *Her2* (*Erb B2*) oncogene is a member of the human epidermal growth factor tyrosine kinase receptor family. *Her2* encodes a 185 kDa transmembrane glycoprotein receptor molecule. Overexpression in human tumors is usually due to gene amplification and is found in 20–30% of human breast cancers (Slamon et al., 1987). Her2 overexpression is associated with aggressive behavior and a poorer prognosis in all stages of breast cancer.

Historically, a number of murine antibodies that bind to Her2 were shown to suppress the growth of Her2-positive cell lines *in vitro* and *in vivo* (Lewis *et al.*, 1993). However, the chronic administration of murine antibodies in man is limited by the development of neutralizing antibodies to the murine immunoglobulin. To overcome this problem the most active of the antibodies, 4D5 was selected for recombinant humanization. Trastuzumab contains 97% human sequences (Carter *et al.*, 1992). It has a binding affinity for Her-2 that is threefold greater than the parent murine antibody ($K_d = 0.1$ nM). The mechanism of trastuzumab action is incompletely defined; however, a number of activities have been observed *in vitro*. Binding of trastuzumab has been shown to result in receptor internalization and enhanced endocytic cleavage (De Santes *et al.*, 1992). This downmodulation disrupts receptor dimerization and signaling. Trastuzumab inhibits the growth of the Her-2 overexpressing breast cancer cell lines, BT-474, and SKBR3 in a dose dependent manner but has little effect on Her-2-negative cell lines. Treatment with trastuzumab results in G1 phase arrest, increased expression of $p27^{kip1}$, increased formation of $p27^{kip1}$-cdk2 complexes, and decreased cell proliferation (reviewed in Sliwkowski *et al.*, 1999). Trastuzumab has also been shown to induce antiangiogenic factors, suppress proangiogenic factors, such as VEGF, and it facilitates ADCC (Clynes *et al.*, 2000; Izumi *et al.*, 2002). *In vitro*, trastuzumab exhibits synergy with a variety of different chemotherapy agents (Pegram *et al.*, 1999).

An early phase I trial studied a weekly schedule of either single-agent trastuzumab or trastuzumab in combination with cisplatin at dose of 10–500 mgs and observed no dose-limiting toxicity due to the antibody. Recommended dosing of trastuzumab is an initial intravenous 4 mg/kg loading dose administered over 90-min followed by weekly maintenance doses of 2 mg/kg as 30-min infusions. At these doses phramacokinetic studies showed a plasma half-life of 5.8 days (range, 1–32 days) indicating that a weekly schedule is appropriate (Baselga *et al.*, 1996). Steady state kinetics is reached between 16 and 32 weeks.

The pivotal phase II trial of single agent trastuzumab enrolled 222 heavily pretreated women with metastatic breast cancer (Cobleigh *et al.*, 1999). All of the patients' tumors overexpressed Her2 by immunohistochemical (IHC) staining (scored as 2+ or 3+). The patients received a loading dose of 4 mg/kg, followed by weekly maintenance doses of 2 mg/kg until progression. The overall response rate was reported as 15% with a median response duration of 9.1 months. A subsequent phase III multiinstitutional trial designed to compare first-line treatment of metastatic breast cancer with chemotherapy or with chemotherapy and trastuzumab entered 469 patients with Her2 overexpressing (2+ or 3+) tumors. Patients were randomized to receive chemotherapy that consisted of an anthracycline and cyclophosphamide, or paclitaxel for those patients that previously received adjuvant therapy with an anthracycline. These treatment arms were compared to either of these chemotherapy regimens and trastuzumab. The results showed a statistically significant improvement in the time to progression for patients receiving the combination of trastuzumab and chemotherapy compared to chemotherapy alone (7.4 versus 4.6 months; $p < 0.001$). The addition of trastuzumab to paclitaxel increased the response rate to 41% compared to 17% for paclitaxel alone ($p < 0.001$), and the addition of trastuzumab to the anthracycline-containing chemotherapy improved the response rate from 42% to 56% for the combination of chemotherapy and trastuzumab ($p = 0.02$). The overall response rate for the combination of trastuzumab and any chemotherapy regimen was 50% versus 32% for any chemotherapy regimen alone ($p < 0.001$). An important observation was the recognition of a significantly higher incidence of serious cardiac dysfunction in patients receiving trastuzumab and the anthracycline/cyclophosphamide combination compared to anthracycline/cyclophosphamide chemotherapy alone (16% versus 3%). The incidence of cardiac dysfunction in patients receiving trastuzumab and paclitaxel was 2% compared to 1% in those treated with paclitaxel alone.

Romond et al. (2005) reported the combined analysis of NSABP Trial B-31 and the North Central Cancer Treatment Group Trial N9831. Both studies treated a combined total of 3351 women with stage II and high-risk stage I (node-negative) breast cancer whose tumors exhibited 3+ overexpression of Her2 using the combination of doxorubicin and cyclophosphamide. Patients were then randomized to treatment with paclitaxel alone, or paclitaxel and trastuzumab. At 3 years there was a 52% improvement in event-free survival and reduction in the risk of developing distant metastatic disease in the trastuzumab treatment arm indicating an important role for the combination of trastuzumab and chemotherapy in the adjuvant treatment of early stage breast cancer.

The level of tumor Her2 overexpression is critical to the selection of patients for trastuzumab therapy. Tumors expressing low levels of Her2 are generally unresponsive to trastuzumab. Even when overexpressed, those patients with high levels (3+) of Her2 expression are more likely to respond and have longer survivals than patients with indeterminate levels (2+) of Her2 overexpression (Cobleigh et al., 1999; Slamon et al., 2001; Vogel et al., 2002). The two clinically approved laboratory techniques used to quantify the level of Her2 expression in breast tumors are IHC staining and fluorescence *in situ* hybridization (FISH) (Dowsett et al., 2003). Immunohistochemical assays, such as the HercepTest (Dako Corporation), measure Her2 protein expression on the surface of tumor cells by antibody binding and subsequent detection by chromogenic staining. Immunohistochemical semiquantitatively reports Her2 expression as 0, 1+, 2+, or 3+. Tumors scored 0 or 1+ are considered negative for overexpression of Her2. Tumors scored as 3+, overexpress Her2, whereas those scored 2+ are considered moderate or indeterminate. In contrast, FISH analysis measures the degree of *Her2* gene amplification. Breast tumors that are IHC 3+ positive show a close correlation with FISH-positivity and response to trastuzumab. FISH analysis may be useful for selecting those IHC 2+ (indeterminate) tumors that are more likely to respond to trastuzumab.

Trastuzumab is generally well tolerated. Commonly reported side effects include mild to moderate chills, fevers, nausea, and respiratory symptoms usually occurring with the initial dose (Cobleigh *et al.*, 1999; Slamon *et al.*, 2001; Vogel *et al.*, 2002). Rare serious infusional reactions have been reported. Abdominal pain, diarrhea, vomiting, headaches, and rash can also occur. The frequency of these events is increased when the antibody is used in combination with chemotherapy. The major serious toxicity associated with trastuzumab has been cardiac. A meta-analysis of seven phase II and III trials revealed higher rates of cardiotoxicity when trastuzumab was combined with an anthracycline and cyclophosphamide (27%) compared with the combination of paclitaxel and trastuzumab (13%), or single agent trastuzumab (3–7%) (Seidman *et al.*, 2002). The majority of these patients had previously received anthracycline therapy. Grazette *et al.* (2004) found that an anti-Her2 antibody induced mitochondrial dysfunction and apoptosis of primary cardiac myocytes.

11.3. Alemtuzumab (Campath™)

Alemtuzumab, a humanized rat monoclonal antibody that defines the CD52 antigen, was approved by the FDA for the treatment of alkylating agent and fludarabine-refractory chronic lymphocytic leukemia (CLL) in 2001. Alemtuzumab is also active in T-cell prolymphocytic leukemia (T-PLL) and cutaneous T-cell lymphoma (CTCL). CD52 is a glycoprotein antigen expressed on normal and malignant T and B cells, NK cells, monocytes, macrophages, eosinophils, and epithelial cells of the male genital tract. Notable exceptions include most granulocytes, erythrocytes, platelets, most $CD34^+$ hematopoietic stem cells, and plasma cells.

The CAMPATH series of anti-CD52 antibodies were developed by Herman Waldmann and colleagues in the early 1980s for T-cell depletion of bone marrow to prevent graft-versus-host disease (Hale *et al.*, 1983). CAMPATH-1M, a rat IgM monoclonal was the first of the series studied. It was followed by the development of CAMPATH-1G, a rat IgG2b that was easier to manufacture, exhibited ADCC with human Fc receptors, as well as the ability to activate complement similar to CAMPATH-1M. CAMPATH-1H (alemtuzumab), a humanized monoclonal with activity similar to CAMPATH-1G generated by fusing the CDR of CAMPATH-1G to a human IgG1 framework was selected for clinical development.

The target antigen, CD52 is a 21–28 kDa glycoprotein molecule with a core peptide of 12 amino acids, an N-glycosylation site at the N-terminus and a glycosphoionostiol (GPI) anchor that is attached to the outer layer of the cell membrane (Treumann et al., 1995). It is expressed at high density (>450,000 molecules per cell) and it is nonmodulating. In vitro, alemtuzumab can initiate complement-mediated lysis, facilitate ADCC, and induce apoptosis of lymphocytes. The epitope recognized by alemtuzumab is the C-terminal peptide and a region of the GPI-anchor. In man, the antibody exhibits a serum half-life of 15–21 days (Rebello et al., 2001).

The first therapeutic use of CAMPATH was reported in 1988 in a patient with refractory B-cell NHL in which a short-lived partial remission was achieved (Hale et al., 1988). Subsequent phase II trials in patients with relapsed and resistant low-grade B-cell NHL reported overall response rates of 14–44%, with few CR (Khorana et al., 2001; Lundin et al., 1998; Uppenkamp et al., 2002). Alemtuzumab showed significantly greater activity in CLL with responses reported in 33–50% of previously treated, relapsed, or chemotherapy refractory patients (Bowen et al., 1997; Keating et al., 2002; Osterborg et al., 1997; Rai et al., 2002). In the CAM-211 study, 93 patients who failed treatment with alkylating agents and fludarabine were treated with alemtuzumab 30 mg intravenously three times per week. An overall response rate of 33% with two CR was observed. An additional 59% of patients had disease stabilization with resolution or improvement of disease-related symptoms. Complete resolution of lymphadenopathy was seen in 64% of patients with lymph nodes <2 cm and in none of the patients with lymph nodes >5 cm in diameter. It is hypothesized that alemtuzumab's lower efficacy in bulky disease is the result of the lower concentrations of the monoclonal antibody achieved in solid tissue or reduced ADCC effector function at the site of bulky disease. Median survival for the entire group was 16 months, which compared very favorably with alternative salvage treatments. For responding patients median survival was improved to 32 months. A small study of the combination of fludarabine and alemtuzumab in heavily pretreated fludarabine-refractory patients reported an 83% response rate with one CR (Kennedy et al., 2002). Response rates in untreated CLL patients are reported as high as 89% with CR's seen in up to one-third of patients (Osterborg et al., 1996). Studies are in progress examining alemtuzumab as consolidation therapy after successful chemotherapy. Interestingly, mutations of the p53 gene in CLL correlate with a likelihood of a poor response to conventional chemotherapy; however, patients with CLL expressing mutant p53 are twice as likely to respond to alemtuzumab than those patients with CLL lacking a p53 mutation (Lozanski et al., 2004).

Alemtuzumab is also under investigation as treatment in various autoimmune diseases including multiple sclerosis, refractory rheumatoid arthritis, and systemic vasculitis. Use of alemtuzumab in the setting of rheumatoid arthritis is associated with a significant incidence of developing neutralizing autoantibodies (Isaacs et al., 1992).

Alemtuzumab treatment is associated with an acute flu-like syndrome of fever, chills, and nausea that rapidly subsides and tends to disappear with repeated dosing. This syndrome is thought to result from cytokine release from the target cells. Alemtuzumab has been shown to induce release of TNFα, and IL-6 in vivo (Wing et al., 1996). Prophylaxis with acetoaminophen and antihistamines are helpful in preventing these reactions. Transient rashes or urticaria occur in about one-third of patients receiving the antibody. Other short-term effects include decreases in granulocyte and platelet counts, and increases in serum liver transaminases. Long-term side effects include profound and prolonged lymphopenia. Depression of peripheral blood $CD4^+$ lymphocytes may last six months or longer. The risks of opportunistic infection appear related to concomitant immunosuppression and the underlying disease. Patients receiving alemtuzumab are usually given antimicrobial prophylaxis that is continued until the peripheral blood $CD4^+$ cell count returns to $\geq 200/mm^3$. Serious opportunistic infections in patients treated with alemtuzumab who receive prophylaxis are uncommon; however, reactivation of cytomegalovirus (CMV) is frequent (Laurenti et al., 2004). Autoimmune thyroiditis (Grave's disease) has been reported in 30% patients with multiple sclerosis who were treated with alemtuzumab, but rarely seen in patients receiving the drug for other disorders (Coles et al., 1999).

11.4. Cetuximab (IM-C225, Erbitux™)

Cetuximab is a chimeric murine–human monoclonal antibody that targets the extracellular domain of the EGFR with high affinity. It was approved by the FDA for the treatment of EGFR-expressing metastatic colorectal cancer as a single agent or for use in combination with irinotecan-based chemotherapy. Cetuximab (C225) consists of the Fv region of the murine monoclonal M225 antibody ligated to a human IgG1 framework (for review see Mendelsohn, 1997). The target of cetuximab, EGFR is a 170-kDa transmembrane glycoprotein tyrosine kinase growth factor receptor. Members of the family are activated by ligand binding and the subsequent interaction of two identical receptor subunits (homodimerization) or different subunits of the same receptor family (heterodimerization). At least six different EGFR ligands are recognized including epidermal growth factor (EGF) and TGFα. Epidermal growth factor receptor is one of the most extensively studied targets in solid tumors. It is overexpressed in many tumors including up to 80% of lung cancers, 90% of head and neck cancers and 50–70% of colorectal cancers. Increased EGFR expression is associated with aggressive behavior and a poorer prognosis in cancers of the lung, breast, colon and rectum, ovary, pancreas, bladder, kidney, and uterine cervix (Mendelsohn and Baselga, 2000).

Cetuximab exhibits tenfold greater affinity for the EGFR than do the natural ligands of EGFR resulting in preferential binding of the antibody and blockade of ligand-induced activation (Goldstein *et al.*, 1995). While permitting receptor dimerization, cetuximab prevents autophosphorylation and signaling. It also promotes receptor internalization reducing the amount of receptor available on the cell surface for dimerization (Sunada *et al.*, 1986). This downregulation of receptor activity appears to be important for the inhibitory action of cetuximab. Cetuximab has multiple effects on EGFR-expressing cells, all of which may contribute to its antitumor action. These include blockade of cell cycle progression, enhanced apoptosis, anti-angiogenesis, inhibition of metastases, and reduced cellular repair after chemotherapy or radiation injury (Herbst *et al.*, 2001). Cetuximab inhibits proliferation of EGFR-expressing human cancer cell lines *in vitro* and *in vivo* (Goldstein *et al.*, 1995). In addition, the Fc portion of the antibody may activate complement and facilitate ADCC. A role for ADCC is suggested by data showing reduced effectiveness of C225 F(ab')$_2$ fragments in inhibiting tumor xenograft growth compared to the intact IgG1 molecule even though both will block ligand binding and receptor activation (Fan *et al.*, 1993).

In phase I trials, cetuximab exhibited pharmacokinetics that are nonlinear with the saturation of drug elimination pathways occurring at weekly doses of 200–400 mg/m^2, and an elimination half-life of 7 days at these dose levels. Based on this, a loading dose of 400 mg/m^2 over 120 min followed by weekly doses of 250 mg/m^2 administered as 1-h infusions is recommended. At these doses the mean circulating levels of cetuximab are sustained above 200 nM.

A series of phase I studies designed to assess cetuximab as a single agent, or in combination with chemotherapy or radiation showed antitumor activity and safety (Baselga *et al.*, 2000; Robert *et al.*, 2001; Shin *et al.*, 2001). Phase II trials in patients with advanced colorectal cancer or squamous cell carcinoma of the head and neck reported overall response rates of 9% and 14% for cetuximab or the combination of cetuximab and cisplatin, respectively (Herbst *et al.*, 2005; Saltz *et al.*, 2004). In the pivotal randomized-controlled trial, 329 patients with metastatic colorectal cancer that had progressed during treatment or within 3 months of receiving irinotecan-based chemotherapy were randomized to receive irinotecan with cetuximab, or cetuximab alone (Cunningham *et al.*, 2004). The objective response rate for the antibody-chemotherapy treatment arm was 22.9% compared to 10.8% for the cetuximab monotherapy. The median response duration was 5.7 months for the combination and 4.2 months in the cetuximab alone arm.

Common adverse events associated with cetuximab treatment include allergic reactions and skin rash. An acne-like folliculitis is seen in less than 20% of patients usually occurring on the upper body. Most rashes have occurred with the initial infusions. Other toxicities include fever, headache, asthenia, anorexia, abdominal pain, constipation, diarrhea, and nausea. A small incidence of life threatening interstitial lung disease has also been reported. The immunogenicity of cetuximab is low and only rarely induces neutralizing anti-chimeric antibodies after treatment.

11.5. Bevacizumab (Avastin)

Bevacizumab is a humanized recombinant IgG1 monoclonal antibody that targets VEGF-A approved for first-line treatment of patients with metastatic colorectal carcinoma in combination with fluorouracil-based chemotherapy. Bevacizumab was derived from the murine anti-VEGF monoclonal antibody A6.4.1 by transferring its CDR to a human IgG1 framework (Kim *et al.*, 1993; Presta *et al.*, 1997). Bevacizumab binds with an affinity of 1.8 nM and neutralizes all biologically active isoforms of VEGF thereby preventing the interaction of VEGF with its receptors. Vascular endothelial growth factor is a 45 kDa heparin-binding glycoprotein and cell-specific mitogen that is the primary regulator of endothelial cell proliferation, migration, permeability, and survival (See Hoeben *et al.*, 2004 for review). Vascular endothelial growth factor-A interacts with at least two receptors, VEGFR-1 (flt-1) and VEGFR-2 (KDR) located predominantly on vascular endothelial cells. Vascular endothelial growth factor is also a multifunctional regulator of immune and inflammatory cells (Gabrilovich *et al.*, 1998). It has been shown to block differentiation of dendritic and other hematopoietic cell lineages and decreased antigen presentation. Elevated levels of VEGF expression are associated with a poorer prognosis in a variety of tumors.

Vascular endothelial growth factor plays a critical role in early tumor vascularization and growth by recruiting bone marrow-derived endothelial stem cells and inducing their differentiation into tumor vessels. Suppression of VEGF by bevacizumab inhibited tumor growth in a number of animal models through inhibition of angiogenesis (Hicklin and Ellis, 2005). Bevacizumab itself exhibits little direct antitumor activity. Bevacizumab's effects are enhanced when it was combined with chemotherapy or radiation (Gerber and Ferrera, 2005; Lee et al., 2000).

A phase I pharmacokinetic analysis of 25 patients treated with bevacizumab 0.1–10 mg/kg on days 0, 28, 35, and 42 found that bevacizumab had a half-life of approximately 21 days (Gordon et al., 2001). Bevacizumab is recommended to be administered at a dose of 5 mg/kg intravenously over 90 min every 14-days in combination with fluorouracil-based chemotherapy. Bevacizumab clearance was found to be unaffected in patients receiving a variety of chemotherapy drugs (Margolin et al., 2001). Bevacizumab in combination with fluorouracil and leucovorin (FU/LV) versus FU/LV alone was evaluated in previously untreated patients with metastatic colorectal cancer (Kabbinavar et al., 2003). One-hundred-four patients were randomized to receive FU/LV alone versus FU/LV and two different doses of bevacizumab (5 mg/kg or 10 mg/kg). The primary endpoint of the trial was objective response rates and the secondary endpoints were survival and response duration. The best overall response was achieved in the patients receiving the lower dose of bevacizumab with FU/LV. These investigators hypothesized that the higher dose of bevacizumab resulted in a rapid vascular collapse in the tumor and impeded the entry of chemotherapy into the tumor. A pivotal placebo-controlled phase III trial randomized 926 patients with metastatic colorectal cancer as initial treatment to the combination of irinotecan, fluorouracil, and leucovorin (IFL) plus bevacizumab or IFL plus placebo (Hurwitz et al., 2004). The addition of bevacizumab to IFL increased the overall response rate (44.8% versus 34.8%; $p = 0.004$), and improved progression free survival (10.6 versus 6.2 months; $p < 0.001$) and overall survival (20.3 versus 15.6 months; $p < 0.001$) compared to IFL chemotherapy with placebo. Yang et al. (2003) evaluated bevacizumab in a randomized double-blind, placebo-controlled phase II trial in 116 patients with metastatic renal cell carcinoma, most of whom had failed to respond to IL-2. Patients were randomized to placebo or treatment with low-dose (3 mg/kg) or high-dose (10 mg/kg) bevacizumab. Patients treated on the high-dose arm had a significantly longer time to progression compared to patients receiving placebo.

Adverse events associated with bevacizumab treatment are difficult to evaluate since the antibody was often administered in combination with other chemotherapy agents. Frequent toxicities include fever, headache, chills, rash, mucosal bleeding, and hypotension. The risk of hypertension was increased in patients with a prior history of high blood pressure and appears to be dose-related with a higher frequency at bevacizumab doses of 10 mg/kg than at 5 mg/kg. Bevacizumab treatment is also associated with increased risk of bowel perforation, impaired wound healing and dehiscence, and should not be initiated within 28-days of major surgery. Less common side effects include nephrosis and proteinuria, thromboembolic events including deep vein thrombosis, pulmonary embolism, pulmonary hemorrhage, and myocardial infarction.

12. Antibodies Armed with Cytokines, Chemotherapeutic Agents, Toxins, and Radionuclides Cytokine Armed Monoclonal Antibodies

Cytokines such as IL-2 have received approval from the FDA for use in the treatment of metastatic renal cancer and malignant melanoma, where it introduced a durable complete response in 5–17% of patients (Rosenberg et al., 1994). Another therapeutic strategy involves the use of cytokines genetically linked to monoclonal antibodies to induce NK- and T-cell proliferation at the tumor site. These immunocytokines create high intratumoral concentrations of cytokines to stimulate the antitumor response and to avoid the toxicities associated with systemic cytokine administration. Cytokines that have been evaluated include IL-2, IL-12, and GM-CSF. Genetically engineered antibody-IL-2 fusion proteins inhibited the growth of hepatic and pulmonary metastases of a human melanoma xenograft in SCID mice (Lode and Reisfeld, 2000). This effect was specific and the survival times of treated animals were more than doubled when compared to those treated with a mixture of antibody and IL-2 at equivalent dose levels. It is possible that IL-15 genetically linked to monoclonal antibodies could be more effective than IL-2 in light of their distinct effects on the immune system (Waldmann et al., 2001). Interleukin-2 has certain undesirable characteristics as an immunomodulatory agent including playing a major role in activation-induced cell death (AICD) wherein there is suicide of T cells reacting with host and perhaps tumor antigens (Lenardo, 1996). Furthermore, IL-2 is pivotal in the induction and survival of T regs that inhibit immune responses (Sakaguchi, 2004). In contrast, IL-15 inhibits AICD and is centrally involved in the induction, maintenance, and activation of NK, NK-T, and CD8 memory phenotype T cells (Marks-Konczalik et al., 2000) (Ku et al., 2000; Waldmann et al., 2001; Zhang et al., 1998).

13. Antibodies Armed with Chemotherapeutic Agents

Another therapeutic strategy is to use the antigen specificity of monoclonal antibodies to deliver chemotherapeutic agents to the surface of the tumor cells. Genetically engineered antibody fragments have been attached to the surface of liposomes for selective tumor targeting. An alternative approach involves the use of antibodies to target prodrugs (Bagshawe, 1995; Denny, 2004). Bagshawe (1995) used antibody-directed enzyme prodrug therapy (ADEPT) to achieve this goal. An antibody conjugated to an enzyme is given intravenously and allowed to localize to a tumor. After the enzyme is cleared a prodrug is administered, which diffuses widely but in the ideal case is activated solely at the tumor following contact with the localized antibody enzyme fusion protein. The benefit of this approach is the ability to kill bystander tumor cells by reducing the ability of tumors to evade therapy by antigen loss. In certain tumor xenograft studies, ADEPT was effective. However, it has been difficult to translate ADEPT into the clinic. Immunogenicity of the chemical conjugates as well as the need for a clearance system to eliminate residual enzyme from the circulation before the prodrug could be administered presented problems. It appears necessary to develop humanized reagents and a more efficient targeting system.

14. Immunotoxins for the Treatment of Cancer

A major limitation in the use of monoclonal antibodies in the treatment of cancer is that most are poor cytocidal agents. To address this issue monoclonal antibodies are being linked to a cytocidal agent, such as a toxin, which is then targeted to the tumor cell by the antibody (Kreitman, 2003). The arming of monoclonal antibodies or cytokines with toxins has been a widely explored strategy for enhancing the efficacy of antitumor antibodies (Kreitman et al., 2000). There are, however, a series of limitations in the use of such oncotoxins. Initial clinical evaluation of toxin-armed antibodies especially those using unmodified toxins yielded unacceptable toxicity in several clinical trials. Furthermore, most toxins are very immunogenic and thus provide only a narrow therapeutic time window before the development of antitoxin antibodies. For effective action against tumor cells, the antigenic target of the antibody must be expressed on all of the malignant cells and the interaction of the antibody with this target must lead to the internalization of the antibody toxin conjugate. Finally, toxin-armed monoclonal antibodies are large molecules, a fact, as noted by Jain (2001) that severely limits their access to central cells in large solid tumors. Despite these limitations, a large number of recombinant immunotoxins have been developed for the treatment of hematological malignancies. Such arming of antibodies with toxins has been stimulated by the approval of the first immunotoxin armed antibody gemtuzumab ozogamicin (Mylotarg^{TM}) that links the toxin calicheamicin to a CD33-specific antibody for the treatment of myelogenous leukemia (see the following section) (Sievers et al., 2001). Furthermore, denileukin diftitox (DAB 389-IL-2, diphtheria toxin linked to IL-2, OnTak^{TM}) to target the IL-2 receptor was approved by the FDA for the treatment of advanced CTCL (Olsen et al., 2001).

A variety of toxins have been linked to receptor directed biological agents including small molecule toxins, such as calicheamicins and maytansinoyds.

Furthermore, protein toxins that kill cells by inhibition of protein synthesis after the toxin fragment enters the cytosol of the cell have been widely utilized. Plant toxins, such as ricin and pokeweed mitogen, work by inactivating ribosomes whereas bacterial toxins, such as diphtheria toxin (DT) and *Pseudomonas* exotoxin (PE), inhibit protein synthesis by ADP ribosylation of elongation factor-2 (Kreitman, 2003). A number of modifications were made in the toxins to address some of the early limitations in oncotoxins. One advance is in the removal of the binding domain of the toxin, which normally leads to its binding by normal tissues. For example, *Pseudomonas* exotoxin is a single-chain protein that is 613 amino acids long and contains 3 major functional domains (Krietman, 2003). Domain Ia (amino acids 1–252) is the binding domain that leads to binding by tissues such as the liver. Domain II (amino acids 253–364) is the translocating domain. Domain III (amino acids 400–613) contains the ADP ribosylating enzyme, which inactivates elongation factor-2 in the cytosol and results in cell death. The PE fragment commonly used in therapy has a deletion of the binding domain and includes amino acids 253–364 plus 381–613. Another advance is the use of genetic engineering rather than chemical linkage to replace the binding domain of the toxin with the targeting element, which is a cytokine, growth factor, or a recombinant single-chain Fv containing only the variable domains of the antibody.

The antigens most successfully targeted by toxin armed antibodies include CD22 that is expressed on mature B cells, including the majority of B-cell lymphomas, CD33 a sialic acid-binding Ig-like lectin that is found on the surface of virtually all acute myelogenous leukemia cells, and CD25 the IL-2R alpha subunit expressed on diverse T cell and other hematopoietic malignant cells. An example of such a genetically engineered toxin armed antibody is LMB-2. It involves the truncated *Pseudomonas* toxin PE38 genetically linked to the murine anti-Tac Fv (anti-CD25) monoclonal antibody (Kreitman *et al.*, 2000). The scientific basis for the use of this antibody is that CD25 is not expressed by resting normal cells other than T regs but by a broad range of hematological malignancies. LMB-2 was administered to 35 patients with chemotherapy resistant leukemia, lymphoma, and Hodgkin's disease (Krietman *et al.*, 2000). Responses include one CR and seven PRs in patients receiving more than 60 mg. Among four patients with hairy cell leukemia (HCL) treated there was one CR and three PRs. The most common toxicities included fever and transaminase elevations.

CD25 is also the target of denileukin diftitox, which represents a chimeric molecule with IL-2 linked to the first 389 amino acids of the diphtheria toxin (Olsen *et al.*, 2001). In phase I clinical trials denileukin diftitox produced five complete remissions and eight partial responses in 35 patients studied with CTCL and one CR and two PRs in 17 patients with NHL evaluated. Toxicities included transaminase elevations without liver failure (62%), hypoalbuminemia (86%), hypotension (32%), the vascular leak syndrome, and in some patients, rashes (32%). In the phase III pivotal trial 7 complete remissions and 14 partial remissions were observed among 71 CTL patients evaluated. Based on these trials denileukin diftitox was approved by the FDA for the treatment of CTCL.

Several chemical conjugates containing plant and bacterial toxins have been constructed to target CD22 on B-cell malignancies (Kreitman, 2003). The BL-22 immunotoxin (truncated *Pseudomonas* toxin PE38 genetically linked to a single chain Fv of anti-CD22 monoclonal antibody RFB4) was administered to 16 patients with HCL (Kreitman *et al.*, 2001). Eleven of the 16 patients (68%) had CRs and 2 patients had PRs (12%). Dose limiting toxicities included a cytokine lysis syndrome in one patient with fever, hypotension, bone pain, and weight gain without pulmonary edema. In addition, two patients had a reversible hemolytic uremic syndrome confirmed by renal biopsy that presented clinically with hematuria and hemoglobinuria.

14.1. Gemtuzumab Ozogamicin (MYLOTARG™; CMA-676)

Gemtuzumab ozogamicin is an immunotoxin composed of a recombinant humanized IgG4 kappa monoclonal anti-CD33 antibody conjugated to the antitumor antibiotic γ_1-calicheamicin. It was FDA approved in 2000 for the treatment of CD33$^+$ acute myeloid leukemia (AML) in patients 60 years of age or older in first relapse and ineligible for further cytotoxic therapy. Gemtuzumab (hP67.6) is derived from the complementarity-determining regions of the murine antibody p67.6 that recognizes CD33 (Hamann *et al.*, 2002). Gemtuzumab is chelated to the *N*-acetyl derivative of γ_1-calicheamicin, an aryltetrasaccharide enediyne antitumor antibiotic isolated from *Micromonospora echinospora calichensis* that is active against a broad spectrum of leukemic and solid tumor cell lines (Hamann *et al.*, 2002; Zein *et al.*, 1988).

CD33 is a 67 kDa glycoprotein silaoadhesin receptor (Freeman *et al.*, 1995). The intracytoplasmic domain of CD33 has two immunoreceptor tyrosine-based inhibitory motifs (ITIM). CD33 is expressed on normal and maturing monomyeloid hematopoietic progenitor cells, but expression is lacking on the earliest normal hematopoietic stem cells and it is not found on nonhematopoietic tissues (Dinndorf *et al.*, 1986). Over 90% of AML patients have blast cells that express the CD33 antigen. On binding to its receptor, the gemtuzumab ozogamicin-CD33 complex is internalized and active γ_1-calicheamicin is liberated by endolysosomal hydrolysis (van Der Velden *et al.*, 2001). Calicheamicin binds to the minor groove of DNA and induces site-specific double-stranded DNA breaks resulting in apoptosis of leukemic cells (Zein et al., 1988). Given that CD33 stimulation is inhibitory, the binding of gentuzumab alone may also exert antileukemic effects, however, this has not been confirmed *in vitro*. As an IgG4, gemtuzumab exhibits little other effector function. *In vitro* studies indicate that gemtuzumab ozogamicin is almost 10^5-fold more toxic to cells expressing CD33 than cells lacking expression, indicating its ability to target CD33$^+$ cells and enhance the uptake of the toxin (Naito et al., 2000). The immunotoxin showed selective cytotoxicity in cultured human HL-60 leukemia cells and in HL-60 murine xenograft models (Hamann et al., 2002).

Since gemtuzumab ozogamicin is composed of the monoclonal antibody hP67.7 and γ_1-calicheamicin, in reality there are two sets of pharmacokinetics for the immunotoxin. At least 85% saturation of CD33 receptor on circulating and bone marrow leukemic blasts is achieved with the initial administration at the maximum tolerated dose of 9 mg/m^2 (van der Velden et al., 2001). Saturating levels of the antibody are thought to enhance efficacy although clinical response has not been correlated with plasma levels of the agent. After a 9 mg/m^2 dose, gentuzumab (hP67.6) achieved a mean peak plasma concentration (C_{max}) of 2.86 ± 1.35 μg/mL and had plasma half-life of 72.4 ± 42.0 h (Dowell et al., 2001). Higher plasma concentrations are observed with second doses and this is thought to be due to reduction of CD33$^+$ tumor burden following the initial dose. Mean C_{max} for γ_1-calicheamicin at this dose was 0.005 μg/mL and its plasma half-life was 101 h. The concentration-time course curve (AUC) for γ_1-calicheamicin mimicked that of gemtuzumab, suggesting that the γ_1-calicheamicin remained conjugated to the antibody after administration.

Acute myeloid leukemia is the most common acute leukemia of adults and its incidence increases with age (Lowenberg et al., 1999). In previously untreated patients, remissions of 50–80% can be achieved with a combination of cytarabine and an anthracycline. For patients achieving a remission, up to three-quarters will relapse and approximately 20% survive 5-years. These numbers are significantly worse for older patients. Therapeutic options are limited for patients over the age of 60 because of lower response rates, increased toxicity from chemotherapy, and frequent comorbidities.

A phase I trial defined the maximum tolerated dose of gemtuzumab ozogamicin administered as a 2-h infusion as 9 mg/m^2 (Sievers et al., 1999). Three combined open-label phase II studies in 277 adults with recurrent CD33$^+$ AML reported an overall response rate of 26% with 13% complete remissions with platelet recovery (Larson et al., 2005). Response rates for patients ≥60 years was 24%, and 28% for those <60 years. Gemtuzumab ozogamicin exhibited significant antileukemic activity as first-line single-agent therapy for AML as well as when it was used as consolidation therapy after a remission is induced with standard chemotherapy for AML (Amadori *et al.*, 2004; Kell *et al.*, 2003; Tsimberidou *et al.*, 2003).

Side effects of gemtuzumab ozogamicin include infusional reactions with chills, fever, nausea, vomiting, tachycardia, headaches, and labile blood pressure. Other toxicities include myelosuppression with granulocytopenia and thrombocytopenia, stomatitis, reversible elevation of serum liver transaminases and bilirubin in 25% of patients, and hepatic veno-occlusive disease. Tumor lysis syndrome and acute adult respiratory distress syndrome (ARDS) have also been reported. Resistance to gemtuzumab ozogamicin has been correlated with expression of the multidrug resistance (MDR-1) p-glycoprotein and its activity on calicheamicin and increased serum levels of CD33 antigen (Linenberger *et al.*, 2001, 2005; van Der Velden *et al.*, 2004).

15. Systemic Radioimmunotherapy with Monoclonal Antibodies

Toxin conjugates do not pass easily from the endosome to the cytosol. In addition, the use of monoclonal antibodies armed with toxins requires the expression of the target antigen by all tumor cells. One advantage in the use of radiolabeled monoclonal antibody conjugates for therapy is that with the appropriate choice of radionuclide, radiolabeled monoclonal antibodies can kill cells from a distance of several cell diameters and may therefore kill antigen-negative cells adjacent to antigen-expressing cells. Furthermore, the radiolabeled antibody need not be internalized to kill the cell. In addition, toxins are immunogenic and thus provide only a short therapeutic window before the development of antibodies toward the toxin. Radiolabled monoclonal antibodies have been developed as alternative immunoconjugates for the delivery of cytotoxic effector agents to target cells (Axworthy *et al.*, 2000; Kaminski *et al.*, 2005; Milenic *et al.*, 2004; Press *et al.*, 1995; Waldmann, 2003a; Witzig *et al.*, 2002a; Zhang *et al.*, 2002). A number of factors need to be considered when designing an optimal radioimmunotherapy strategy: (1) the choice of the monoclonal antibody and thus the antigenic target; (2) the choice of delivery system used to target the radionuclide to the tumor cell; and (3) the choice of radionuclide. As the effectiveness of monoclonal antibodies increases it becomes critical to ensure that the target antigen is necessary for the survival of the tumor cell but is not expressed by cells vital to normal functioning. The two radioimmunoconjugates most widely studied to date and those that are approved by the FDA have been developed for use in the treatment of indolent B-cell lymphomas. Monoclonal antibodies directed toward CD20: Ibritumomab tiuxetan (the murine parent of rituximab linked to tiuxetan) conjugated to ^{90}Y (Zevalin^{TM}) and tositumomab conjugated to ^{131}I (Bexxar^{TM}) (Kaminski et al., 2005; Press et al., 1995). These radiolabeled monoclonal antibodies are discussed more extensively below. Other targets for systemic radioimmunotherapy include YM-I specific for human leukocyte antigen (HLA-DR) expressed on B-cell tumors and the CD33 antigen expressed on most myeloid leukemic-blasts and leukemic progenitor cells. The humanized antibody HuM-195 directed toward CD33 has been employed as a vehicle for radioimmunotherapy conjugated with ^{131}I and^{90}Y in the therapy of patients with acute and chronic myelogenous leukemia (Burke et al., 2003). Furthermore, it has been conjugated to ^{213}Bi in the first use of α particles for systemic radioimmunotherapy in human clinical trials (Jurcic et al., 2002).

Our own studies involving systemic radioimmunotherapy have focused on CD25, the IL-2 receptor alpha subunit (Waldmann et al., 1995; Zhang et al., 2002). The scientific basis for targeting CD25 is that in contrast to most normal resting cells certain tumor cells, such as adult T-cell leukemia (ATL), HCL, Hodgkin's lymphoma, and anaplastic large cell lymphoma express high levels of IL-2R alpha (Waldmann, 2003a). The initial focus of the therapeutic clinical trials was on patients with ATL and aggressive malignancy associated with infection by the retrovirus human T-cell lymphotropic virus I (HTLV-I). Patients with the acute form of the disease have a median survival duration of 9 months. Currently no chemotherapeutic regimen has been successful in increasing disease free survival. Utilizing murine anti-Tac (anti-CD25) armed with the radionuclide ^{90}Y produced responses in 9 of 16 evaluable patients (seven PRs and two CRs) (Waldmann et al., 1995).

A second issue in designing an optimal radioimmunotherapy regimen is the choice of the method used to deliver the radionuclide to the tumor cell. In most clinical trials intact monoclonal antibodies have been employed to deliver the radionuclide. There are however a number of limitations in this approach. There are physiological and structural barriers that limit the delivery of high-molecular molecules, such as intact antibodies, to tumor cells especially those of solid tumors. Meaningful tumor uptake of antibody may not occur until 24–48 h after injection. Unfortunately the long serum half-lives of the monoclonal antibodies prolong radiation exposure to normal organs including the radiosensitive bone marrow, which limits the radiation that can be safely administered and delivered to the tumor cell. Finally, because of the slow equilibration of intact monoclonal antibodies with the cells in a tumor mass, such therapy is limited to relatively long-lived β-emitting rather than short-lived α-emitting radionuclides. The low dose of radiation delivered by β-emitting radionuclides may be insufficient to overcome the continual proliferation and repair of tumor cells.

To circumvent some of the obstacles encountered by radioimmunotherapy with intact radiolabeled antibodies, a series of multistep strategies have been described to decouple the administration of the radionuclide from that of the antibody (Axworthy et al., 2000, Press et al., 2001; Zhang et al., 2002). The strategy proposed by Axworthy et al. involves a pretargeting approach using Streptavidin-conjugated antibody followed 24–48 h later by the administration of a "clearing agent" to remove unbound antibody from the bloodstream. This procedure is followed 1–3 h later with radiolabed Biotin. The fundamental advantages of this pretargeting approach over conventional radioimmunotherapy are that the uptake of the therapeutic radionuclide by the tumor is high and rapid and any excess radioactivity is efficiently eliminated from the body in the urine. We used the pretargeting technique to treat a nonobese diabetic/severe combined immunodeficient (NOD/SCID) xenograft model of human ATL with an anti-Tac antibody Streptavidin conjugate, which binds to CD25 expressed on the tumor cell followed by DOTA-biotin armed with ^{213}Bi (Zhang et al., 2002). Prolongation of survival was observed with this approach. The best results were obtained with combined therapy that involved a pretargeting technique with ^{213}Bi-DOTA-biotin supplemented by doses of unlabeled humanized anti-Tac (daclizumab). Weiden et al. (2000) demonstrated the efficacy and safety of the pretargeting approach in patients with B-cell lymphoma. Rituximab conjugated to Streptavidin was administered to 10 patients with relapsed or refractory NHL; 6 of 7 patients who received 30 or 50 mCi/m^2 ^{90}Y DOTA-Biotin experienced tumor regression including three CRs and one PR. Five patients experienced transient grade 3 hematologic toxicity. The pretargeting strategy allowed delivery of substantially higher doses of radioactivity to the tumor than could be achieved with nonpretargeted radioimmunoconjugates. Furthermore, there was an exceedingly rapid delivery of the radionuclide following the intravenous administration of the radiolabeled biotin permitting the use of α-emitting radionuclides that have a short physical half-life. This approach should lead to a significant increase in the number of patients with lymphoma achieving complete responses (CRs) and in the duration of these remissions with less toxicity than is observed under current regimens.

The third component of an optimal radioimmunotherapy regimen to consider is the nature of the radionuclide used. A variety of radionuclides are available that differ in terms of their emission type, energy/range of emission, and half-life. Historically β particles have received the most use. The two β-emitting radionuclides most commonly used at present for radioimmunotherapy are ^{90}Y and ^{131}I. Other clinically relevant β-emitters include ^{67}Cu, ^{186}Re, and ^{177}Lu. ^{90}Y has become the dominant β-emitting radionuclide in recent studies in light of its pure β-emission and the fact that it delivers to the tumor approximately 4.5 times more radiation per mCi than does ^{131}I. The emission path lengths of β-emitters are relatively long (mean range of 275 μm) with linear-energy transfer (LET). Energy deposition takes place at some distance from the actual decay event. Therapeutic benefit results from crossfire on cells at a distance. In light of the crossfire effect, therapy with monoclonal antibodies linked to β-emitting radionuclides is most effective with a large tumor mass as is seen in lymphoma. However, the use of β-emitting radionuclides has a number of limitations. As the tumor mass decreases so does the benefit of the crossfire effect. When used with small tumors, micrometastases or individual tumor cells as in leukemia the relatively long path length of β-irradiation compared to α irradiation may result in high-energy β-emission outside of the tumor target volume. In addition, it may not be possible to achieve the number of β-emission traversals that are required to kill the cells in small tumors. Future development of isotopic monoclonal antibodies for the treatment of leukemia or micrometastases may focus on α-emitting radionuclides, which may be most effective at killing tumor targets without damaging distant normal tissues (Mulford et al., 2005). Radionuclides emitting α particles release high-energy emissions (6–9 MeV) ten times as great as β-emitters over a short distance (40–80 μm) and are efficient at killing individual target cells such as those found at leukemia. Suitable α-emitting nuclides available for immunotherapy include ^{212}Bi, ^{213}Bi, ^{211}At, and generators based on ^{225}Ac. The limitation of α-emitters is that their short physical half-lives limit their use to cells such as leukemic cells in rapid equilibrium with the circulation or require the use of a pretargeting approach such as that described above. In general, systemic radioimmunotherapy employing therapeutic monoclonal antibodies may represent relatively nonimmunogenic agents that are effective in eliminating malignant cells when used alone or as part of a multimodality treatment with conventional chemotherapy.

15.1. ^{131}I-Tositumomab (BEXXAR™) and ^{90}Y-Ibritumomab Tiuxetan (ZEVALIN™)

Tositumomab and ibritumomab tiuxetan are two different murine monoclonal antibodies that are approved for the radioimmunotherapy of B-cell lymphoma. Both antibodies target CD20 similar to rituximab. Tositumomab is armed with radio-emitting iodine-131 (^{131}I) and ibritumomab is chelated to yttrium-90 (^{90}Y). Yttrium-90 ibritumomab tiuxetan and ^{131}I-tositumomab were approved for use in the clinic in 2002 and 2003, respectively. They are indicated for the treatment of patients with CD20$^+$ follicular NHL, with and without transformation, whose disease is refractory to rituximab and has relapsed following chemotherapy. The indication for ^{131}I-tositumomab was recently expanded to include rituximab naïve patients.

Tositumomab is anti-B1, a murine IgG2a lamba monoclonal antibody that targets CD20 (Nadler et al., 1981). Ibritumomab is 2B8, the murine IgG1 kappa monoclonal antibody that was used to generate the chimeric antibody rituximab. Radiolabeled tositumomab is generated by direct covalent linkage of ^{131}I to tyrosine residues on the immunoglobulin molecule (Zalutsky et al., 1990). Iodine-131 offers the advantages of easy conjugation to protein, is inexpensive, and can be used for imaging binding of the antibody to the target. Yttrium-90 on the other hand is chelated to the linker tiuxetan ({N-[2-bis (carboxymethyl) amino]-3-p-isothiocyanatophenyl}-propyl-{N-[2-bis(carboxymethyl) amino-2-methyl-ethyl] glycine}), which is covalently bonded to ibritumomab (Chinn et al., 1999). Iodine-131 emits β particles and γ rays, whereas ^{90}Y is a high-energy β-emitter (Press et al., 1996). Iodine-131 has a half-life of 8 days compared to approximately 2.7 days for ^{90}Y. Yttrium-90, however, exhibits a favorable dosimetry and safety profile. In contrast to unlabeled antibodies, agents used for radioimmunotherapy are administered in much smaller doses. The goal is to use the smallest amounts of the antibody that will result in favorable targeting and dosimetry.

Yttrium-90 ibritumomab tiuxetan is dosed according to body weight, and ^{131}I-tositumomab is administered based on dosimetry to achieve a maximum tolerated whole body dose. Both agents are administered in a two-step process. In the initial "cold" phase for ^{131}I-tositumomab, unlabeled tositumomab 450 mg, or rituximab 250 mg/m^2 in the case of ^{90}Y-ibritumomab tiuxetan are administered along with nontherapeutic doses of 5 mCi ^{131}I-tositumomab or 5 mCi ^{111}In-ibritumomab tiuxetan respectively. These "cold doses" are used to clear B cells from the circulation and bone marrow in order to optimize the biodistribution and subsequent targeting of the therapeutic dose of "hot" antibody. The small amounts of radioactive ^{131}I-tositumomab or ^{111}In-ibritumomab tiuxetan are used for imaging or for dosimetry based on the calculation of ^{131}I clearance. The whole body ^{131}I clearance is determined from images obtained at 3-time points following injection of imaging dose of ^{131}I-tositumomab. Iodine-131 clearance varies significantly between patients and the therapeutic dose of ^{131}I-tositumomab is determined from this information (Wahl, 2005). For each of these agents, 1–2 weeks later, a second dose of "cold" antibody (tositumomab 450 mg or rituximab 250 mg/m^2) is administered followed by the therapeutic "hot" antibody. Iodine-131 tositumomab is dosed to deliver a total body dose of 75 cGy or for ^{90}Y-ibritumomab tiuxetan 0.4 mCi/kg is administered (Kaminski et al., 1996; Witzig et al., 2003). For patients with marginal platelet counts defined as 100,000–149,000/mm^3, 0.3 mCi/kg ^{90}Y-ibritumomab tiuxetan, ^{131}I-tositumomab total body dose, of 65 cGy are recommended. Treatment is not recommended at platelet levels below these or in those patients with more than 25% bone marrow involvement with lymphoma due to the increased bone marrow radiation dose. The dose of "cold" antibody saturates CD20 on the surface of tumors and facilitates penetration of the radiolabeled antibodies deeper into the tumor mass. The tissue penetrating effects of radiation also allows for treatment of bulky or poorly vascularized tumors because tumor cells can be killed at a distance by ionizing radiation directed to the tumor by the monoclonal antibody. This "cross-fire" effect also allows the killing of antigen-negative tumor cells in proximity to the targeted cells (Essand et al., 1995). In addition to the effects of radiation, the doses of "cold" tositumomab or rituximab may have therapeutic activity (Davis et al., 2004).

Phase I and II trials for both radioantibodies have focused primarily on treatment of patients with relapsed or refractory low grade NHL. A number of phase II trials using either agent in patients with rituximab-refractory follicular, small B cell, and mantle cell NHL reported overall response rates of 57–83% (Davies et al., 2004; Horning et al., 2005; Vose et al., 2000; Wiseman et al., 2002; Witzig et al., 1999, 2002a). Both ^{131}I-tositumomab and ^{90}Y-ibritumomab tiuxetan have been compared to unlabeled tositumomab and rituximab, respectively in randomized trials. In a trial in which almost half the patients were deemed to be unresponsive to their immediate prior treatment, ^{90}Y-ibritumomab tiuxetan and rituximab 250 mg/m^2 × 2 doses was compared to rituximab 375 mg/m^2 weekly × 4 doses (Witzig et al., 2002b). Eighty percent of the patients treated with ^{90}Y-ibritumomab tiuxetan and rituximab responded compared to 56% of patients treated with rituximab alone ($p = 0.002$). The complete response rate was 30% in the ibritumomab tiuxetan group versus 16% in those patients treated with rituximab alone ($p = 0.04$). Iodine-131 tositumomab and tositumomab was compared to tositumomab alone (Davis et al., 2004). Two doses of unlabeled tositumomab were administered to patients in both arms of the trial. The overall response rate was higher for the radiolabeled antibody treated group, 55% versus 19% ($p = 0.002$) including CR, 33% versus 8% ($p = 0.012$). A recent trial of ^{131}I-tositumomab demonstrated remarkable activity in 76 previously untreated patients with stage III/IV follicular lymphoma with a response rate of 95%, with 75% CR and a median progression-free survival of 6.1 years (Kaminski et al., 2005).

Adverse events associated with both agents include infusion-related symptoms, cytokine release syndrome, and tumor lysis syndrome, especially in patients with high circulating B-cell counts. The major toxicity of both radiopharmaceuticals is bone marrow suppression especially thrombocytopenia and granulocytopenia usually occurring 5–7 weeks after treatment. Another concern is the induction of neutralizing HAMA since both agents are unmodified murine antibodies. The induction of HAMA can restrict patients to a single cycle of treatment, however, patients have undergone more than one treatment with either agent. Induction of HAMA is more frequent with ^{131}I-tositumomab and may be dose related. Patients treated with ^{90}Y-ibritumomab tiuxetan receive less than 100 mg of murine antibody, because the chimerized antibody rituximab is used in the cold phase of treatment. Patients treated with ^{131}I-tositumomab receive nearly 1000 mg of the unmodified murine antibody in a single treatment cycle. Induction of HAMA seen in up to 10% of ^{131}I-tositumomab treated patients compared to about 1% of patients receiving ^{90}Y-ibritumomab tiuxetan. The frequency of HAMA induction is also related to the amount of prior chemotherapy that a patient has received, occurring less frequently in heavily pretreated patients. A late effect of ^{131}I-tositumomab, is hypothyroidism that occurs in a small number of patients from the accumulation of ^{131}I in the thyroid. Myelodysplasia and secondary leukemias have been reported after treatment with either agent, but it is unclear if the incidence is increased over that already seen in NHL patients (Bennett et al., 2005; Witzig et al., 1999).

16. Conclusions and Future Prospects

Monoclonal antibodies have come of age and are being incorporated into the standard care of patients with cancer. Eight monoclonal antibodies have been approved by the FDA for the treatment of cancer. In addition, it has been reported that over 400 monoclonal antibodies or fragments are under clinical evaluation (Gura, 2002). In addition to the approved antibodies, a number of promising antibodies directed against novel targets including the insulin like growth factor receptor pathway, the IL-6 receptor, and CD2, CD4, CD22, and CD30 are being evaluated. Diverse approaches are being used to define additional cancer-associated antigens that could become the targets of new therapeutic monoclonal antibodies. For example, the technique of serologic identification by recombinant expression cloning (SEREX) is being used in cancer patients to identify circulating IgG antibodies that are specific for tumor antigens (Krackhardt et al., 2002). Screening cDNA libraries from tumor tissues using tumor reactive T-cell lines and clones from cancer patients is another approach that may lead to the identification of tumor antigenic targets. An alternative approach is to characterize tumor-associated peptides bound to Class I MHC molecules by mass spectrometry. Furthermore, the present intense effort in molecular profiling of cancer should provide additional useful antigenic targets for immunotherapy. One drawback in the use of monoclonal antibodies to date has been that they attach to proteins on the cell surface and only small quantities of the antibodies enter the cells. Future platforms that combine site-specific chemical conjugation and genetically engineered fusion proteins could be used to promote the intracellular transit of monoclonal antibodies. Combining a synthetic peptide membrane-translocator sequence to a monoclonal antibodies might allow the antibody to penetrate cells and target intracellular antigens (Zhao et al., 2003).

Promising new targets for antibody therapy of cancer include benign host cells and tissues. One advantage of this approach is that there is easier access for the very large monoclonal antibodies to such tissues than is provided by tumor cells within large tumor cell masses. An additional advantage is that normal tissue antigens are less likely to undergo a mutation of the epitope identified by the monoclonal antibody than are tumor cell antigens. Major efforts are being employed to target tumor neo-angiogenesis. Bevacizumab, a recombinant humanized monoclonal antibody to VEGF, has been approved by the FDA. In addition, antibodies to the VEGF receptor and the VEGF-TRAP composed of VEGF receptors fused to the Fc portion of human IgG are under development. Another anticancer strategy employs antibodies directed toward host-immune cells or proteins that act as checkpoints on the immune system. Agents under development include antibodies to CTLA-4 and PD1 inhibitory receptors to eliminate negative T-cells signaling pathways. Unmodified antibodies, anti-CD25 monoclonal antibody toxin fusion proteins and IL-2 toxin fusion chimeric molecules are focused on eliminating $CD4^+$ $CD25^+$, IL-2R alpha expressing Tregs (suppressor T cells). Furthermore, monoclonal antibodies and receptor Ig fusion chimeric molecules are being used to target the inhibitory cytokines IL-13 and TGF-beta.

A major contributor to the present optimism concerning monoclonal antibodies in cancer therapy reflects the results of genetic engineering that has been employed to increase the efficacy of monoclonal antibodies (Fig. 1). Humanized and fully human monoclonal antibodies have replaced murine monoclonal antibodies for cancer therapy thereby reducing immunogenicity, increasing effector action, and prolonging *in vivo* survival. Furthermore, the amino acid sequences of the antibody CDR have been altered to increase affinity of the antibody for its target. In addition, the Fc element of the monoclonal antibody has been modified to augment binding to the FcγRIII agonist receptor while reducing binding to the FcRγII inhibitory Fc receptor to ADCC toxic killing of the tumor cell. In addition, the Fc element of the IgG molecule has been modified to change binding of the antibody to the FcRn receptor to alter the *in vivo* pharmacokinetics of the antibody.

To circumvent the limitation that monoclonal antibodies have been relatively poor cytocidal agents, they are being armed with cytokines, chemotherapeutic agents, toxins, and radionuclides. Antibody toxin conjugates involving calicheamicin, maytansine, and auristatin molecules linked to antibodies directed to CD22, CD30, CD33, CD56, CD70, and the prostate antigen PSMA are under development. Radiolabeled monoclonal antibodies have also been developed as alternative immunoconjugates for the delivery of cytotoxic effector agents to target cells. There are radioimmunotherapy strategies being developed that address the major problem inherent in the use of intact monoclonal antibodies in systemic radioimmunotherapy—their limited ability to penetrate large solid tumor masses. A pretargeting approach that decouples the administration of the radionuclide from that of the antibody that involves a Streptavidin-A conjugated antibody, followed by the administration of DOTA-biotin armed with a radionuclide. This approach that permits an approximately tenfold increase in the dose of radionuclide that can be delivered safely to the tumor cells when compared to systemic radioimmunotherapy may represent a major alternative approach for future systemic radioimmunotherapy.

A number of clinical dosing strategies are being developed in the use of monoclonal antibodies. First of all, monoclonal antibodies are most effective when used in the adjuvant setting when there is a limited residual tumor burden (Riethmuller *et al.*, 1998). In conventional chemotherapeutic regimens the use of different cytotoxic drugs is a standard strategy that increases the response rate. A similar paradigm is emerging with the use of monoclonal antibodies. Clinical trials as well as preclinical tumor xenograft studies have demonstrated the superior efficacy of the combination of monoclonal antibodies with chemotherapeutic agents when compared with each drug used in isolation (Baselga *et al.*, 1998; Slamon *et al.*, 2001). It is probable with their low incidence of toxicities, which do not overlap those of chemotherapeutic agents, that the standard of care with virtually all monoclonal antibodies will involve combining them with anticancer drugs that have a different mode of action.

In summary, 30 years after their initial development, monoclonal antibodies have become established elements in the therapy of neoplasia. Articles characterizing this situation have reflected the present optimism by the use of such titles as "Therapeutic antibodies: magic bullets hit the target" and "Therapeutic mAbs: saving lives and making billions" (Gura, 2002; Stacy, 2005). We are approaching the vision of Paul Ehrlich of the "magic bullet" for cancer therapy by developing antibodies and chimeric molecules that are effective in cancer immunotherapy.

Acknowledgments

This research was supported by the Intramural Program of the NIH, NCI.

References

Adams, G. P., Schier, R., McCall, A. M., *et al.* (1998). Prolonged *in vivo* tumour retention of a human diabody targeting the extracellular domain of human HER2/neu. *Br. J. Cancer* **77**, 1405–1412.

Adams, G. P., and Weiner, L. M. (2005). Monoclonal antibody therapy of cancer. *Nat. Biotechnol.* **23**, 1147–1157.

Amadori, S., Suciu, S., Willemze, R., *et al.* (2004). Sequential administration of gemtuzumab ozogamicin and conventional chemotherapy as first line therapy in elderly patients with acute myeloid leukemia: A phase II study (AML-15) of the EORTC and GIMEMA leukemia groups. *Haematologica* **89**, 950–956.

Axworthy, D. B., Reno, J. M., Hylarides, M. D., *et al.* (2000). Cure of human carcinoma xenografts by a single dose of pretargeted yttrium-90 with negligible toxicity. *Proc. Natl. Acad. Sci. USA* **97**, 1802–1807.

Bagshawe, K. D. (1995). Antibody-directed enzyme prodrug therapy for cancer: Its theoretical basis and application. *Mol. Med. Today* **1**, 424–431.

Baselga, J., Norton, L., Albanell, J., *et al.* (1998). Recombinant humanized anti-HER2 antibody (Herceptin™) enhances the antitumor activity of paclitaxel and doxorubicin against HER2/neu overexpressing human breast cancer xenografts. *Cancer Res.* **58**, 2825–2831.

Baselga, J., Tripathy, D., Mendelsohn, J., *et al.* (1996). Phase II study of weekly intravenous recombinant humanized anti-p185HER2 monoclonal antibody in patients with HER2/neu-overexpressing metastatic breast cancer. *J. Clin. Oncol.* **14**, 737–744.

Baselga, J., Pfister, D., Cooper, M. R., *et al.* (2000). Phase I studies of anti-epidermal growth factor receptor chimeric antibody C225 alone and in combination with cisplatin. *J. Clin. Oncol.* **18**, 904–914.

Bennett, J. M., Kaminski, M. S., Leonard, J. P., *et al.* (2005). Assessment of treatment-related myelodysplastic syndromes and acute myeloid leukemia in patients with non-Hodgkin lymphoma treated with tositumomab and iodine I131 tositumomab. *Blood* **105**, 4576–4582.

Berinstein, N. L., Grillo-Lopez, A. J., White, C. A., *et al.* (1998). Association of serum rituximab (IDEC-C2B8) concentration and anti-tumor response in the treatment of recurrent low-grade or follicular non-Hodgkin's lymphoma. *Ann. Oncol.* **9**, 995–1001.

Bielekova, B., Richert, N., Howard, T., *et al.* (2004). Humanized anti-CD25 (daclizumab) inhibits disease activity in multiple sclerosis patients failing to respond to interferon beta. *Proc. Natl. Acad. Sci. USA* **101**, 8705–8708.

Bowen, A. L., Zomas, A., Emmett, E., *et al.* (1997). Subcutaneous CAMPATH-1H in fludarabine-resistant/relapsed chronic lymphocytic and B-prolymphocytic leukaemia. *Br. J. Haematol.* **96**, 617–619.

Burke, J. M., Caron, P. C., Papadopoulos, E. B., *et al.* (2003). Cytoreduction with iodine-131-anti-CD33 antibodies before bone marrow transplantation for advanced myeloid leukemias. *Bone Marrow Transplant.* **32**, 549–556.

Carter, P. (2001). Improving the efficacy of antibody-based cancer therapies. *Nat. Rev. Cancer* **1**, 118–129.

Carter, P., and McDonagh, C. F. (2005). Designer antibody-based therapeutics for oncology. *In* 7th International Congress on monoclonal antibodies. Physicians Education Publisher, Dallas, Texas, pp. 147–154.

Carter, P., Presta, L., Gorman, C. M., *et al.* (1992). Humanization of an anti-p185HER2 antibody for human cancer therapy. *Proc. Natl. Acad. Sci. USA* **89**, 4285–4289.

Cartron, G., Dacheux, L., Salles, G., *et al.* (2002). Therapeutic activity of humanized anti-CD20 monoclonal antibody and polymorphism in IgG Fc receptor FcgammaRIIIa gene. *Blood* **99**, 754–758.

Chester, K., Pedley, B., Tolner, B., et al. (2004). Engineering antibodies for clinical applications in cancer. *Tumor Biol.* **25**, 91–98.

Chinn, P. C., Leonard, J. E., Rosenberg, J., et al. (1999). Preclinical evaluation of 90Y-labeled anti-CD20 monoclonal antibody for treatment of non-Hodgkin's lymphoma. *Int. J. Oncol.* **15**, 1017–1025.

Clynes, R. A., Towers, T. L., Presta, L. G., et al. (2000). Inhibitory Fc receptors modulate *in vivo* cytotoxicity against tumor targets. *Nat. Med.* **6**, 443–446.

Cobleigh, M. A., Vogel, C. L., Tripathy, D., et al. (1999). Multinational study of the efficacy and safety of humanized anti-HER2 monoclonal antibody in women who have HER2-overexpressing metastatic breast cancer that has progressed after chemotherapy for metastatic disease. *J. Clin. Oncol.* **17**, 2639–2648.

Coiffier, B., Lepage, E., Briere, J., et al. (2002). CHOP chemotherapy plus rituximab compared with CHOP alone in elderly patients with diffuse large-B-cell lymphoma. *N. Engl. J. Med.* **346**, 235–242.

Coles, A. J., Wing, M., Smith, S., et al. (1999). Pulsed monoclonal antibody treatment and autoimmune thyroid disease in multiple sclerosis. *Lancet* **354**, 1691–1695.

Cunningham, D., Humblet, Y., Siena, S., et al. (2004). Cetuximab monotherapy and cetuximab plus irinotecan in irinotecan-refractory metastatic colorectal cancer. *N. Engl. J. Med.* **351**, 337–345.

Davies, A. J., Rohatiner, A. Z., Howell, S., et al. (2004). Tositumomab and iodine I 131 tositumomab for recurrent indolent and transformed B-cell non-Hodgkin's lymphoma. *J. Clin. Oncol.* **22**, 1469–1479.

Davis, T. A., Grillo-Lopez, A. J., White, C. A., et al. (2000). Rituximab anti-CD20 monoclonal antibody therapy in non-Hodgkin's lymphoma: Safety and efficacy of re-treatment. *J. Clin. Oncol.* **18**, 3135–3143.

Davis, T. A., Kaminski, M. S., Leonard, J. P., et al. (2004). The radioisotope contributes significantly to the activity of radioimmunotherapy. *Clin. Cancer Res.* **10**, 7792–7798.

Denny, W. A. (2004). Tumor-activated prodrugs—a new approach to cancer therapy. *Cancer Invest.* **22**, 604–619.

De Santes, K., Slamon, D., Anderson, S. K., et al. (1992). Radiolabeled antibody targeting of the HER-2/neu oncoprotein. *Cancer Res.* **52**, 1916–1923.

Di Gaetano, N., Cittera, E., Nota, R., et al. (2003). Complement activation determines the therapeutic activity of rituximab *in vivo*. *J. Immunol.* **171**, 1581–1587.

Dinndorf, P. A., Andrews, R. G., Benjamin, D., et al. (1986). Expression of normal myeloid-associated antigens by acute leukemia cells. *Blood* **67**, 1048–1053.

Dong, H., Strome, S. E., Salomao, D. R., et al. (2002). Tumor-associated B7-H1 promotes T-cell apoptosis: A potential mechanism of immune evasion. *Nat. Med.* **8**, 793–800.

Dowell, J. A., Korth-Bradley, J., Liu, H., et al. (2001). Pharmacokinetics of gemtuzumab ozogamicin, an antibody-targeted chemotherapy agent for the treatment of patients with acute myeloid leukemia in first relapse. *J. Clin. Pharmacol.* **41**, 1206–1214.

Dowsett, M., Bartlett, J., Ellis, I. O., et al. (2003). Correlation between immunohistochemistry (HercepTest) and fluorescence *in situ* hybridization (FISH) for HER-2 in 426 breast carcinomas from 37 centres. *J. Pathol.* **199**, 418–423.

Dranoff, G. (2004). Cytokines in cancer pathogenesis and cancer therapy. *Nat. Rev. Cancer* **4**, 11–22.

Dranoff, G. (2005). CTLA-4 blockade: Unveiling immune regulation. *J. Clin. Oncol.* **23**, 662–664.

Dupont, J., Rothenberg, M., Springs, D., et al. (2005). Safety and pharmacokinetics of intravenous VEGF trap in a Phase I clinical trial of patients with advanced solid tumors. *J. Clin. Oncol.* **23** (Suppl. 16S), 3029.

Ehrlich, P. (1956). On immunity with special reference to cell life: Croonian lecture. In "The Collected Papers of Paul Ehrlich" (B. Himmelweir, Ed.), Vol. II, pp. 148–192, 195–196. Immunology and Cancer Research, Pergammon, London.

Essand, M., Gronvik, C., Hartman, T., et al. (1995). Radioimmunotherapy of prostatic adenocarcinomas: Effects of 131I-labelled E4 antibodies on cells at different depth in DU 145 spheroids. Int. J. Cancer **63**, 387–394.

Fan, Z., Masui, H., Altas, I., and Mendelsohn, J. (1993). Blockade of epidermal growth factor receptor function by bivalent and monovalent fragments of 225 anti-epidermal growth factor receptor monoclonal antibodies. Cancer Res. **53**, 4322–4328.

Flavell, R. A., and Gorelik, L. (2002). Transforming growth factor-B in T cell biology. Nat. Rev. Immunol. **2**, 46–53.

Freeman, G. J., Long, A. J., Iwai, Y., et al. (2000). Engagement of the PD-1 immunoinhibitory receptor by a novel B7 family member leads to negative regulation of lymphocyte activation. J. Exp. Med. **192**, 1027–1034.

Freeman, S. D., Kelm, S., Barber, E. K., et al. (1995). Characterization of CD33 as a new member of the sialoadhesin family of cellular interaction molecules. Blood **85**, 2005–2012.

Gabrilovich, D., Ishida, T., Oyama, T., et al. (1998). Vascular endothelial growth factor inhibits the development of dendritic cells and dramatically affects the differentiation of multiple hematopoietic lineages in vivo. Blood **92**, 4150–4166.

Gerber, H. P., and Ferrara, N. (2005). Pharmacology and pharmacodynamics of bevacizumab as monotherapy or in combination with cytotoxic therapy in preclinical studies. Cancer Res. **65**, 671–680.

Goldstein, G. (1986). An overview of Orthoclone OKT3 transplantation proceedings. In "Proceedings of an International Symposium on Monoclonal Antibody Therapy with Orthoclone OKT3 in Renal Transplantation." Transplant. Proc. **18**, 927–930.

Goldstein, N. I., Prewett, M., Zuklys, K., et al. (1995). Biological efficacy of a chimeric antibody to the epidermal growth factor receptor in a human tumor xenograft model. Clin. Cancer Res. **1**, 1311–1318.

Gordon, M. S., Margolin, K., Talpaz, M., et al. (2001). Phase I safety and pharmacokinetic study of recombinant human anti-vascular endothelial growth factor in patients with advanced cancer. J. Clin. Oncol. **19**, 843–850.

Gorelik, L., and Flavell, R. A. (2001). Immune-mediated eradication of tumors through the blockade of transforming growth factor-beta signaling in T cells. Nat. Med. **7**, 1118–1122.

Grazette, L. P., Boecker, W., Matsui, T., et al. (2004). Inhibition of ErbB2 causes mitochondrial dysfunction in cardiomyocytes: Implications for herceptin-induced cardiomyopathy. J. Am. Coll. Cardiol. **44**, 2231–2238.

Gura, T. (2002). Therapeutic antibodies: Magic bullets hit the target. Nature **417**, 584–586.

Hale, G., Bright, S., Chumbley, G., et al. (1983). Removal of T cells from bone marrow for transplantation: A monoclonal antilymphocyte antibody that fixes human complement. Blood **62**, 873–882.

Hale, G., Dyer, M. J., Clark, M. R., et al. (1988). Remission induction in non-Hodgkin lymphoma with reshaped human monoclonal antibody CAMPATH-1H. Lancet **2**, 1394–1399.

Hamann, P. R., Hinman, L. M., Hollander, I., et al. (2002). Gemtuzumab ozogamicin, a potent and selective anti-CD33 antibody-calicheamicin conjugate for treatment of acute myeloid leukemia. Bioconjug. Chem. **13**, 47–58.

Herbst, R. S., Arquette, M., Shin, D. M., et al. (2005). Phase II multicenter study of the epidermal growth factor receptor antibody cetuximab and cisplatin for recurrent and refractory squamous cell carcinoma of the head and neck. J. Clin. Oncol. **23**, 5578–5587.

Herbst, R. S., Kim, E. S., and Harari, P. M. (2001). IMC-C225, an anti-epidermal growth factor receptor monoclonal antibody, for treatment of head and neck cancer. *Expert Opin. Biol. Ther.* **1**, 719–732.

Hericourt, J., and Richet, C. (1895). Physologie pathologique'—de la serotherapie dans la traitement du cancer. *C.R. Hebd. Seanc. Acad. Sci.* **121**, 567.

Hicklin, D. J., and Ellis, L. M. (2005). Role of the vascular endothelial growth factor pathway in tumor growth and angiogenesis. *J. Clin. Oncol.* **23**, 1011–1027.

Hinton, P. R., Johlfs, M. G., Xiong, J. M., et al. (2004). Engineered human IgG antibodies with longer serum half-lives in primates. *J. Biol. Chem.* **279**, 6213–6216.

Hodi, F. S., Mihm, M. C., Soiffer, R. J., et al. (2003). Biologic activity of cytotoxic T lymphocyte-associated antigen 4 antibody blockade in previously vaccinated metastatic melanoma and ovarian carcinoma patients. *Proc. Natl. Acad. Sci. USA* **100**, 4712–4717.

Hoeben, A., Landuyt, B., Highley, M. S., et al. (2004). Vascular endothelial growth factor and angiogenesis. *Pharmacol. Rev.* **56**, 549–580.

Horning, S. J., Younes, A., Jain, V., et al. (2005). Efficacy and safety of tositumomab and iodine-131 tositumomab (Bexxar) in B-cell lymphoma, progressive after rituximab. *J. Clin. Oncol.* **23**, 712–719.

Hudson, P. J., and Souriau, C. (2003). Engineered antibodies. *Nat. Med.* **9**, 129–134.

Hurwitz, A. A., Foster, B. A., Kwon, E. D., et al. (2000). Combination immunotherapy of primary prostate cancer in a transgenic mouse model using CTLA-4 blockade. *Cancer Res.* **60**, 2444–2448.

Hurwitz, H., Fehrenbacher, L., Novotny, W., et al. (2004). Bevacizumab plus irinotecan, fluorouracil, and leucovorin for metastatic colorectal cancer. *N. Engl. J. Med.* **350**, 2335–2342.

Isaacs, J. D., Watts, R. A., Hazleman, B. L., et al. (1992). Humanised monoclonal antibody therapy for rheumatoid arthritis. *Lancet* **340**, 748–752.

Iwai, Y., Ishida, M., Tanaka, Y., et al. (2002). Involvement of PD-L1 on tumor cells in the escape from host immune system and tumor immunotherapy by PD-L1 blockade. *Proc. Natl. Acad. Sci. USA* **99**, 12293–12297.

Izumi, Y., Xu, L., di Tomaso, E., et al. (2002). Tumour biology: Herceptin acts as an anti-angiogenic cocktail. *Nature* **416**, 279–280.

Jain, R. K. (2001). Delivery of molecular and cellular medicine to solid tumors. *Adv. Drug Deliv. Rev.* **46**, 149–168.

Junghans, R. P., and Anderson, C. L. (1996). The protection receptor for IgG catabolism is the beta2-microglobulin-containing neonatal intestinal transport receptor. *Proc. Natl. Acad. Sci. USA* **93**, 5512–5516.

Jurcic, J. G., Larson, S. M., Sgouros, G., et al. (2002). Targeted alpha particle immunotherapy for myeloid leukemia. *Blood* **100**, 1233–1239.

Kabbinavar, F., Hurwitz, H. I., Fehrenbacher, L., et al. (2003). Phase II, randomized trial comparing bevacizumab plus fluorouracil (FU)/leucovorin (LV) with FU/LV alone in patients with metastatic colorectal cancer. *J. Clin. Oncol.* **21**, 60–65.

Kaminski, M. S., Zasadny, K. R., Francis, I. R., et al. (1996). Iodine-131-anti-B1 radioimmunotherapy for B-cell lymphoma. *J. Clin. Oncol.* **14**, 1974–1981.

Kaminski, M. S., Tuck, M., Estes, J., et al. (2005). ^{131}I-tositumomab therapy as initial treatment for follicular lymphoma. *N. Engl. J. Med.* **352**, 441–449.

Keating, M. J., Flinn, I., Jain, V., et al. (2002). Therapeutic role of alemtuzumab (Campath-1H) in patients who have failed fludarabine: Results of a large international study. *Blood* **99**, 3554–3561.

Kell, W. J., Burnett, A. K., Chopra, R., et al. (2003). A feasibility study of simultaneous administration of gemtuzumab ozogamicin with intensive chemotherapy in induction and consolidation in younger patients with acute myeloid leukemia. *Blood* **102**, 4277–4283.

Kennedy, B., Rawstron, A., Carter, C., et al. (2002). Campath-1H and fludarabine in combination are highly active in refractory chronic lymphocytic leukemia. *Blood* **99**, 2245–2247.

Khorana, A., Bunn, P., McLaughlin, P., et al. (2001). A phase II multicenter study of CAMPATH-1H antibody in previously treated patients with nonbulky non-Hodgkin's lymphoma. *Leuk. Lymphoma* **41**, 77–87.

Kim, K. J., Li, B., Winer, J., et al. (1993). Inhibition of vascular endothelial growth factor-induced angiogenesis suppresses tumour growth *in vivo*. *Nature* **362**, 841–844.

Koene, H. R., Kleijer, M., Algra, J., et al. (1997). Fc gammaRIIIa-158V/F polymorphism influences the binding of IgG by natural killer cell Fc gammaRIIIa, independently of the Fc gammaRIIIa-48L/R/H phenotype. *Blood* **90**, 1109–1114.

Köhler, G., and Milstein, C. (1975). Continuous cultures of fused cells secreting antibody of predefined specificity. *Nature* **256**, 495–497.

Krackhardt, A. M., Witzens, M., Harig, S., et al. (2002). Identification of tumor-associated antigens in chronic lymphocytic leukemia by SEREX. *Blood* **100**, 2123–2131.

Kreitman, R. J. (2003). Recombinant toxins for the treatment of cancer. *Curr. Opin. Mol. Ther.* **5**, 44–51.

Kreitman, R. J., Wilson, W. H., White, J. D., et al. (2000). Phase I trial of recombinant immunotoxin anti-Tac(Fv)-PE38 (LMB-2) in patients with hematologic malignancies. *J. Clin. Oncol.* **18**, 1622–1636.

Kreitman, R. J., Wilson, W. H., Bergeron, K., et al. (2001). Efficacy of the anti-CD22 recombinant immunotoxin BL22 in chemotherapy-resistant hairy-cell leukemia. *N. Engl. J. Med.* **345**, 241–247.

Ku, C. C., Murakami, M., Sakamoto, A., et al. (2000). Control of homeostasis of $CD8^+$ memory T cells by opposing cytokines. *Science* **288**, 675–678.

Kwon, E. D., Foster, B. A., Hurwitz, A. A., et al. (1999). Elimination of residual metastatic prostate cancer after surgery and adjunctive cytotoxic T lymphocyte-associated antigen 4 (CTLA-4) blockade immunotherapy. *Proc. Natl. Acad. Sci. USA* **96**, 15074–15079.

Larson, R. A., Sievers, E. L., Stadtmauer, E. A., et al. (2005). Final report of the efficacy and safety of gemtuzumab ozogamicin (mylotarg) in patients with CD33 positive acute myeloid leukemia in first recurrence. *Cancer* **104**, 1442–1452.

Laurenti, L., Piccioni, P., Cattani, P., et al. (2004). Cytomegalovirus reactivation during alemtuzumab therapy for chronic lymphocytic leukemia: Incidence and treatment with oral ganciclovir. *Haematologica* **89**, 1248–1252.

Leach, D. R., Krummel, M. F., and Allison, J. P. (1996). Enhancement of antitumor immunity by CTLA-4 blockade. *Science* **271**, 1734–1736.

Lee, C. G., Heijn, M., di Tomaso, E., et al. (2000). Anti-vascular endothelial growth factor treatment augments tumor radiation response under normoxic or hypoxic conditions. *Cancer Res.* **60**, 5565–5570.

Lenardo, M. J. (1996). Fas and the art of lymphocyte maintenance. *J. Exp. Med.* **183**, 721–724.

Lewis, G. D., Figari, I., Fendly, B., et al. (1993). Differential responses of human tumor cell lines to anti-p185HER2 monoclonal antibodies. *Cancer Immunol. Immunother.* **37**, 255–263.

Linenberger, M. L. (2005). CD33-directed therapy with gemtuzumab ozogamicin in acute myeloid leukemia: Progress in understanding cytotoxicity and potential mechanisms of drug resistance. *Leukemia* **19**, 176–182.

Linenberger, M. L., Hong, T., Flowers, D., et al. (2001). Multidrug-resistance phenotype and clinical responses to gemtuzumab ozogamicin. *Blood* **98**, 988–994.

Lode, H. N., and Reisfeld, R. A. (2000). Targeted cytokines for cancer immunotherapy. *Immunol. Res.* **21**, 279–288.

Lowenberg, B., Downing, J. R., and Burnett, A. (1999). Acute myeloid leukemia. *N. Engl. J. Med.* **341**, 1051–1062.

Lozanski, G., Heerema, N. A., Flinn, I. W., *et al.* (2004). Alemtuzumab is an effective therapy for chronic lymphocytic leukemia with p53 mutations and deletions. *Blood* **103**, 3278–3281.

Lundin, J., Osterborg, A., Brittinger, G., *et al.* (1998). CAMPATH-1H monoclonal antibody in therapy for previously treated low-grade non-Hodgkin's lymphomas: A phase II multicenter study. European Study Group of CAMPATH-1H Treatment in Low-Grade Non-Hodgkin's Lymphoma. *J. Clin. Oncol.* **16**, 3257–3263.

Maloney, D. G., Liles, T. M., Czerwinski, D. K., *et al.* (1994). Phase I clinical trial using escalating single-dose infusion of chimeric anti-CD20 monoclonal antibody (IDEC-C2B8) in patients with recurrent B-cell lymphoma. *Blood* **84**, 2457–2466.

Maloney, D. G., Grillo-Lopez, A. J., Bodkin, D. J., *et al.* (1997). IDEC-C2B8: Results of a phase I multiple-dose trial in patients with relapsed non-Hodgkin's lymphoma. *J. Clin. Oncol.* **15**, 3266–3274.

Margolin, K., Gordon, M. S., Holmgren, E., *et al.* (2001). Phase Ib trial of intravenous recombinant humanized monoclonal antibody to vascular endothelial growth factor in combination with chemotherapy in patients with advanced cancer: Pharmacologic and long-term safety data. *J. Clin. Oncol.* **19**, 851–856.

Marks-Konczalik, J., Dubois, S., Losi, J. M., *et al.* (2000). IL-2-induced activation-induced cell death is inhibited in IL-15 transgenic mice. *Proc. Natl. Acad. Sci. USA* **97**, 11445–11450.

McLaughlin, P., Grillo-Lopez, A. J., Link, B. K., *et al.* (1998). Rituximab chimeric anti-CD20 monoclonal antibody therapy for relapsed indolent lymphoma: Half of patients respond to a four-dose treatment program. *J. Clin. Oncol.* **16**, 2825–2833.

Mendelsohn, J. (1997). Epidermal growth factor receptor inhibition by a monoclonal antibody as anticancer therapy. *Clin. Cancer Res.* **3**, 2703–2707.

Mendelsohn, J., and Baselga, J. (2000). The EGF receptor family as targets for cancer therapy. *Oncogene* **19**, 6550–6565.

Milenic, D. E., Brady, E. D., and Brechbiel, M. W. (2004). Antibody-targeted radiation cancer therapy. *Nat. Rev. Drug. Discov.* **3**, 488–499.

Miller, R. A., Maloney, D. G., Warnke, R., *et al.* (1982). Treatment of B-cell lymphoma with monoclonal anti-idiotype antibody. *N. Engl. J. Med.* **306**, 517–522.

Mir, S. S., Richter, B. W., and Duckett, C. S. (2000). Differential effects of CD30 activation in anaplastic large cell lymphoma and Hodgkin disease cells. *Blood* **96**, 4307–4312.

Morris, J. C., and Waldmann, T. A. (2000). Advances in interleukin 2 receptor targeted treatment. *Ann. Rheum. Dis.* **59**(Suppl. 1), i109–i114.

Mulford, D. A., Scheinberg, D. A., and Jurcic, J. G. (2005). The promise of targeted (alpha)-particle therapy. *J. Nucl. Med.* **46**(suppl. 1), 199S–204S.

Nadler, L. M., Ritz, J., Hardy, R., *et al.* (1981). A unique cell surface antigen identifying lymphoid malignancies of B cell origin. *J. Clin. Invest.* **67**, 134–140.

Naito, K., Takeshita, A., Shigeno, K., *et al.* (2000). Calicheamicin-conjugated humanized anti-CD33 monoclonal antibody (gemtuzumab zogamicin, CMA-676) shows cytocidal effect on CD33-positive leukemia cell lines, but is inactive on P-glycoprotein-expressing sublines. *Leukemia* **14**, 1436–1443.

Nimmerjahn, F., Bruhns, P., Horiuchi, K., *et al.* (2005). FcgammaRIV: A novel FcR with distinct IgG subclass specificity. *Immunity* **23**, 41–51.

Nussenblatt, R. B., Fortin, E., Schiffman, R., *et al.* (1999). Treatment of noninfectious intermediate and posterior uveitis with the humanized anti-Tac mAb: A phase I/II clinical trial. *Proc. Natl. Acad. Sci. USA* **96**, 7462–7466.

Olafsen, T., Tan, G. J., Cheung, C. W., et al. (2004). Characterization of engineered anti-p185^{HER-2} (scFv-CH3)$_2$ antibody fragments for tumor targeting. *Protein Eng. Des. Sel.* **17**, 315–323.

Olsen, E., Duvic, M., Frankel, A., et al. (2001). Pivotal phase III trial of two dose levels of denileukin diftitox for the treatment of cutaneous T-cell lymphoma. *J. Clin. Oncol.* **19**, 376–388.

Osterborg, A., Dyer, M. J., Bunjes, D., et al. (1997). Phase II multicenter study of human CD52 antibody in previously treated chronic lymphocytic leukemia. European Study Group of CAMPATH-1H Treatment in Chronic Lymphocytic Leukemia. *J. Clin. Oncol.* **15**, 1567–1574.

Osterborg, A., Fassas, A. S., Anagnostopoulos, A., et al. (1996). Humanized CD52 monoclonal antibody Campath-1H as first-line treatment in chronic lymphocytic leukaemia. *Br. J. Haematol.* **93**, 151–153.

Pegram, M., Hsu, S., Lewis, G., et al. (1999). Inhibitory effects of combinations of HER-2/neu antibody and chemotherapeutic agents used for treatment of human breast cancers. *Oncogene* **18**, 2241–2251.

Piro, L. D., White, C. A., Grillo-Lopez, A. J., et al. (1999). Extended Rituximab (anti-CD20 monoclonal antibody) therapy for relapsed or refractory low-grade or follicular non-Hodgkin's lymphoma. *Ann. Oncol.* **10**, 655–661.

Phan, G. Q., Yang, J. C., Sherry, R. M., et al. (2003). Cancer regression and autoimmunity induced by cytotoxic T lymphocyte-associated antigen 4 blockade in patients with metastatic melanoma. *Proc. Natl. Acad. Sci. USA* **100**, 8372–8377.

Press, O. W., Corcoran, M., Subbiah, K., et al. (2001). A comparative evaluation of conventional and pretargeted radioimmunotherapy of CD20-expressing lymphoma xenografts. *Blood* **98**, 2535–2543.

Press, O. W., Eary, J. F., Appelbaum, F. R., et al. (1995). Phase II trial of ^{131}I-B1 (anti-CD20) antibody therapy with autologous stem cell transplantation for relapsed B cell lymphomas. *Lancet* **346**, 336–340.

Press, O. W., Shan, D., Howell-Clark, J., et al. (1996). Comparative metabolism and retention of iodine-125, yttrium-90, and indium-111 radioimmunoconjugates by cancer cells. *Cancer Res.* **56**, 2123–2129.

Presta, L. G., Chen, H., O'Connor, S. J., et al. (1997). Humanization of an anti-vascular endothelial growth factor monoclonal antibody for the therapy of solid tumors and other disorders. *Cancer Res.* **57**, 4593–4599.

Queen, C., Schneider, W. P., Selick, H. E., et al. (1989). A humanized antibody that binds to the interleukin 2 receptor. *Proc. Natl. Acad. Sci. USA* **86**, 10029–10033.

Rai, K. R., Freter, C. E., Mercier, R. J., et al. (2002). Alemtuzumab in previously treated chronic lymphocytic leukemia patients who also had received fludarabine. *J. Clin. Oncol.* **20**, 3891–3897.

Ravetch, J. V., and Lanier, L. L. (2000). Immune inhibitory receptors. *Science* **290**, 84–89.

Rebello, P., Cwynarski, K., Varughese, M., et al. (2001). Pharmacokinetics of CAMPATH-1H in BMT patients. *Cytotherapy* **3**, 261–267.

Reff, M. E., Carner, K., Chambers, K. S., et al. (1994). Depletion of B cells in vivo by a chimeric mouse human monoclonal antibody to CD20. *Blood* **83**, 435–445.

Riechmann, L., Clark, M., Waldmann, H., et al. (1988). Reshaping human antibodies for therapy. *Nature* **332**, 323–327.

Riethmuller, G., Holz, E., Schlimok, G., et al. (1998). Monoclonal antibody therapy for resected Dukes' C colorectal cancer: Seven-year outcome of a multicenter randomized trial. *J. Clin. Oncol.* **16**, 1788–1794.

Robert, F., Ezekiel, M. P., Spencer, S. A., et al. (2001). Phase I study of anti-epidermal growth factor receptor antibody cetuximab in combination with radiation therapy in patients with advanced head and neck cancer. *J. Clin. Oncol.* **19,** 3234–3243.

Romond, E. H., Perez, E. A., Bryant, J., et al. (2005). Trastuzumab plus adjuvant chemotherapy for operable HER-2 positive breast cancer. *N. Engl. J. Med.* **353,** 1673–1684.

Rosenberg, S. A., Yang, J. C., Topalian, S. L., et al. (1994). Treatment of 283 consecutive patients with metastatic melanoma or renal cell cancer using high-dose bolus interleukin-2. *JAMA* **271,** 907–913.

Sakaguchi, S. (2004). Naturally arising CD4+ regulatory T cells for immunologic self-tolerance and negative control of immune responses. *Annu. Rev. Immunol.* **22,** 531–562.

Saltz, L. B., Meropol, N. J., Loehrer, P. J., Sr., et al. (2004). Phase II trial of cetuximab in patients with refractory colorectal cancer that expresses the epidermal growth factor receptor. *J. Clin. Oncol.* **22,** 1201–1208.

Schwartzentruber, D. J., Restifo, N. P., Haworth, L. R., et al. (2003). Cancer regression induced by cytotoxic T-lymphocytes associated antigen 4-blockade in patients with metastatic melanoma. *Proc. Natl. Acad. Sci. USA* **100,** 8372–8377.

Segal, D. M., Weiner, G. J., and Weiner, L. M. (2001). Introduction: Bispecific antibodies. *J. Immunol. Methods* **248,** 1–6.

Seidman, A., Hudis, C., Pierri, M. K., et al. (2002). Cardiac dysfunction in the trastuzumab clinical trials experience. *J. Clin. Oncol.* **20,** 1215–1221.

Shevach, E. M. (2000). Regulatory T cells in autoimmmunity. *Annu. Rev. Immunol.* **18,** 423–449.

Shields, R. L., Namenuk, A. K., Hong, K., et al. (2001). High resolution mapping of the binding site on human IgG1 for Fc gamma RI, Fc gamma RII, Fc gamma RIII, and FcRn and design of IgG1 variants with improved binding to the Fc gamma R. *J. Biol. Chem.* **276,** 6591–6604.

Shimizu, J., Yamazaki, S., and Sakaguchi, S. (1999). Induction of tumor immunity by removing CD25+CD4+ T cells: A common basis between tumor immunity and autoimmunity. *J. Immunol.* **163,** 5211–5218.

Shin, D. M., Donato, N. J., Perez-Soler, R., et al. (2001). Epidermal growth factor receptor targeted therapy with C225 and cisplatin in patients with head and neck cancer. *Clin. Cancer Res.* **7,** 1204–1213.

Shinkawa, T., Nakamura, K., Yamane, N., et al. (2003). The absence of fucose but not the presence of galactose or bisecting N-acetylglucosamine of human IgG1 complex-type oligosaccharides shows the critical role of enhancing antibody-dependent cellular cytotoxicity. *J. Biol. Chem.* **278,** 3466–3473.

Sievers, E. L., Appelbaum, F. R., Spielberger, R. T., et al. (1999). Selective ablation of acute myeloid leukemia using antibody-targeted chemotherapy: A phase I study of an anti-CD33 calicheamicin immunoconjugate. *Blood* **93,** 3678–3684.

Sievers, E. L., Larson, R. A., Stadtmauer, E. A., et al. (2001). Efficacy and safety of gemtuzumab ozogamicin in patients with CD33-positive acute myeloid leukemia in first relapse. *J. Clin. Oncol.* **19,** 3244–3254.

Slamon, D. J., Clark, G. M., Wong, S. G., et al. (1987). Human breast cancer: Correlation of relapse and survival with amplification of the HER-2/neu oncogene. *Science* **235,** 177–182.

Slamon, D. J., Leyland-Jones, B., Shak, S., et al. (2001). Use of chemotherapy plus a monoclonal antibody against HER2 for metastatic breast cancer that overexpresses HER2. *N. Engl. J. Med.* **344,** 783–792.

Sliwkowski, M. X., Lofgren, J. A., Lewis, G. D., et al. (1999). Nonclinical studies addressing the mechanism of action of trastuzumab (Herceptin). *Semin. Oncol.* **26,** 60–70.

Smith, M. R. (2003). Rituximab (monoclonal anti-CD20 antibody): Mechanisms of action and resistance. *Oncogene* **22,** 7359–7368.

Stacy, K. (2005). Therapeutic MAbs: Saving lives and making billions. *The Scientist* **19**, 17–19.
Staerz, U. D., Kanagawa, O., and Bevan, M. J. (1985). Hybrid antibodies can target sites for attack by T cells. *Nature* **314**, 628–631.
Stashenko, P., Nadler, L. M., Hardy, R., et al. (1981). Expression of cell surface markers after human B lymphocyte activation. *Proc. Natl. Acad. Sci. USA* **78**, 3848–3852.
Sunada, H., Magun, B. E., Mendelsohn, J., et al. (1986). Monoclonal antibody against epidermal growth factor receptor is internalized without stimulating receptor phosphorylation. *Proc. Natl. Acad. Sci. USA* **83**, 3825–3829.
Sutmuller, R. P., van Duivenvoorde, L. M., van Elsas, A., et al. (2001). Synergism of cytotoxic T lymphocyte-associated antigen 4 blockade and depletion of CD25(+) regulatory T cells in antitumor therapy reveals alternative pathways for suppression of autoreactive cytotoxic T lymphocyte responses. *J. Exp. Med.* **194**, 823–832.
Terabe, M., Matsui, S., Noben-Trauth, N., et al. (2000). NKT cell-mediated repression of tumor immunosurveillance by IL-13 and the IL-4R-STAT6 pathway. *Nat. Immunol.* **1**, 515–520.
Thornton, A. M., and Shevach, E. M. (2000). Suppressor effector function of CD4+CD25+ immunoregulatory T cells is antigen nonspecific. *J. Immunol.* **164**, 183–190.
Treumann, A., Lifely, M. R., Schneider, P., et al. (1995). Primary structure of CD52. *J. Biol. Chem.* **270**, 6088–6099.
Tsimberidou, A., Estey, E., Cortes, J., et al. (2003). Gemtuzumab, fludarabine, cytarabine, and cyclosporine in patients with newly diagnosed acute myelogenous leukemia or high-risk myelodysplastic syndromes. *Cancer* **97**, 1481–1487.
Uppenkamp, M., Engert, A., Diehl, V., et al. (2002). Monoclonal antibody therapy with CAMPATH-1H in patients with relapsed high- and low-grade non-Hodgkin's lymphomas: A multicenter phase I/II study. *Ann. Hematol.* **81**, 26–32.
van der Velden, V. H., Boeckx, N., Jedema, I., et al. (2004). High CD33-antigen loads in peripheral blood limit the efficacy of gemtuzumab ozogamicin (Mylotarg) treatment in acute myeloid leukemia patients. *Leukemia* **18**, 983–988.
van Der Velden, V. H., te Marvelde, J. G., Hoogeveen, P. G., et al. (2001). Targeting of the CD33-calicheamicin immunoconjugate Mylotarg (CMA-676) in acute myeloid leukemia: In vivo and in vitro saturation and internalization by leukemic and normal myeloid cells. *Blood* **97**, 3197–3204.
Vincenti, F., Kirkman, R., Light, S., et al. (1998). Interleukin-2-receptor blockade with daclizumab to prevent acute rejection in renal transplantation. Daclizumab Triple Therapy Study Group. *N. Engl. J. Med.* **338**, 161–165.
Vogel, C. L., Cobleigh, M. A., Tripathy, D., et al. (2002). Efficacy and safety of trastuzumab as a single agent in first-line treatment of HER2-overexpressing metastatic breast cancer. *J. Clin. Oncol.* **20**, 719–726.
von Behring, E., and Kitasato, S. (1890). The mechanism of immunity in animals to diphtheria and tetanus. In "Milestones in Microbiology" (T. Brock, Ed.), pp. 138–140. Prentice-Hall Int., London.
von Mehren, M., Adams, G. P., and Weiner, L. M. (2003). Monoclonal antibody therapy for cancer. *Annu. Rev. Med.* **54**, 343–369.
Vose, J. M., Wahl, R. L., Saleh, M., et al. (2000). Multicenter phase II study of iodine-131 tositumomab for chemotherapy-relapsed/refractory low-grade and transformed low-grade B-cell non-Hodgkin's lymphomas. *J. Clin. Oncol.* **18**, 1316–1323.
Wahl, R. L. (2005). Tositumomab and (131) I therapy in non-Hodgkin's lymphoma. *J. Nucl. Med.* **46**(Suppl. 1), 165–175.
Waldmann, T. A. (1991). Monoclonal antibodies in diagnosis and therapy. *Science* **252**, 1657–1662.
Waldmann, T. (2003a). ABCsv of radioisotopes used for radioimmunotherapy: Alpha- and beta-emitters. *Leuk. Lymphoma* **44**(suppl. 3), S107–S113.

Waldmann, T. (2003b). Immunotherapy: Past, present and future. *Nat. Med.* **9**, 269–277.

Waldmann, T. A., and Strober, W. (1969). Metabolism of immunoglobulins. *Prog. Allergy* **13**, 1–110.

Waldmann, T. A., White, J. D., Goldman, C. K., et al. (1993). The interleukin-2 receptor: A target for monoclonal antibody treatment of human T-cell lymphotropic I virus induced adult T-cell leukemia. *Blood* **82**, 1701–1712.

Waldmann, T. A., Dubois, S., and Tagaya, Y. (2001). Contrasting roles of IL-2 and IL-15 in the life and death of lymphocytes: Implications for immunotherapy. *Immunity* **14**, 105–110.

Waldmann, T. A., White, J. D., Carrasquillo, J. C., et al. (1995). Radioimmunotherapy of interleukin-2R alpha expressing adult T-cell leukemia with yttrium-90-labeled anti-Tac. *Blood* **86**, 4063–4075.

Weiden, P. L., Breitz, H. B., Press, O., et al. (2000). Pretargeted radioimmunotherapy (PRIT) for treatment of non-Hodgkin's lymphoma (NHL): Initial phase I/II study results. *Cancer Biother. Radiopharm.* **15**, 15–29.

Weinblatt, M. E., Keystone, E. C., Furst, D. E., et al. (2003). Adalimumab, a fully human antitumor necrosis factor alpha monoclonal antibody, for the treatment of rheumatoid arthritis in patients taking concomitant methotrexate: The ARMADA trial. *Arthritis. Rheum.* **48**, 35–45.

Weng, W. K., and Levy, R. (2003). Two immunoglobulin G fragment C receptor polymorphisms independently predict response to rituximab in patients with follicular lymphoma. *J. Clin. Oncol.* **21**, 3940–3947.

Wing, M. G., Moreau, T., Greenwood, J., et al. (1996). Mechanism of first-dose cytokine-release syndrome by CAMPATH 1-H: Involvement of CD16 (FcgammaRIII) and CD11a/CD18 (LFA-1) on NK cells. *J. Clin. Invest.* **98**, 2819–2826.

Winter, G., and Milstein, C. (1991). Man made antibodies. *Nature* **349**, 293–299.

Wiseman, G. A., Gordon, L. I., Multani, P. S., et al. (2002). Ibritumomab tiuxetan radioimmunotherapy for patients with relapsed or refractory non-Hodgkin lymphoma and mild thrombocytopenia: A phase II multicenter trial. *Blood* **99**, 4336–4342.

Witzig, T. E., White, C. A., Wiseman, G. A., et al. (1999). Phase I/II trial of IDEC-Y2B8 radioimmunotherapy for treatment of relapsed or refractory CD20(+) B-cell non-Hodgkin's lymphoma. *J. Clin. Oncol.* **17**, 3793–3803.

Witzig, T. E., Flinn, I. W., Gordon, L. I., et al. (2002a). Treatment with ibritumomab tiuxetan radioimmunotherapy in patients with rituximab-refractory follicular non-Hodgkin's lymphoma. *J. Clin. Oncol.* **20**, 3262–3269.

Witzig, T. E., Gordon, L. I., Cabanillas, F., et al. (2002b). Randomized controlled trial of yttrium-90-labeled ibritumomab tiuxetan radioimmunotherapy versus rituximab immunotherapy for patients with relapsed or refractory low-grade, follicular, or transformed B-cell non-Hodgkin's lymphoma. *J. Clin. Oncol.* **20**, 2453–2463.

Witzig, T. E., White, C. A., Gordon, L. I., et al. (2003). Safety of yttrium-90 ibritumomab tiuxetan radioimmunotherapy for relapsed low-grade, follicular, or transformed non-Hodgkin's lymphoma. *J. Clin. Oncol.* **21**, 1263–1270.

Yang, J. C., Haworth, L., Sherry, R. M., et al. (2003). A randomized trial of bevacizumab, an antivascular endothelial growth factor antibody, for metastatic renal cancer. *N. Engl. J. Med.* **349**, 427–434.

Zalutsky, M. R., Garg, P. K., and Narula, A. S. (1990). Labeling monoclonal antibodies with halogen nuclides. *Acta Radiol. Suppl.* **374**, 141–145.

Zein, N., Sinha, A. M., McGahren, W. J., et al. (1988). Calicheamicin gamma 1I: An antitumor antibiotic that cleaves double-stranded DNA site specifically. *Science* **240**, 1198–1201.

Zhang, M., Yao, Z., Garmestani, K., *et al.* (2002). Pretargeting radioimmunotherapy of a murine model of adult T-cell leukemia with the alpha-emitting radionuclide, bismuth 213. *Blood* **100,** 208–216.

Zhang, M., Zhang, Z., Garmestani, K., *et al.* (2004). Activating Fc receptors are required for antitumor efficacy of the antibodies directed toward CD25 in a murine model of adult T-cell leukemia. *Cancer Res.* **64,** 5825–5829.

Zhang, X., Sun, S., Hwang, I., *et al.* (1998). Potent and selective stimulation of memory-phenotype CD8+ T cells *in vivo* by IL-15. *Immunity* **8,** 591–599.

Zhao, Y., Brown, T. L., Kohler, H., *et al.* (2003). MTS-conjugated-antiactive caspase 3 antibodies inhibit actinomycin D-induced apoptosis. *Apoptosis* **8,** 631–637.

Induction of Tumor Immunity Following Allogeneic Stem Cell Transplantation

Catherine J. Wu and Jerome Ritz

*Cancer Vaccine Center, Department of Medical Oncology,
Dana-Farber Cancer Institute,
Boston, Massachusetts*

Abstract 133
1. Introduction 134
2. Reconstitution of Donor Hematopoiesis Following Allogeneic HSCT 134
3. Sequence of Immune Reconstitution Following Allogeneic HSCT 136
4. The Graft-Versus-Leukemia Effect 138
5. Donor Lymphocyte Infusions Induce GVL Responses After
   Allogeneic HSCT 141
6. The Central Role of Donor T Cells as Mediators of GVL 143
7. Target Antigens of Donor T Cells After Allogeneic HSCT 146
8. Donor Natural Killer Cells as Mediators of GVL 150
9. Donor B Cells as Mediators of GVL 154
10. Future Directions 158
    References 160

Abstract

The curative potential of allogeneic hematopoietic stem cell transplantation (allo-HSCT) for many hematologic malignancies derives in large part from reconstitution of normal donor immunity and the development of a potent graft-versus-leukemia (GVL) immune response capable of rejecting tumor cell in vivo. Elucidation of the mechanisms of GVL by studies of animal models and analysis of clinical data has yielded important insights into how clinically effective tumor immunity is generated following allo-HSCT. These studies have identified NK cells and B cells as well as T cells as important mediators of the GVL response. A variety of antigenic targets of the GVL response have also been identified, and include tumor-associated antigens as well as minor histocompatibility antigens. The principles of effective GVL can now be applied to the development of novel therapies that enhance the therapeutic benefit of allogeneic HSCT while minimizing the toxicities associated with treatment. Moreover, many components of this approach that result in elimination of tumor cells following allogeneic HSCT can potentially be adapted to enhance the effectiveness of tumor immunity in the autologous setting.

1. Introduction

Allogeneic hematopoietic stem cell transplantation (HSCT) is a well-established curative treatment approach for many hematologic malignancies. In preparation for conventional allogeneic HSCT, patients first receive high-dose myeloablative chemotherapy with or without total body irradiation to eradicate residual tumor cells and to suppress host immunity preventing rejection of allogeneic cells. Subsequently, donor hematopoietic stem cells are transplanted through intravenous infusion and migrate to bone marrow where they engraft and reconstitute all elements of the hematopoietic and immune systems. While the intensity and composition of the conditioning regimen are important to successful HSCT, the reconstitution of donor immune cells plays a critical role in the elimination of recipient tumor cells, a process termed graft-versus-leukemia (GVL). Over the past two decades, a large body of clinical experience and laboratory studies has contributed to a better understanding of the targets and effectors responsible for GVL. As will be reviewed in this chapter, several unique features of allogeneic HSCT contribute to its ability to generate effective tumor immunity *in vivo*. First, engraftment of normal multilineage donor hematopoietic cells results in the establishment of nontolerant immune cells that can reject recipient tumor cells. Second, the expression by tumor cells of polymorphic peptides that distinguish recipient from donor [minor histocompatibility antigens (mHA)] represents an entire class of host-specific targets, which, in addition to tumor-associated antigens, may directly result in tumor lysis. Full understanding of the range of antigenic targets and the precise cellular subsets that mediate antitumor immunity in the allogeneic setting are still incomplete and several clinical factors [i.e., graft-versus-host disease (GVHD), concurrent immunosuppressive therapy] can limit the ability of donor immune cells to respond to recipient tumor cells following transplant. Nevertheless, elucidation of the mechanisms of GVL by studies of animal models and analysis of clinical data has yielded important insights into how clinically effective tumor immunity is generated following HSCT. These principles can now be applied to the development of therapies that enhance the therapeutic benefit of allogeneic transplantation while minimizing the risks and toxicities associated with treatment. Moreover, many of the components of this approach that result in elimination of tumor cells following allogeneic HSCT can potentially be adapted to enhance the effectiveness of tumor immunity in the autologous setting.

2. Reconstitution of Donor Hematopoiesis Following Allogeneic HSCT

For patients with malignant disease, the goal of allogeneic HSCT is long-lasting elimination of recipient tumor cells and disease cure. Critical to this goal is the replacement of the patient's immune system that has become tolerant to tumor cells with an immune system from a normal donor that is capable of recognizing tumor-associated antigens, mounting an effective rejection response, and maintaining a sufficient memory response to prevent disease relapse. In this setting, immunologic control of recipient tumor cells is critically dependent on the pace and extent to which donor immunity reconstitutes following transplant.

As summarized in Fig. 1, many variables can affect donor immune reconstitution following transplant. Variables in the transplant recipient include: (1) underlying conditions in the host such as age, intensity of prior treatment, and disease status; (2) the intensity of the transplant preparative regimen and toxicities associated with different agents; (3) intensity and duration of immunosuppressive medications used for prevention and treatment of GVHD; and (4) the extent of engraftment of donor hematopoietic stem cells and their differentiation into distinct myeloid and lymphoid lineages. For example, recovery of T-cell immunity occurs more rapidly in pediatric recipients, and this likely reflects the higher level of thymic function in these patients (Mackall *et al*., 1995; Weinberg *et al*., 2001). In contrast, older patients who have previously received intensive chemotherapy and have minimal thymic tissue experience more prolonged periods of immune deficiency and are at increased risk of infectious complications following transplant (Hakim *et al*., 1997, 2005). Some patients have markedly abnormal marrow microenvironments, particularly those with

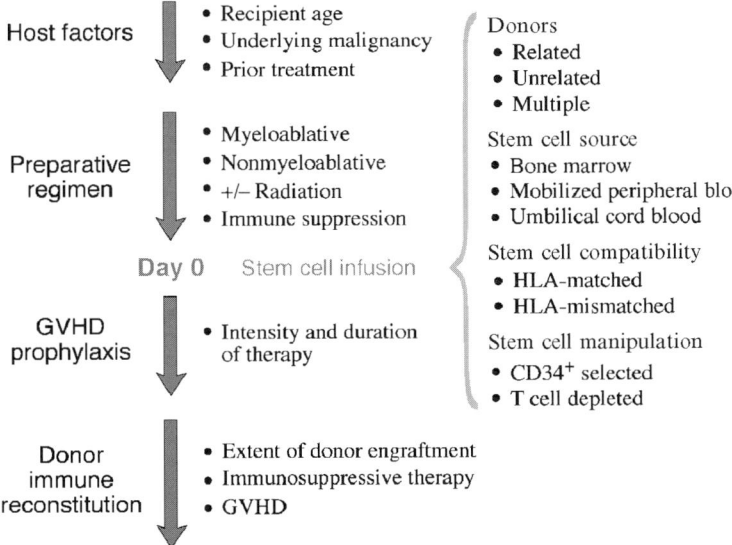

Figure 1 The complexity of variables that influence the outcome of allogeneic HSCT.

myelodysplasia (MDS) (Duhrsen et al., 1995; Payne et al., 1987; Tauro et al., 2001). As a result, donor stem cell engraftment is often delayed in patients with MDS, but successful engraftment with normal hematopoietic stem cells subsequently leads to normalization of the marrow microenvironment and establishment of normal hematopoietic function (Oblon et al., 1983). In patients who receive high-dose myeloablative therapy in preparation for HSCT, both early engraftment and long-term maintenance of hematopoiesis are almost entirely derived from donor stem cells. In contrast, patients who receive less intensive conditioning regimens can develop mixed hematopoietic chimerism following transplant (Baron et al., 2005; Sykes et al., 1999). The use of less intensive conditioning regimens is associated with less toxicity, but patients with chimeric immune systems following transplant may be tolerant to recipient cells and may not be able to develop effective tumor immunity.

Many variables in the allogeneic stem cell graft can also influence immune reconstitution in the recipient. These graft-associated variables include: (1) genetic relationship of the donor and recipient, (2) the number and quality of hematopoietic stem cells as well as other cells contained within the graft, (3) the degree of human leukocyte antigen (HLA) compatibility with the recipient, and (4) effects of procedures used to manipulate the stem cell graft *in vitro* prior to infusion. Each of these factors can have a profound influence on immune reconstitution in individual patients and can therefore directly affect the ability of donor cells to develop effective tumor immunity. For example, hematopoietic stem cell grafts can be obtained from HLA-identical siblings, HLA-matched unrelated donors, partially HLA-mismatched related or unrelated adults, or partially HLA-mismatched umbilical cord blood. In these instances, the degree of HLA-matching influences the frequency and severity of GVHD following transplant and also affects the reconstitution of T-cell immunity. The rapidity of engraftment and reconstitution of immune function is also dependent on the total number of hematopoietic stem cells in the graft as well as on the large numbers of other donor cells in the product (Zubair et al., 2004). Grafts with small numbers of hematopoietic stem cells (e.g., cord blood products) or highly purified $CD34^+$ cells are capable of engraftment and long-term maintenance of all hematopoietic and immune functions. However, engraftment is often delayed in these individuals and the slow rate of immune reconstitution frequently leads to severe infectious complications following transplant (Platzbecker et al., 2004; Vose et al., 2001).

3. Sequence of Immune Reconstitution Following Allogeneic HSCT

Mature T, B, and natural killer (NK) cells present in the stem cell product contribute to immune function in the early posttransplant period, but long-lasting immune reconstitution following myeloablative therapy is primarily dependent on the differentiation of new immune cells from undifferentiated hematopoietic progenitor cells. The sequence of cellular reconstitution that occurs following myeloablative stem cell transplantation is summarized schematically in Fig. 2. In most patients, NK cells are the first lymphoid population to recover. In the first month posttransplant, NK cells often represent the predominant lymphoid cell in peripheral blood, especially in patients who receive marrow depleted of mature T cells (Soiffer et al., 1990). T cells typically reconstitute more slowly, with $CD4^+$ cells lagging behind the $CD8^+$ population. This results in inversion of the normal CD4/CD8 ratio for prolonged periods post-HSCT (Atkinson, 1990; Forman et al., 1982; Keever et al., 1989). $CD8^+$ T cells reach normal numbers by 3–4 months after HSCT, whereas CD4 plus; numbers do not normalize until 6–12 months after HSCT. Peripheral blood B cells typically recover very slowly, achieving normal numbers by 12 months posttransplant. Whereas T cells in the first 3 to 6 months posttransplant primarily reflect expansion of mature donor cells within the stem cell graft, late T cells are naïve cells and are derived from differentiation of donor-derived hematopoietic progenitor cells (T-cell neogenesis) (Hochberg et al., 2001; Patel et al., 2000; Weinberg et al., 2001).

Although thymic function declines with age, normal adults are able to maintain a highly diverse T cell receptor (TCR) repertoire (Douek et al., 1998). Without a highly diverse T cell repertoire, the ability of foreign antigens to escape detection increases and the subsequent development of an effective T-cell response to external pathogens decreases. The ability to develop specific T cell-responses to tumor-associated antigens would be similarly affected by loss of TCR repertoire diversity. The complexity of the TCR repertoire in an individual can be measured by quantifying the use of various TCR

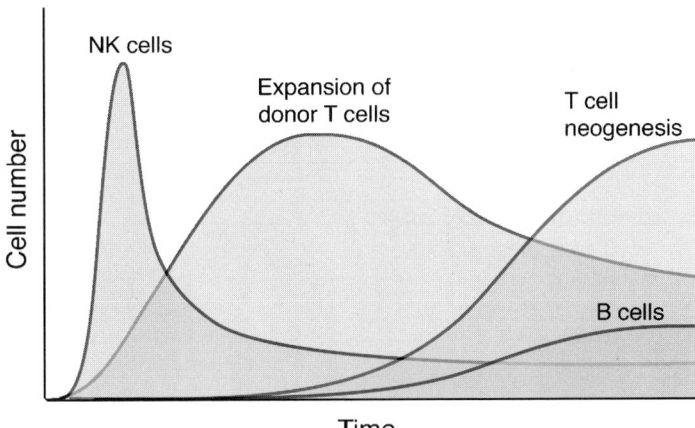

Figure 2 Schematic sequence of immune reconstitution following allogeneic HSCT.

Vβ genes in peripheral T cells (Rowen et al., 1996). Moreover, the diversity of the CDR3 regions generated within populations of T cells can be measured by the method of spectratyping (Genevee et al., 1992; Gorski et al., 1994). These methods have been used in our laboratory and by others to directly examine reconstitution of T-cell repertoire following myeloablative therapy and HSCT (Bomberger et al., 1998; Wu et al., 2000a). In these studies, TCR repertoire diversity was found to be very limited in the early posttransplant period. TCR repertoire gradually improves and often recovers to relatively normal levels by 1 year following HSCT in patients who have engrafted completely with donor cells and have no posttransplant complications. This occurs more rapidly in pediatric patients, presumably because of a higher level of thymic function in these individuals (Roux et al., 2000; Small et al., 1999). Reconstitution of normal TCR repertoire appears to be delayed in patients who have posttransplant complications, such as GVHD, and who have mixed hematopoietic chimerism rather than complete donor hematopoiesis (Verfuerth et al., 2000; Wu et al., 2000a). Reduced TCR repertoire diversity has also been noted in patients with relapsed disease after allogeneic HSCT, and recovery of a highly diverse TCR repertoire is associated with effective immune response to tumor cells and disease remission (Claret et al., 1997).

4. The Graft-Versus-Leukemia Effect

Many clinical studies in patients with hematologic malignancies have demonstrated that reconstitution of donor immunity after allogeneic HSCT can lead to immune-mediated suppression of recipient tumor cells. This immunologic effect has generally been termed GVL, and a variety of clinical and laboratory studies have been undertaken to elucidate the precise immunologic mechanisms involved in the recognition and subsequent elimination of malignant recipient cells *in vivo*. A large series of clinical studies published over the last 30 years provide convincing evidence for the existence of GVL. These studies also document the remarkable effectiveness of GVL and its contribution to the long-lasting immunologic rejection of malignant cells in patients with overt disease. Various types of clinical observations supporting the existence of GVL are summarized in Table 1.

In the 1970s and 1980s, clinical studies first began to reveal that the risk of disease relapse after HSCT was highly correlated with immunologic variables in the recipient. For example, Weiden et al. demonstrated that leukemia relapse was 2.5 times more likely in recipients of syngeneic stem cells compared to HLA-matched allogeneic recipients who developed GVHD (Weiden et al., 1979). In several large studies, patients who experienced GVHD were less likely to relapse, and this appeared to be related to the extent of HLA

Table 1 Clinical Evidence for GVL Activity Following Allogeneic HSCT

Clinical observations

Lower relapse rate after transplantation of allogeneic stem cells compared to autologous or syngeneic stem cells

Positive correlation between GVHD and GVL
    Temporal association of leukemia remission with episodes of acute or chronic GVHD
    Disease remission after stopping immunosuppressive medications
    Decreased relapse associated with GVHD

T-cell depletion of donor stem cell graft is associated with higher relapse rates

Allogeneic HSCT after nonmyeloablative conditioning induces remission of hematologic malignancies and some nonhematologic malignancies

---

matching between recipient and donor (Fefer *et al.*, 1987; Sullivan *et al.*, 1989; Weiden *et al.*, 1981). This observation was subsequently confirmed by other investigators (Butturini *et al.*, 1987; Gale *et al.*, 1994; Jones *et al.*, 1991; Weisdorf *et al.*, 1987). It was also observed that leukemia remission could occur in association with worsening GVHD (Odom *et al.*, 1978; Tricot *et al.*, 1996). Finally, several investigators reported that disease remission could occur after stopping immunosuppressive medications used for prevention of GVHD (Collins *et al.*, 1992; Libura *et al.*, 1999). Following single-institution reports describing a positive correlation between GVHD and GVL, several large registry studies in North America (Horowitz *et al.*, 1990) and Europe (Ringden *et al.*, 1996) subsequently confirmed these findings. In these studies, decreased relapse was consistently observed in patients with acute and/or chronic GVHD when compared with similar patients without GVHD. Some patients in these retrospective studies had received stem cells grafts from which T cells had been depleted *in vitro* to prevent GVHD. T-cell depletion effectively prevented severe GVHD, but patients who received T-cell depleted stem cells from HLA-identical allogeneic donors grafts had higher rates of relapse than recipients of non-T cell depleted stem cells. This effect of T-cell depletion was most often noted in patients with chronic myelocytic leukemia (CML). Patients who receive stem cells from identical twins do not develop GVHD, and similar increased rates of leukemia relapse were seen in these patients. Taken together, these studies demonstrated that GVHD was associated with a highly significant GVL effect. Moreover, this effect appeared to be mediated by donor T cells in the stem cell products (Champlin *et al.*, 1990; Goldman *et al.*, 1988; Horowitz *et al.*, 1990; Martin *et al.*, 1988).

In patients who undergo allogeneic HSCT for treatment of hematologic malignancy, intensive myeloablative conditioning administered prior to stem cell infusion was previously felt to play a major role in the elimination of recipient tumor cells. With the ability to monitor minimal residual disease in patients with CML using polymerase chain reaction (PCR) for *bcr-abl* transcripts, a study from the Dana-Farber Cancer Institute and Hôpital Maisonneuve-Rosemont (Pichert *et al.*, 1995) examined the relative contributions of the transplant preparative regimen and immunologic mechanisms posttransplant on the elimination of leukemia cells in the recipient. In 92 patients that received conventional myeloablative conditioning regimens, >80% continued to have detectable bcr-abl positive cells in the first 6 months posttransplant. Between 6 and 12 months posttransplant, 88% of patients receiving T-cell depleted marrow remained PCR positive compared to 30% of patients who received unmodified marrow ($p = 0.001$). During this period, elimination of PCR-detectable CML cells was highly correlated with the development of GVHD. However, a substantial subset of patients (approximately 40%) appeared to be able to mediate disease suppression without clinically evident GVHD. Laboratory studies indicated that the bcr-abl positive cells detected in these individuals represented early progenitor cells derived from the CML clone (Pichert *et al.*, 1994). The persistence of these CML cells in the vast majority of patients who received myeloablative therapy, therefore, suggested that high-dose conditioning regimens, by themselves, did not effectively eliminate leukemia cells. In contrast, immunologic mechanisms mediated by donor T cells appeared to be more important for suppressing leukemia cells after transplant and preventing leukemia relapse.

With the demonstration that GVL plays an important role in the elimination of leukemia cells following transplant, many studies began to examine the feasibility of using less intensive, nonmyeloablative conditioning regimens to prepare patients for allogeneic HSCT. A variety of nonmyeloablative conditioning regimens have been developed and a large number of clinical studies have demonstrated the effectiveness of this approach, especially in patients who are not eligible for more intensive conditioning (Khouri *et al.*, 1998; McSweeney *et al.*, 2001). As expected, reduced intensity conditioning regimens are associated with substantially less toxicity but nevertheless provide sufficient immune suppression of the recipient to prevent rejection of allogeneic hematopoietic stem cells. Since donor hematopoiesis is not completely eradicated, achievement of full donor hematopoiesis is dependent on donor immune recognition of residual host cells. Similarly, nonmyeloablative conditioning regimens are not sufficient to eliminate leukemia cells in the recipient and long-term remissions are primarily dependent on immunologic mechanisms mediated by donor cells. The effectiveness of this approach has now been demonstrated in many studies in patients with various hematologic malignancies (Alyea *et al.*, 2005; Morris *et al.*, 2004). As in patients who receive myeloablative conditioning, GVL post nonmyeloablative transplant is often associated with GVHD. For example, a recent analysis of 229 patients with multiple myeloma, who had undergone reduced intensity allogeneic HSCT treated at 33 centers within the European Group for Blood and Marrow Transplantation (EBMT) found that development of chronic GVHD was associated with better overall survival (OS) and progression free survival (PFS); patients with limited chronic GVHD experienced 84% OS and 46% PFS, whereas patients without chronic GVHD had 29% OS and 12% PFS (Crawley et al., 2005). Taken together, the ability to markedly reduce the intensity of the transplant conditioning regimen while maintaining therapeutic control of malignant cells provides further evidence for the ability of allogeneic immune cells to provide effective tumor immunity *in vivo*. This effect is most evident in patients with hematologic malignancies, but similar clinical trials in patients with solid tumors suggest that graft versus tumor responses can be observed in at least some of these patients (Childs et al., 2000; Tykodi et al., 2004; Ueno et al., 2003).

5. Donor Lymphocyte Infusions Induce GVL Responses After Allogeneic HSCT

The use of donor lymphocyte infusions (DLI) as a therapeutic approach for patients with relapsed hematologic malignancy after allogeneic HSCT grew directly from clinical observations demonstrating that GVL was mediated by unstimulated donor T cells present in the allogeneic stem cell product. Kolb et al. (1990) reported that DLI in three patients with relapsed CML after allogeneic HSCT resulted in dramatic clinical responses. The clinical observation that DLI alone, in the absence of further chemotherapy or radiation, was able to induce disease remission, directly demonstrated that immune effector cells derived from the donor were responsible for generating potent tumor immunity.

Since this initial report, many studies have confirmed the efficacy of DLI for inducing GVL. Kolb et al. (1995) reported the experience of 27 centers participating in the EBMT, and noted durable responses to DLI, especially in patients with myeloid leukemias. Collins et al. (1997) reported the experience in 140 patients from multiple centers across North America. From these clinical studies, a number of findings have been consistently observed. First, DLI appears to be especially effective in the treatment of CML where durable responses occur in 75–80% of patients. Other diseases are responsive to DLI as well, but to a lesser degree (Lokhorst et al., 1997; Mandigers et al., 2003; Rondon et al., 1996; Tricot et al., 1996). Collins et al. (1997) reported response rates of 50% and 40% in patients with multiple myeloma and CLL, respectively. In contrast, response rates in patients with acute leukemia are relatively low (10–15%). Consistent with these observations, DLI is generally more effective in patients with lower burdens of disease and less acute disease progression (van Rhee et al., 1994). Response rates in patients with cytogenetic evidence of relapse CML without overt hematologic relapse are generally >90%. Whereas stable phase CML relapse is highly responsive to DLI, only 5–10% of patients with advanced CML (blast crisis/accelerated phase) respond to DLI. Second, clinical responses following DLI are often delayed until 2–4 months after a single infusion. This prolonged interval may reflect the time required to mount an effective response when the frequency of naïve T cells capable of responding is very low. Alternatively, delayed responses may reflect the time required to demonstrate the impact of lysing the large number of cells comprising the malignant clone. Finally, DLI responses for at least some diseases are quite durable (Mattei et al., 2001; Shimoni et al., 2001). Porter et al. (1999) reported the long-term follow-up of 66 patients who achieved complete remission after DLI (39 with CML, 27 with other diseases). In patients with CML, the probability of survival at 1, 2, and 3 years was 83%, 76%, and 73%, respectively. The durability of these responses appears to be linked to achievement of molecular remission, suggesting that the effectiveness of DLI results from immunologic elimination of the malignant stem cell clone (Dazzi et al., 2000).

Given the effectiveness of DLI in some patients with relapsed disease, several studies have examined alternate approaches for using DLI as preemptive therapy to prevent relapse of malignant disease. For example, Ferra et al. (2001) administered DLI after transplantation of purified $CD34^+$ peripheral blood stem cells, a method to reduce the number of T cells in the stem cell graft. Barrett et al. (1998) have similarly infused donor T cells at defined intervals following T-cell depleted BMT as a method to limit acute GVHD while conserving a GVL effect. Such approaches have become particularly important with increasing use of nonmyeloablative preparative regimens, which rely primarily on GVL effects to suppress residual malignancy (Bethge et al., 2004; Dey et al., 2003; Marks et al., 2002; Morris et al., 2004; Peggs et al., 2004). Taken together, these studies have identified several approaches for the clinical use of DLI to promote tumor immunity and prevent relapse after allogeneic HSCT. Many of these approaches are currently being evaluated in clinical trials.

As expected, the most common toxicity of DLI is GVHD, and a variety of approaches have been developed to limit this toxicity while maintaining the effectiveness of GVL. One approach tested at the Dana-Farber Cancer Institute has been to deplete $CD8^+$ cells from the DLI product and infuse defined numbers of $CD4^+$ donor cells (Alyea et al., 1998). Several studies have demonstrated that CD8 depleted DLI retain GVL activity while reducing the risk of GVHD following infusion (Alyea et al., 1998; Shimoni et al., 2001). In a prospective trial, patients who received myeloablative conditioning and T-cell depleted stem cell grafts were randomized to subsequently receive either unmodified or CD8-depleted DLI (Soiffer et al., 2002). Patients who received CD8-depleted DLI had a significantly reduced risk of GVHD without increased risk of relapse. Importantly, infusion of $CD4^+$ donor T cells has been found to induce a variety of clinical and immunologic effects *in vivo*. These include the conversion of mixed hematopoietic chimerism to complete donor hematopoiesis (Orsini et al., 2000), increased T-cell neogenesis (Hochberg et al., 2001) and improvement in TCR repertoire diversity (Bellucci et al., 2002; Claret et al., 1997; Orsini et al., 2000). Moreover, tumor-reactive $CD8^+$ donor T-cell clones have been isolated from patients who have responded to $CD4^+$ DLI (Orsini et al., 2003; Zorn et al., 2002). Taken together, these trials and others suggest that $CD4^+$ donor T cells play a critical role as mediators of GVL and that it may also be possible to target malignant recipient cells *in vivo* without also inducing severe GVHD. However, the mechanisms whereby donor $CD4^+$ cells induce GVL are not yet well understood and likely involve the induction of $CD8^+$ effector T cells *in vivo*.

6. The Central Role of Donor T Cells as Mediators of GVL

Having demonstrated the important role of GVL in eliminating malignant recipient cells after transplant, many clinical and laboratory studies have begun to define the immunologic mechanisms that contribute to GVL. Although DLI products contain a variety of mononuclear cell types, including NK cells, B cells, and dendritic cells, T cells comprise the predominant effector cells in these products and are presumed to be the primary cells responsible for the efficacy of this approach. In murine models, both $CD4^+$ and $CD8^+$ T-cell populations have been shown to contribute to GVL activity *in vivo* (Truitt and Atasoylu, 1991). When either of these T-cell populations was removed, GVL reactivity was compromised, indicating that an optimal GVL response requires both $CD4^+$ and $CD8^+$ T cells. In patients who have undergone allogeneic HSCT, both $CD4^+$ and $CD8^+$ leukemia-reactive T cells have also been identified. However, few GVL T-cell clones have thus far been isolated from patients after allogeneic HSCT and the precise role that various T-cell populations play as mediators of GVL has not been determined.

In general, laboratory studies to isolate and characterize T-cell clones that mediate GVL and GVHD have utilized one of the two approaches schematically represented in Fig. 3. One approach shown in sequence **A**, begins with stimulation of donor T cells with recipient target cells and subsequent selection of T-cell lines or clones for their ability to specifically recognize recipient cells without also responding to normal donor cells (Faber et al., 1995, 1992; Warren et al., 1998b). The initial population of responding T cells can be obtained from the normal donor or from patient peripheral blood after the individual has engrafted with donor cells. Once T-cell clones that specifically react with either normal or malignant cells from the recipient have been

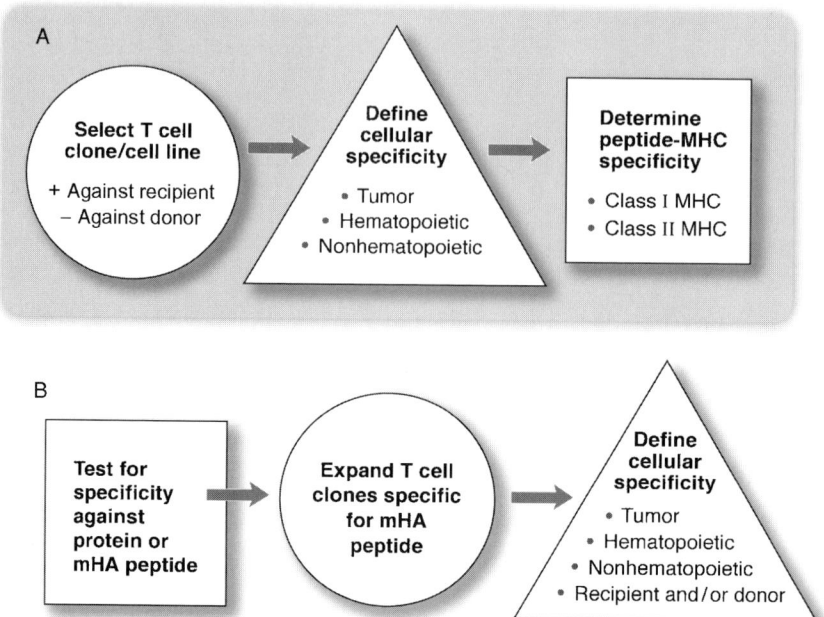

Figure 3 Alternative approaches for characterizing donor T cells following allogeneic HSCT.

isolated and expanded *in vitro*, the spectrum of tissue specificity is defined by testing for reactivity with tumor cells as well as with a variety of normal hematopoietic and nonhematopoietic cell types. Once patterns of tissue restriction are defined, further studies can determine whether the target antigen is presented by either class I or class II major histocompatibility complex (MHC) molecules, and specific MHC restricting alleles can be identified. In a limited number of cases, further studies have been carried out to define the peptide epitope recognized by the donor T-cell clone and to characterize the genetic polymorphism that underlies recognition by donor T cells (den Haan *et al.*, 1995; Dolstra *et al.*, 1999; Murata *et al.*, 2003; Warren *et al.*, 2000). Once the peptide epitopes recognized by these T-cell clones has been identified, further experiments using peptide-MHC tetramers and peptide ELISPOT assays can be used to better characterize the specific T-cell clone in peripheral blood and tissue samples from the patient (Marijt *et al.*, 2003; Takami *et al.*, 2004). In addition, molecular sequencing of the rearranged TCR genes in specific clones can also be used to develop PCR-based approaches to detect and quantify individual clones in serial samples obtained from the patient after transplant (McHeyzer-Williams and Davis, 1995; Zorn *et al.*, 2002). Using this approach, a variety of interesting T-cell clones have been characterized and the precise target specificity of these cells has been well documented.

An alternate approach to characterizing GVL and GVHD T cells is shown in sequence **B** of Fig. 3. This approach begins with the selection of a target protein or panel of peptides. These targets are used as stimulating antigens to detect and expand antigen-specific T-cell clones *in vitro* (Zorn *et al.*, 2004). Once antigen-specific T-cell clones are expanded, further studies can define the MHC-restricting allele and determine which recipient tissues express sufficient target peptide to allow recognition by the donor T-cell clone. Target tissues from the recipient as well as from other individuals can also be tested to better define the reactivity of the T-cell clone. Although both approaches have provided interesting results that have helped clarify the role of T cells in GVL and GVHD after allogeneic HSCT, it is evident that each approach has inherent limitations. Since the first approach is based on selection of clones that are reactive with recipient cells and not donor cells, it is primarily useful for the identification of mHA that reflect genetic polymorphisms that are disparate in these 2 individuals. "Autoreactive" clones that recognize antigens expressed on donor cells as well as recipient cells would not be identified using this approach. Since the second approach is based on the prior selection of a target protein, this method is better suited to characterize *in vivo* responses to known tumor-associated antigens or mHA after transplant. However, this approach is not suited to the identification of new mHA or new tumor-associated antigens.

Using these general approaches, various investigators have identified a variety of immunogenic peptide epitopes that are recognized by donor T cells after allogeneic HSCT and leukemia-reactive clones have been isolated from responding patients. For example, Falkenburg *et al.* (1999) isolated cytotoxic T lymphocytes (CTL) clones directed against mHA from patients with GVHD after allogeneic HSCT that are capable of antigen-specific lysis of freshly obtained leukemic cells and inhibition of leukemic precursor cells *in vitro*. Bonnet *et al.* (1999) further demonstrated that human CTL clones specific for mHA could preferentially target leukemia stem cells and that T-cell clones with this type of specificity could effectively eliminate transplanted leukemia cells in NOD/SCID mice. Leukemia-reactive CTL have also been isolated from patients following DLI. For example, Zorn *et al.* (2002) reported the expansion of $CD8^+$ donor T cells from patients with relapsed CML with cytolytic activity directed against recipient hematopoietic cells. Orsini *et al.* (2003) reported similar findings in a patient with myeloma who responded to DLI. In both of these studies patients had received CD8-depleted DLI, suggesting that infusion of $CD4^+$ donor T cells are able to stimulate $CD8^+$ effector activity in the recipient. CTL clones specific for mHA, such as HA-1, have also been identified as GVL effectors after DLI (Kircher *et al.*, 2002).

Finally, CTL clones specific for mHA have been isolated and expanded *in vitro* and subsequently infused in patients with relapsed leukemia after allogeneic HSCT (Falkenburg *et al.*, 1999). Although not effective in most cases, clinical responses have been noted in some of these individuals. Taken together, these studies and others clearly demonstrate that both $CD4^+$ and $CD8^+$ donor T cells play a central role in mediating GVL and suppressing residual tumor cells in patients who have undergone allogeneic HSCT.

7. Target Antigens of Donor T Cells After Allogeneic HSCT

A great deal of effort has been directed toward the precise identification of the target antigens of donor T cells after allogeneic HSCT. Since donor T cells are the primary mediators of GVL and GVHD, a better characterization of the precise peptide epitopes recognized by T cells will likely lead to a better understanding of these immunologic mechanisms and the optimization of strategies to distinguish these effects *in vivo*. Clinically, GVL and GVHD are often tightly linked, but GVHD represents one of the primary toxicities of allogeneic HSCT while GVL represents one of the major benefits of treatment. Being able to distinguish the target antigens of GVL and GVHD would greatly facilitate the ability to develop new methods to improve patient outcome after HSCT. Moreover, a better understanding of the mechanisms of GVL will also be helpful in determining whether similar mechanisms can be applied to the induction of autologous tumor immunity or whether these mechanisms are restricted to the setting of allogeneic HSCT.

When the transplant recipient and donor are not HLA-identical, MHC antigens themselves become targets of donor T cells and are responsible for increased GVHD after transplant. However, as methods for HLA typing have improved and the number of volunteer stem cell donors has increased, the majority of allogeneic stem cell transplants occur between recipients and related or unrelated donors that are HLA-matched. In this setting, mHA become the primary antigenic targets of donor T cells that are responsible for GVHD (Hambach and Goulmy, 2005; Warren *et al.*, 1998a).

Unlike major histocompatibility antigens, which are encoded by a discrete set of genes on chromosome 6, mHA occur as a result of genetic polymorphisms that exist throughout the human genome. During normal T cell differentiation in the thymus, T cells expressing rearranged high-affinity receptors reactive with self-peptides expressed by self-MHC molecules are deleted in a process termed negative selection. Although still incompletely understood, a highly diverse array of self-proteins are expressed and processed within the thymus, and peptides derived from these proteins are presented on MHC class I and class II molecules. Negative selection of T cells reactive with any of these self-peptides results in apoptosis of auto-reactive T cells and deletion of the great majority of T cells undergoing maturation in the thymus. Mature $CD4^+$ and $CD8^+$ T cells that survive thymic selection nevertheless exhibit a highly diverse TCR repertoire that remains capable of recognizing "nonself" human peptides as well as foreign peptides. As a consequence of genetic diversity within any outbred population, each individual in a population expresses a diverse set of polymorphic proteins in different cell types. These polymorphic proteins are subject to proteasomal processing resulting in the presentation of a unique set of polymorphic peptides by individual MHC molecules. Except for syngeneic twins, each individual, including HLA-identical siblings, presents a unique set of diverse self-peptides on their own cell surface MHC molecules. Since each cell type expresses different proteins at distinct stages of maturation and functional activation, there is a high degree of diversity of peptide presentation and each cell type is capable of expressing a unique set of self-peptides. Minor histocompatibility antigens are a reflection of those polymorphic self-peptides that distinguish any two individuals and transplantation of mature T cells during allogeneic HSCT results in the transfer of large numbers of cells capable of recognizing these mHA. In contrast, donor T cells that differentiate from hematopoietic stem cells after transplantation undergo negative selection resulting in depletion of T-cell clones reactive with recipient mHA. This explains the lack of GVHD in patients who receive T-cell depleted stem cell grafts despite full reconstitution of donor T-cell immunity. This process occurs in adult as well as pediatric patients even though the thymus has undergone involution in these individuals.

Based on work from many laboratories, a large number of human mHA summarized in Table 2 have already been defined. Although estimates for the total number of mHA vary widely, this list likely represents only a small fraction of the human mHA that exist. Since single nucleotide polymorphisms (SNP) represent the most common manifestation of genetic diversity, (Cargill et al., 1999; Wang et al., 1998) almost all of the autosomal mHA listed in Table 2 represent consequences of SNP expression. In these instances SNP can lead to creation of alternate transcripts, differences in proteasomal processing (Brickner et al., 2001; Spierings et al., 2003a) and distinct posttranslational modifications (Meadows et al., 1997) as well as simple substitution of single amino acids in the antigenic peptide (den Haan et al., 1998; Mommaas et al., 2002; Pierce et al., 2001; Vogt et al., 2000b). Recently described gene deletion polymorphisms may also play an important role in the generation of mHA (Murata et al., 2003). In all cases described thus far, genetically defined mHA do not appear to represent clinically significant differences that result in altered protein function. Rather, the clinical consequences of mHA appear to result entirely from their expression in different cell types and the recognition of these antigens by donor T cells (Akatsuka et al., 2003; Dickinson et al., 2002; Kloosterboer et al., 2005).

Table 2 Human Minor Histocompatibility Antigens

Antigen	Tissue distribution	Peptide sequence	MHC restriction	Reference
Y-encoded (HY) mHA				
SMCY	Hematopoietic and nonhematopoietic tissue	SP **S/A** VDKA **R/Q** AEL	B7	(Wang et al., 1995)
DFFRY	Hematopoietic and nonhematopoietic tissue	FI **D/E** SYLVC **Q/R V/M**	A2	(Meadows et al., 1997)
		IVD **C/S** LTEMY	A1	(Pierce et al., 1999; Vogt et al., 2000a)
UTY	Hematopoietic and nonhematopoietic tissue	LPHN **H/R** T **D/N** L	B8	(Warren et al., 2000)
DBY	Ubiquitous	**R/G** ESEE **E/A** S **V/P** SL	B60	(Vogt et al., 2000b)
		HIE **N/S** FSD **I/V D/E** MGE	DQ5	(Vogt et al., 2002)
		ASTASKGRYIPPHLRNKEA	DRB1°1501	(Zorn et al., 2004)
RPS4Y	Ubiquitous	**V/L** IKVNDT **V/I** QI	DRB3°0301	(Spierings et al., 2003b)
TMSB4Y	Hematopoietic and nonhematopoietic tissue	E V/T L FL/LR PGLHFR	A33	(Torikai et al., 2004)
Autosomal mHA				
HA-1	Hematopoietic and nonhematopoietic tissue	VL **R/H** DDLLEA	A2	(den Haan et al., 1995)
HA-2	Hematopoietic tissue	KECVLHDDL	B60	(Mommaas et al., 2002)
HA-3	Ubiquitous	YIGEVLVS **V/M**	A2	(Pierce et al., 2001)
HA-8	Ubiquitous	V **T/M** EPGTAQY	A1	(Spierings et al., 2003a)
HB-1	B-ALL, EBV cells	**R/P** TLDKVLEV	A2	(Brickner et al., 2001)
BCL2A1	Hematopoietic and nonhematopoietic tissue	EEKRGSL **H/Y** VW	B44	(Dolstra et al., 1999)
		DYLQ **Y/C** VLQI	A24	(Akatsuka et al., 2003)
UGT2B17	Hematopoietic and nonhematopoietic tissue	KEFED **D/G** IINW	B44	
		AELLNIPFLY/null	A29	(Murata et al., 2003)
PANE1	B-lymphoid cells	RVWDLPGVLK/null	A3	(Brickner et al., 2006)
LRH-1	Hematopoietic cells	TP **N/T Q/S R/G Q/R N/T V/S C/V**	B7	(de Rijke et al., 2005)

As summarized in Table 2, many of the mHA identified thus far are encoded by genes on the Y chromosome, which contains a relatively small set of genes that are widely expressed and also have expressed X chromosome homologues (Foote *et al.*, 1992; Wang *et al.*, 1995). Males are tolerant to these Y proteins (HY antigens), but T cells reactive with HY peptides are not deleted in normal females. Females exposed to HY antigens through pregnancy or blood transfusion can develop long-lived T-cell responses to these mHA (James *et al.*, 2003; Verdijk *et al.*, 2004). Similarly engraftment of female T cells in male recipients can lead to the expansion of HY specific donor T cells (Pierce *et al.*, 1999; Takami *et al.*, 2004; Vogt *et al.*, 2000a). Several studies have documented the increased incidence of GVHD in male recipients of stem cell grafts from female donors (Atkinson *et al.*, 1986; Flowers *et al.*, 1990; Gratwohl *et al.*, 2001; Randolph *et al.*, 2004) and this is presumed to be due to the broad tissue and cellular expression of HY proteins and the immunogenicity of these antigens. As shown in Table 2, many of the HY mHA contain multiple disparate amino acids when compared to their X-homologues and these peptide epitopes are presented by both MHC class I and class II molecules (Spierings *et al.*, 2003b; Torikai *et al.*, 2004; Vogt *et al.*, 2002). Both of these factors likely contribute to the high level of immunogenicity of these antigens.

The clinical significance of mHA is highly dependent on the tissues and cell types that express the target antigen. Most of the human mHA identified thus far have broad tissue expression and the targeting of these varied cell types by donor T cells represents one of the initiating events of GVHD (Dickinson *et al.*, 2002). In contrast, mHA with very limited tissue expression are not likely to lead to clinically significant toxicity after allogeneic HSCT (Nishida *et al.*, 2004). Expression of several mHA in Table 2 has been found to be restricted to hematopoietic cells. In these instances, targeting of these mHA can suppress recipient hematopoiesis and facilitate engraftment of donor stem cells and the establishment of complete donor hematopoiesis. To the extent that mHA are expressed on malignant cells in the recipient, targeting of these antigenic epitopes by donor T cells can also contribute to GVL (Fig. 4). In instances where mHA are expressed by both malignant and normal hematopoietic cells in the recipient but not other tissues, targeting of these antigens will contribute to GVL and conversion to full donor hematopoiesis but will not contribute to GVHD. For this reason, targeting mHA with restricted hematopoietic expression has been proposed as an important mechanism for distinguishing GVL from GVHD following allogeneic HSCT and DLI (Hambach and Goulmy, 2005; Mutis and Goulmy, 2002; Riddell *et al.*, 2003).

After allogeneic HSCT, mHA expressed by recipient tumor cells represent a unique opportunity to target malignant cells for immune destruction (Bleakley and Riddell, 2004). These antigens play an important role as GVL targets but normal donor T cells are also able to initiate immune responses against other

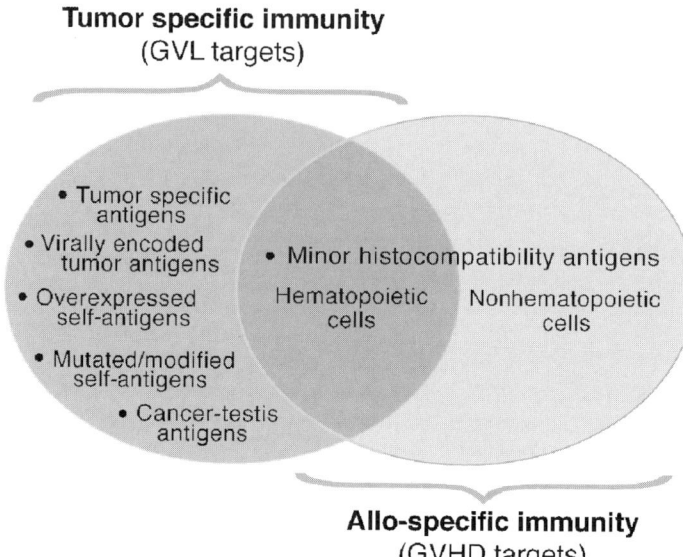

Figure 4 Spectrum of target antigens associated with tumor immunity and allo-immunity after allogeneic HSCT.

tumor-associated antigens. As summarized in Fig. 4, a large variety of such antigens have been identified. This includes tumor-specific antigens, virally encoded tumor antigens, overexpressed self-antigens, mutated or modified self-antigens, and cancer-testis antigens. For hematopoietic malignancies, there are many potentially important antigens in these categories, including chimeric BCR-ABL (Bocchia et al., 1995; Cathcart et al., 2004) and PML/ RARα (Bocchia et al., 1995) proteins, latent EBV antigens, proteinase-3 (Molldrem et al., 2000), WT-1 (Azuma et al., 2002), survivin (Reker et al., 2004), ML-IAP (Schmollinger et al., 2003) and cancer-testes antigens such as SLLP1 (Wang et al., 2004). In these instances, the immunogenicity of these targets is not dependent on genetic disparity between recipient and donor. However, recipients with leukemia may have become tolerant to these antigens, whereas normal donors may not be tolerant to the antigens and remain capable of developing effective immune responses after transplantation.

8. Donor Natural Killer Cells as Mediators of GVL

The human NK cell repertoire is defined by the combination of NK cell receptors, either MHC class I specific killer inhibitory receptors (KIR) or receptors, such as CD94/NKG2, that are specific for nonclassical HLA molecules such as

HLA-E and NK cell ligands (Lanier, 2005; Norman and Parham, 2005; Uhrberg, 2005). The genes for KIR, CD94/NKG2, and HLA are located on different chromosomes, and therefore expression of NK cell receptors and ligands segregate independently. Although NK receptors do not undergo molecular rearrangements, individual KIR genes exhibit a high degree of allelic polymorphism and this contributes to the expression of a diverse repertoire of NK receptors. Every mature NK cell in the repertoire expresses at least one KIR for self-HLA class I molecules and each NK cell is therefore inhibited from killing autologous cells. However, within the NK cell pool, individual NK cells are capable of detecting autologous cells that have lost expression of even a single HLA class I allele. Loss of HLA expression occurs most often as a result of viral infection and in some cases of malignant transformation.

Engagement of NK cell receptors results in stimulation or inhibition of NK cell effector function, depending on intracellular signaling mediated through the cytoplasmic tail or adaptor molecules associated with each receptor (Chiesa *et al.*, 2005; Moretta and Moretta, 2004). Although the NK cell response to a target depends on the net effect of activating and inhibitory receptors, it is predominantly negatively regulated by KIRs. As shown schematically in Fig. 5, adequate expression of appropriate inhibitory NK receptor ligands protects healthy "self" cells against NK cell lysis. However, in the absence of this inhibitory pathway, targets become susceptible to NK mediated lysis. In the setting of allogeneic HSCT, the results of NK activity depend on the directionality of lysis (Hsu and Dupont, 2005; Ruggeri *et al.*, 2005a). When the NK cells are donor-derived and recipient cells lack expression of the cognate KIR ligand, the donor NK cell lysis of recipient target cells can result in GVL and/or GVHD, depending on the tissue origin of the NK target. However, if the target cell is of donor origin, and the NK effector cell is of recipient origin, NK cell lysis can result in graft rejection. It has been estimated that NK cell alloreactivity can be expected to occur in about 50% of unrelated donor transplants with one or more HLA allele level mismatches.

Several lines of evidence have implicated donor NK cells as potential mediators of GVL. NK cells are the first of lymphoid lineage cells to reconstitute following allogeneic transplantation, and adequate recovery of NK cell number in the early posttransplant period has been associated with improved relapse-free outcome (Jiang *et al.*, 1997). Hercend *et al.* (1986) isolated and cloned lymphoid cells displaying cytotoxicity against leukemic blasts in the early transplant period. Characterization of these cells revealed them to be NK cells of donor origin that did not express T-cell antigens. This study demonstrated that at least some clones with antileukemia activity after HSCT are cells with NK cell function and phenotype. Hauch *et al.* (1990) also examined NK cell lytic function in the early posttransplant period in patients with CML

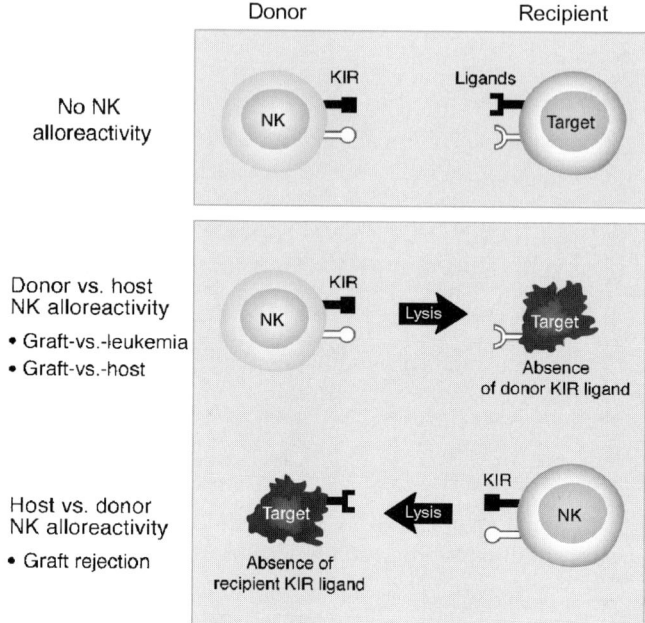

Figure 5 KIR regulate alloreactivity mediated by NK cells.

undergoing allogeneic HSCT. This study detected NK cell lysis of CML targets as early as 3 weeks following transplant and improved survival in those patients who were capable of generating NK-lytic activity against host-derived CML targets.

The strongest clinical evidence supporting a role for NK cells as mediators of GVL has been found in patients who receive stem cell transplants from HLA-mismatched donors. In this setting, KIR on donor NK cells are potentially mismatched with their inhibiting HLA-ligands and, as shown in Fig. 5, are capable of recognizing and killing recipient leukemia cells. For example, several studies by Ruggeri et al. (1999, 2002, 2005b) examined the impact of NK alloreactivity in patients who received myeloablative conditioning followed by transplantation of T-cell depleted stem cells from HLA haplotype-mismatched donors. In these studies, NK alloreactivity was predicted on the basis of HLA-B and HLA-C typing, and donor–recipient pairs were divided into two groups: those with KIR ligand incompatibility in the donor versus host direction, and those without. In a large clinical trial that included 112 patients with high-risk acute leukemia, predicted NK alloreactivity was highly correlated with transplant outcome in patients with acute myelogenous leukemia (AML). Notably, event-free survival for AML patients in the KIR ligand incompatible group was 60%, compared to only 5% in the compatible group. Moreover, screening donor-derived NK clones for lysis against recipient cells confirmed that KIR ligand incompatibility correlated closely with the detection of donor NK clones killing recipient targets. KIR ligand incompatibility did not influence outcome in patients with acute lymphoblastic leukemia (ALL), but NK cell alloreactivity in the donor versus host direction appeared to protect patients with AML against graft rejection, GVHD, and leukemia relapse.

Since national and international registries have successfully increased the number of healthy volunteers willing to anonymously donate hematopoietic stem cells, it is increasingly possible to identify unrelated HLA-matched donors for patients who do not have HLA-identical sibling donors. In this setting, it is potentially possible to identify donors with disparity at specific MHC class I alleles and to select donors that would provide a favorable mismatch for NK cell alloreactivity. However, retrospective studies of patients who have had partially HLA-mismatched unrelated donors have not consistently found that KIR ligand incompatibility has been associated with improved outcome. In one study, Giebel et al. (2003) evaluated 130 patients with hematologic malignancies who received transplants from unrelated donors. Overall survival was 87% in patients with KIR ligand incompatible donors compared to 48% who did not have KIR ligand incompatibility. However, two other studies did not find any correlation between KIR ligand incompatibility and transplant outcome in patients with partially HLA-mismatched unrelated donors (Bornhauser et al., 2001; Davies et al., 2002). Moreover, a follow-up study by Aversa et al. (2005), in 101 patients with HLA-mismatched related donors, did not observe a significant impact of NK alloreactivity on relapse in patients with AML. Notably, these studies utilized different conditioning regimens, different immune suppressive medications for GVHD prophylaxis and different methods for T-cell depletion of donor stem cells. These factors likely affect the degree to which NK alloreactivity can effectively mediate GVL after transplant and further clinical trials will be necessary to optimize clinical protocols that facilitate donor versus host NK alloreactivity.

Another approach to better characterize the role of NK cells as mediators of GVL is to specifically determine KIR genotype in individual donors (Leung et al., 2004). Population KIR genotyping studies have revealed that significant KIR diversity exists between individuals, and that one or more inhibitory KIR may be lacking in some individuals (Hsu et al., 2002; Norman and Parham, 2005). Thus, KIR-driven alloreactivity in the transplant setting may be more accurately assessed if the donor KIR genotype were known in addition to the

HLA genotype of the recipient. In contrast to assessment of NK alloreactivity based entirely on KIR ligand incompatibility, which is only present when recipient and donor are HLA-mismatched, KIR alloreactivity can also be demonstrated when recipient and donor are HLA-matched. To address this issue, Hsu et al. (2005) examined 178 patients who received T-cell depleted stem cells from HLA-identical siblings. When KIR and HLA genotypes were determined for each donor recipient pair, it was found that 63% of patients lacked an HLA ligand for donor inhibitory KIR ("missing KIR ligand"). While the absence of KIR ligand did not affect transplant outcomes in patients with CML or ALL, KIR/HLA-ligand mismatch contributed significantly to improved disease free survival in AML and MDS. Notably, patients lacking 2 HLA ligands for donor-inhibitory KIR had the best disease free survival but donor-activating KIR did not contribute to transplant outcome. These observations suggest that there may be a dose effect of inhibitory NK receptors, but activating NK receptors do not appear to play an important role in GVL after allogeneic HSCT. Now that methods for determining KIR genotype are becoming available, further studies will be able to define the role of these receptors in the ability of NK cells to mediate GVL.

9. Donor B Cells as Mediators of GVL

While substantial clinical and laboratory evidence indicates that donor T cells and NK cells are important mediators of GVL, few studies have examined whether antibodies produced by donor B cells might also contribute to tumor immunity following allogeneic HSCT. Nevertheless, several recent studies suggest that B cells are also likely to play an important role in GVL. As part of the adaptive immune response, B cells can enhance immunogenicity of tumors by secretion of cytokines and chemokines and antigen-antibody immune complexes facilitate antigen delivery to antigen presenting cells (APC) and can thereby enhance antigen-specific T-cell activation. When directed against cell surface molecules, antigen-specific antibodies that can directly lyse tumor cells through antibody-dependent cellular cytotoxicity (ADCC) and complement-mediated lysis.

As described previously for T cells and summarized in Fig. 4, both mHA and tumor-associated antigens are potential targets of donor B cells that can contribute to GVL following allogeneic HSCT. To determine whether mHA could elicit antibody responses following allogeneic HSCT, Miklos et al. (2004) tested posttransplant serum from 150 patients for the presence of antibodies specific for DBY protein, a known target of T-cell responses after allogeneic HSCT. Remarkably, 50% of male patients who received stem cell grafts from female donors developed antibody responses to recombinant DBY protein compared to 5% of male patients with male donors. Antibodies to DBY were also detected in 17% of healthy women, but not in healthy men. Very few of the patients developed antibodies against the X-encoded homologue, DBX, and antibody responses were directed primarily against areas of amino acid disparity between DBY and DBX. Further studies extended this analysis to detect antibodies to a panel of 5 recombinant HY proteins (DBY, UTY, ZFY, RPS4Y, and EIF1AY) and their HX homologues in a cohort of 75 male patients who had engrafted with stem cells from female donors (Miklos et al., 2005). Although DBY was the most immunogenic protein, antibody responses were detected against each of the HY proteins, including several that had not previously been documented to be targets of T-cell responses. IgG antibodies generally developed 4–12 months after transplant and persisted for several years after HSCT. HY antibodies were not associated with acute GVHD, but as shown in Fig. 6, 89% of patients with at least one HY antibody developed chronic GVHD compared to only 31% of patients without antibodies to this panel ($p < 0.0001$). Also shown in Fig. 6, 48% of patients without HY antibodies relapsed compared to 0% of patients with HY antibodies ($p < 0.0001$). Thus far, all mHA identified have been intracellular proteins and the mechanisms whereby antibodies to these proteins might contribute to GVHD and GVL have not been elucidated. The role of preexisting antibody responses to HY antigens in healthy female stem cell donors, presumably resulting from previous exposure to male cells during pregnancy or blood transfusion, is also unknown (Verdijk et al., 2004). Detailed studies in one transplant patient with both T and B cell responses to DBY suggested that these responses are directed against distinct epitopes and that the antibody response is primarily responsible for discriminating between recipient and

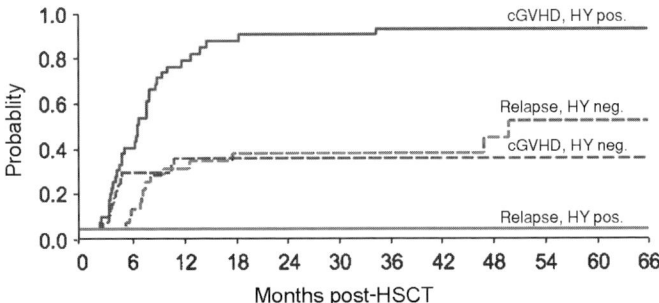

Figure 6 Cumulative incidence of chronic GVHD (cGVHD-blue lines) and relapse (red lines) as competing risk after allogeneic HSCT. All patients are males who engrafted with stem cells from female donors. Patients who developed antibodies to at least one HY antigen (solid lines) are compared to patients without detectable HY antibodies (broken lines).

donor alleles in this individual with persistent chronic GVHD (Zorn et al., 2004). If antibodies to mHA contribute to the immunopathology of GVHD, B cell directed therapy with agents, such as rituximab, might represent a new therapeutic modality for severe chronic GVHD. Clinical studies at our center and others have suggested that rituximab may improve some of the clinical manifestations of chronic GVHD and larger trials evaluating this approach have been initiated (Ratanatharathorn et al., 2003). However, inhibition of B cell responses may also reduce GVL activity and this should be closely monitored in these patients.

Antibody responses against tumor-associated antigens have also been identified in association with GVL activity after allogeneic HSCT (Bellucci et al., 2004; Hishizawa et al., 2005; Wu et al., 2000b). In previous studies from our laboratory, we characterized the repertoire of GVL-associated antibody responses by focusing on a group of patients with CML who achieved durable remission following $CD4^+$ DLI. Since these patients achieved a clinically well-defined tumor response in the absence of GVHD or any other therapy, they provided a unique opportunity to characterize the immunologic events associated with this effective GVL response in vivo. Using an antibody-based cDNA expression cloning strategy, post-DLI responder sera was used to screen a CML cDNA library, and clones specifically reactive with post-DLI but neither pre-DLI nor pre-BMT sera were isolated and identified (Sahin et al., 1997; Wu et al., 2000b). Using serial samples from 3 patients, we initially identified a group of 13 antigens, encoding a variety of known and novel genes involved in various cellular functions, including gene transcription, cell cycle, and cell signaling. Each of these antigens elicited high-titer antibody responses that were temporally correlated with clinical responses after DLI. An illustration of antibody responses specific for two of the novel CML-associated antigens in this group, CML66 and CML28, are shown in Fig. 7. Antibody responses to both of these targets were not present before transplant or before DLI. High-titer antibodies developed 2–3 months after DLI coincident with the achievement of cytogenetic and molecular remission of CML (Yang et al., 2001, 2002). Unlike HY genes, neither of these genes appears to encode polymorphisms that distinguish the alleles expressed in the transplant donor and recipient. Moreover, antibodies to CML66 and CML28 were not present in patients with chronic GVHD; patients with CML who underwent T-cell depleted allogeneic HSCT or normal donors. Remarkably, antibodies to these 2 antigens were also present in patients with CML who had responded to treatment with interferon-α, but not in patients treated with hydroxyurea or imatinib. Taken together with experiments demonstrating high-level expression of these antigens in leukemia cells, these studies suggest that the

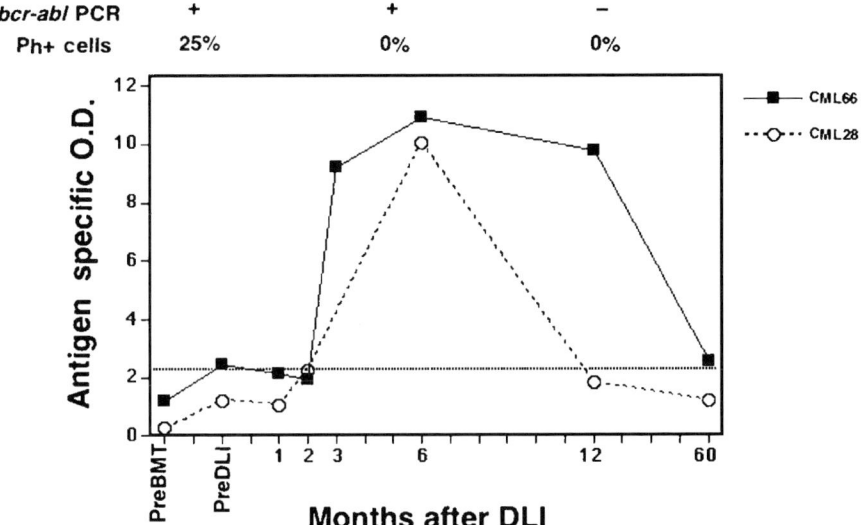

Figure 7 Antibody titers specific for 2 CML-associated tumor antigens following allogeneic HSCT. CML66—solid line; CML28—broken line; and upper limit of normal—dotted line.

immunogenicity of both of these proteins derives from their high-level expression in leukemia cells and not because they represent novel alloantigens.

A similar cloning strategy has been applied to the identification of tumor-associated antigens in other hematologic malignancies (Bellucci et al., 2004; Hishizawa et al., 2005). Bellucci et al. (2004) examined antibody responses in patients with multiple myeloma who responded to CD4$^+$ DLI and identified a series of target antigens in which antibody responses correlated with clinical response. Individual patients with CML and myeloma generally appear to demonstrate their own unique patterns of antibody responses. However, some antigens, such as RBP-J$_k$, RAFTK, BCMA, ROCK-1, Homer-3, and dihydrolipoamide acetyltransferase, are recognized in common by several DLI responders. In general, these antibody-defined target antigens are highly expressed in hematopoietic tumors and some are widely expressed in different solid tumors. Expression of these antigens in normal tissues is also highly variable. Some have very restricted expression in normal tissues, similar to cancer-testes antigens whereas others are expressed in many cell types. Interestingly, CML66 and CML28 are highly expressed in myeloid progenitor cells but not in more mature myeloid cells (Wu et al., 2005). This restricted pattern of expression for CML28 and CML66 is particularly relevant since effective GVL responses in this disease must target antigens present in self-renewing malignant progenitor populations (Jamieson et al., 2004; Passegue et al., 2003).

The great majority of antigens identified by serological screening are intracellular proteins. Antibodies targeting these antigens cannot initiate direct lysis of leukemia cells through complement activation or ADCC. However, antibodies to intracellular antigens are able to facilitate cross-presentation of target antigens through an FcγR mediated pathway in dendritic cells resulting in the stimulation of $CD8^+$ T-cell responses to peptide epitopes within the target protein (Amigorena, 2002; Dhodapkar et al., 2002; Kita et al., 2002). In some instances, serologically defined antigens after allogeneic HSCT are expressed on the surface membrane of tumor cells. In particular, one of the myeloma-associated antigens identified by Bellucci et al. (2005) was B cell maturation antigen (BCMA). This membrane receptor of the tumor necrosis factor (TNF) receptor superfamily is selectively expressed on the surface of mature B cells and myeloma cells. In this instance, antibodies that developed in vivo after DLI were reactive with cell surface domain of BCMA. When tested in functional assays, these IgG antibodies in patient serum were able to mediate complement-induced lysis and ADCC of stably transfected BCMA expressing cells or primary BCMA expressing myeloma cells. These antibodies were detected in 2 of 9 DLI responders and persisted for long periods after DLI. Taken together, these observations suggest several mechanisms whereby B cell responses to leukemia-associated likely contribute to GVL activity in vivo.

10. Future Directions

Worldwide, over 10,000 patients with hematologic malignancies undergo allogeneic HSCT each year. Ongoing clinical research continues to reduce the toxicity of treatment, and increased availability of unrelated stem cell products from adult volunteer donors and from cryopreserved umbilical cord blood banks continues to make allogeneic HSCT available to larger numbers of patients each year. This increased utilization of allogeneic HSCT is based entirely on the clinical utility of this approach for elimination of tumor cells in vivo in patients with a variety of hematologic malignancies. The previous sections of this review have summarized a large body of data demonstrating that the effectiveness of this approach is largely based on the immunologic elimination and long-term control of malignant cells by the donor immune system. Although this treatment continues to be associated with significant toxicity and disease control is not achieved in all patients, allogeneic HSCT represents an excellent example of the power of effective tumor immunity and the clinical results that can be achieved through this mechanism.

Many aspects of GVL after allogeneic HSCT are not well understood, but remarkable progress in this area has begun to elucidate many important target antigens of this response and the immunologic mechanisms responsible for this effect *in vivo*. Interestingly, characterization of the GVL targets of T and B cell responses has revealed that clinically effective immune responses appear to be polyclonal, directed at a wide variety of both alloantigens and tumor-associated antigens. While some immune responses against specific target antigens are shared among different patients, many immune targets appear to be individualized and dependent on the variable expression of these antigens by tumor cells as well as genetic polymorphisms and diversity of MHC molecules. There also appears to be compelling evidence that effective tumor rejection involves a coordinated response that includes cellular, humoral, and innate immunity. Each of these responses appears to play a significant role in tumor rejection and long lasting prevention of relapse. Finally, clinical responses are more easily generated in the setting of minimal residual disease and slowly proliferating tumor cells, especially when less intensive chemotherapy and radiation therapy are used to prepare patients for allogeneic HSCT.

These insights suggest several ways in which new therapies can be developed in the allogeneic setting to further enhance GVL. To the extent that these new therapies target antigens that are widely expressed in recipient tissues, these new approaches may increase the risk of GVHD. However, directing new therapies against mHA with very restricted distribution or against tumor-associated antigens may reduce the risk of GVHD. For example, DLI has been shown to be effective in some patients with relapsed disease and has also been used to prevent relapse following transplant. More effective ways of using donor cells are being developed (Barge *et al.*, 2003; Riddell, 2004). These include the selection of specific donor cells for infusion or the expansion of specific T-cell populations *in vitro* that target either mHA or tumor-associated antigens in the recipient (Bleakley and Riddell, 2004; Marijt *et al.*, 2003). Donor NK cells or subsets of NK cells can also be selected and expanded *in vitro* to target leukemia cells in the recipient (Miller *et al.*, 2005). Another approach to enhance immunologic targeting of malignant cells after transplant is to incorporate active vaccination of the recipient after engraftment of donor cells to either induce or enhance responses to mHA or tumor-associated antigens. Model systems have suggested that this approach is feasible and potentially effective (Anderson *et al.*, 2000; Luznik *et al.*, 2003; Teshima *et al.*, 2002), but the selection of methods for vaccination as well as timing and dosing of vaccines must take into consideration the ability of the reconstituting donor immune system to respond to antigenic challenge and a variety of patient factors that were summarized in Fig. 1.

Once GVL responses have been initiated, persistence of the effector response and the generation of long-lived memory appear to be highly regulated *in vivo*. Multiple mechanisms for inhibiting tumor immunity have been identified in patients with cancer and it is likely that similar mechanisms also play an important role in downregulating GVL after allogeneic HSCT. Methods to enhance or suppress regulatory cells or regulatory pathways are now being evaluated in clinical trials in patients with solid tumors. These include infusions of anti-CTLA-4 monoclonal antibody either alone or following administration of tumor vaccine (Hodi *et al.*, 2003; Sanderson *et al.*, 2005). Similar approaches may also be useful for enhancing GVL after allogeneic HSCT. In this setting, it will be important to consider that negative immune regulatory pathways also contribute to control of GVHD (Hanash and Levy, 2005; Taylor *et al.*, 2005; Zorn *et al.*, 2005). In animal models, regulatory T cells appear to be more effective in controlling GVHD than GVL (Trenado *et al.*, 2003), and approaches that eliminate regulatory T cells *in vivo* may therefore induce both GVL and GVHD.

Although GVL provides an excellent practical example of the potential clinical effectiveness of tumor immunity, this treatment approach continues to be associated with significant toxicities resulting from intensive chemotherapy, allo-immunity, and immune deficiency. Progress is being made in all of these areas, and this promises to further reduce the toxicity of this treatment. Moreover, as further studies continue to elucidate the immune mechanisms that contribute to GVL, it is likely that investigators in this field will be able to develop new and effective strategies for improving the elimination of malignant cells after allogeneic HSCT. The overall goal of these studies is to enhance GVL without also increasing GVHD, and significant improvements in patient outcome will result if this can be accomplished. Better understanding of the mechanisms required for tumor rejection after allogeneic HSCT will also be applicable to the development of autologous approaches to induce effective tumor immunity *in vivo*.

References

Akatsuka, Y., Nishida, T., Kondo, E., Miyazaki, M., Taji, H., Iida, H., Tsujimura, K., Yazaki, M., Naoe, T., Morishima, Y., *et al.* (2003). Identification of a polymorphic gene, BCL2A1, encoding two novel hematopoietic lineage-specific minor histocompatibility antigens. *J. Exp. Med.* **197,** 1489–1500.

Alyea, E. P., Kim, H. T., Ho, V., Cutler, C., Gribben, J., DeAngelo, D. J., Lee, S. J., Windawi, S., Ritz, J., Stone, R. M., *et al.* (2005). Comparative outcome of nonmyeloablative and myeloablative allogeneic hematopoietic cell transplantation for patients older than 50 years of age. *Blood* **105,** 1810–1814.

Alyea, E. P., Soiffer, R. J., Canning, C., Neuberg, D., Schlossman, R., Pickett, C., Collins, H., Wang, Y., Anderson, K. C., and Ritz, J. (1998). Toxicity and efficacy of defined doses of CD4(+) donor lymphocytes for treatment of relapse after allogeneic bone marrow transplant. *Blood* **91,** 3671–3680.

Amigorena, S. (2002). Fc gamma receptors and cross-presentation in dendritic cells. *J. Exp. Med.* **195,** F1–F3.

Anderson, L. D., Jr., Savary, C. A., and Mullen, C. A. (2000). Immunization of allogeneic bone marrow transplant recipients with tumor cell vaccines enhances graft-versus-tumor activity without exacerbating graft-versus-host disease. *Blood* **95,** 2426–2433.

Atkinson, K. (1990). Reconstruction of the haemopoietic and immune systems after marrow transplantation. *Bone Marrow Transplant.* **5,** 209–226.

Atkinson, K., Farrell, C., Chapman, G., Downs, K., Penny, R., and Biggs, J. (1986). Female marrow donors increase the risk of acute graft-versus-host disease: Effect of donor age and parity and analysis of cell subpopulations in the donor marrow inoculum. *Br. J. Haematol.* **63,** 231–239.

Aversa, F., Terenzi, A., Tabilio, A., Falzetti, F., Carotti, A., Ballanti, S., Felicini, R., Falcinelli, F., Velardi, A., Ruggeri, L., *et al.* (2005). Full haplotype-mismatched hematopoietic stem-cell transplantation: A phase II study in patients with acute leukemia at high risk of relapse. *J. Clin. Oncol.* **23,** 3447–3454.

Azuma, T., Makita, M., Ninomiya, K., Fujita, S., Harada, M., and Yasukawa, M. (2002). Identification of a novel WT1-derived peptide which induces human leucocyte antigen-A24-restricted anti-leukaemia cytotoxic T lymphocytes. *Br. J. Haematol.* **116,** 601–603.

Barge, R. M., Osanto, S., Marijt, W. A., Starrenburg, C. W., Fibbe, W. E., Nortier, J. W., Falkenburg, J. H., and Willemze, R. (2003). Minimal GVHD following *in-vitro* T cell-depleted allogeneic stem cell transplantation with reduced-intensity conditioning allowing subsequent infusions of donor lymphocytes in patients with hematological malignancies and solid tumors. *Exp. Hematol.* **31,** 865–872.

Baron, F., Little, M. T., and Storb, R. (2005). Kinetics of engraftment following allogeneic hematopoietic cell transplantation with reduced-intensity or nonmyeloablative conditioning. *Blood Rev.* **19,** 153–164.

Barrett, A. J., Mavroudis, D., Tisdale, J., Molldrem, J., Clave, E., Dunbar, C., Cottler-Fox, M., Phang, S., Carter, C., Okunnieff, P., Young, N. S., and Read, E. J. (1998). T cell-depleted bone marrow transplantation and delayed T cell add-back to control acute GVHD and conserve a graft-versus-leukemia effect. *Bone Marrow Transplant.* **21,** 543–551.

Bellucci, R., Alyea, E. P., Chiaretti, S., Wu, C. J., Zorn, E., Weller, E., Wu, B., Canning, C., Schlossman, R., Munshi, N. C., Anderson, K. C., and Ritz, J. (2005). Graft-versus-tumor response in patients with multiple myeloma is associated with antibody response to BCMA, a plasma-cell membrane receptor. *Blood* **105,** 3945–3950.

Bellucci, R., Alyea, E. P., Weller, E., Chillemi, A., Hochberg, E., Wu, C. J., Canning, C., Schlossman, R., Soiffer, R. J., Anderson, K. C., and Ritz, J. (2002). Immunologic effects of prophylactic donor lymphocyte infusion after allogeneic marrow transplantation for multiple myeloma. *Blood* **99,** 4610–4617.

Bellucci, R., Wu, C. J., Chiaretti, S., Weller, E., Davies, F. E., Alyea, E. P., Dranoff, G., Anderson, K. C., Munshi, N. C., and Ritz, J. (2004). Complete response to donor lymphocyte infusion in multiple myeloma is associated with antibody responses to highly expressed antigens. *Blood* **103,** 656–663.

Bethge, W. A., Hegenbart, U., Stuart, M. J., Storer, B. E., Maris, M. B., Flowers, M. E., Maloney, D. G., Chauncey, T., Bruno, B., Agura, E., Forman, S. J., Blume, K. G., *et al.* (2004). Adoptive immunotherapy with donor lymphocyte infusions after allogeneic hematopoietic cell transplantation following nonmyeloablative conditioning. *Blood* **103,** 790–795.

Bleakley, M., and Riddell, S. R. (2004). Molecules and mechanisms of the graft-versus-leukaemia effect. *Nat. Rev. Cancer* **4,** 371–380.

Bocchia, M., Wentworth, P. A., Southwood, S., Sidney, J., McGraw, K., Scheinberg, D. A., and Sette, A. (1995). Specific binding of leukemia oncogene fusion protein peptides to HLA class I molecules. *Blood* **85,** 2680–2684.

Bomberger, C., Singh-Jairam, M., Rodey, G., Guerriero, A., Yeager, A. M., Fleming, W. H., Holland, H. K., and Waller, E. K. (1998). Lymphoid reconstitution after autologous PBSC transplantation with FACS-sorted CD34+ hematopoietic progenitors. *Blood* **91,** 2588–2600.

Bonnet, D., Warren, E. H., Greenberg, P. D., Dick, J. E., and Riddell, S. R. (1999). CD8(+) minor histocompatibility antigen-specific cytotoxic T lymphocyte clones eliminate human acute myeloid leukemia stem cells. *Proc. Natl. Acad. Sci. USA* **96,** 8639–8644.

Bornhauser, M., Thiede, C., Platzbecker, U., Jenke, A., Helwig, A., Plettig, R., Freiberg-Richter, J., Rollig, C., Geissler, G., Lutterbeck, K., Oelshlagel, U., and Ehninger, G. (2001). Dose-reduced conditioning and allogeneic hematopoietic stem cell transplantation from unrelated donors in 42 patients. *Clin. Cancer Res.* **7,** 2254–2262.

Brickner, A. G., Evans, A. M., Mito, J. K., Xuereb, S., Feng, X., Nishida, T., Fairfull, L., Ferrell, R. E., Foon, K. A., Hunt, D. F., Shahanowitz, J., Engelhard, V. H., et al. (2006). The PANE1 gene encodes novel human minor histocompatibility antigen that is selectively expressed in B-lymphoid cells and B-cell. *Blood* (in press).

Brickner, A. G., Warren, E. H., Caldwell, J. A., Akatsuka, Y., Golovina, T. N., Zarling, A. L., Shabanowitz, J., Eisenlohr, L. C., Hunt, D. F., Engelhard, V. H., and Riddell, S. R. (2001). The immunogenicity of a new human minor histocompatibility antigen results from differential antigen processing. *J. Exp. Med.* **193,** 195–206.

Butturini, A., Bortin, M. M., and Gale, R. P. (1987). Graft-versus-leukemia following bone marrow transplantation. *Bone Marrow Transplant.* **2,** 233–242.

Cargill, M., Altshuler, D., Ireland, J., Sklar, P., Ardlie, K., Patil, N., Shaw, N., Lane, C. R., Lim, E. P., Kalyanaraman, N., Nemesh, J., Ziangra, L., et al. (1999). Characterization of single-nucleotide polymorphisms in coding regions of human genes. *Nat. Genet.* **22,** 231–238.

Cathcart, K., Pinilla-Ibarz, J., Korontsvit, T., Schwartz, J., Zakhaleva, V., Papadopoulos, E. B., and Scheinberg, D. A. (2004). A multivalent bcr-abl fusion peptide vaccination trial in patients with chronic myeloid leukemia. *Blood* **103,** 1037–1042.

Champlin, R., Ho, W., Gajewski, J., Feig, S., Burnison, M., Holley, G., Greenberg, P., Lee, K., Schmid, I., Giorgi, J., Yam, P., Petz, L., et al. (1990). Selective depletion of CD8$^+$ T lymphocytes for prevention of graft-versus-host disease after allogeneic bone marrow transplantation. *Blood* **76,** 418–423.

Chiesa, S., Tomasello, E., Vivier, E., and Vely, F. (2005). Coordination of activating and inhibitory signals in natural killer cells. *Mol. Immunol.* **42,** 477–484.

Childs, R., Chernoff, A., Contentin, N., Bahceci, E., Schrump, D., Leitman, S., Read, E. J., Tisdale, J., Dunbar, C., Linehan, W. M., Young, N. S., and Barrett, A. J. (2000). Regression of metastatic renal-cell carcinoma after nonmyeloablative allogeneic peripheral-blood stem-cell transplantation. *N. Engl. J. Med.* **343,** 750–758.

Claret, E. J., Alyea, E. P., Orsini, E., Pickett, C. C., Collins, H., Wang, Y., Neuberg, D., Soiffer, R. J., and Ritz, J. (1997). Characterization of T cell repertoire in patients with graft-versus-leukemia after donor lymphocyte infusion. *J. Clin. Invest.* **100,** 855–866.

Collins, R. H., Jr., Rogers, Z. R., Bennett, M., Kumar, V., Nikein, A., and Fay, J. W. (1992). Hematologic relapse of chronic myelogenous leukemia following allogeneic bone marrow transplantation: Apparent graft-versus-leukemia effect following abrupt discontinuation of immunosuppression. *Bone Marrow Transplant.* **10,** 391–395.

Collins, R. H., Jr., Shpilberg, O., Drobyski, W. R., Porter, D. L., Giralt, S., Champlin, R., Goodman, S. A., Wolff, S. N., Hu, W., Verfaillie, C., List, A., Dalton, W., *et al.* (1997). Donor leukocyte infusions in 140 patients with relapsed malignancy after allogeneic bone marrow transplantation. *J. Clin. Oncol.* **15,** 433–444.

Crawley, C., Lalancette, M., Szydlo, R., Gilleece, M., Peggs, K., Mackinnon, S., Juliusson, G., Ahlberg, L., Nagler, A., Shimoni, A., Sureda, A., Boiron, J. M., *et al.* (2005). Outcomes for reduced-intensity allogeneic transplantation for multiple myeloma: An analysis of prognostic factors from the Chronic Leukaemia Working Party of the EBMT. *Blood* **105,** 4532–4539.

Davies, S. M., Ruggieri, L., DeFor, T., Wagner, J. E., Weisdorf, D. J., Miller, J. S., Velardi, A., and Blazar, B. R. (2002). Evaluation of KIR ligand incompatibility in mismatched unrelated donor hematopoietic transplants. Killer immunoglobulin-like receptor. *Blood* **100,** 3825–3827.

Dazzi, F., Szydlo, R. M., Cross, N. C., Craddock, C., Kaeda, J., Kanfer, E., Cwynarski, K., Olavarria, E., Yong, A., Apperley, J. F., and Goldman, J. M. (2000). Durability of responses following donor lymphocyte infusions for patients who relapse after allogeneic stem cell transplantation for chronic myeloid leukemia. *Blood* **96,** 2712–2716.

de Rijke, B., van Horssen-Zoetbrod, A., Beekman, J. M., Otterud, B., Maas, F., Woestenenk, R., Kester, M., Leppert, M., Schattenberg, A. V., Witte, T., Van de Wiel-van Kemenade, E., and Dolstra, H. (2005). A frameshift polymorphism in P2X5 elicits an allogeneic cytotoxic T lymphocyte response associated with remission of chronic myeloid leukemia. *J. Clin. Invest.* **115,** 3506–3516.

den Haan, J. M., Meadows, L. M., Wang, W., Pool, J., Blokland, E., Bishop, T. L., Reinhardus, C., Shabanowitz, J., Offringa, R., Hunt, D. F., Engelhard, V. H., and Goulmy, E. (1998). The minor histocompatibility antigen HA-1: A diallelic gene with a single amino acid polymorphism. *Science* **279,** 1054–1057.

den Haan, J. M., Sherman, N. E., Blokland, E., Huczko, E., Koning, F., Drijfhout, J. W., Skipper, J., Shabanowitz, J., Hunt, D. F., Engelhard, V. H., and Goulmy, E. (1995). Identification of a graft versus host disease-associated human minor histocompatibility antigen. *Science* **268,** 1476–1480.

Dey, B. R., McAfee, S., Colby, C., Sackstein, R., Saidman, S., Tarbell, N., Sachs, D. H., Sykes, M., and Spitzer, T. R. (2003). Impact of prophylactic donor leukocyte infusions on mixed chimerism, graft-versus-host disease, and antitumor response in patients with advanced hematologic malignancies treated with nonmyeloablative conditioning and allogeneic bone marrow transplantation. *Biol. Blood Marrow Transplant.* **9,** 320–329.

Dhodapkar, K. M., Krasovsky, J., Williamson, B., and Dhodapkar, M. V. (2002). Antitumor monoclonal antibodies enhance cross-presentation ofcCellular antigens and the generation of myeloma-specific killer T cells by dendritic cells. *J. Exp. Med.* **195,** 125–133.

Dickinson, A. M., Wang, X. N., Sviland, L., Vyth-Dreese, F. A., Jackson, G. H., Schumacher, T. N., Haanen, J. B., Mutis, T., and Goulmy, E. (2002). In situ dissection of the graft-versus-host activities of cytotoxic T cells specific for minor histocompatibility antigens. *Nat. Med.* **8,** 410–414.

Dolstra, H., Fredrix, H., Maas, F., Coulie, P. G., Brasseur, F., Mensink, E., Adema, G. J., de Witte, T. M., Figdor, C. G., and van de Wiel-van Kemenade, E. (1999). A human minor histocompatibility antigen specific for B cell acute lymphoblastic leukemia. *J. Exp. Med.* **189,** 301–308.

Douek, D. C., McFarland, R. D., Keiser, P. H., Gage, E. A., Massey, J. M., Haynes, B. F., Polis, M. A., Haase, A. T., Feinberg, M. B., Sullivan, J. L., Jamieson, B. O., Zack, J. A., *et al.* (1998). Changes in thymic function with age and during the treatment of HIV infection. *Nature* **396,** 690–695.

Duhrsen, U., Knieling, G., Beecken, W., Neumann, S., and Hossfeld, D. K. (1995). Chimaeric cultures of human marrow stroma and murine leukaemia cells: Evidence for abnormalities in the haemopoietic microenvironment in myeloid malignancies and other infiltrating marrow disorders. *Br. J. Haematol.* **90,** 502–511.

Faber, L. M., van Luxemburg-Heijs, S. A., Veenhof, W. F., Willemze, R., and Falkenburg, J. H. (1995). Generation of CD4+ cytotoxic T-lymphocyte clones from a patient with severe graft-versus-host disease after allogeneic bone marrow transplantation: Implications for graft-versus-leukemia reactivity. *Blood* **86**, 2821–2828.

Faber, L. M., van Luxemburg-Heijs, S. A., Willemze, R., and Falkenburg, J. H. (1992). Generation of leukemia-reactive cytotoxic T lymphocyte clones from the HLA-identical bone marrow donor of a patient with leukemia. *J. Exp. Med.* **176**, 1283–1289.

Falkenburg, J. H., Wafelman, A. R., Joosten, P., Smit, W. M., van Bergen, C. A., Bongaerts, R., Lurvink, E., van der Hoorn, M., Kluck, P., Landegent, J. E., Kluin-Nelemans, H. C., Fibbe, W. E., et al. (1999). Complete remission of accelerated phase chronic myeloid leukemia by treatment with leukemia-reactive cytotoxic T lymphocytes. *Blood* **94**, 1201–1208.

Fefer, A., Sullivan, K. M., Weiden, P., Buckner, C. D., Schoch, G., Storb, R., and Thomas, E. D. (1987). Graft versus leukemia effect in man: The relapse rate of acute leukemia is lower after allogeneic than after syngeneic marrow transplantation. *Prog. Clin. Biol. Res.* **244**, 401–408.

Ferra, C., Rodriguez-Luaces, M., Gallardo, D., Encuentra, M., Martin-Henao, G. A., Peris, J., Ancin, I., Sarra, J., Berlanga, J. J., Garcia, J., and Granena, A. (2001). Individually adjusted prophylactic donor lymphocyte infusions after CD34-selected allogeneic peripheral blood stem cell transplantation. *Bone Marrow Transplant.* **28**, 963–968.

Flowers, M. E., Pepe, M. S., Longton, G., Doney, K. C., Monroe, D., Witherspoon, R. P., Sullivan, K. M., and Storb, R. (1990). Previous donor pregnancy as a risk factor for acute graft-versus-host disease in patients with aplastic anaemia treated by allogeneic marrow transplantation. *Br. J. Haematol.* **74**, 492–496.

Foote, S., Vollrath, D., Hilton, A., and Page, D. C. (1992). The human Y chromosome: Overlapping DNA clones spanning the euchromatic region. *Science* **258**, 60–66.

Forman, S. J., Nocker, P., Gallagher, M., Zaia, J., Wright, C., Bolen, J., Mills, B., and Hecht, T. (1982). Pattern of T cell reconstitution following allogeneic bone marrow transplantation for acute hematological malignancy. *Transplantation* **34**, 96–98.

Gale, R. P., Horowitz, M. M., Ash, R. C., Champlin, R. E., Goldman, J. M., Rimm, A. A., Ringden, O., Stone, J. A., and Bortin, M. M. (1994). Identical-twin bone marrow transplants for leukemia. *Ann. Intern. Med.* **120**, 646–652.

Genevee, C., Diu, A., Nierat, J., Caignard, A., Dietrich, P. Y., Ferradini, L., Roman-Roman, S., Triebel, F., and Hercend, T. (1992). An experimentally validated panel of subfamily-specific oligonucleotide primers (V alpha 1-w29/V beta 1-w24) for the study of human T cell receptor variable V gene segment usage by polymerase chain reaction. *Eur. J. Immunol.* **22**, 1261–1269.

Giebel, S., Locatelli, F., Lamparelli, T., Velardi, A., Davies, S., Frumento, G., Maccario, R., Bonetti, F., Wojnar, J., Martinetti, M., Frassoni, F., Giorgiani, G., et al. (2003). Survival advantage with KIR ligand incompatibility in hematopoietic stem cell transplantation from unrelated donors. *Blood* **102**, 814–819.

Goldman, J. M., Gale, R. P., Horowitz, M. M., Biggs, J. C., Champlin, R. E., Gluckman, E., Hoffmann, R. G., Jacobsen, S. J., Marmont, A. M., McGlave, P. B., Messner, H. A., Rimin, A. A., et al. (1988). Bone marrow transplantation for chronic myelogenous leukemia in chronic phase. Increased risk for relapse associated with T-cell depletion. *Ann. Intern. Med.* **108**, 806–814.

Gorski, J., Yassai, M., Zhu, X., Kissela, B., Kissella, B., Keever, C., and Flomenberg, N. (1994). Circulating T cell repertoire complexity in normal individuals and bone marrow recipients analyzed by CDR3 size spectratyping. Correlation with immune status. *J. Immunol.* **152**, 5109–5119.

Gratwohl, A., Hermans, J., Niederwieser, D., van Biezen, A., van Houwelingen, H. C., and Apperley, J. (2001). Female donors influence transplant-related mortality and relapse incidence in male recipients of sibling blood and marrow transplants. *Hematol. J.* **2,** 363–370.

Hakim, F. T., Cepeda, R., Kaimei, S., Mackall, C. L., McAtee, N., Zujewski, J., Cowan, K., and Gress, R. E. (1997). Constraints on CD4 recovery postchemotherapy in adults: Thymic insufficiency and apoptotic decline of expanded peripheral CD4 cells. *Blood* **90,** 3789–3798.

Hakim, F. T., Memon, S. A., Cepeda, R., Jones, E. C., Chow, C. K., Kasten-Sportes, C., Odom, J., Vance, B. A., Christensen, B. L., Mackall, C. L., and Gress, R. E. (2005). Age-dependent incidence, time course, and consequences of thymic renewal in adults. *J. Clin. Invest.* **115,** 930–939.

Hambach, L., and Goulmy, E. (2005). Immunotherapy of cancer through targeting of minor histocompatibility antigens. *Curr. Opin. Immunol.* **17,** 202–210.

Hanash, A. M., and Levy, R. B. (2005). Donor CD4+CD25+ T cells promote engraftment and tolerance following MHC-mismatched hematopoietic cell transplantation. *Blood* **105,** 1828–1836.

Hauch, M., Gazzola, M. V., Small, T., Bordignon, C., Barnett, L., Cunningham, I., Castro-Malaspinia, H., O'Reilly, R. J., and Keever, C. A. (1990). Anti-leukemia potential of interleukin-2 activated natural killer cells after bone marrow transplantation for chronic myelogenous leukemia. *Blood* **75,** 2250–2262.

Hercend, T., Takvorian, T., Nowill, A., Tantravahi, R., Moingeon, P., Anderson, K. C., Murray, C., Bohuon, C., Ythier, A., and Ritz, J. (1986). Characterization of natural killer cells with antileukemia activity following allogeneic bone marrow transplantation. *Blood* **67,** 722–728.

Hishizawa, M., Imada, K., Sakai, T., Ueda, M., and Uchiyama, T. (2005). Identification of APOBEC3B as a potential target for the graft-versus-lymphoma effect by SEREX in a patient with mantle cell lymphoma. *Br. J. Haematol.* **130,** 418–421.

Hochberg, E. P., Chillemi, A. C., Wu, C. J., Neuberg, D., Canning, C., Hartman, K., Alyea, E. P., Soiffer, R. J., Kalams, S. A., and Ritz, J. (2001). Quantitation of T-cell neogenesis *in vivo* after allogeneic bone marrow transplantation in adults. *Blood* **98,** 1116–1121.

Hodi, F. S., Mihm, M. C., Soiffer, R. J., Haluska, F. G., Butler, M., Seiden, M. V., Davis, T., Henry-Spires, R., MacRae, S., Willman, A., Padera, R., Jaklitsch, M. T., *et al.* (2003). Biologic activity of cytotoxic T lymphocyte-associated antigen 4 antibody blockade in previously vaccinated metastatic melanoma and ovarian carcinoma patients. *Proc. Natl. Acad. Sci. USA* **100,** 4712–4717.

Horowitz, M. M., Gale, R. P., Sondel, P. M., Goldman, J. M., Kersey, J., Kolb, H. J., Rimm, A. A., Ringden, O., Rozman, C., Speck, B., Truitt, R. L., Zwaan, F. E., *et al.* (1990). Graft-versus-leukemia reactions after bone marrow transplantation. *Blood* **75,** 555–562.

Hsu, K. C., and Dupont, B. (2005). Natural killer cell receptors: Regulating innate immune responses to hematologic malignancy. *Semin. Hematol.* **42,** 91–103.

Hsu, K. C., Keever-Taylor, C. A., Wilton, A., Pinto, C., Heller, G., Arkun, K., O'Reilly, R. J., Horowitz, M. M., and Dupont, B. (2005). Improved outcome in HLA-identical sibling hematopoietic stem-cell transplantation for acute myelogenous leukemia predicted by KIR and HLA genotypes. *Blood* **105,** 4878–4884.

Hsu, K. C., Liu, X. R., Selvakumar, A., Mickelson, E., O'Reilly, R. J., and Dupont, B. (2002). Killer Ig-like receptor haplotype analysis by gene content: Evidence for genomic diversity with a minimum of six basic framework haplotypes, each with multiple subsets. *J. Immunol.* **169,** 5118–5129.

James, E., Chai, J. G., Dewchand, H., Macchiarulo, E., Dazzi, F., and Simpson, E. (2003). Multiparity induces priming to male-specific minor histocompatibility antigen, HY, in mice and humans. *Blood* **102,** 388–393.

Jamieson, C. H., Ailles, L. E., Dylla, S. J., Muijtjens, M., Jones, C., Zehnder, J. L., Gotlib, J., Li, K., Manz, M. G., Keating, A., Sawyers, C. L., and Weissman, J. L. (2004). Granulocyte-macrophage progenitors as candidate leukemic stem cells in blast-crisis CML. *N. Engl. J. Med.* **351,** 657–667.

Jiang, Y. Z., Barrett, A. J., Goldman, J. M., and Mavroudis, D. A. (1997). Association of natural killer cell immune recovery with a graft-versus-leukemia effect independent of graft-versus-host disease following allogeneic bone marrow transplantation. *Ann. Hematol.* **74,** 1–6.

Jones, R. J., Ambinder, R. F., Piantadosi, S., and Santos, G. W. (1991). Evidence of a graft-versus-lymphoma effect associated with allogeneic bone marrow transplantation. *Blood* **77,** 649–653.

Keever, C. A., Small, T. N., Flomenberg, N., Heller, G., Pekle, K., Black, P., Pecora, A., Gillio, A., Kernan, N. A., and O'Reilly, R. J. (1989). Immune reconstitution following bone marrow transplantation: Comparison of recipients of T-cell depleted marrow with recipients of conventional marrow grafts. *Blood* **73,** 1340–1350.

Khouri, I. F., Keating, M., Korbling, M., Przepiorka, D., Anderlini, P., O'Brien, S., Giralt, S., Ippoliti, C., von Wolff, B., Gajewski, J., Donato, M., Claxton, D., *et al.* (1998). Transplant-lite: Induction of graft-versus-malignancy using fludarabine-based nonablative chemotherapy and allogeneic blood progenitor-cell transplantation as treatment for lymphoid malignancies. *J. Clin. Oncol.* **16,** 2817–2824.

Kircher, B., Stevanovic, S., Urbanek, M., Mitterschiffthaler, A., Rammensee, H. G., Grunewald, K., Gastl, G., and Nachbaur, D. (2002). Induction of HA-1-specific cytotoxic T-cell clones parallels the therapeutic effect of donor lymphocyte infusion. *Br. J. Haematol.* **117,** 935–939.

Kita, H., Lian, Z. X., Van de Water, J., He, X. S., Matsumura, S., Kaplan, M., Luketic, V., Coppel, R. L., Ansari, A. A., and Gershwin, M. E. (2002). Identification of HLA-A2-restricted CD8(+) cytotoxic T cell responses in primary biliary cirrhosis: T cell activation is augmented by immune complexes cross-presented by dendritic cells. *J. Exp. Med.* **195,** 113–123.

Kloosterboer, F. M., van Luxemburg-Heijs, S. A., van Soest, R. A., van Egmond, H. M., Willemze, R., and Falkenburg, J. H. (2005). Upregulated expression in non-hematopoietic tissues of the BCL2A1-derived minor histocompatibility antigens in response to inflammatory cytokines: Relevance for allogeneic immunotherapy of leukemia. *Blood* **106,** 3955–3957.

Kolb, H. J., Mittermuller, J., Clemm, C., Holler, E., Ledderose, G., Brehm, G., Heim, M., and Wilmanns, W. (1990). Donor leukocyte transfusions for treatment of recurrent chronic myelogenous leukemia in marrow transplant patients. *Blood* **76,** 2462–2465.

Kolb, H. J., Schattenberg, A., Goldman, J. M., Hertenstein, B., Jacobsen, N., Arcese, W., Ljungman, P., Ferrant, A., Verdonck, L., Niederwieser, D., van Rhee, F., Mittermueller, J., *et al.* (1995). Graft-versus-leukemia effect of donor lymphocyte transfusions in marrow grafted patients. *Blood* **86,** 2041–2050.

Lanier, L. L. (2005). NK cell recognition. *Annu. Rev. Immunol.* **23,** 225–274.

Leung, W., Iyengar, R., Turner, V., Lang, P., Bader, P., Conn, P., Niethammer, D., and Handgretinger, R. (2004). Determinants of antileukemia effects of allogeneic NK cells. *J. Immunol.* **172,** 644–650.

Libura, J., Hoffmann, T., Passweg, J., Gregor, M., Favre, G., Tichelli, A., and Gratwohl, A. (1999). Graft-versus-myeloma after withdrawal of immunosuppression following allogeneic peripheral stem cell transplantation. *Bone Marrow Transplant.* **24,** 925–927.

Lokhorst, H. M., Schattenberg, A., Cornelissen, J. J., Thomas, L. L., and Verdonck, L. F. (1997). Donor leukocyte infusions are effective in relapsed multiple myeloma after allogeneic bone marrow transplantation. *Blood* **90,** 4206–4211.

Luznik, L., Slansky, J. E., Jalla, S., Borrello, I., Levitsky, H. I., Pardoll, D. M., and Fuchs, E. J. (2003). Successful therapy of metastatic cancer using tumor vaccines in mixed allogeneic bone marrow chimeras. *Blood* **101,** 1645–1652.

Mackall, C. L., Fleisher, T. A., Brown, M. R., Andrich, M. P., Chen, C. C., Feuerstein, I. M., Horowitz, M. E., Magrath, I. T., Shad, A. T., Steinberg, S. M., Wexler, L. H., and Greos, R. E. (1995). Age, thymopoiesis, and CD4$^+$ T-lymphocyte regeneration after intensive chemotherapy. *N. Engl. J. Med.* **332,** 143–149.

Mandigers, C. M., Verdonck, L. F., Meijerink, J. P., Dekker, A. W., Schattenberg, A. V., and Raemaekers, J. M. (2003). Graft-versus-lymphoma effect of donor lymphocyte infusion in indolent lymphomas relapsed after allogeneic stem cell transplantation. *Bone Marrow Transplant.* **32,** 1159–1163.

Marijt, W. A., Heemskerk, M. H., Kloosterboer, F. M., Goulmy, E., Kester, M. G., van der Hoorn, M. A., van Luxemburg-Heys, S. A., Hoogeboom, M., Mutis, T., Drijfhout, J. W., van Rood, J. J., Wollenze, R., *et al.* (2003). Hematopoiesis-restricted minor histocompatibility antigens HA-1- or HA-2-specific T cells can induce complete remissions of relapsed leukemia. *Proc. Natl. Acad. Sci. USA* **100,** 2742–2747.

Marks, D. I., Lush, R., Cavenagh, J., Milligan, D. W., Schey, S., Parker, A., Clark, F. J., Hunt, L., Yin, J., Fuller, S., vanden Bergne, E., Marsh, J., *et al.* (2002). The toxicity and efficacy of donor lymphocyte infusions given after reduced-intensity conditioning allogeneic stem cell transplantation. *Blood* **100,** 3108–3114.

Martin, P. J., Clift, R. A., Fisher, L. D., Buckner, C. D., Hansen, J. A., Appelbaum, F. R., Doney, K. C., Sullivan, K. M., Witherspoon, R. P., Storb, R., and Thomas, E. D. (1988). HLA-identical marrow transplantation during accelerated-phase chronic myelogenous leukemia: Analysis of survival and remission duration. *Blood* **72,** 1978–1984.

Mattei, D., Saglio, G., Gottardi, E., Gallamini, A., Mordini, N., and Bacigalupo, A. (2001). Persisting molecular remission ten years after donor lymphocyte infusion for hematologic relapse in chronic myeloid leukemia. *Haematologica* **86,** 545–546.

McHeyzer-Williams, M. G., and Davis, M. M. (1995). Antigen-specific development of primary and memory T cells *in vivo*. *Science* **268,** 106–111.

McSweeney, P. A., Niederwieser, D., Shizuru, J. A., Sandmaier, B. M., Molina, A. J., Maloney, D. G., Chauncey, T. R., Gooley, T. A., Hegenbart, U., Nash, R. A., Radich, J., Wagner, J. L., *et al.* (2001). Hematopoietic cell transplantation in older patients with hematologic malignancies: Replacing high-dose cytotoxic therapy with graft-versus-tumor effects. *Blood* **97,** 3390–3400.

Meadows, L., Wang, W., den Haan, J. M., Blokland, E., Reinhardus, C., Drijfhout, J. W., Shabanowitz, J., Pierce, R., Agulnik, A. I., Bishop, C. E., Hunt, D. F., Goulmy, E., *et al.* (1997). The HLA-A°0201-restricted H-Y antigen contains a posttranslationally modified cysteine that significantly affects T cell recognition. *Immunity* **6,** 273–281.

Miklos, D. B., Kim, H. T., Miller, K. H., Guo, L., Zorn, E., Lee, S. J., Hochberg, E. P., Wu, C. J., Alyea, E. P., Cutler, C., Ho, V., Soitter, R. J., *et al.* (2005). Antibody responses to H-Y minor histocompatibility antigens correlate with chronic graft-versus-host disease and disease remission. *Blood* **105,** 2973–2978.

Miklos, D. B., Kim, H. T., Zorn, E., Hochberg, E. P., Guo, L., Mattes-Ritz, A., Viatte, S., Soiffer, R. J., Antin, J. H., and Ritz, J. (2004). Antibody response to DBY minor histocompatibility antigen is induced after allogeneic stem cell transplantation and in healthy female donors. *Blood* **103,** 353–359.

Miller, J. S., Soignier, Y., Panoskaltsis-Mortari, A., McNearney, S. A., Yun, G. H., Fautsch, S. K., McKenna, D., Le, C., Defor, T. E., Burns, L. J., Orchard, P. J., Blazar, B. R., *et al.* (2005). Successful adoptive transfer and *in vivo* expansion of human haploidentical NK cells in patients with cancer. *Blood* **105,** 3051–3057.

Molldrem, J. J., Lee, P. P., Wang, C., Felio, K., Kantarjian, H. M., Champlin, R. E., and Davis, M. M. (2000). Evidence that specific T lymphocytes may participate in the elimination of chronic myelogenous leukemia. *Nat. Med.* **6,** 1018–1023.

Mommaas, B., Kamp, J., Drijfhout, J. W., Beekman, N., Ossendorp, F., Van Veelen, P., Den Haan, J., Goulmy, E., and Mutis, T. (2002). Identification of a novel HLA-B60-restricted T cell epitope of the minor histocompatibility antigen HA-1 locus. *J. Immunol.* **169,** 3131–3136.

Moretta, L., and Moretta, A. (2004). Unravelling natural killer cell function: Triggering and inhibitory human NK receptors. *EMBO J.* **23,** 255–259.

Morris, E., Thomson, K., Craddock, C., Mahendra, P., Milligan, D., Cook, G., Smith, G. M., Parker, A., Schey, S., Chopra, R., Hatton, C., Tigne, J., et al. (2004). Outcomes after alemtuzumab-containing reduced-intensity allogeneic transplantation regimen for relapsed and refractory non-Hodgkin lymphoma. *Blood* **104,** 3865–3871.

Murata, M., Warren, E. H., and Riddell, S. R. (2003). A human minor histocompatibility antigen resulting from differential expression due to a gene deletion. *J. Exp. Med.* **197,** 1279–1289.

Mutis, T., and Goulmy, E. (2002). Targeting alloreactive T cells to hematopoietic system specific minor histocompatibility antigens for cellular immunotherapy of hematological malignancies after stem cell transplantation. *Ann. Hematol.* **81**(Suppl. 2), S38–S39.

Nishida, T., Akatsuka, Y., Morishima, Y., Hamajima, N., Tsujimura, K., Kuzushima, K., Kodera, Y., and Takahashi, T. (2004). Clinical relevance of a newly identified HLA-A24-restricted minor histocompatibility antigen epitope derived from BCL2A1, ACC-1, in patients receiving HLA genotypically matched unrelated bone marrow transplant. *Br. J. Haematol.* **124,** 629–635.

Norman, P. J., and Parham, P. (2005). Complex interactions: The immunogenetics of human leukocyte antigen and killer cell immunoglobulin-like receptors. *Semin. Hematol.* **42,** 65–75.

Oblon, D. J., Elfenbein, G. J., Braylan, R. C., Jones, J., and Weiner, R. S. (1983). The reversal of myelofibrosis associated with chronic myelogenous leukemia after allogeneic bone marrow transplantation. *Exp. Hematol.* **11,** 681–685.

Odom, L. F., August, C. S., Githens, J. H., Humbert, J. R., Morse, H., Peakman, D., Sharma, B., Rusnak, S. L., and Johnson, F. B. (1978). Remission of relapsed leukaemia during a graft-versus-host reaction. A "graft-versus-leukaemia reaction" in man? *Lancet* **2,** 537–540.

Orsini, E., Alyea, E. P., Chillemi, A., Schlossman, R., McLaughlin, S., Canning, C., Soiffer, R. J., Anderson, K. C., and Ritz, J. (2000). Conversion to full donor chimerism following donor lymphocyte infusion is associated with disease response in patients with multiple myeloma. *Biol. Blood Marrow Transplant.* **6,** 375–386.

Orsini, E., Bellucci, R., Alyea, E. P., Schlossman, R., Canning, C., McLaughlin, S., Ghia, P., Anderson, K. C., and Ritz, J. (2003). Expansion of tumor-specific CD8$^+$ T cell clones in patients with relapsed myeloma after donor lymphocyte infusion. *Cancer Res.* **63,** 2561–2568.

Passegue, E., Jamieson, C. H., Ailles, L. E., and Weissman, I. L. (2003). Normal and leukemic hematopoiesis: Are leukemias a stem cell disorder or a reacquisition of stem cell characteristics? *Proc. Natl. Acad. Sci. USA* **100**(Suppl. 1), 11842–11849.

Patel, D. D., Gooding, M. E., Parrott, R. E., Curtis, K. M., Haynes, B. F., and Buckley, R. H. (2000). Thymic function after hematopoietic stem-cell transplantation for the treatment of severe combined immunodeficiency. *N. Engl. J. Med.* **342,** 1325–1332.

Payne, C. M., Greenberg, B., Cromey, D., and Woo, L. (1987). Morphological evidence of an altered bone marrow microenvironment in patients with acute nonlymphoblastic leukemia and myelodysplastic disorders. *Exp. Hematol.* **15,** 143–153.

Peggs, K. S., Thomson, K., Hart, D. P., Geary, J., Morris, E. C., Yong, K., Goldstone, A. H., Linch, D. C., and Mackinnon, S. (2004). Dose-escalated donor lymphocyte infusions following reduced intensity transplantation: Toxicity, chimerism, and disease responses. *Blood* **103,** 1548–1556.

Pichert, G., Alyea, E. P., Soiffer, R. J., Roy, D. C., and Ritz, J. (1994). Persistence of myeloid progenitor cells expressing BCR-ABL mRNA after allogeneic bone marrow transplantation for chronic myelogenous leukemia. *Blood* **84,** 2109–2114.

Pichert, G., Roy, D. C., Gonin, R., Alyea, E. P., Belanger, R., Gyger, M., Perreault, C., Bonny, Y., Lerra, I., Murray, C., Soiffer, R. J., and Ritz, J. (1995). Distinct patterns of minimal residual disease associated with graft-versus-host disease after allogeneic bone marrow transplantation for chronic myelogenous leukemia. *J. Clin. Oncol.* **13,** 1704–1713.

Pierce, R. A., Field, E. D., den Haan, J. M., Caldwell, J. A., White, F. M., Marto, J. A., Wang, W., Frost, L. M., Blokland, E., Reinhardus, C., Shabanowitz, J., Hunt, D. F., *et al.* (1999). Cutting edge: The HLA-A°0101-restricted HY minor histocompatibility antigen originates from DFFRY and contains a cysteinylated cysteine residue as identified by a novel mass spectrometric technique. *J. Immunol.* **163,** 6360–6364.

Pierce, R. A., Field, E. D., Mutis, T., Golovina, T. N., Von Kap-Herr, C., Wilke, M., Pool, J., Shabanowitz, J., Pettenati, M. J., Eisenlohr, L. C., *et al.* (2001). The HA-2 minor histocompatibility antigen is derived from a diallelic gene encoding a novel human class I myosin protein. *J. Immunol.* **167,** 3223–3230.

Platzbecker, U., Ehninger, G., and Bornhauser, M. (2004). Allogeneic transplantation of CD34+ selected hematopoietic cells – clinical problems and current challenges. *Leuk. Lymphoma* **45,** 447–453.

Porter, D. L., Collins, R. H., Jr., Shpilberg, O., Drobyski, W. R., Connors, J. M., Sproles, A., and Antin, J. H. (1999). Long-term follow-up of patients who achieved complete remission after donor leukocyte infusions. *Biol. Blood Marrow Transplant.* **5,** 253–261.

Randolph, S. S., Gooley, T. A., Warren, E. H., Appelbaum, F. R., and Riddell, S. R. (2004). Female donors contribute to a selective graft-versus-leukemia effect in male recipients of HLA-matched, related hematopoietic stem cell transplants. *Blood* **103,** 347–352.

Ratanatharathorn, V., Ayash, L., Reynolds, C., Silver, S., Reddy, P., Becker, M., Ferrara, J. L., and Uberti, J. P. (2003). Treatment of chronic graft-versus-host disease with anti-CD20 chimeric monoclonal antibody. *Biol. Blood Marrow Transplant.* **9,** 505–511.

Reker, S., Meier, A., Holten-Andersen, L., Svane, I. M., Becker, J. C., thor Straten, P., and Andersen, M. H. (2004). Identification of novel survivin-derived CTL epitopes. *Cancer Biol. Ther.* **3,** 173–179.

Riddell, S. R. (2004). Finding a place for tumor-specific T cells in targeted cancer therapy. *J. Exp. Med.* **200,** 1533–1537.

Riddell, S. R., Berger, C., Murata, M., Randolph, S., and Warren, E. H. (2003). The graft versus leukemia response after allogeneic hematopoietic stem cell transplantation. *Blood Rev.* **17,** 153–162.

Ringden, O., Labopin, M., Gluckman, E., Reiffers, J., Vernant, J. P., Jouet, J. P., Harrousseau, J. L., Fiere, D., Bacigalupo, A., Frassoni, F., and Gorin, N. C. (1996). Graft-versus-leukemia effect in allogeneic marrow transplant recipients with acute leukemia is maintained using cyclosporin A combined with methotrexate as prophylaxis. Acute Leukemia Working Party of the European Group for Blood and Marrow Transplantation. *Bone Marrow Transplant.* **18,** 921–929.

Rondon, G., Giralt, S., Huh, Y., Khouri, I., Andersson, B., Andreeff, M., and Champlin, R. (1996). Graft-versus-leukemia effect after allogeneic bone marrow transplantation for chronic lymphocytic leukemia. *Bone Marrow Transplant.* **18,** 669–672.

Roux, E., Dumont-Girard, F., Starobinski, M., Siegrist, C. A., Helg, C., Chapuis, B., and Roosnek, E. (2000). Recovery of immune reactivity after T-cell-depleted bone marrow transplantation depends on thymic activity. *Blood* **96,** 2299–2303.

Rowen, L., Koop, B. F., and Hood, L. (1996). The complete 685-kilobase DNA sequence of the human beta T cell receptor locus. *Science* **272,** 1755–1762.

Ruggeri, L., Capanni, M., Casucci, M., Volpi, I., Tosti, A., Perruccio, K., Urbani, E., Negrin, R. S., Martelli, M. F., and Velardi, A. (1999). Role of natural killer cell alloreactivity in HLA-mismatched hematopoietic stem cell transplantation. *Blood* **94,** 333–339.

Ruggeri, L., Capanni, M., Mancusi, A., Martelli, M. F., and Velardi, A. (2005a). The impact of donor natural killer cell alloreactivity on allogeneic hematopoietic transplantation. *Transpl. Immunol.* **14,** 203–206.

Ruggeri, L., Capanni, M., Urbani, E., Perruccio, K., Shlomchik, W. D., Tosti, A., Posati, S., Rogaia, D., Frassoni, F., Aversa, F., Martelli, M. F., and Velardi, A. (2002). Effectiveness of donor natural killer cell alloreactivity in mismatched hematopoietic transplants. *Science* **295,** 2097–2100.

Ruggeri, L., Mancusi, A., Perruccio, K., Burchielli, E., Martelli, M. F., and Velardi, A. (2005b). Natural killer cell alloreactivity for leukemia therapy. *J. Immunother.* **28,** 175–182.

Sahin, U., Tureci, O., and Pfreundschuh, M. (1997). Serological identification of human tumor antigens. *Curr. Opin. Immunol.* **9,** 709–716.

Sanderson, K., Scotland, R., Lee, P., Liu, D., Groshen, S., Snively, J., Sian, S., Nichol, G., Davis, T., Keler, T., Yellin, M., and Weber, J. (2005). Autoimmunity in a phase I trial of a fully human anti-cytotoxic T-lymphocyte antigen-4 monoclonal antibody with multiple melanoma peptides and Montanide ISA 51 for patients with resected stages III and IV melanoma. *J. Clin. Oncol.* **23,** 741–750.

Schmollinger, J. C., Vonderheide, R. H., Hoar, K. M., Maecker, B., Schultze, J. L., Hodi, F. S., Soiffer, R. J., Jung, K., Kuroda, M. J., Letvin, N. L., Greenfield, E. A., Mihm, M., et al. (2003). Melanoma inhibitor of apoptosis protein (ML-IAP) is a target for immune-mediated tumor destruction. *Proc. Natl. Acad. Sci. USA* **100,** 3398–3403.

Shimoni, A., Gajewski, J. A., Donato, M., Martin, T., O'Brien, S., Talpaz, M., Cohen, A., Korbling, M., Champlin, R., and Giralt, S. (2001). Long-term follow-up of recipients of CD8-depleted donor lymphocyte infusions for the treatment of chronic myelogenous leukemia relapsing after allogeneic progenitor cell transplantation. *Biol. Blood Marrow Transplant.* **7,** 568–575.

Small, T. N., Papadopoulos, E. B., Boulad, F., Black, P., Castro-Malaspina, H., Childs, B. H., Collins, N., Gillio, A., George, D., Jakubowski, A., Heller, G., Fazzari, M., et al. (1999). Comparison of immune reconstitution after unrelated and related T-cell-depleted bone marrow transplantation: Effect of patient age and donor leukocyte infusions. *Blood* **93,** 467–480.

Soiffer, R. J., Alyea, E. P., Hochberg, E., Wu, C., Canning, C., Parikh, B., Zahrieh, D., Webb, I., Antin, J., and Ritz, J. (2002). Randomized trial of CD8$^+$ T-cell depletion in the prevention of graft-versus-host disease associated with donor lymphocyte infusion. *Biol. Blood Marrow Transplant.* **8,** 625–632.

Soiffer, R. J., Bosserman, L., Murray, C., Cochran, K., Daley, J., and Ritz, J. (1990). Reconstitution of T-cell function after CD6-depleted allogeneic bone marrow transplantation. *Blood* **75,** 2076–2084.

Spierings, E., Brickner, A. G., Caldwell, J. A., Zegveld, S., Tatsis, N., Blokland, E., Pool, J., Pierce, R. A., Mollah, S., Shabanowitz, J., Eisenlohr, L. C., van Veelen, P., et al. (2003). The minor histocompatibility antigen HA-3 arises from differential proteasome-mediated cleavage of the lymphoid blast crisis (Lbc) oncoprotein. *Blood* **102,** 621–629.

Spierings, E., Vermeulen, C. J., Vogt, M. H., Doerner, L. E., Falkenburg, J. H., Mutis, T., and Goulmy, E. (2003). Identification of HLA class II-restricted H-Y-specific T-helper epitope evoking CD4$^+$ T-helper cells in H-Y-mismatched transplantation. *Lancet* **362,** 610–615.

Sullivan, K. M., Weiden, P. L., Storb, R., Witherspoon, R. P., Fefer, A., Fisher, L., Buckner, C. D., Anasetti, C., Appelbaum, F. R., Badger, C., Beatty, P., Bensinger, W., et al. (1989). Influence of acute and chronic graft-versus-host disease on relapse and survival after bone marrow transplantation from HLA-identical siblings as treatment of acute and chronic leukemia. *Blood* **73,** 1720–1728.

Sykes, M., Preffer, F., McAfee, S., Saidman, S. L., Weymouth, D., Andrews, D. M., Colby, C., Sackstein, R., Sachs, D. H., and Spitzer, T. R. (1999). Mixed lymphohaemopoietic chimerism and graft-versus-lymphoma effects after non-myeloablative therapy and HLA-mismatched bone-marrow transplantation. *Lancet* **353,** 1755–1759.

Takami, A., Sugimori, C., Feng, X., Yachie, A., Kondo, Y., Nishimura, R., Kuzushima, K., Kotani, T., Asakura, H., Shiobara, S., and Nakao, S. (2004). Expansion and activation of minor histocompatibility antigen HY-specific T cells associated with graft-versus-leukemia response. *Bone Marrow Transplant.* **34,** 703–709.

Tauro, S., Hepburn, M. D., Bowen, D. T., and Pippard, M. J. (2001). Assessment of stromal function, and its potential contribution to deregulation of hematopoiesis in the myelodysplastic syndromes. *Haematologica* **86,** 1038–1045.

Taylor, P. A., Panoskaltsis-Mortari, A., Freeman, G. J., Sharpe, A. H., Noelle, R. J., Rudensky, A. Y., Mak, T. W., Serody, J. S., and Blazar, B. R. (2005). Targeting of inducible costimulator (ICOS) expressed on alloreactive T cells down-regulates graft-versus-host disease (GVHD) and facilitates engraftment of allogeneic bone marrow (BM). *Blood* **105,** 3372–3380.

Teshima, T., Liu, C., Lowler, K. P., Dranoff, G., and Ferrara, J. L. (2002). Donor leukocyte infusion from immunized donors increases tumor vaccine efficacy after allogeneic bone marrow transplantation. *Cancer Res.* **62,** 796–800.

Torikai, H., Akatsuka, Y., Miyazaki, M., Warren, E. H., 3rd, Oba, T., Tsujimura, K., Motoyoshi, K., Morishima, Y., Kodera, Y., Kuzushima, K., and Takahashi, T. (2004). A novel HLA-A°3303-restricted minor histocompatibility antigen encoded by an unconventional open reading frame of human TMSB4Y gene. *J. Immunol.* **173,** 7046–7054.

Trenado, A., Charlotte, F., Fisson, S., Yagello, M., Klatzmann, D., Salomon, B. L., and Cohen, J. L. (2003). Recipient-type specific CD4+CD25+ regulatory T cells favor immune reconstitution and control graft-versus-host disease while maintaining graft-versus-leukemia. *J. Clin. Invest.* **112,** 1688–1696.

Tricot, G., Vesole, D. H., Jagannath, S., Hilton, J., Munshi, N., and Barlogie, B. (1996). Graft-versus-myeloma effect: Proof of principle. *Blood* **87,** 1196–1198.

Truitt, R. L., and Atasoylu, A. A. (1991). Contribution of CD4$^+$ and CD8$^+$ T cells to graft-versus-host disease and graft-versus-leukemia reactivity after transplantation of MHC-compatible bone marrow. *Bone Marrow Transplant.* **8,** 51–58.

Tykodi, S. S., Warren, E. H., Thompson, J. A., Riddell, S. R., Childs, R. W., Otterud, B. E., Leppert, M. F., Storb, R., and Sandmaier, B. M. (2004). Allogeneic hematopoietic cell transplantation for metastatic renal cell carcinoma after nonmyeloablative conditioning: Toxicity, clinical response, and immunological response to minor histocompatibility antigens. *Clin. Cancer Res.* **10,** 7799–7811.

Ueno, N. T., Cheng, Y. C., Rondon, G., Tannir, N. M., Gajewski, J. L., Couriel, D. R., Hosing, C., de Lima, M. J., Anderlini, P., Khouri, I. F., Booser, D. J., Hortobagyi, G. N., *et al.* (2003). Rapid induction of complete donor chimerism by the use of a reduced-intensity conditioning regimen composed of fludarabine and melphalan in allogeneic stem cell transplantation for metastatic solid tumors. *Blood* **102,** 3829–3836.

Uhrberg, M. (2005). Shaping the human NK cell repertoire: An epigenetic glance at KIR gene regulation. *Mol. Immunol.* **42,** 471–475.

van Rhee, F., Lin, F., Cullis, J. O., Spencer, A., Cross, N. C., Chase, A., Garicochea, B., Bungey, J., Barrett, J., and Goldman, J. M. (1994). Relapse of chronic myeloid leukemia after allogeneic bone marrow transplant: The case for giving donor leukocyte transfusions before the onset of hematologic relapse. *Blood* **83,** 3377–3383.

Verdijk, R. M., Kloosterman, A., Pool, J., van de Keur, M., Naipal, A. M., van Halteren, A. G., Brand, A., Mutis, T., and Goulmy, E. (2004). Pregnancy induces minor histocompatibility antigen-specific cytotoxic T cells: Implications for stem cell transplantation and immunotherapy. *Blood* **103,** 1961–1964.

Verfuerth, S., Peggs, K., Vyas, P., Barnett, L., O'Reilly, R. J., and Mackinnon, S. (2000). Longitudinal monitoring of immune reconstitution by CDR3 size spectratyping after T-cell-depleted allogeneic bone marrow transplant and the effect of donor lymphocyte infusions on T-cell repertoire. *Blood* **95,** 3990–3995.

Vogt, M. H., de Paus, R. A., Voogt, P. J., Willemze, R., and Falkenburg, J. H. (2000a). DFFRY codes for a new human male-specific minor transplantation antigen involved in bone marrow graft rejection. *Blood* **95,** 1100–1105.

Vogt, M. H., Goulmy, E., Kloosterboer, F. M., Blokland, E., de Paus, R. A., Willemze, R., and Falkenburg, J. H. (2000b). UTY gene codes for an HLA-B60-restricted human male-specific minor histocompatibility antigen involved in stem cell graft rejection: Characterization of the critical polymorphic amino acid residues for T-cell recognition. *Blood* **96,** 3126–3132.

Vogt, M. H., van den Muijsenberg, J. W., Goulmy, E., Spierings, E., Kluck, P., Kester, M. G., van Soest, R. A., Drijfhout, J. W., Willemze, R., and Falkenburg, J. H. (2002). The DBY gene codes for an HLA-DQ5-restricted human male-specific minor histocompatibility antigen involved in graft-versus-host disease. *Blood* **99,** 3027–3032.

Vose, J. M., Bierman, P. J., Lynch, J. C., Atkinson, K., Juttner, C., Hanania, C. E., Bociek, G., and Armitage, J. O. (2001). Transplantation of highly purified CD34+Thy-1+ hematopoietic stem cells in patients with recurrent indolent non-Hodgkin's lymphoma. *Biol. Blood Marrow Transplant.* **7,** 680–687.

Wang, D. G., Fan, J. B., Siao, C. J., Berno, A., Young, P., Sapolsky, R., Ghandour, G., Perkins, N., Winchester, E., Spencer, J., Kruglyak, L., Stein, L., *et al.* (1998). Large-scale identification, mapping, and genotyping of single-nucleotide polymorphisms in the human genome. *Science* **280,** 1077–1082.

Wang, W., Meadows, L. R., den Haan, J. M., Sherman, N. E., Chen, Y., Blokland, E., Shabanowitz, J., Agulnik, A. I., Hendrickson, R. C., Bishop, C. E., Hunt, D. F., Goulmy, E., *et al.* (1995). Human H-Y: A male-specific histocompatibility antigen derived from the SMCY protein. *Science* **269,** 1588–1590.

Wang, Z., Zhang, Y., Mandal, A., Zhang, J., Giles, F. J., Herr, J. C., and Lim, S. H. (2004). The spermatozoa protein, SLLP1, is a novel cancer-testis antigen in hematologic malignancies. *Clin. Cancer Res.* **10,** 6544–6550.

Warren, E. H., Gavin, M., Greenberg, P. D., and Riddell, S. R. (1998). Minor histocompatibility antigens as targets for T-cell therapy after bone marrow transplantation. *Curr. Opin. Hematol.* **5,** 429–433.

Warren, E. H., Gavin, M. A., Simpson, E., Chandler, P., Page, D. C., Disteche, C., Stankey, K. A., Greenberg, P. D., and Riddell, S. R. (2000). The human UTY gene encodes a novel HLA-B8-restricted H-Y antigen. *J. Immunol.* **164,** 2807–2814.

Warren, E. H., Greenberg, P. D., and Riddell, S. R. (1998). Cytotoxic T-lymphocyte-defined human minor histocompatibility antigens with a restricted tissue distribution. *Blood* **91,** 2197–2207.

Weiden, P. L., Flournoy, N., Thomas, E. D., Prentice, R., Fefer, A., Buckner, C. D., and Storb, R. (1979). Antileukemic effect of graft-versus-host disease in human recipients of allogeneic-marrow grafts. *N. Engl. J. Med.* **300,** 1068–1073.

Weiden, P. L., Sullivan, K. M., Flournoy, N., Storb, R., and Thomas, E. D. (1981). Antileukemic effect of chronic graft-versus-host disease: Contribution to improved survival after allogeneic marrow transplantation. *N. Engl. J. Med.* **304,** 1529–1533.

Weinberg, K., Blazar, B. R., Wagner, J. E., Agura, E., Hill, B. J., Smogorzewska, M., Koup, R. A., Betts, M. R., Collins, R. H., and Douek, D. C. (2001). Factors affecting thymic function after allogeneic hematopoietic stem cell transplantation. *Blood* **97,** 1458–1466.

Weisdorf, D. J., Nesbit, M. E., Ramsay, N. K., Woods, W. G., Goldman, A. I., Kim, T. H., Hurd, D. D., McGlave, P. B., and Kersey, J. H. (1987). Allogeneic bone marrow transplantation for acute lymphoblastic leukemia in remission: Prolonged survival associated with acute graft-versus-host disease. *J. Clin. Oncol.* **5,** 1348–1355.

Wu, C. J., Biernacki, M., Kutok, J. L., Rogers, S., Chen, L., Yang, X. F., Soiffer, R. J., and Ritz, J. (2005). Graft-versus-leukemia target antigens in chronic myelogenous leukemia are expressed on myeloid progenitor cells. *Clin. Cancer Res.* **11,** 4504–4511.

Wu, C. J., Chillemi, A., Alyea, E. P., Orsini, E., Neuberg, D., Soiffer, R. J., and Ritz, J. (2000a). Reconstitution of T-cell receptor repertoire diversity following T-cell depleted allogeneic bone marrow transplantation is related to hematopoietic chimerism. *Blood* **95,** 352–359.

Wu, C. J., Yang, X. F., McLaughlin, S., Neuberg, D., Canning, C., Stein, B., Alyea, E. P., Soiffer, R. J., Dranoff, G., and Ritz, J. (2000b). Detection of a potent humoral response associated with immune-induced remission of chronic myelogenous leukemia. *J. Clin. Invest.* **106,** 705–714.

Yang, X. F., Wu, C. J., Chen, L., Alyea, E. P., Canning, C., Kantoff, P., Soiffer, R. J., Dranoff, G., and Ritz, J. (2002). CML28 is a broadly immunogenic antigen, which is overexpressed in tumor cells. *Cancer Res.* **62,** 5517–5522.

Yang, X. F., Wu, C. J., McLaughlin, S., Chillemi, A., Wang, K. S., Canning, C., Alyea, E. P., Kantoff, P., Soiffer, R. J., Dranoff, G., and Ritz, J. (2001). CML66, a broadly immunogenic tumor antigen, elicits a humoral immune response associated with remission of chronic myelogenous leukemia. *Proc. Natl. Acad. Sci. USA* **98,** 7492–7497.

Zorn, E., Kim, H. T., Lee, S. J., Floyd, B. H., Litsa, D., Arumugarajah, S., Bellucci, R., Alyea, E. P., Antin, J. H., Soiffer, R. J., and Ritz, J. (2005). Reduced frequency of FOXP3+ CD4+CD25+ regulatory T cells in patients with chronic graft-versus-host disease. *Blood* **106,** 2903–2911.

Zorn, E., Miklos, D. B., Floyd, B. H., Mattes-Ritz, A., Guo, L., Soiffer, R. J., Antin, J. H., and Ritz, J. (2004). Minor histocompatibility antigen DBY elicits a coordinated B and T cell response after allogeneic stem cell transplantation. *J. Exp. Med.* **199,** 1133–1142.

Zorn, E., Wang, K. S., Hochberg, E. P., Canning, C., Alyea, E. P., Soiffer, R. J., and Ritz, J. (2002). Infusion of CD4$^+$ donor lymphocytes induces the expansion of CD8$^+$ donor T cells with cytolytic activity directed against recipient hematopoietic cells. *Clin. Cancer Res.* **8,** 2052–2060.

Zubair, A. C., Zahrieh, D., Daley, H., Schott, D., Gribben, J. G., Alyea, E. P., Schlossman, R., Freedman, A., Antin, J. H., Soiffer, R. J., *et al.* (2004). Engraftment of autologous and allogeneic marrow HPCs after myeloablative therapy. *Transfusion* **44,** 253–261.

Vaccination for Treatment and Prevention of Cancer in Animal Models

Federica Cavallo,* Rienk Offringa,[†] Sjoerd H. van der Burg,[†] Guido Forni,* and Cornelis J. M. Melief[†]

*Department of Clinical and Biological Sciences, University of Torino, Torino, Italy
[†]Leiden University Medical Center, Leiden, The Netherlands

Abstract 175
1. Introduction 176
2. Synthetic Exact MHC Class I Binding Peptide Vaccines for Induction of Protective CD8[+] Cytotoxic T-Cell Responses in Mouse Models 177
3. Therapy of Established Mouse Tumors by Treatment with Synthetic Vaccines, in Particular Long Peptides 178
4. Clinical Trials with Synthetic Peptide-Based Cancer Vaccines 181
5. DC Immunotherapy 182
6. Therapeutic Interventions Counteracting Tumor-Induced Immunoregulation 183
7. Genetically Modified Mice that Develop Tumors 185
8. Mice Transgenic for Her2 Oncogene 186
9. BALB-neuT Mice as a Study Model for Mammary Cancer 188
10. DNA Vaccination Inhibits Her2 Mammary Carcinogenesis 191
11. The Mode of EC-TM Plasmid Delivery is Decisive for Vaccine Efficacy 193
12. The Limitations of DNA Vaccination and How They Can Be Overcome 196
13. Coordinated Low-Avidity Mechanisms 199
14. Cure Versus Control of Her2 Lesions 204
15. Conclusions 205
    References 206

Abstract

Two approaches to immunological intervention in tumor–host interactions in mouse models are discussed in this review. The first is described with reference to experiments in which CD8[+] T lymphocytes are used to kill established transplantable tumors. Peptides and their optimal presentation by dendritic cells and intervention in immune regulatory mechanisms are the key issues for efficient induction of T-killer cell-mediated tumor eradication. The time frame of tumor therapy and the threat imposed by tumor growth in transplantable models and cancer patients require the induction of a robust T-cell reaction. Prevention of the progression of small preneoplastic lesions, on the other hand, requires the significant and prolonged immune protection sought in the second approach. This is based on antibody production and the coordinated activation of multiple low-avidity cell-mediated mechanisms elicited by DNA vaccination *in genetically modified cancer-prone mice, transgenic for a mutant Her-2/neu growth factor receptor expressed at the plasma membrane surface of preneoplastic mammary gland epithelial cells. Vaccination with appropriate DNA formulations results in prolonged immune inhibition of the progression of preneoplastic mammary lesions but is ineffective against established tumors. The use of molecularly defined adjuvants and intervention in immune regulatory mechanisms are critical in both the elicitation of an effective T-cell mediated reaction required for tumor debulking in the first set of models and the induction by vaccination of a sustained immune memory able to prevent the expansion of preneoplastic lesions in genetically cancer-prone mice.*

1. Introduction

Experimental models are valuable since they allow a quick and sagacious penetration into the true essence of complex immunological problems. When a model is commonly used, the consensus on its experimental data spreads freely, influences what is believed, and provides the foundation for clinical trials. Often models are so widely used and accepted that one must resist the temptation to view data derived from them as the true gospel. The danger here lies in the fact that the design of a model may influence the experimental results and thus bias a concept based on it. Experimental mouse tumors are hardly a true illustration of a patient's complex and variable tumor–host immune relationship, or even of natural mouse tumors. They do, however, provide a basic picture and simplification of the situation can be used to tease apart a few features of a complex reality.

These considerations should be taken into account in evaluating the information provided by the mouse models described here. Tumors transplanted in syngeneic mice are attractive because they grow quickly and provide prompt answers. Details of the antigenic profile and growth features of the numerous transplantable tumors are readily available and fine modulation of the immune system of recipient mice can be induced. This unique combination furnishes well-defined premises for the testing of an experimental hypothesis or even a series of successive hypotheses.

In the last 20 years, a large variety of tumors have been transplanted into mice variously immunized and selectively immunosuppressed. Almost all the information available on the tumor–host immune relationship rests on the data from these experimental systems. In the first part of this review, the results obtained in such models in the laboratory of R. Offringa, S. van der Burg, and C. J. M. Melief on the subject of peptide vaccination combined with fine modulation of the host's immune reactivity are reviewed. The second part of the review is devoted to the results obtained by F. Cavallo and G. Forni from mice transgenic for the Her-2/neu (Her2, also known as ErbB-2 in humans) oncogene that develop autochthonous mammary carcinomas. Tumors developing as a natural consequence of an artificial gene defect inserted in transgenic mice provide a useful alternative to transplantable tumor models. Since such tumors progress slowly, these models mirror a few additional features of human cancer. Nonetheless, they are cumbersome. A single experiment may last more than 1 year and several fine questions cannot be explored in depth. In essence, therefore, transplantable and transgenic tumor models constitute highly complementary approaches in the analysis of the interaction between tumor and immune system and the development of immune intervention strategies against cancer.

2. Synthetic Exact MHC Class I Binding Peptide Vaccines for Induction of Protective $CD8^+$ Cytotoxic T-Cell Responses in Mouse Models

Quite soon after it was found that $CD8^+$ cytotoxic T-cells recognize small protein fragments presented by MHC class I molecules at the cell surface, it proved to be possible to achieve protective T-cell immunity by vaccinating with synthetic peptides representing these 9–11 amino acid long sequences and formulated in incomplete Freund's adjuvant (IFA) (Kast et al., 1991; Schultz et al., 1991). In both studies preventive vaccination with these exact MHC class I binding peptides protected mice against a subsequent challenge with lymphocytic choriomeningitis virus or Sendai virus, respectively. Similar results were achieved with a recombinant vaccinia virus incorporating a single murine cytomegalovirus cytotoxic T-cell lymphocytes (CTL) epitope (Del Val et al., 1991). Thus, vaccination with a strong CTL epitope was found to cause protection by preventive vaccination in three independent virus infections. Subsequently, the principle of preventive vaccination with a minimal 9-mer peptide representing an epitope of human papilloma virus type 16 (HPV16) proved also applicable to prevent outgrowth of an HPV16 induced mouse tumor (Feltkamp et al., 1993). These early results are in many ways surprising, if only because we now know that robust $CD8^+$ CTL responses are dependent on $CD4^+$ T cell help (Ossendorp et al., 1998) and antigen presentation by activated dendritic cells (DC) (Bennett et al., 1998; Schoenberger et al., 1998, 2000). $CD4^+$ T helper cells deliver help for $CD8^+$ CTL in part by signaling of CD40 ligand (CD40L) on activated helper cells to CD40 on DC, leading to DC activation (Bennett et al., 1998; Schoenberger et al., 1998; Schuurhuis et al., 2000).

Prevention of subsequent infections with viruses or outgrowth of tumor inocula is not a rigorous criterion of vaccine potency. It did not take us long to realize that vaccination with exact MHC class I binding peptides is far from optimal. Two completely different CTL epitopes of adenovirus type 5, one encoded by E1A, the other by E1B, when injected as exact MHC class I binding peptides in IFA, instead of protecting against outgrowth of subsequently inoculated adenovirus E1 transformed tumor cells, caused specific CTL tolerance, associated with enhanced tumor outgrowth instead of protection (Toes et al., 1996a,b). Cytotoxic T-cell lymphocyte tolerization could only be avoided and turned into protective immunity by injecting these peptides on bone marrow DC that had been loaded *ex vivo* with either of these two peptides (Toes et al., 1998) or by addition of anti-CD40 agonist antibody to the vaccine (Diehl et al., 1999). Protection mediated by the HPV peptide was found to be correlated with slower release from the IFA depot but a long half-life, once released, in comparison with the tolerizing E1A peptide (Weijzen et al., 2001), thus attributing an important role to the pharmacokinetics of peptide delivery to T cells. We have identified two aspects of exact MHC class I binding peptides that seriously call into question the wisdom of delivering CTL epitopes this way for $CD8^+$ CTL induction in a therapeutic setting. The first of these is our observation that upon injection in phosphate buffered saline (PBS) or IFA, with or without DC activating agents, exact MHC class I binding peptides become rapidly loaded exogenously onto nonprofessional antigen presenting cells (APC), in particular T and B cells. These cells recirculate through the lymphoid system, and depending on their need for costimulation either cause a (short-lived) $CD8^+$ CTL effector response (HPV peptide, Sendai peptide, little need for costimulation) or $CD8^+$ CTL tolerance (adeno E1 peptides). Injection of long peptides (in PBS or IFA) comprising the same epitopes with additional flanking amino acids are efficiently presented *in vivo* by DC only because these professional APC are uniquely capable of efficiently processing the long peptides for presentation by MHC class I molecules (Fig. 1).

The second flaw in the design of exact MHC class I binding peptides as (tumor) vaccines is the lack of induction of $CD4^+$ T-cell help. Although exact MHC class I binding peptides formulated in IFA can sometimes cause a short burst of $CD8^+$ CTL effector expansion, these responses are: (1) suboptimal and (2) short-lived, both because of lack of $CD4^+$ T-helper cells that need to properly signal through DC (Fig. 2). Both the rather disastrous pharmacokinetics of these short peptides, in particular their loading onto nonprofessional APC with insufficient costimulatory properties, and the equally calamitous lack of proper T-cell help concern unpublished observations of M. Bijker, R. Offringa, C. J. M. Melief, and S. H. van der Burg. These general conclusions are strongly supported by the finding that not only the generation of $CD8^+$ effector CTL is $CD4^+$ T-helper dependent, but also the generation of memory $CD8^+$ CTL, both operating through DC licensing (Janssen et al., 2003, 2005; Smith et al., 2004; Toka et al., 2005).

3. Therapy of Established Mouse Tumors by Treatment with Synthetic Vaccines, in Particular Long Peptides

Based on the flaws in the design of exact MHC class I binding peptide vaccines discussed in the previous paragraph, it is not surprising that such vaccines have

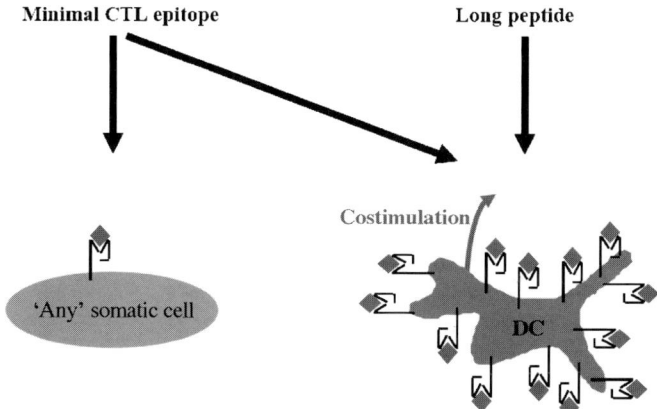

Figure 1 Differential loading of MHC class I after immunization with minimal epitope and long peptide vaccines. Upon injection of a minimal epitope peptide vaccine, the peptides can be exogenously loaded onto any somatic cells that expresses MHC class I at its surface. This includes dendritic cells, but also various nonprofessional APC that present the epitope in the absence of the costimulatory signals essential for activation of the CTL immune response. Consequently, minimal epitope vaccines result in a suboptimal blend of immunostimulatory and tolerogenic signals. In contrast, antigen presentation after injection of long peptide vaccines will be focused on the dendritic cells, as these are uniquely capable of efficiently processing exogenous antigen into MHC class I. Consequently, a more optimal immunostimulatory signal is obtained. (**See Plate 4 in color insert at the end of the book.**)

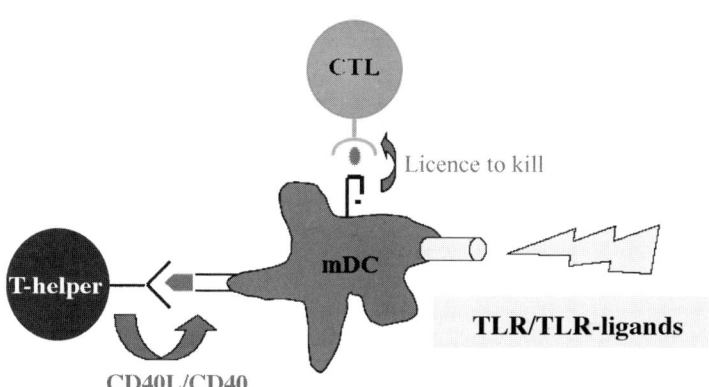

Figure 2 Exploitation of two independent pathways for DC activation. Dendritic cells can only provide $CD8^+$ T cells with strong costimulatory signals, constituting a "licence to kill" as well as an important requirement for memory cell formation, if they are themselves activated. This activation can be achieved by two complementary pathways, involving CD40L–CD40-mediated interaction with $CD4^+$ T-helper cells and triggering by TLR ligands, respectively. When applied together in a vaccine, T-cell help and TLR-ligands can act synergistically. (**See Plate 5 in color insert at the end of the book.**)

not been reported to efficiently eradicate established murine tumors. To rigorously compare the therapeutic potency of an exact MHC class I binding peptide with that of a long peptide incorporating the same HPV16 E7 CTL epitope but in addition HPV16 T helper epitope, we tested these short and long peptide vaccines in a therapeutic setting (Zwaveling et al., 2002). Prime-boost vaccinations with the HPV16-derived 35 amino acid long peptide E7 (43–77) resulted in the induction of far more robust E7-specific $CD8^+$ CTL responses than vaccinations with the short peptide containing only the minimal CTL epitope. We showed that two distinct mechanisms are responsible for this. First, the level of the induced E7-specific $CD8^+$ CTL responses by the long peptide was dependent on interactions of E7-specific $CD4^+$ T-helper cells with professional APC through CD40L–CD40 interactions (Zwaveling et al., 2002). Second, we showed that vaccination with the long peptide and DC activating agents, in particular the Toll-like receptor (TLR) 9 ligand unmethylated deoxycytidyl-deoxyguanosine (CpG), resulted in a superior induction of E7-specific $CD8^+$ T cells, even when T-cell help was excluded by performing the experiments in MHC class II knockout (KO) animals (Zwaveling et al., 2002). The efficacy of the induced HPV-specific T-cell responses was demonstrated in therapeutic prime-boost vaccinations in which the long peptide admixed with CpG resulted in the eradication of large established HPV16-expressing tumors. The advantage of using CpG in the vaccine was that it induced a strong $CD8^+$ CTL response after only one injection, confirming that TLR ligands are potent adjuvants for priming peptide-specific CTL responses (Fig. 2). Dendritic cell activation dependent on CD40L–CD40 interactions was shown to operate only upon boosting with long peptides in the absence of TLR ligands (Zwaveling et al., 2002). Subsequent studies in our laboratory have extended and confirmed these observations. Of many TLR ligands tested, CpG deoxyoligonucleotide is best at inducing therapeutic $CD8^+$ CTL responses in combination with long peptide vaccines. Certain combinations of TLR agonist, such as CpG, and CD40 agonist antibody, despite clear-cut synergism in DC activation and $CD8^+$ expansion, as also reported by others (Napolitani et al., 2005), were not more effective in tumor eradication because these expanded T-cell effector populations accumulated only in the draining lymph nodes and did not emigrate into the blood (M. Schoenmaekers-Welters, R. Offringa, C. Melief, and S. H. van der Burg, submitted for publication).

Interestingly, in therapeutic vaccination with overlapping 32–35 amino acid long peptides, together spanning the E6 and E7 protein sequences of cottontail rabbit papilloma virus (CRPV), of established CRPV-induced warts in rabbits, marked suppression of wart growth was observed and abrogation of latent CRPV infection (Vambutas et al., 2005).

4. Clinical Trials with Synthetic Peptide-Based Cancer Vaccines

In a survey of the status of melanoma vaccines, the overall objective response rate in a series of 440 patients treated with various melanoma-specific vaccines was only 2.6% and comparable to the response rates observed by other types of treatment (Rosenberg et al., 2004). A substantial proportion of these vaccines was based on injection of melanoma associated peptides. This is very disappointing, and the authors concluded that the immunotherapeutic approaches need drastic improvement. Considering the fact that most peptide vaccination trials to date were carried out by injecting exact MHC class I binding peptides, often without TLR ligand, this evaluation is certainly justified. Measures for improved clinical results with melanoma and other cancer peptide-based vaccines include use of long peptides incorporating both HLA class I and II tumor associated epitopes. Linking class I and II epitopes is more effective than mixing class I and II epitopes (reviewed in Zwaveling et al., 2002). Additionally, the choice of TLR ligands for obtaining optimal efficacy of human DC activation therapy may differ from that in the mouse. Notably, the CpG receptor TLR9 in human beings is only expressed on plasmacytoid DC and not, like in the mouse, also on myeloid DC. Nonetheless rapid and robust $CD8^+$ CTL responses were induced by combining MART1/Melan-A HLA-A2 peptide vaccination with CpG oligodeoxynucleotides (ODN) 7909 (Speiser et al., 2005), in line with our results in mice. In the future conjugates of TLR ligands and peptides for vaccination need to be considered (Daftarian et al., 2005). Also in our hands such conjugates are more effective than mixtures of peptides and TLR ligands (S. Khan, F. Ossendorp, M. Bijker, M. Schoenmaekers-Welters, R. Offringa, C. Melief, and S. van der Burg, unpublished observations). Addition of the cytokines IL-12 or IL-15, or of anti-CD40 agonist antibody can help to further promote $CD8^+$ T-cell memory formation by peptide/CpG vaccination (Toka et al., 2005), provided the lymph node shutdown observed in our laboratory upon vaccination combined with both anti-CD40 and CpG (see Section 3) can be avoided.

In conclusion, synthetic peptide-based cancer vaccines can be improved drastically by improvement of the antigen-specific component of the vaccine. Exact MHC class I binding peptides, which not only tend to cause tolerance and, by lack of CD4 help, fail to induce proper memory, but also have the disadvantage that their application is restricted to subjects expressing the relevant MHC molecules. By comparison long peptides offer a better alternative. Long peptides can incorporate multiple MHC class I and II epitopes in linked fashion, which is important for optimal cellular interactions between DC, $CD4^+$, and $CD8^+$ T cells (Zwaveling et al., 2002). The proper class I and II epitopes are efficiently processed from injected long peptides by

DC. Optimization of adjuvants, including TLR ligands, is also important to properly activate these DC.

Other therapeutic maneuvers that can help to increase the efficiency of long peptide vaccines and cancer vaccines in general will be discussed in Section 6. Finally, it must be remembered that even if T-cell expansions induced by clinical peptide or recombinant canary pox vaccines are small, this can be associated with substantial tumor regressions, for example, in the case of melanoma (Karanikas et al., 2003; Lonchay et al., 2004) possibly due to epitope spreading (Lurquin et al., 2005).

5. DC Immunotherapy

Ever since murine DC loaded *ex vivo* with CD8 CTL epitope peptides were shown to serve as efficient inducers of tumor immunity (Mayordomo et al., 1995; Ossevoort et al., 1995), DC have attracted much attention as vaccine carriers for human cancer immunotherapy (reviewed in Figdor et al., 2004). The difference with the directly injected peptides reviewed in Sections 3 (animal models) and 4 (patients) is that, instead of activating the DC *in vivo*, the DC maturation required for optimal effector T-cell induction is performed *ex vivo*, either from immature monocyte-derived DC, following GM-CSF and IL-4 treatment, or from bone marrow $CD34^+$ stem cell derived DC. The advantage is that the properties of the injected DC, particularly with regard to maturation parameters and cytokine secretion can be exactly controlled and monitored. Repeated immunization of patients with established melanoma with $CD34^+$ progenitor-derived DC loaded with a mix of exact HLA-A°0201 binding melanoma associated peptides led to considerable expansion of peptide-specific $CD8^+$ CTL, but repeated boosting was necessary (Palucka et al., 2005). $CD4^+$ melanoma-specific cytolytic $CD4^+$ T cells could be generated by vaccination with monocyte-derived DC loaded with an HLA class II (DP4)-binding MAGE-3 peptide (Schultz et al., 2004). For reasons outlined in Sections 3 and 4, it seems wise to load DCs with immunogens, for example, long peptides, that express both HLA class I and II epitopes because, TLR ligands or CD40 agonists cannot completely replace all of the beneficial effects of specific $CD4^+$ T cells, particularly interferon (IFN)γ-producing specific T-helper 1 cells, on the vaccine-induced antitumor immune response (Melief et al., 2000, 2002; Toes et al., 1999). Much can be learned from the clinical study of cancer immunotherapy with *ex vivo* tumor antigen loaded and properly activated DC. This could even become common clinical practice if properly standardized and implemented as a blood transfusion-like cell product (Figdor et al., 2004). However, such therapy is likely to be laborious and expensive. No a priori reasons exist why similar therapeutic results could not be achieved by direct antigen targeting and activation of DC *in vivo* as outlined in Sections 3 and 4. Regardless of the mode of vaccination (peptides, antigen-loaded DC, and other modalities such as viral vectors), additional therapeutic interventions are likely to be needed for full therapeutic efficacy of cancer vaccines. This is largely due to the immunoregulatory influence exerted by growing tumors. How some deleterious aspects of immunoregulation can be addressed therapeutically will be addressed in Section 6.

6. Therapeutic Interventions Counteracting Tumor-Induced Immunoregulation

Tumors masquerade to a large extent as self-tissues. Accordingly tumors are likely to only cause DC activation to the extent that the tumors alert the DC sentinel system by sending out endogenous danger signals, such as stress proteins and type I IFN (Melief *et al.*, 2000, 2005). Even cancer viruses and virus-induced cancers very often do not send out proper DC activation signals causing persistent virus infection and carcinogenesis by viruses such as hepatitis B virus (HBV), hepatitis C virus (HCV), and high-risk HPV. In the case of high-risk HPV16 infection, the development of cancer is associated with failure to induce IFN-γ-producing T cells, whereas efficient immunosurveillance operates in resistant people (de Jong *et al.*, 2004).

Sporadic tumors, not caused by infectious agents, are even more likely to fail in arousing proper effector T-cell responses by failing to cause DC maturation/activation (Melief, 2005). A very striking case in point is the report by Willimsky and Blankenstein (2005), who reported that sporadic tumors in mice caused by sporadic expression of transgenic SV40 large T viral oncoprotein, to which the immune system initially is not tolerant, nevertheless manage to grow out by causing $CD8^+$ CTL tolerance. Nonetheless, even so-called sporadic tumors very often cause sufficient DC activation and consequently T-cell effector cell expansion to be subject to so-called immunoediting (Dunn *et al.*, 2002; Khong and Restifo, 2002; Melief, 2005). Also the Her2 induced tumors in the transgenic mouse model discussed further in this chapter (Sections 7–14) are immunogenic because appropriate DNA vaccination against this oncogenic protein can induce protection against the development of breast cancer. Virus-induced or sporadic tumors rarely cause the type of DC activation associated with and necessary for the robust effector T-cell responses associated with clearance of acute infectious agents such as influenza virus. As a result the T-cell response in the tumor-bearing host is usually far from optimal. In many instances various types of regulatory T cells, either preexistent as $CD4^+$ $CD25^+$ regulatory T cells against tumor-expressed self-antigens, or tumor induced, often producing the immunosuppressive cytokines interleukin-10 (IL-10) or transforming growth factor β (TGFβ), counteract whichever tumoricidal T-cell activity coexists with these regulatory T cells (reviewed in Sutmuller et al., 2004). After the discovery of $CD4^+$ $CD25^+$ regulatory T cells as a distinct $CD4^+$ T-cell subset in naïve individuals (Sakaguchi et al., 1995), these cells were shown to be a highly important T-cell subset in the maintenance of self-tolerance (reviewed in Fehérvari and Sakaguchi, 2004; Sakaguchi, 2004), a clearly beneficial physiological function. However, in tumor immunity, these cells clearly counteract efficacy of therapeutic immune interventions. In our own work, depletion of $CD25^+$ regulatory T cells and cytotoxic T lymphocyte-associated antigen 4 (CTLA4) blockade synergistically augmented the result of tumor vaccination against a very aggressive murine melanoma cell, associated with enhanced $CD8^+$ CTL effector function (Sutmuller et al., 2001) and depletion of $CD4^+$ $CD25^+$ naïve T cells and CTLA4 were shown to act synergistically in this study. CTLA-4 blockade takes away the brakes of costimulation through the CD80/86 → CD28 costimulation pathway (reviewed in Egen et al., 2002) and has already shown considerable clinical activity in patients with metastatic melanoma in conjunction with peptide vaccination, however, at the expense of severe autoimmunity in a high proportion of patients (Phan et al., 2003). While CTLA4 blockade can be expected to indiscriminately augment effector T-cell responses regardless of fine specificity, depletion of $CD4^+$ $CD25^+$ regulatory T cells is likely to preferentially augment effector T-cell responses against self-antigens overexpressed on tumors such as those detected by SEREX serology (Nishikawa et al., 2005). A problem with the $CD25^+$ marker on the $CD4^+$ $C25^+$ T-regulatory subset is that this marker is only discriminatory enough for this subset in tumor-free naïve mice or people and not in tumor-bearing animals (Sutmuller et al., 2001) or patients because recently activated tumor-specific effector cells also express the CD25 IL-2 receptor. This limits clinical applicability of $CD25^+$ T-cell depletion at present, but undoubtedly better surface markers for depleting this subset for clinical cancer therapy will become available. Other, often tumor induced, subsets of regulatory T cells have been shown variously to produce IL-10 or TGFβ (reviewed in Sutmuller et al., 2004) and therapeutic benefits can be expected in the clinic by interfering with the function of these cells, for example, by blockade of the receptors for these cytokines. In one study, tumor-induced DC paralysis in a murine tumor model was reverted by the simultaneous injection of CpG ODN and anti-IL-10 receptor antibody (Vicari et al., 2002). The potential benefits for cancer therapy of these antibodies are also evident from their effects on the immune response against infectious agents (Murray et al., 2003; Rigopoulou et al., 2005).

Similar beneficial effects are reported of TGFβ receptor blockade in murine or xenogenic tumor models (Suzuki et al., 2004; Zhang et al., 2005). Transforming growth factor β appears to act, at least in part, by suppressing T helper type 1 development through regulation of natural killer cell IFN-γ (Laouar et al., 2005).

A novel mode of action of the established chemotherapeutic agent cyclophosphamide was reported in mouse or rat studies. In three independent studies, low-dose cyclophosphamide selectively eliminated and suppressed $CD4^+$ $C25^+$ regulatory T cells (Ercolini et al., 2005; Ghiringhelli et al., 2004; Lutsiak et al., 2005). In one of these (Ercolini et al., 2005) low-dose cyclophosphamide treatment allowed the activation of high-avidity Her2-specific $CD8^+$ T-cells in Her2 transgenic mice, comparable to those generated from non-transgenic mice. In the noncyclophosphamide treated transgenic mice such $CD8^+$ T cells capable of tumor rejection were found to be suppressed by $CD4^+$ $CD25^+$ regulatory T cells. In particular cycling $CD4^+$ $CD25^+$ regulatory T cells were found to be depleted by the cyclophosphamide. Similar beneficial effects in human cancer treatment are likely (Gomez et al., 2001). Also the beneficial effects of lymphodepletion practised by Dudley et al. (2005) to augment the beneficial effects of adoptive effector T-cell transfer in the clinic are likely to be partly due to depletion of various types of regulatory T cells. In our hands, the deleterious effects of regulatory T cells in tumor-bearing hosts sometimes outweigh the beneficial effects. In a murine model of adenovirus E1-induced tumors, depletion of all $CD4^+$ T cells spontaneously unleashed strong $CD8^+$ T-cell immunity capable of tumor eradication without the need for tumor-specific vaccination (den Boer et al., 2005). The deleterious effects of $CD4^+$ T cells in tumor-bearing hosts on tumor rejection could also be overcome by treatment with CD40 agonist antibody or CpG (den Boer et al., 2005). This confirms another report stating that CD40 ligation releases immature DC from the control of regulatory $CD4^+$ $CD25^+$ T cells (Serra et al., 2003).

Finally, self-tissues can express B7-H1 (PD-L1), a cell surface molecule of the B7 family with strong regulatory effects on T- and B-cell responses. A mouse tumor model study shows that blockade of the B7-H1 → PD-1 pathway can potentiate tumor regression mediated by anti-CD137 triggered $CD8^+$ CTL (Hirano et al., 2005).

7. Genetically Modified Mice that Develop Tumors

Mice that naturally develop a tumor as a consequence of a defined gene alteration artificially inserted in their genome constitute a relatively new experimental model. This alteration usually takes the form of over expression of defined oncogenes, whereas a few models are based on the loss of function of onco-suppressor genes or their KO, or on a combination of such overexpression and loss of function. In these mice, tumors become evident by stages, whereas their relationship with the surrounding tissues is preserved (Spadaro *et al.*, 2004). The genetic predestination to develop a specific cancer, the slowness of tumor progression and its reproduction of the development of natural tumors, the natural occurrence of invasion and metastasis, and the presence of a long-lasting interaction between the evolving tumor and the host immune system are the appealing features of these models. Yet despite these substantial similarities with human cancer, these models are not devoid of subtle pitfalls that, if overlooked, may lead to major conceptual mistakes. Some models are too artificial, since the tumor arises as the result of a gene alteration foreign to the human setting. In others, the pathogenic alteration has no exact equivalent in human tumors, and several subtle and curious phenomena occurring in transgenic mice may lead to misleading conclusions.

Genetic instability is a hallmark of cancer cells, whereas the lifespan of a mouse is too short to produce the degree of genetic heterogeneity observed in human cancer (Rangarajan and Weinberg, 2003). Long telomeres and promiscuous telomerase may defend a transgenic cancer against a telomere "crisis." No such protection is evident in humans and transition through this crisis seems to be the source of many of the genomic aberrations found in advanced cancers.

In addition, because of the peculiarities of the transgene promoter, the genetic alteration may not follow the same developmental expression pattern as those leading to human cancer. Moreover, genetic aberrations may be overexpressed throughout a whole organ resulting in the parallel progression of several regions toward cancer.

The timing of the first expression of an oncogene is also of crucial importance since it may influence the kind and intensity of the immune tolerance to the oncogene protein product. When the transgene is xenogeneic, the question becomes even more critical: Is the tolerance to transgene-encoded proteins comparable to that of tumor associated antigens in humans? Are vaccination strategies that succeed in breaking tolerance to xenogeneic transgene proteins equally able to break human tolerance to tumor antigens? (Lollini *et al.*, 2005). Finally, a few transgenic models are devoid of practical utility simply because the tumor arises after a very long latency, or only in a small percentage of mice or in particular conditions such as pregnancy.

8. Mice Transgenic for Her2 Oncogene

As with transplantable tumors, the choice of a genetic model of cancer represents a delicate compromise between its features, its handiness and the specific problem it permits one to address. Because the Her2 oncogene is directly involved in cell carcinogenesis, mice transgenic for the Her2 oncogene allow assessment of the potential of immunity in preventing the onset of mammary carcinoma or curing its progressive stages (Forni et al., 2000; Lollini et al., 2005).

The protein product coded by *Her2* ($p185^{neu}$) is a member of the epidermal growth factor receptor (EGFR) family endowed with a potent tyrosine kinase activity. Receptor tyrosine kinases are central components of cell signaling networks and play crucial roles in normal physiological processes, such as embryogenesis, cell proliferation, and apoptosis. Malfunction of these receptors is a leading cause of major human diseases, such as developmental defects, cancer, and diabetes, and several new drugs that target these receptors (e.g., Herceptin, Cetuximab, Iressa, and Gleevec) have been approved in the last few years (Yarden and Sliwkowski, 2001).

Because of the conformation of its first cysteinic domain, $p185^{neu}$ does not bind a specific ligand, while its fixed open structure enables it to act as a coreceptor and interact with other EGFRs when complexed with their specific ligands (Garret et al., 2003). By forming both heterodimers and $p185^{neu}$–$p185^{neu}$ homodimers (when it is overexpressed or mutated), it activates a cascade of intracellular signals that deregulate apoptosis and cell survival as well as the cell cycle (Yarden and Sliwkowski, 2001).

Apart from its direct involvement in tumor pathogenesis, many other features make $p185^{neu}$ an ideal target. Its overexpression in tumors compared with normal tissues confers selectivity on treatments for which $p185^{neu}$ is the target. EGFRs are involved in various stages of mammary gland development as shown by impairment of mammary development in mice with some defects in these receptors. *Her2* also plays a fundamental role in development of other organs such as the heart and central nervous system. However, its role is confined to embryonic differentiation, unlike the mammary gland, which continues to develop even in adult life following hormone stimulation. Thus, an immunological response induced against $p185^{neu}$ is expected to perturb mammary gland development but not the heart or nervous system (Pupa et al., 2005). On the other hand, in patients *Her2* amplification and overexpression are associated with tumorigenesis in 20–30% of breast, ovary, brain, and prostate carcinomas, a more aggressive course, greater invasiveness, and greater resistance to both chemotherapy and hormone therapy. Moreover, the percentage of $p185^{neu}$ positive cells is usually high in preneoplastic lesions, primary tumors and metastases (Garrett et al., 2003; Pupa et al., 2005; Yarden and Sliwkowski, 2001).

Thanks to the work of W. J. Muller (1988), there are several lines of mice transgenic for the rat (r-) Her2 oncogene. Females of these lines overexpress the transgenic r-Her2 at a distinct period of their life and develop mammary carcinomas whose progression mirrors that of their human counterparts. The latency time of the first palpable tumor and the cumulative number of independent tumors (tumor multiplicity) is characteristic of each transgenic line. Mice transgenic for the transforming (activated) *r-Her2* oncogene typically have more and earlier tumors than those transgenic for the proto-oncogene. The single-point mutation at position 664 in the transmembrane domain of p185^{neu} coded by the transforming *r-Her2* leads to replacement of valine with glutamic acid. On the cell membrane, the negative charge of glutamic acid results in the formation of an H-bond with an alanine at position 661 of another p185^{neu} molecule, as well as with other EGFRs (Bargmann *et al.*, 1986). These homo- and heterodimers spontaneously transduce the proliferative signals responsible for the aggressive neoplastic behavior of the cell. Investigators have thus an ample choice in terms of tumor models and carcinoma aggressiveness.

9. BALB-*neu*T Mice as a Study Model for Mammary Cancer

Probably the most aggressive and consistent model of r-Her2 mammary carcinogenesis is provided by BALB-*neu*T mice (H-2^d) transgenic for the transforming *r-Her2* oncogene under the transcriptional control of a long terminal repeat sequence from mammary tumor virus (http://cancermodels.nci.nih.gov/mmhcc/index.jsp). We bred these mice starting from a noninbred transgenic male mouse (#1330) generated by Dr. L. Clerici, Euratom, Ispra, Italy (Lucchini *et al.*, 1992). We have mated this male with regular BALB/c females, and their r-Her2$^+$ male offspring were genotyped and backcrossed with regular BALB/c females. As this genotyping and mating has been performed for more than 42 generations, we have generated syngeneic mice whose virgin females inexorably display a palpable invasive carcinoma in all their 10 mammary glands around the 33rd week of age. The progression of these lesions is consistent. Around the nipple, epithelial nodular neoformations (side buds) stemming from the main and secondary mammary ducts are already evident in 4-week-old mice (Di Carlo *et al.*, 1999) (Fig. 3A). Histologically, these buds are the foci of atypical hyperplasia in carcinomatous progression. A thick network of microvessels expressing αvβ3 integrin associated with these lesions suggests a close connection between the increased epithelial cell proliferation of hyperplastic lesions and activation of angiogenesis. At 8 weeks, most side buds have progressed to *in situ* carcinomas, while an increasing number of hyperplastic foci are evident all over the gland. Between the 10th and the 20th week, the *in situ* carcinomas become invasive and metastasize to the bone marrow and lungs. This progression is similar in all the mammary

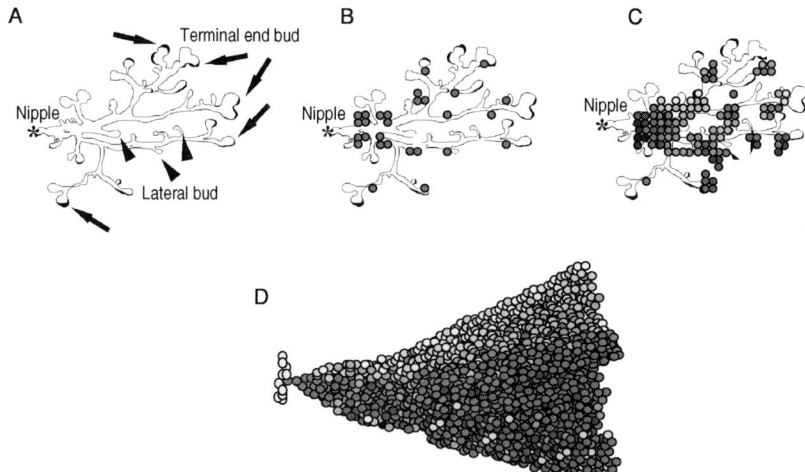

Figure 3 Schematic representation of the progression of r-Her2 lesions in a mammary gland of BALB-*neu*T mice. (A) In a 4-week-old wild-type BALB/c mice ducts and ductules branching off from the nipple (*) give rise to small protuberances (lateral buds) (arrowheads) and display terminal end buds. (B) In the BALB-*neu*T mice, Her2 lesions appear as multiple epithelial nodular neoformations (in red) disseminated along the mammary tree. (C) Her2 lesions become progressively more numerous, fuse and enlarge (modified from Pannellini *et al.*, 2004). As in the human monoclonal disease (D), these multiple cell clones share Her2 overexpression as the same first mutational lesion (in red) while their independent progression (C) may replicate the clonal diversification that takes place in human cancer over the decades of its progression. (**See Plate 6 in color insert at the end of the book.**)

glands. The cells of the hyperplastic, neoplastic, and metastatic lesions constantly highly overexpress r-Her2 receptor in both their cytoplasm and their membrane (Boggio *et al.*, 1998; Pannellini *et al.*, 2004).

The gene expression signatures of carcinomas progressing in BALB-*neu*T mice are also similar to those of human Her2 positive tumors. Genes that characterize human breast cancer and predict clinical outcome differentiate neoplastic mammary glands, whereas genes differently expressed in normal and neoplastic glands of BALB-*neu*T mice separate human Her2 positive tumors from normal mammary tissue (Astolfi *et al.*, 2005). BALB-*neu*T mice thus neatly model the progression of human breast tumor in terms of gene expression.

Despite these substantial analogies with human mammary cancer, BALB-*neu*T mice are not exempt from some of the concerns that make transgenic models far from perfect. Whether their immunological tolerance to xenogeneic r-p185^{neu} coded by the transforming *r-Her2* oncogene driven by an engineered promoter is comparable with that of patients with Her2 carcinomas is a crucial question to which an unconditional answer cannot be provided (Lollini et al., 2005). Even so, several facts point toward a substantial tolerance analogy. First, r-p185^{neu} shares 94.8% sequence homology with mouse p185^{neu} (Nagata et al., 1997). Moreover, in FVB mice transgenic for r-Her2 it has been shown that transgenic r-p185^{neu} is expressed in the thymic stroma by newborn mice (Reilly et al., 2000). In BALB-neuT mice we have shown that r-p185^{neu} is markedly and diffusely overexpressed in multiple epithelial tissues during weaning. This early overexpression of r-p185^{neu} along with the absence of a cellular and humoral reactivity against the tissue cells overexpressing it (Rovero et al., 2000) poses a significant challenge to the induction of protective immunity. While in wild-type BALB/c mice various forms of vaccination elicit strong cellular and humoral immunity and confer full protection against challenge by transplantable r-p185^{neu+} tumor cells (Curcio et al., 2003), in BALB-neuT mice the same vaccines fail to elicit the strong and rapid reactivity required for the rejection of r-p185^{neu+} transplantable tumor (Rovero et al., 2000). Immunoscope investigation (Ria et al., 2001) of their T-cell repertoire shows the absence of the high-affinity anti-r-p185^{neu} CD8$^+$ T-cell clones dominant in anti-r-Her2 immunized wild-type BALB/c mice (Rolla, manuscript in preparation).

An increase of Gr-1 (Ly6G), Mac-1 (CD11b), and ER-MP12 (CD31) immature myeloid cells in the peripheral blood and spleen goes along with the progression of mammary lesions. Their expansion rests on vascular endothelial growth factor (VEGF) as well as on other factors released by tumor cells, and progressively inhibits T lymphocytes that fail to respond to alloantigens and CD3 triggering (Melani et al., 2003). In BALB-neuT mice the expansion of mammary lesions also leads to progressive expansion of the CD4$^+$ CD25$^+$, Foxp3$^+$, and GITR$^+$ population of T-regulatory (Treg) cells. These Treg cells appear to hamper the anti-r-Her2 immune reactivity naturally triggered by tumor progression and markedly limit vaccine efficacy (Ambrosino and Wei-Zen Wei, manuscript in preparation).

In BALB-neuT mice the mammary lesions are multifocal and scattered all over the gland (Di Carlo et al., 1999; Pannellini et al., 2004) (Fig. 3B and C). This is not a feature of their most common human counterparts, even if several human mammary carcinomas (especially the nodular forms) are multifocal and/or multicentric. However, as in the human monoclonal disease, these multiple cell clones share the same first mutational lesion. Their independent progression may replicate the clonal diversification that takes place in human cancer over the decades of its progression, and thus reproduce another key issue of human tumors (Fig. 3D).

The inexorability of the development by all BALB-*neu*T mice of a palpable mammary tumor by week 20 allows evaluation of the protection afforded, as measured by both the extension of the disease-free survival and the percentage of tumor-free mice as time progresses. Moreover, as a tumor is palpable in all 10 mammary glands around week 33, the tumor multiplicity can also be evaluated and increases in the size of each lesion can be measured. The *r-Her2* oncogene is embedded in the genome of these mice, and therefore an immune response cannot eradicate the cells that will eventually produce another lesion. Immunized mice are engaged in a long-lasting confrontation between the r-Her2 signals and the sustained inhibitory potential of their immune reactions. This means that to be of significance, the immune control of cancer progression must last for long periods sometimes exceeding 1 year. This unusual length calls for induction and maintenance of a long-lasting immune memory, whereas it hampers precise study of immunological functions and makes it hard to decide when they should be assessed. Long experiments are demanding and expensive. Their reward lies in their modeling of the length of the human tumor–host relationship. Time, a crucial variable too often neglected in tumor immunology experiments, thus gets its revenge.

10. DNA Vaccination Inhibits Her2 Mammary Carcinogenesis

In view of the strong protection of Her2 FVB transgenic mice conferred by DNA vaccination (Amici *et al.*, 1998), its preventive effect on the progression of mammary lesions and its therapeutic potency against invasive tumors in BALB-*neu*T mice have been systematically explored. DNA vaccines are molecularly defined reagents that are easy to construct and modify. They can elicit a long-lasting cellular and immune response to a variety of antigens in experimental animals and human volunteers. The consistent and long-lasting progression of mammary lesions in BALB-*neu*T provide an unique experimental system with which to both assess the ability of DNA vaccination to inhibit the progression of precancerous lesions and cure more advanced stages of the tumor and identify the requirements for maintaining protection during the aging of mice.

First, we observed that expression on the cell membrane of the protein coded by the DNA vaccine is an important issue. The protective potential of vaccination with a plasmid coding for the transmembrane and extracellular domain of r-p185^{neu} but lacking the intracellular kinase domain (EC-TM plasmid) (Rovero *et al.*, 2000) was stronger than that elicited by a plasmid coding the soluble extracellular domain only (Rovero *et al.*, 2001). In mice, bearing diffuse areas of atypical hyperplasia in all their mammary glands, intramuscular injection of 100 µg of EC-TM plasmid in the surgically exposed left quadriceps when mice display mammary atypical hyperplasia (6 weeks of age) and repeated at 6-week intervals keeps all mice free of a palpable tumor at week 22, when control mice vaccinated with the empty plasmid all display at least one palpable tumor. However, starting from week 27 this protection decreases progressively and all immunized animals develop a tumor by week 42 (Di Carlo et al., 2001; Rovero et al., 2000, 2001). Empty plasmid administrations delayed carcinoma onset only slightly. These findings illustrate the concept that active specific immunity can efficiently block the progression of early Her2 precancerous lesions (Forni et al., 2000) and encourage the search for ways of improving their efficacy and inducing long-lasting protection.

Longer protection was sought by combining EC-TM plasmid inoculation with that of soluble mouse lymphocyte activation gene-3/CD223 (LAG-3) generated by fusing the extracellular domain of murine LAG-3 to a murine IgG2a Fc portion (mLAG-3Ig) (Cappello et al., 2003). LAG-3 is a type I transmembrane protein associated with the T-cell receptor-CD3 complex and binds MHC class II molecules in a manner similar to and more efficaciously than CD4. It is expressed in all subsets of T and NK cells after activation, and its expression is upregulated by IL-2 and IL-12. By triggering the functional maturation of DC, LAG-3 permits the optimal priming of native CD4 or CD8 T cells. For this reason, soluble mLAG-3Ig has been used as a vaccine adjuvant for both conventional and tumor antigens (Triebel, 2003).

Injection of mLAG-3Ig leads to the recruitment of APC expressing CD86, granulocytes, NK cells, $CD4^+$ T lymphocytes, and $CD8^+$ IFN-γ-expressing cells. Infiltrating cells release IFN-γ, TNFα, and IL-1β, and chemokines, namely CXCL5, CXCL9, CXCL10, CXCL11, CCL5, and CCL2 (Di Carlo et al., 2005). BALB-neuT mice first received EC-TM plasmids injected intramuscularly and a few seconds later 1 µg of either mouse LAG-3Ig or a nonspecific isotype-matched purified control mouse Ig in the same area. At 1 year of age, 70% of those vaccinated with EC-TM plasmid and LAG-3Ig on weeks 4 and 7, and 20% of those vaccinated with EC-TM plasmid only were still free from palpable tumors. Assessment of effector/memory CD8 cells in the spleen showed that $CD11b^+/CD28^+$ double positive lymphocytes were more numerous in mice vaccinated with EC-TM plasmid and LAG-3Ig. This difference was already evident 1 week after the last vaccination and doubled after 10 weeks (Cappello et al., 2003).

This further indication of the central role of DC cross presentation in EC-TM plasmid vaccination (Sumida et al., 2004) spurred exploitation of the possibility of directly exploiting DC ability to present the protein coded by the EC-TM plasmid. Dendritic cells, from 10-day bone marrow cultures infected with a recombinant adenovirus containing the EC-TM plasmid showed both the EC-TM mRNA transcript and EC-TM protein expression on the cell surface and in the cytoplasm (DC^{EC-TM}). Irradiated DC^{EC-TM} cultured in various ratios stimulated the proliferation of spleen lymphocytes from the nonimmunized BALB-*neu*T mice. Vaccination of BALB-*neu*T mice bearing a mammary atypical hyperplasia (5–6 week of age) with weekly subcutaneous injections of DC^{EC-TM} significantly improved tumor-free survival compared with mice treated with controls. Over 65% of vaccinated mice remained tumor free at 28 weeks of age, whereas all of the mice in the control group developed tumors. Importantly, the efficacy of antitumor vaccination with adenovirus-infected DC was unaffected by preexisting immunity to adenovirus (Sakai *et al.*, 2004).

11. The Mode of EC-TM Plasmid Delivery is Decisive for Vaccine Efficacy

The amount of protein expressed following plasmid administration, the persistence of this production, and the kind of APC involved are key variables on which the efficiency of DNA vaccination rests. They are markedly affected by the way in which plasmid is administered. In wild-type BALB/c mice, intradermal shots of EC-TM plasmid with a gene gun at 1-week intervals elicit a completely protective immunity against a subsequent lethal challenge of r-Her2$^+$ tumor cells, while the reaction thus triggered is strong enough to eradicate large established r-Her2$^+$ transplantable tumors. This successful eradication is the result of a robust coordinated response involving CD4$^+$ and CD8$^+$ T cells, antibodies, Fc receptors, CD1d-restricted NKT cells, macrophages, neutrophils, perforin, and IFN-γ (Curcio *et al.*, 2003) (Table 1).

Therefore, it was surprising to discover that the same vaccination regimen is ineffective in Her2 tolerant BALB-*neu*T mice displaying widespread areas of atypical hyperplasia and multiple foci of *in situ* carcinomas in all mammary glands (weeks 10 and 12) (Fig. 4). By contrast, EC-TM plasmid injection into the surgically exposed quadriceps delays the progression of the lesions and maintains 20% of mice free of palpable tumors at 1 year of age. Cross-presentation of the plasmid-coded protein is dominant in muscle, whereas direct transfection may be of greater importance when plasmids are delivered to the skin (Sumida *et al.*, 2004). It is therefore possible that the way of EC-TM protein presentation following intradermal shots are effective in not-tolerant wild-type BALB/c mice but are unable to trigger the immune mechanisms that acquire a critical importance in BALB-*neu*T mice.

A much more delayed occurrence of the first palpable tumor and about 50% of mice tumor free at 1 year of age were observed when BALB-*neu*T mice received EC-TM plasmid injected intramuscularly and a few seconds later two short electric pulses generated by a square wave pulse generator, delivered by electrodes placed on the shaved skin covered with a conducting gel around the

Table 1 Distinct Mechanisms of Specific Immunity Induced by EC-TM Vaccination are Required for the Rejection of a Challenge of r-Her2 Tumor Cells and the Eradication of an Established r-Her2 Tumor by Wild-Type BALB/c Mice, and for the Protection of BALB-*neu*T Mice Against the Development of Autochthonous r-Her2 Carcinomas

	Immune mechanisms elicited by EC-TM plasmid vaccine and required by		
	BALB/c mice to reject a r-Her2 cell challenge	BALB/c mice to eradicated an r-Her2 tumor	BALB-*neu*T mice to control mammary carcinogenesis
DC mobilization	Not tested	Not tested	Induced and required (Curcio and Hirsch, unpublished observations)
CD4$^+$ T cell activation[a]	Elicited and required[b]	Elicited and required[b]	Elicited and required[c,d,e,f]
CD8$^+$ T cell activation[a]	Elicited but dispensable[b]	Elicited and required[b]	Elicited but dispensable[c,d,e,g]
CTL activation	Elicited but dispensable[b]	Elicited and required[b]	Not induced[c,d,e,f,h,i]
IFN-γ production	Elicited and required[b]	Induced and required[b]	Induced and required[c,e]
Anti-r-Her2 IgG2a	Induced and dispensable[b]	Induced and required[b]	Induced and required[c,e,f]
Activation of FcγRI/III	Induced and dispensable[b]	Induced and required[b]	Induced and required (Mastini and Clynes, unpublished observations)

[a] EC-TM plasmid: shoot in the dermis by gene gun[b]; electroporated intramuscularly[c] assessed as IFN-γ production.
[b] Curcio et al., 2003.
[c] Quaglino et al., 2004a.
[d] Sakai et al., 2004.
[e] Nanni et al., 2004.
[f] Park et al., 2005.
[g] Lo Iacono et al., 2005.
[h] Rovero et al., 2000.
[i] Cappello et al., 2003.

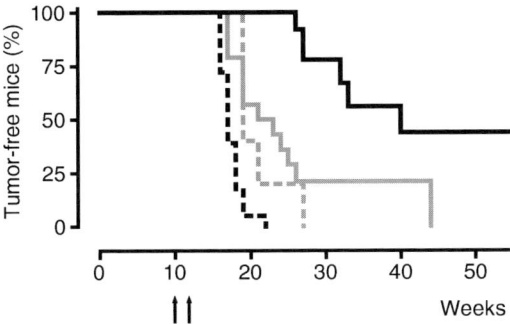

Figure 4 The way in which EC-TM plasmid is administered to BALB-*neu*T mice decides the amplitude of the protection. Mice bearing widespread areas of atypical hyperplasia and numerous multifocal *in situ* carcinomas in all mammary glands were immunized at weeks 10 and 12 (arrows) with the optimal dose of EC-TM plasmid: 1.2 µg for gene gun administration (dotted grey); 100 µg for intramuscular administration (grey), 50 µg for intramuscular electroporation (black). Dotted black line, untreated mice. Results show the time of appearance of the first palpable tumor. Groups of at least 12 mice. Tumor incidence in mice receiving EC-TM plasmid electroporation was significantly lower than that in control mice ($p < 0.0001$, Mantel-Henszel log-rank test).

injection site. In these mice tumor multiplicity, too, was significantly reduced (Quaglino *et al.*, 2004a).

Short high-voltage pulses that surpass the capacitance of the cell membrane induce a transient permeabilization that permits plasmids to better overcome this barrier. Whereas pore formation happens in microseconds, membrane resealing happens over a range of minutes (Gehl, 2003). As compared with simple intramuscular injection, vaccination by electroporation provides a greater and more persistent mass of antigen available for the induction of immune responses. Transfection of other cells, such as DC, may also be facilitated. Direct application of an electric field to the tissue could result in an inflammatory response that may further enhance the immunogenicity of the plasmid-coded antigen. Electroporation was shown to induce cellular infiltration (Babiuk *et al.*, 2004; Sumida *et al.*, 2004), and the different electroporation conditions might influence the quality and quantity of subsequent antigen cross-presentation. Our observations with BALB-*neu*T mice KO for the phosphoinositide 3-kinase (PI3Kγ) gene (BALB-*neu*T/PI3Kγ KO mice) further point to the central role played by DC infiltration in the induction of immunity following EC-TM plasmid electroporation. The gamma isoform of PI3K plays a nonreductant role in DC migration *in vivo*. The reduced ability of antigen-loaded DC to travel is responsible for the impaired ability of PI3Kγ KO mice to mount a T-cell-mediated immune responses (Del Prete *et al.*, 2004).

Experiments in progress in BALB-*neu*T/PI3Kγ KO mice show that EC-TM plasmid vaccine is unable to elicit a protective response in these mice (Curcio and Hirsch, unpublished observations). As our comparative studies showed that EC-TM plasmid electroporation provides a straightforward method for inducing a strong protection in BALB-*neu*T mice with advanced and multifocal preneoplastic lesions, we decided to use DNA electroporation as our standard vaccination procedure. The smaller amount of DNA required as compared with intramuscular DNA vaccination, the positive results obtained in large animals, along with the availability of devices for electroporation in humans, endorse our choice.

The significant but temporary protection elicited by EC-TM plasmid electroporation prompts exploration of the signals that enable the protective immune memory to be prolonged once it is established. In immunoprevention experiments, the significance of the results is a function of the length of the follow-up. Additional EC-TM plasmid electroporation courses performed at 10-week intervals extended tumor-free survival (Quaglino *et al*., 2004a). Ongoing experiments with repeated electroporations show that almost all mice are still free of mammary tumors at 75 weeks of age. The inexorably slow progression of r-Her2 carcinogenesis in nonvaccinated BALB-*neu*T mice make this persistent inhibition of advanced precancerous lesions a significant finding. Studies are in progress to evaluate the point of time to which significant protection can be prolonged by repeated boosting. A comparable sustained and total protection is also obtained when mice first receive EC-TM plasmid electroporation at 10–12 weeks of age and are then boosted every 10 weeks with empty plasmids containing 4 CpG motifs (ODN 1760). In the absence of a specific priming by EC-TM plasmid, injections of plasmids containing CpG do not provide any significant protection.

12. The Limitations of DNA Vaccination and How They Can Be Overcome

The consistency of r-Her2 mammary carcinogenesis progression in BALB-*neu*T mice as well as its similarities with human cancer enable an assessment to be made of the ability of EC-TM plasmid electroporation to protect against pathologically defined stages of mammary cancer. In mice bearing diffuse areas of atypical hyperplasia, vaccination through EC-TM plasmid electroporation significantly extends the disease-free interval and keeps about 50% of mice tumor-free at 1 year of age. However, the same vaccination provides a decreasing protection as the mice bear more advanced lesions and is ineffective in mice with invasive cancer, even if this is only microscopically detectable (Fig. 5A).

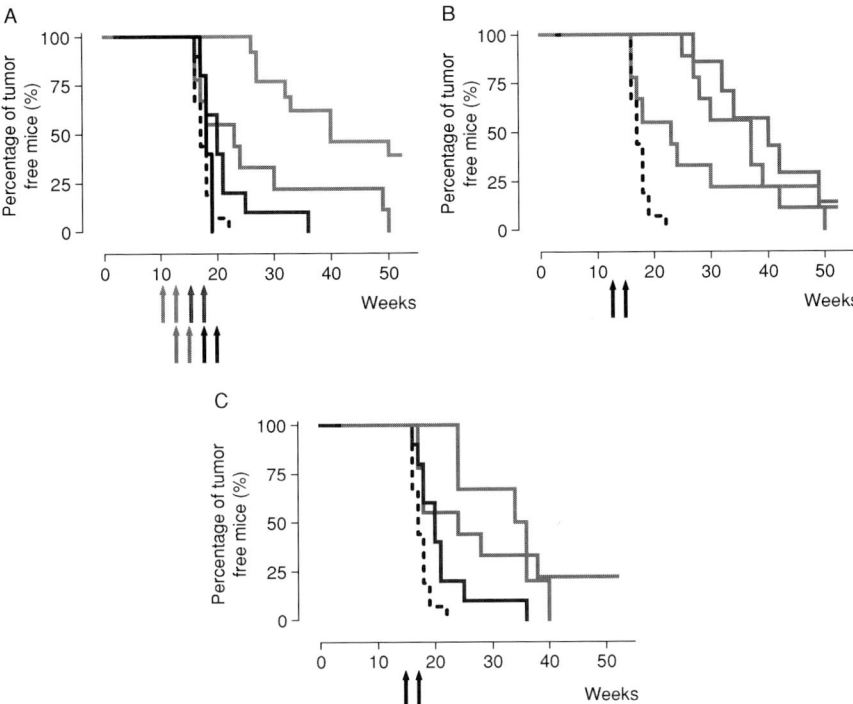

Figure 5 Ability of EC-TM plasmid electroporation to protect against progressive stages of mammary lesions of BALB-*neu*T mice. (A) Mice bearing widespread areas of atypical hyperplasia and numerous multifocal *in situ* carcinomas (week 10) (red), with more advanced *in situ* carcinomas (week 12) (green), with larger multifocal lesions (week 14) (blue), and with early invasive carcinomas (week 18) (black) received two courses of EC-TM plasmid electroporations administered with an interval of 14 days (arrows). Dotted line, untreated mice. Mice bearing advanced *in situ* carcinomas (B) (green) and larger multifocal lesions (C) (blue) received EC-TM electroporations (arrows) combined with the subsequent intramuscular injection of 1 μg mLAG-3Ig (Cappello *et al.*, 2003) (purple) or 10 μg of BAT monoclonal antibodies (brown) injected intravenously 1 week after electroporation (Quaglino *et al.*, 2005). Dotted line, untreated mice. Results show the time of appearance of the first palpable tumor in groups of al least 12 mice. (**See Plate 7 in color insert at the end of the book.**)

These results endorse the concept that immunological prevention of tumor progression is an appropriate and rational goal for active immunotherapy, perhaps more sensible than the cure of an established tumor (Forni *et al.*, 2000; Lollini and Forni, 2003; Lollini *et al.*, 2005). Nevertheless, in the hope that vaccination could also be made to cure the more advanced stages of mammary cancer, we explored whether combinations of EC-TM plasmid electroporation with other signals might increase vaccine curative potential. mLAG-3 proved capable of extending the efficacy of vaccination of mice bearing diffuse atypical hyperplasia (Cappello et al., 2003). Its combination with EC-TM plasmid electroporation also extended the disease-free survival of mice already harboring large multifocal *in situ* carcinomas in all mammary glands, while providing only limited protection of mice with more advanced lesions (Fig. 5B and C).

A T-cell stimulatory monoclonal antibody (BAT) was obtained by immunization of BALB/c mice with membranes from a human Burkitt lymphoma cell line (Daudi cells). BAT binds T cells and elevates their proliferation and antitumor cytotoxicity *in vitro* in a way similar to that of anti-CTLA-4 antibodies, but its binding to lymphocytes displays a different profile (Raiter et al., 1999). A significant extension of the disease-free survival was observed when EC-TM plasmid electroporation was combined with costimulation with BAT IgG3 monoclonal antibody administered intravenously (Quaglino et al., 2005). However, this combination was ineffective in mice with more advanced lesions (Fig. 5B and C).

We also explored the therapeutic protection stemming from EC-TM plasmid electroporation combined with IL-12. While neo-adjuvant therapy is emerging as a treatment option in early primary breast cancer, almost no data are available on the use of antiangiogenic and immunomodulatory agents in a neoadjuvant setting. Interleukin-12 is a promising adjunct for cancer and other vaccines since it activates potent antiangiogenic mechanisms, mainly through the induction of IFN-γ and a cascade of secondary and tertiary cytokines. Systemic IL-12 administered alone to BALB-*neu*T mice delayed carcinogenesis, extended the disease-free survival and reduced tumor multiplicity (Boggio et al., 1998, 2000; Cavallo et al., 2001; Cifaldi et al., 2001). Significant protection, however, was only obtained when this treatment was started during the early phases of tumor growth, and even when it was significant, the inhibition of carcinogenesis was only temporary. Besides its ability to stimulate numerous functions of innate immunity, IL-12 appears to be effective in both inhibiting the formation of new capillary sprouts that accompanies the shift from the preneoplastic to the neoplastic condition (Cifaldi et al., 2001) and modulating the gene expression patterns in Her2 tumor cells from proangiogenic to antiangiogenic (Cavallo et al., 2001). Moreover, in BALB-*neu*T mice bearing initial atypical mammary hyperplasia IL-12 was an important component of an allogeneic r-p185^{neu+} cell vaccine that led to almost complete prevention of Her2 mammary tumorigenesis (Nanni et al., 2001).

To investigate whether early neo-adjuvant stimulation of innate immunity by IL-12 could render EC-TM plasmid electroporation effective after the onset of carcinomas, when it is ineffective on its own, BALB-*neu*T mice with lesions equivalent to atypical hyperplasia and *in situ* carcinoma received four weekly injections of IL-12 followed by a 3-week rest. This course given four times markedly delayed the progression of mammary lesions but no mice remained tumor free. By contrast, IL-12 treated mice that received additional EC-TM plasmid electroporation at weeks 16 and 18 displayed tumor regression and 63% were tumor free at week 35 (Spadaro *et al.*, 2005). Moreover, all mice were tumor free at 1 year of age when IL-12 was followed by EC-TM plasmid electroporation at weeks 16, 18, 23, and 25.

13. Coordinated Low-Avidity Mechanisms

Our data suggest that EC-TM plasmid electroporation is a straightforward way for eliciting preventive immunity against preneoplastic Her2 lesions (Fig. 6). By contrast, cure of invasive carcinomas seems to require vaccination with another form of treatment. Attempts to combine distinct antitumor strategies provide a glimpse of the therapeutic possibilities. They also raise the question of why EC-TM plasmid vaccination is no longer enough when invasive carcinoma is present. A straightforward answer is barred because this failure is the outcome of several factors. The tumor burden may be too large and widespread to be controlled by the immune system alone. It also impairs the ability of the immune system to mount an effective response because suppressor factors are released by the tumor, and because of the expansion of immature myeloid cells and Treg lymphocytes, and improper tumor recognition. Furthermore, its genetic instability increases as a tumor expands. Clones no longer dependent on *Her2* transduction pathways or no longer susceptible to the effector mechanisms of the immune system are likely to be selected by a late-induced immune response. Large tumors in BALB-*neu*T mice may thus model what happens when patients no longer respond to Herceptin.

As these conclusions call for determination of the mechanisms that lead to tumor prevention of r-Her2 tumors, we have devoted much attention to teasing apart and weighing the importance of the pathways of effector immunity elicited by EC-TM plasmid electroporation.

As reported in Table 1, in nontolerant wild-type BALB/c mice, EC-TM plasmid vaccination elicits a robust coordinated response that leads to both the rejection of a subsequent tumor transplant and the cure of fast growing established transplantable r-Her2 tumors. In the prophylactic immunization, $CD4^+$ cells were essential for immune priming but not tumor rejection. $CD8^+$ T cells partially contributed to tumor prevention, neutrophils were absolutely required, whereas antibodies were dispensable. By contrast, rejection of established tumors required the coordinated action of $CD4^+$ and $CD8^+$

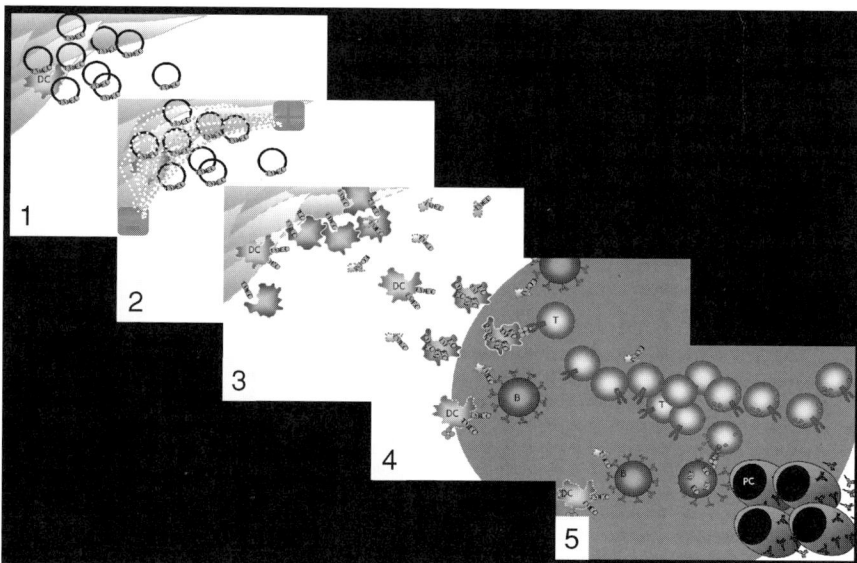

Figure 6 Steps and mechanisms of critical importance for the protection against r-Her2 lesions in BALB-*neu*T mice. (1) Intramuscular injection of plasmids. The way of DNA plasmid delivery (Quaglino *et al.*, 2004a) and the possibility that the plasmid-coded proteins are being expressed on the cell membrane increase the intensity of the protection elicited (Lollini and Forni, 2003); (2) electroporation of muscle and APC cells. The transient permeabilization of the cell membrane following the electric pulses leads to a more persistent and enhanced expression of the plasmid coded protein (Geninatti Crich *et al.*, 2005); (3) recruitment of an inflammatory infiltrate. Fresh data with BALB-*neu*T mice with impaired mobilization of DC (Del Prete *et al.*, 2004) shows that an inflammatory infiltrate plays a key role in the elicitation of a protective response (Curcio and Hirsch, manuscript in preparation); (4) activation of B and C4$^+$ T cells. The plasmid-coded protein expressed by muscle cell debris and transfected DC should directly activate B cells, while peptides cross-presented by DC are required for the activation of CD4$^+$ T cells; (5) induction of effector mechanisms. The protection elicited rests on the combined action of antiap185^{neu} antibodies (mainly IgG2a) and IFN-γ releasing T cells (Nanni *et al.*, 2004; Quaglino *et al.*, 2004a). (**See Plate 8 in color insert at the end of the book.**)

T cells, antibodies, Fc receptors, CD1d-restricted NKT cells, macrophages, neutrophils, perforin, and IFN-γ (Curcio *et al.*, 2003).

Since the same EC-TM plasmid was used for immunization, these data from wild-type BALB/c mice may be used as a standard against which to measure the immune mechanisms leading to inhibition of early Her2 lesions in BALB-*neu*T mice. At first, we were surprised to discover that the protection against preneoplastic Her2 lesions elicited by EC-TM plasmid electroporation was not related to the activation of CD8 CTL (Rovero *et al.*, 2000). When this issue was investigated extensively, no major CTL activity was detected in the spleen, lymph nodes, and blood of EC-TM plasmid immunized and protected mice in both a 4-h *in vitro* test and longer and different tests (Cappello *et al.*, 2003; Quaglino *et al.*, 2004a; Rovero *et al.*, 2000; Sakai *et al.*, 2004; Spadaro *et al.*, 2005). As a consequence of the early and diffuse tissue overexpression of r-Her2, vaccinated BALB-*neu*T mice are unable to activate the high-avidity $CD8^+$ CTL that recognize the TYVPANASL dominant r-Her2 peptide presented by the $H-2K^d$ glycoproteins of the major histocompatibility complex (Nagata *et al.*, 1997). Data show that no significant cytotoxicity is evident in EC-TM plasmid electroporated BALB-*neu*T mice, both *in vitro* and *in vivo* against target cells pulsed with TYVPANASL peptide. By contrast, a cytotoxic response is clearly evident in wild-type BALB/c mice vaccinated with EC-TM plasmid either by gene gun or electroporation (Curcio *et al.*, 2003).

Therefore, the immunity elicited by EC-TM plasmid in BALB-*neu*T lacks a critical component, such as the high-avidity $CD8^+$ CTL response. Even so, EC-TM plasmid immunization induces an immune response effective in the sustained clearance of precancerous lesions and inhibition of carcinogenesis. Adoptive transfer experiments (Quaglino *et al.*, 2004a; Spadaro *et al.*, 2005) and experiments with BALB-*neu*T mice rendered deficient in various immune components through gene targeting or antibody-mediated depletion of selected lymphocyte populations (Cappello *et al.*, 2003; Quaglino *et al.*, 2004a,b, 2005; Rovero *et al.*, 2000; Sakai *et al.*, 2004; Spadaro *et al.*, 2005) made it clear that anti-r-$p185^{neu}$ antibodies are both necessary and sufficient for protection, and the IgG2a isotype is the most effective. For the T-cell chauvinism of experimental immunologists induced by myriads of experiments with transplantable tumors to believe that T-cell reactivity is the only way to inhibit tumor growth, this was an uncomfortable finding, only partially soothed by the new data from monoclonal antibodies in the management of patients with Her2 tumors (Garrett *et al.*, 2003; Yarden and Sliwkowski, 2001).

As $p185^{neu}$ is both a cell surface receptor regulating cell growth and the target tumor antigen, antibodies can play both a direct role and trigger a more complex response. These two roles are not mutually exclusive, and may depend on the epitope recognized and the isotype of the antibody produced (Yarden and Sliwkowski, 2001). By directly downregulating r-$p185^{neu}$ expression, and impeding the formation of homo- or heterodimers that transduce proliferative signals, the antibody impedes neoplastic proliferation. The membrane downmodulation of r-$p185^{neu}$, its intracytoplasmic confinement, and the morphological features of inhibited proliferation associated with diminished nuclear positivity of proliferating cell nuclear antigen in the mammary glands of EC-TM plasmid electroporated mice endorse this direct and noncytotoxic role of the anti-r-185^{neu} antibody (Quaglino *et al.*, 2004a,b; Rovero *et al.*,

2000). However, data in progress show that the protective immunity elicited in BALB-neuT by EC-TM plasmid electroporation requires the presence of FcR I/III positive cells (Mastini, manuscript in preparation). Anti-r-p185^{neu} antibodies induced by EC-TM plasmid electroporation may also activate complement-mediated lysis, as suggested by their isotype, and the importance of this effector mechanism must be explored.

The inability of EC-TM plasmid electroporation to protect BALB-neuT KO for the IFN-γ gene points to a critical role of IFN-γ. IgG2a is by far the most predominant isotype of the anti-r-p185^{neu} antibody elicited, and T-cell released IFN-γ is the main IgG2a switch factor (Nanni et al., 2001, 2004; Quaglino et al., 2004a,b). An expanded population of both CD4$^+$ and CD8$^+$ cells specifically releasing IFN-γ following in vitro stimulation with r-Her2 tumor cells is present in the spleen of EC-TM plasmid electroporated mice. The role played by these cells may be not restricted to induction of the most effective antibody isotype. Adoptive transfer experiments show that a better protection is transferred when the recipient gets both antibody and T cells from EC-TM plasmid immunized BALB-neuT mice (Quaglino et al., 2004a). Moreover, the clearance of mammary lesions in EC-TM plasmid electroporated BALB-neuT mice is associated with a massive infiltration of IFN-γ-releasing T cells that penetrate the basement membrane and interact with tumor cells. Intratumor IFN-γ may trigger many downstream proinflammatory and antitumor factors, directly impair the proliferation of tumor cells and their production of proangiogenic factors (Cavallo et al., 2001), and thus significantly contribute to tumor inhibition.

Progression of a preneoplastic lesion is a lengthy process that may be hampered by mechanisms that are not efficacious when confronted with the high speed of transplantable tumors. Highly proliferating invasive carcinomas easily evade the weakly efficient immune response elicited in BALB-neuT mice. Transplantable r-Her2 carcinomas are poorly inhibited by immunized BALB-neuT mice in which the autochthonous carcinogenesis is blocked (Rovero et al., 2000). The importance of the proliferative kinetics of the tumor is also made evident by experiments in which the proliferative ability of invasive cancers in BALB-neuT mice is reduced by repeated IL-12 administrations (Spadaro et al., 2005). The IL-12-induced inhibition of angiogenesis and the resulting slowing down of tumor proliferation make invasive cancers susceptible to low-avidity effector mechanisms.

As a whole these findings reinforce the concept that in the absence of a dominant high-avidity CTL response sustained inhibition of slowly progressing early r-Her2 lesions rests on antibodies and IFN-γ. They trigger diverse direct and indirect mechanisms that reduce tumor proliferation and lead to the death of tumor cells. Each mechanism is endowed with a different weight in the protection as a whole. In transgenic tolerant mice it is probably naïve to try and single out a dominant immune mechanism on which sustained protection rests.

Immunizations with EC-TM plasmid overcomes tolerance to rat and mouse Her2, since the anti-r-p185^{neu} antibodies induced cross-react with mouse p185^{neu} (Lo Iacono et al., 2005). Even so, EC-TM plasmid electroporated BALB-neuT mice necroscopied at 1 year of age were free from overt signs of autoimmune lesions in the heart, kidney, and liver, even if the induced anti-r-p185^{neu} antibodies cross-reacted with mouse p185^{neu} (Lo Iacono et al., 2005; Quaglino et al., 2004a). This absence of overt lesions is attributable to the combination of the poor expression of p185^{neu} by the tissues of adult mice and the inability of BALB-neuT mice to generate a high-affinity immune response to the r-p185^{neu} protein. Both wild-type BALB/c mice and BALB-neuT mice are naturally tolerant to self-expressed p185^{neu} and the immune response elicited is of low avidity. A low-avidity response may be critical in discriminating between quantitative differences in the expression of the target antigen. The response generated by EC-TM plasmid electroporation appears enough to successfully control the slow but devastating progression of multiple preneoplastic lesions without causing evident autoimmune aggression of the normal tissues, where p185^{neu} is expressed at a much lower level (Quaglino et al., 2004a). By contrast with high-avidity monoclonal antibodies, the immune response elicited by immunization in naturally tolerant mice (and patients?) is not expected to attack heart or nervous system. Following immunization signs of autoimmunity were only found in the mammary gland (Lo Iacono et al., 2005). Mammary gland continues to develop in adult life after hormone stimulation and differentiating cells overexpressing p185^{neu} are present and play an important role in maintaining the normal structure of the gland. The immune control of r-p185^{neu} cells is associated with a major alteration of the normal branching of ductules and the formation of lobular structures (Lo Iacono et al., 2005; Pannellini et al., 2004). This limited alteration of the mammary gland structure could be an acceptable price for carcinoma prevention. Generation of tissue-restricted autoimmune responses may even be an additional approach to cancer immunotherapy that will allow treatment of cancers arising from nonessential organs, such as breast, prostate, thyroid, and testis. This issue is of practical importance for young women at hereditary risk of breast cancers, especially those with mutations in the BRCA1 or BRCA2 gene, for whom an "immunological mastectomy" would represent a great improvement over double surgical prophylactic mastectomy (Pupa et al., 2005).

14. Cure Versus Control of Her2 Lesions

Sequential histology, whole-mount analysis, and transcriptional gene profiling concordantly show that as long as the protection lasts, the mammary lesions present at the time of vaccination remain unchanged or display a slow but progressive clearance. While the lesions may remain "frozen" for more than 1 year, as the immunity fades they progress again. In the mesenchymal tissue and in the stroma surrounding the "frozen" lesions, morphological examination reveals the presence of numerous plasma cells (Quaglino et al., 2004a,b). This indication of local antibody production also fits in well with the upregulation of a group of genes generically pertinent to the humoral response and encoding antibody-related genes. The gene coding for the Ig J polypeptide is one of those selectively upregulated and suggests a local production of IgA (Astolfi et al., 2005; Lo Iacono et al., 2005).

In addition, gene expression profiles show that genes related to the $p185^{neu}$ signal transduction pathways, such as *ras, cyclin D1, cdk4 cyclin-dependent kinase, jun transcription factor, protein kinase C,* and *PI3K* are downregulated. By contrast, transcription of the *Cbl, endophilin,* and *ubiquitin* genes related to the Her2 degradation pathway is upregulated. The inhibited *Her2* transduction pathway results in a reduction of the proliferative activity (Quaglino et al., 2004b). Moreover, immunohistochemistry observations show a marked decrease of membrane expression of $r\text{-}p185^{neu}$ that is confined to the cytoplasm and is faint even there. These data suggest that the role of the humoral response is so prominent because of the double role of $r\text{-}p185^{neu}$ in BALB-*neu*T mice, which is both the target tumor antigen and a membrane-exposed tyrosine kinase receptor regulating neoplastic proliferation (Lollini and Forni, 2003).

While the immune reaction elicited by EC-TM plasmid does not eradicate the neoplastic lesions, it controls their progression and maintains both the morphological appearance and transcriptional profile of the mammary glands at the stage when vaccination was started. When in most mice this controls last as long as their natural life, it coincides with a cancer cure.

In the absence of its continuous offsetting by neoplastic stem cells, the slow but progressive clearance of neoplastic lesions would coincide with a definitive cure. By contrast, the continuous regrowth of neoplastic stem cells challenges the protective potential of immunity by building a dynamic equilibrium. Several interfering factors may tip the scales and arouse "frozen" lesions. Time and aging of the immune system lead to the progressive loss of the immune memory, whereas repeated EC-TM plasmid recalls help to maintain an effective protection (Quaglino et al., 2004a). However, the lack of high-affinity lymphocytes along with the expansion of immature myeloid cells and

T suppressor cells that takes place as the lesions progress makes any kind of immune intervention a delicate balancing act.

As a whole, the data from vaccinated mice provide novel proof of concept, as they show that it is possible to block the progression of early neoplastic lesions by DNA vaccination provided one targets the right antigen. However, it is not clear to what extent these findings can be generalized beyond this particular model, for example, to clinical human ductal *in situ* carcinomas (DCIS) of the breast, since 34–60% overexpress Her2 (Quaglino *et al.*, 2004b). A category of patients for whom this approach may be desirable could be those who cannot undergo surgery due to concomitant, unrelated conditions. Rather than in newly diagnosed, clinically detectable DCIS, this approach may be more useful to control clinically undetectable DCIS lesions in a postsurgical setting (i.e., as secondary prevention) or as a way to generate an endogenous "Herceptin-like" effect in patients with advanced Her2 positive lesions. This could still be advantageous compared to exogenous antibodies because plasma cells releasing anti-p185^{neu} antibodies may be very close to the target cells.

15. Conclusions

At first sight, it may seem that the cure of transplantable tumors and tumor prevention in transgenic mice lead to contradictory results. Each, of course, has its own specific features. The differences between them, however, are primarily determined by the time frame within which an antitumor reaction must be elicited. In the cure of established tumors, this is dramatically short because of their generally rapid and life-threatening growth. A fast and robust antitumor reaction is the only way to block such growth and achieve eradication. A reaction of this kind rests mostly, if not solely on T-killer cell reactivity directed toward MHC-bound peptides presented by DC optimally activated for induction of this response. By contrast, time is not of the essence in the generation of an immune reaction against indolent precancerous lesions. What is required is a persistent and possibly lifelong reaction. Low-avidity reaction mechanisms ineffective in the control of fast-growing tumors can coordinately lead to a sustained blockade of carcinogenesis in conjunction with antibodies against the Her2-expressing preneoplastic cells. Unlike most tumor associated antigens recognized by T cells, in fact, Her2 is expressed on the cell surface.

The combination of appropriate antigen stimulation with appropriate adjuvant and costimulatory signals is required for the induction of both a fast and effective tumor cure and long-lasting prevention of carcinogenesis. Another common issue of critical importance is modulation of regulatory mechanisms. The apparently contradictory information emerging from the two approaches is thus found to be highly complementary and illustrates the significant progress achieved in our understanding of the interplay between tumors and a vaccine-alerted immune system. These insights can be used to elaborate better antitumor vaccination strategies.

References

Amici, A., Venanzi, F. M., and Concetti, A. (1998). Genetic immunization against neu/erbB2 transgenic breast cancer. *Cancer Immunol. Immunother.* **47,** 183–190.

Astolfi, A., Landuzzi, L., Nicoletti, G., De Giovanni, C., Croci, S., Paladini, A., Ferrini, S., Iezzi, M., Musiani, P., Cavallo, F., Forni, G., Nanni, P., et al. (2005). Gene expression analysis of immune-mediated arrest of tumorigenesis in a transgenic mouse model of HER-2/neu-positive basal-like mammary carcinoma. *Am. J. Pathol.* **166,** 1205–1216.

Babiuk, S., Baca-Estrada, M. E., Foldvari, M., Middleton, D. M., Rabussay, D., Widera, G., and Babiuk, L. A. (2004). Increased gene expression and inflammatory cell infiltration caused by electroporation are both important for improving the efficacy of DNA vaccines. *J. Biotechnol.* **110,** 1–10.

Bargmann, C. I., Hung, M. C., and Weinberg, R. A. (1986). Multiple independent activations of the neu oncogene by a point mutation altering the transmembrane domain of p185. *Cell* **45,** 649–657.

Bennett, S. R. M., Carbone, F. R., Karamalis, F., Flavell, R. A., Miller, J. F. A. P., and Heath, W. R. (1998). Help for cytotoxic-T-cell responses is mediated by CD40 signalling. *Nature* **393,** 478–480.

den Boer, A. Th., van Mierlo, G. J. D., Fransen, M. F., Melief, C. J. M., Offringa, R., and Toes, R. E. M. (2005). CD4$^+$ T cells are able to promote tumor growth through inhibition of tumor-specific CD8$^+$ T-cell responses in tumor-bearing hosts. *Cancer Res.* **65,** 6984–6989.

Boggio, K., Di Carlo, E., Rovero, S., Cavallo, F., Quaglino, E., Lollini, P.-L., Nanni, P., Nicoletti, G., Wolf, S., Musiani, P., and Forni, G. (2000). Ability of systemic interleukin-12 to hamper progressive stages of mammary carcinogenesis in HER2/neu transgenic mice. *Cancer Res.* **60,** 359–364.

Boggio, K., Nicoletti, G., Di Carlo, E., Cavallo, F., Landuzzi, L., Melani, C., Giovarelli, M., Rossi, I., Nanni, P., De Giovanni, C., Bouchard, P., Wolf, S., et al. (1998). Interleukin 12-mediated prevention of spontaneous mammary adenocarcinomas in two lines of Her-2/neu transgenic mice. *J. Exp. Med.* **188,** 589–596.

Cappello, P., Triebel, F., Iezzi, M., Caorsi, C., Quaglino, E., Lollini, P.-L., Amici, A., Di Carlo, E., Musiani, P., Giovarelli, M., and Forni, G. (2003). LAG-3 enables DNA vaccination to persistently prevent mammary carcinogenesis in HER-2/neu transgenic BALB/c mice. *Cancer Res.* **63,** 2518–2525.

Cavallo, F., Quaglino, E., Cifaldi, L., Di Carlo, E., Andre, A., Bernabei, P., Musiani, P., Forni, G., and Calogero, R. A. (2001). Interleukin 12-activated lymphocytes influence tumor genetic programs. *Cancer Res.* **61,** 3518–3523.

Cifaldi, L., Quaglino, E., Di Carlo, E., Musiani, P., Spadaro, M., Lollini, P.-L., Wolf, S., Boggio, K., Forni, G., and Cavallo, F. (2001). A light, nontoxic interleukin 12 protocol inhibits HER-2/neu mammary carcinogenesis in BALB/c transgenic mice with established hyperplasia. *Cancer Res.* **61,** 2809–2812.

Curcio, C., Di Carlo, E., Clynes, R., Smyth, M. J., Boggio, K., Quaglino, E., Spadaro, M., Colombo, M. P., Amici, A., Lollini, P. L., Musiani, P., and Forni, G. (2003). Nonredundant roles of antibody, cytokines, and perforin in the eradication of established Her-2/neu carcinomas. *J. Clin. Invest.* **111,** 1161–1170.

Daftarian, P., Sharan, R., Haq, W., Ali, S., Longmate, J., Termini, J., and Diamond, D. J. (2005). Novel conjugates of epitope fusion peptides with CpG-ODN display enhanced immunogenicity and HIV recognition. *Vaccine* **23**, 3453–3468.

Del Prete, A., Vermi, W., Dander, E., Otero, K., Barberis, L., Luini, W., Bernasconi, S., Sironi, M., Santoro, A., Garlanda, C., Facchetti, F., Wymann, M. P., et al. (2004). Defective dendritic cell migration and activation of adaptive immunity in PI3Kgamma-deficient mice. *EMBO J.* **23**, 3505–3515.

Del Val, M., Schlicht, H. J., Volkmer, H., Messerle, M., Reddehase, M. J., and Koszinowski, U. H. (1991). Protection against lethal cytomegalovirus infection by a recombinant vaccine containing a single nonameric T-cell epitope. *J. Virol.* **65**, 3641–3646.

Di Carlo, E., Cappello, P., Sorrentino, C., D'Antuono, T., Pellicciotta, A., Giovarelli, M., Forni, G., Musiani, P., and Triebel, F. (2005). Immunological mechanisms elicited at the tumour site by lymphocyte activation gene-3 (LAG-3) versus IL-12: Sharing a common Th1 anti-tumour immune pathway. *J. Pathol.* **205**, 82–91.

Di Carlo, E., Diodoro, M. G., Boggio, K., Modesti, A., Modesti, M., Nanni, P., Forni, G., and Musiani, P. (1999). Analysis of mammary carcinoma onset and progression in HER-2/neu oncogene transgenic mice reveals a lobular origin. *Lab. Invest.* **79**, 1261–1269.

Di Carlo, E., Rovero, S., Boggio, K., Quaglino, E., Amici, A., Smorlesi, A., Forni, G., and Musiani, P. (2001). Inhibition of mammary carcinogenesis by systemic interleukin 12 or p185neu DNA vaccination in Her-2/neu transgenic BALB/c mice. *Clin. Cancer Res.* **7**, 830s–837s.

Diehl, L., den Boer, A. Th., Schoenberger, S. P., van der Voort, E. I. H., Schumacher, T. N. M., Melief, C. J. M., Offringa, R., and Toes, R. E. M. (1999). CD40 activation *in vivo* overcomes peptide-induced peripheral cytotoxic T-lymphocyte tolerance and augments anti-tumor vaccine efficacy. *Nat. Med.* **5**, 774–779.

Dudley, M. E., Wunderlich, J. R., Yang, J. C., Sherry, R. M., Topalian, S. L., Restifo, N. P., Royal, R. E., Kammula, U., White, D. E., Mavroukakis, S. A., Rogers, L. J., Gracia, G. J., et al. (2005). Adoptive cell transfer therapy following non-myeloablative but lymphodepleting chemotherapy for the treatment of patients with refractory metastatic melanoma. *J. Clin. Oncol.* **23**, 2346–2357.

Dunn, G. P., Bruce, A. T., Ikeda, H., Old, L. J., and Schreiber, R. D. (2002). Cancer immunoediting: From immuno-surveillance to tumor escape. *Nat. Immunol.* **3**, 991–998.

Egen, J. G., Kuhns, M. S., and Allison, J. P. (2002). CTLA-4: New insights into its biological function and use in tumor immunotherapy. *Nat. Immunol.* **3**, 611–618.

Ercolini, A. M., Ladle, B. H., Manning, E. A., Pfannenstiel, L. W., Armstrong, T. D., Machiels, J.-P. H., Bieler, J. G., Emens, L. A., Reilly, R. T., and Jaffee, E. M. (2005). Recruitment of latent pools of high-avidity $CD8^+$ T cells to the antitumor immune response. *J. Exp. Med.* **201**, 1591–1602.

Fehérvari, Z., and Sakaguchi, S. (2004). $CD4^+$ Tregs and immune control. *J. Clin. Invest.* **114**, 1209–1217.

Feltkamp, M. C., Smits, H. L., Vierboom, M. P., Minnaar, R. P., de Jongh, B. M., Drijfhout, J. W., ter Schegget, J., Melief, C. J., and Kast, W. M. (1993). Vaccination with cytotoxic T lymphocyte epitope-containing peptide protects against a tumor induced by human papillomavirus type 16-transformed cells. *Eur. J. Immunol.* **23**, 2242–2249.

Figdor, C. G., de Vries, J. M., Lesterhuis, W. J., and Melief, C. J. M. (2004). Dendritic cell immunotherapy: Mapping the way. *Nat. Med.* **10**, 475–480.

Forni, G., Lollini, P.-L., Musiani, P., and Colombo, M. P. (2000). Immunoprevention of cancer: Is the time ripe? *Cancer Res.* **60**, 2571–2575.

Garrett, T. P., McKern, N. M., Lou, M., Elleman, T. C., Adams, T. E., Lovrecz, G. O., Kofler, M., Jorissen, R. N., Nice, E. C., Burgess, A. W., and Ward, C. W. (2003). The crystal structure of a truncated ErbB2 ectodomain reveals an active conformation, poised to interact with other ErbB receptors. *Mol. Cell.* **11**, 495–505.

Gehl, J. (2003). Electroporation: Theory and methods, perspectives for drug delivery, gene therapy and research. *Acta Physiol. Scand.* **177**, 437–447.

Geninatti Crich, S. G., Lanzardo, S., Barge, A., Esposito, G., Tei, L., Forni, G., and Aime, S. (2005). Visualization through magnetic resonance imaging of DNA internalized following "*in vivo*" electroporation. *Mol. Imaging* **4**, 7–17.

Ghiringhelli, F., Larmonier, N., Schmitt, E., Parcellier, A., Cathelin, D., Garrido, C., Chauffert, B., Solary, E., Bonnotte, B., and Martin, F. (2004). $CD4^+$ $CD25^+$ regulatory T cells suppress tumor immunity but are sensitive to cyclophosphamide which allows immunotherapy of established tumors to be curative. *Eur. J. Immunol.* **34**, 336–344.

Gomez, G. G., Hutchison, R. B., and Kruse, C. A. (2001). Chemo-immunotherapy and chemo-adoptive immunotherapy of cancer. *Cancer Treat. Rev.* **6**, 375–402.

Janssen, E. M., Lemmens, E. E., Wolfe, T., Christen, U., von Herrath, M. G., and Schoenberger, S. P. (2003). CD4(+) T cells are required for secondary expansion and memory in CD8(+) T lymphocytes. *Nature* **421**, 852–856.

Hirano, F., Kaneko, K., Tamura Dong, H., Wang, S., Ichikawa, M., Rietz, C., Flies, D. B., Lau, J. S., Zhu, G., Tamada, K., and Chen, L. (2005). Blockade of B7-H1 and PD-1 by monoclonal antibodies potentiates cancer therapeutic immunity. *Cancer Res.* **65**, 1089–1096.

Janssen, E. M., Droin, N. M., Lemmens, E. E., Pinkoski, J. J., Bensinger, S. J., Ehst, B. D., Griffith, T. S., Green, D. R., and Schoenberger, S. P. (2005). CD4(+) T-cell help controls CD8(+) T-cell memory via TRAIL-mediated activation-induced cell death. *Nature* **434**, 88–93.

De Jong, A., van Poelgeest, M. I. E., van der Hulst, J. M., Drijfhout, J. W., Fleuren, G. J., Melief, C. J. M., Kenter, G., Offringa, R., and van der Burg, S. H. (2004). Human papillomavirus type 16-positive cervical cancer is associated with impaired $CD4^+$ T-cell immunity against early antigens E2 and E6. *Cancer Res.* **64**, 5449–5455.

Karanikas, V., Lurquin, C., Colau, D., van Baren, N., De Smet, C., Lethé, B., Connerotte, T., Corbière, Demoitié, M.-A., Liénard, D., Dréno, B., Velu, T., *et al.* (2003). Monoclonal anti-MAGE-3 CTL responses in melanoma patients displaying tumor regression after vaccination with a recombinant canarypox virus. *J. Immunol.* **171**, 4898–4904.

Kast, W. M., Roux, L., Curren, J., Blom, H. J. J., Voordouw, A. C., Meloen, R. H., Kolakofsky, D., and Melief, C. J. M. (1991). Protection against lethal Sendai virus-infection by *in vivo* priming of virus-specific cytotoxic lymphocytes-T with a free synthetic peptide. *Proc. Natl. Acad. Sci. USA* **88**, 2283–2287.

Khong, H. T., and Restifo, N. P. (2002). Natural selection of tumor variants in the generation of "tumor escape" phenotypes. *Nat. Immunol.* **3**, 999–1005.

Laouar, Y., Sutterwala, F. S., Gorelik, L., and Flavell, R. A. (2005). Transforming growth factor-β controls T helper type 1 cell development through regulation of natural killer cell interferon-γ. *Nat. Immunol.* **6**, 600–607.

Lo Iacono, M., Cavallo, F., Quaglino, E., Rolla, S., Iezzi, M., Pupa, S. M., De Giovanni, C., Lollini, P.-L., Musiani, P., Forni, G., and Calogero, R. A. (2005). A limited autoimmunity to p185neu elicited by DNA and allogeneic cell vaccine hampers the progression of preneoplastic lesions in HER-2/NEU transgenic mice. *Int. J. Immunopathol. Pharmacol.* **18**, 351–363.

Lollini, P.-L., and Forni, G. (2003). Cancer immunoprevention: Tracking down persistent tumor antigens. *Trends Immunol.* **24**, 62–66.

Lollini, P.-L., De Giovanni, C., Pannellini, T., Cavallo, F., Forni, G., and Nanni, P. (2005). Cancer immunoprevention. *Future Oncol.* **1**, 57–66.

Lonchay, C., van der Bruggen, P., Connerotte, T., Hanagiri, T., Coulie, P., Colau, D., Lucas, S., van Pel, A., Thielemans, K., van Baren, N., and Boon, T. (2004). Correlation between tumor regression and T cell responses in melanoma patients vaccinated with a MAGE antigen. *Proc. Natl. Acad. Sci. USA* **101**, 14631–14638.

Lucchini, F., Sacco, M. G., Hu, N., Villa, A., Brown, J., Cesano, L., Mangiarini, L., Rindi, G., Kindl, S., Sessa, F., Vezzoni, P., and Clerici, L. (1992). Early and multifocal tumors in breast, salivary, harderian and epididymal tissues developed in MMTV-Neu transgenic mice. *Cancer Lett.* **64**, 203–209.

Lurquin, C., Lethé, B., de Plaen, E., Corbière, V., Théate, I., van Baren, N., Coulie, P. G., and Boon, T. (2005). Contrasting frequencies of antitumor and anti-vaccine T cells in metastases of a melanoma patient vaccinated with a MAGE tumor antigen. *J. Exp. Med.* **201**, 249–257.

Lutsiak, M. E. C., Semnani, R. T., De Pascallis, R., Kashmiri, S. V. S., Schlom, J., and Sabzevari, H. (2005). Inhibition of CD4+25+ T regulatory cell function implicated in enhanced immune response by low-dose cyclophosphamide. *Blood* **105**, 2862–2868.

Mayordomo, J. I., Zorina, T., Storkus, W. J., Zitvogel, L., Celluzzi, C., Falo, L. D., Melief, C. J., Ildstad, S. T., Kast, W. M., and Deleo, A. B. (1995). Bone marrow-derived dendritic cells pulsed with synthetic tumour peptides elicit protective and therapeutic antitumour immunity. *Nat. Med.* **1**, 1297–1302.

Melani, C., Chiodoni, C., Forni, G., and Colombo, M. P. (2003). Myeloid cell expansion elicited by the progression of spontaneous mammary carcinomas in c-erbB-2 transgenic BALB/c mice suppresses immune reactivity. *Blood* **102**, 2138–2145.

Melief, C. J. M., Toes, R. E. M., Medema, J. P., van der Burg, S. H., Ossendorp, F., and Offringa, R. (2000). Strategies for immunotherapy of cancer. *Adv. Immunol.* **75**, 235–282.

Melief, C. J. M., van der Burg, S. H., Toes, R. E. M., Ossendorp, F., and Offringa, R. (2002). Effective therapeutic anticancer vaccines based on precision guiding of cytolytic T lymphocytes. *Immunol. Rev.* **188**, 177–182.

Melief, C. J. M. (2005). Cat and mouse games of immune response and tumours. *Nature* **437**, 41–42.

Muller, W. J., Sinn, E., Pattengale, P. K., Wallace, R., and Leder, P. (1988). Single-step induction of mammary adenocarcinoma in transgenic mice bearing the activated c-neu oncogene. *Cell* **54**, 105–115.

Murray, H. W., Moreira, A. L., Lu, C. M., DeVecchio, J. L., Matsuhashi, M., Ma, X., and Heinzel, F. P. (2003). Determinants of response to interleukin-10 receptor blockade immunotherapy in experimental visceral leishmaniasis. *J. Infect. Dis.* **188**, 458–464.

Nagata, Y., Furugen, R., Ikeda, H., Otha, N., Forukawa, K., Nakamura, H., Furukawa, K., Kanematsu, T., and Siku, H. (1997). Peptides derived from a wild-type murine proto-oncogene c-erbB-2/HER2/neu can induce CTL and tumor suppression in syngeneic hosts. *J. Immunol.* **159**, 1336–1340.

Nanni, P., Landuzzi, L., Nicoletti, G., De Giovanni, C., Rossi, I., Croci, S., Astolfi, A., Iezzi, M., Di Carlo, E., Musiani, P., Forni, G., and Lollini, P.-L. (2004). Immunoprevention of mammary carcinoma in HER-2/neu transgenic mice is IFN-gamma and B cell dependent. *J. Immunol.* **173**, 2288–2296.

Nanni, P., Nicoletti, G., De Giovanni, C., Landuzzi, L., Di Carlo, E., Cavallo, F., Pupa, S. M., Rossi, I., Colombo, M. P., Ricci, C., Astolfi, A., Musiani, P., *et al.* (2001). Combined allogeneic tumor cell vaccination and systemic interleukin 12 prevents mammary carcinogenesis in HER-2/neu transgenic mice. *J. Exp. Med.* **194**, 1195–1205.

Napolitani, G., Rinaldi, A., Bertoni, F., Sallusto, F., and Lanzavecchia, A. (2005). Selected Toll-like receptor agonist combinations synergistically trigger a T helper type 1-polarizing program in dendritic cells. *Nat. Immunol.* **6**, 769–776.

Nishikawa, H., Kato, T., Tawara, I., Saito, K., Ikeda, H., Kuribayashi, K., Allen, P. M., Schreiber, R. D., Sakaguchi, S., Old, L. J., and Shiku, H. (2005). Definition of targets antigens for naturally occurring $CD4^+$ $CD25^+$ regulatory T cells. *J. Exp. Med.* **201**, 681–686.

Ossendorp, F., Mengede, E., Camps, M., Filius, R., and Melief, C. J. M. (1998). Specific T helper cell requirement for optimal induction of cytotoxic T lymphocytes against major histocompatibility class II negative tumors. *J. Exp. Med.* **187,** 693–702.

Ossevoort, M. A., Feltkamp, M. C., van Veen, K. J., Melief, C. J., and Kast, W. M. (1995). Dendritic cells as carriers for a cytotoxic T-lymphocyte epitope-based peptide vaccine in protection against a human papillomavirus type 16-induced tumor. *J. Immunother.* **18,** 86–94.

Palucka, A. K., Dhodapkar, M. V., Paczesny, S., Ueno, H., Fay, J., and Banchereau, J. (2005). Boosting vaccinations with peptide-pulsed CD34$^+$ progenitor-derived dendritic cells can expand long-lived melanoma peptide-specific CD8$^+$ T-cells in patients with metastatic melanoma. *J. Immunother.* **28,** 158–168.

Pannellini, T., Forni, G., and Musiani, P. (2004). Immunobiology of her-2/neu transgenic mice. *Breast Dis.* **20,** 33–42.

Park, J. M., Terabe, M., Sakai, Y., Munasinghe, J., Forni, G., Morris, J. C., and Berzofsky, J. A. (2005). Early role of CD4$^+$ Th1 cells and antibodies in HER-2 adenovirus vaccine protection against autochthonous mammary carcinomas. *J. Immunol.* **174,** 4228–4236.

Phan, G. Q., Yang, J. C., Sherry, R. M., Hwu, P., Topalian, S. L., Schwartzentruber, D. J., Restifo, N. P., Haworth, L. R., Seipp, C. A., Freezer, L. J., Morton, K. E., Mavroukakis, S. A., *et al.* (2003). Cancer regression and autoimmunity induced by cytotoxic T lymphocyte-associated antigen 4 blockades in patients with metastatic melanoma. *Proc. Natl. Acad. Sci. USA* **100,** 8372–8377.

Pupa, S., Iezzi, M., Di Carlo, E., Invernizzi, A. M., Cavallo, F., Meazza, R., Comes, A., Ferrini, S., Musiani, P., and Menard, S. (2005). Inhibition of mammary carcinoma development in HER-2/neu transgenic mice through induction of autoimmunity by xenogeneic DNA vaccination. *Cancer Res.* **65,** 10171–10178.

Quaglino, E., Iezzi, M., Mastini, C., Amici, A., Pericle, F., Di Carlo, E., Pupa, S. M., De Giovanni, C., Spadaro, M., Curcio, C., Lollini, P. L., Musiani, P., *et al.* (2004a). Electroporated DNA vaccine clears away multifocal mammary carcinomas in her-2/neu transgenic mice. *Cancer Res.* **64,** 2858–2864.

Quaglino, E., Rolla, S., Iezzi, M., Spadaro, M., Musiani, P., De Giovanni, C., Lollini, P.-L., Lanzardo, S., Forni, G., Sanges, R., Crispi, S., Deluca, P., Calogero, R., and Cavallo, F. (2004b). Concordant morphologic and gene expression data show that a vaccine halts HER-2/neu preneoplastic lesions. *J. Clin. Invest.* **113,** 707–717.

Quaglino, E., Mastini, C., Iezzi, M., Forni, G., Musiani, P., Klapper, L. N., Hardy, B., and Cavallo, F. (2005). The adjuvant activity of BAT antibody enables DNA vaccination to inhibit the progression of established autochthonous Her-2/neu carcinomas in BALB/c mice. *Vaccine* **23,** 3280–3287.

Raiter, A., Novogrodsky, A., and Hardy, B. (1999). Activation of lymphocytes by BAT and anti CTLA-4: Comparison of binding to T and B cells. *Immunol. Lett.* **69,** 247–251.

Rangarajan, A., and Weinberg, R. A. (2003). Opinion: Comparative biology of mouse versus human cells: Modelling human cancer in mice. *Nat. Rev. Cancer* **3,** 952–959.

Reilly, R. T., Gottlieb, M. B., Ercolini, A. M., Machiels, J. P., Kane, C. E., Okoye, F. I., Muller, W. J., Dixon, K. H., and Jaffee, E. M. (2000). HER-2/neu is a tumor rejection target in tolerized HER-2/neu transgenic mice. *Cancer Res.* **60,** 3569–3576.

Ria, F., van den Elzen, P., Madakamutil, L. T., Miller, J. E., Maverakis, E., and Sercarz, E. E. (2001). Molecular characterization of the T cell repertoire using immunoscope analysis and its possible implementation in clinical practice. *Curr. Mol. Med.* **1,** 297–304.

Rigopoulou, E. I., Abbot, W. G. H., Haigh, P., and Naoumov, N. V. (2005). Blocking of interleukin-10 receptor—a novel approach to stimulate T-helper cell type 1 responses to hepatitis C virus. *Clin. Immunol.* **117,** 57–64.

Rosenberg, S. A., Yang, J. C., and Restifo, N. P. (2004). Cancer immunotherapy: Moving beyond current vaccines. *Nat. Med.* **10,** 909–915.

Rovero, S., Amici, A., Di Carlo, E., Bei, R., Nanni, P., Quaglino, E., Porcedda, P., Boggio, K., Smorlesi, A., Lollini, P.-L., Landuzzi, L., Colombo, M. P., *et al.* (2000). DNA vaccination against rat her-2/Neu p185 more effectively inhibits carcinogenesis than transplantable carcinomas in transgenic BALB/c mice. *J. Immunol.* **165,** 5133–5142.

Rovero, S., Boggio, K., Di Carlo, E., Amici, A., Quaglino, E., Porcedda, P., Musiani, P., and Forni, G. (2001). Insertion of the DNA for the 163–171 peptide of IL1beta enables a DNA vaccine encoding p185(neu) to inhibit mammary carcinogenesis in Her-2/neu transgenic BALB/c mice. *Gene Ther.* **8,** 447–452.

Sakai, Y., Morrison, B. J., Burke, J. D., Park, J.-M., Terabe, M., Janik, J. E., Forni, G., Berzofsky, J. A., and Morris, J. C. (2004). Vaccination by genetically modified dendritic cells expressing a truncated neu oncogene prevents development of breast cancer in transgenic mice. *Cancer Res.* **64,** 8022–8028.

Sakaguchi, S., Sakaguchi, N., Asano, M., Itoh, M., and Toda, M. (1995). Immunologic Self-Tolerance Maintained by Activated T Cells Expressing IL-2 Receptor α-Chains (CD25). *J. Immunol.* **155,** 1151–1164.

Sakaguchi, S. (2004). Naturally arising $CD4^+$ regulatory t cells for immunologic self-tolerance and negative control of immune responses. *Ann. Rev. Immunol.* **22,** 531–562.

Schoenberger, S. P., Toes, R. E. M., van der Voort, E. I. H., Offringa, R., and Melief, C. J. M. (1998). T-cell help for cytotoxic T lymphocytes is mediated by CD40-CD40L interactions. *Nature* **393,** 480–483.

Schultz, M., Zinkernagel, R. M., and Hengartner, H. (1991). Peptide-induced antiviral protection by cytotoxic T-cells. *Proc. Natl. Acad. Sci. USA* **88,** 991–993.

Schultz, E. S., Schuler-Thurner, B., Stroobant, V., Jenne, L., Berger, T. G., Thielemanns, K., van der Bruggen, P., and Schuler, G. (2004). Functional analysis of tumor-specific Th cell responses detected in melanoma patients after dendritic cell-based immunotherapy. *J. Immunol.* **172,** 1304–1310.

Schuurhuis, D. H., Laban, S., Toes, R. E. M., Ricciardi-Castagnoli, P., Kleijmeer, M. J., van der Voort, E. I. H., Rea, D., Offringa, R., Geuze, H. J., Melief, C. J. M., and Ossendorp, F. (2000). Immature dendritic cells acquire $CD8^+$ cytotoxic T lymphocyte priming capacity upon activation by T helper cell-independent or—dependent stimuli. *J. Exp. Med.* **192,** 145–150.

Smith, C. M., Wilson, N. S., Waithman, J., Villadangos, J. A., Carbone, F. R., Heath, W. R., and Belz, G. T. (2004). Cognate CD4(+) T cell licensing of dendritic cells in CD°(+) T cell immunity. *Nat. Immunol.* **5,** 1143–1148.

Serra, P., Amrani, A., Yamanouchi, J., Han, B., Thiessen, S., Utsugi, T., Verdaguer, J., and Santamaria, P. (2003). CD40 ligation releases immature dendritic cells from the control of regulatory CD4+CD25+ T cells. *Immunity* **19,** 877–889.

Spadaro, M., Ambrosino, E., Iezzi, M., Di Carlo, E., Sacchetti, P., Curcio, C., Amici, A., Wei, W. Z., Musiani, P., Lollini, P.-L., Forni, G., and Cavallo, F. (2005). *Clin. Cancer Res.* **11,** 1941–1952.

Spadaro, M., Lanzardo, S., Curcio, C., Forni, G., and Cavallo, F. (2004). Cure of mammary carcinomas in Her-2 transgenic mice through sequential stimulation of innate (neoadjuvant interleukin-12) and adaptive (DNA vaccine electroporation) immunity. *Cancer Immunol. Immunother.* **53,** 204–216.

Speiser, D. E., Liénard, D., Rufer, N., Rubio-Godoy, V., Rimoldi, D., Lejeune, F., Krieg, A. M., Cerottini, J.-C., and Romero, P. (2005). Rapid and strong human $CD8^+$ T cell responses to vaccination with peptide, IFA, and CpG oligodeoxynucleotide 7909. *J. Clin. Invest.* **115**, 739–746.

Sumida, S. M., McKay, P. F., Truitt, D. M., Kishko, M. G., Arthur, J. C., Seaman, M. S., Jackson, S. S., Gorgonie, D. A., Lifton, M. A., Letvin, N. L., and Barouch, D. H. (2004). Recruitment and expansion of dendritic cells *in vivo* potentiate the immunogenicity of plasmid DNA vaccines. *J. Clin. Invest.* **14**, 1334–1342.

Sutmuller, R. P. M., Offringa, R., and Melief, J. M. (2004). Revival of the regulatory T cell: New targets for drug development. *Drug Discov. Today* **9**, 310–316.

Sutmuller, R. P. M., van Duivenvoorde, L. M., van Elsas, A., Schumacher, T. N. M., Wildenberg, M. E., Allison, J. P., Toes, R. E. M., Offringa, R., and Melief, C. J. M. (2001). Synergism of cytotoxic T lymphocyte-associated antigen 4 blockade and depletion of $CD25^+$ regulatory T cells in antitumor therapy reveals alternative pathways for suppression of autoreactive cytotoxic T lymphocyte responses. *J. Exp. Med.* **194**, 823–832.

Suzuki, E., Kapoor, V., Cheung, H. K., Ling, L. E., DeLong, P. A., Kaiser, L. R., and Albelda, S. M. (2004). Soluble type II transforming growth factor-β receptor inhibits established murine malignant mesothelioma tumor growth by augmenting host antitumor immunity. *Clin. Cancer Res.* **10**, 5907–5918.

Toes, R. E. M., Blom, R. J. J., Offringa, R., Kast, W. M., and Melief, C. J. M. (1996a). Enhanced tumor outgrowth after peptide vaccination. *J. Immunol.* **156**, 3911–3918.

Toes, R. E. M., Offringa, R., Blom, R. J. J., Melief, C. J. M., and Kast, W. M. (1996b). Peptide vaccination can lead to enhanced tumor growth through specific T-cell tolerance induction. *Proc. Natl. Acad. Sci. USA* **93**, 7855–7860.

Toes, R. E. M., van der Voort, E. I. H., Schoenberger, S. P., Drijfhout, J. W., van Bloois, L., Storm, G., Kast, W. M., Offringa, R., and Melief, C. J. M. (1998). Enhancement of tumor outgrowth through CTL tolerization after peptide vaccination is avoided by peptide presentation on dendritic cells. *J. Immunol.* **160**, 4449–4456.

Toes, R. E. M., Ossendorp, F., Offringa, R., and Melief, C. J. M. (1999). CD4 T cells and their role in antitumor immune responses. *J. Exp. Med.* **189**, 753–756.

Toka, F. N., Gierynska, M., Suvas, S., Schoenberger, S. P., and Rouse, B. T. (2005). Rescue of memory $CD8^+$ T cell reactivity in peptide/TLR9 ligand immunization by codelivery of cytokines or CD40 ligation. *Virology* **331**, 151–158.

Triebel, F. (2003). LAG-3: A regulator of T-cell and DC responses and its use in therapeutic vaccination. *Trends Immunol.* **24**, 619–622.

Vambutas, A., DeVoti, J., Nouri, M., Drijfhout, J. W., Lipford, G. B., Bonagura, V. R., van der Burg, S. H., and Melief, C. J. M. (2005). Therapeutic vaccination with papillomavirus E6 and E7 long peptides results in the control of both established virus-induced lesions and latently infected sites in a pre-clinical cottontail rabbit papillomavirus model. *Vaccine* **23**, 5271–5280.

Vicari, A. P., Chiodoni, C., Vaure, C., Aït-Yahia, S., Dercamp, C., Matsos, F., Reynard, O., Taverne, C., Merle, P., Colombo, M. P., O'Garra, A., Trinchieri, G., *et al.* (2002). Reversal of tumor-induced dendritic cell paralysis by CpG immunostimulatory oligonucleotide and anti-interleukin 10 receptor antibody. *J. Exp. Med.* **196**, 541–549.

Weijzen, S., Meredith, S. C., Velders, M. P., Elmishad, A. G., Schreiber, H., and Kast, W. M. (2001). Pharmacokinetic differences between a T cell-tolerizing and a T cell-activating peptide. *J. Immunol.* **166**, 7151–7157.

Willimsky, G., and Blankenstein, T. (2005). Sporadic immunogenic tumours avoid destruction by inducing T cell tolerance. *Nature* **437**, 141–146.

Yarden, Y., and Sliwkowski, M. X. (2001). Untangling the ErbB signalling network. *Nature Rev. Mol. Cell. Biol.* **2**, 127–137.

Zhang, F., Lee, J., Lu, S., Pettaway, C. A., and Dong, Z. (2005). Blockade of transforming growth factor-β signaling suppresses progression of androgen-independent human prostate cancer in nude mice. *Clin. Cancer Res.* **11,** 4512–4520.

Zwaveling, S., Ferreira Mota, S. C., Nouta, J., Johnson, M., Lipford, G. B., Offringa, R., van der Burg, S. H., and Melief, C. J. M. (2002). Established human papillomavirus type 16-expressing tumors are effectively eradicated following vaccination with long peptides. *J. Immunol.* **169,** 350–358.

Unraveling the Complex Relationship Between Cancer Immunity and Autoimmunity: Lessons from Melanoma and Vitiligo

Hiroshi Uchi,* Rodica Stan,* Mary Jo Turk,[†]
Manuel E. Engelhorn,* Gabrielle A. Rizzuto,*[,‡]
Stacie M. Goldberg,* Jedd D. Wolchok,*[,‡] and
Alan N. Houghton*[,‡]

*Swim Across America Laboratory, Memorial Sloan-Kettering Cancer Center,
1275 York Avenue, New York, New York
[†]Dartmouth-Hitchcock Medical Center, Lebanon, New Hampshire
[‡]Weill Medical and Graduate Schools of Cornell University,
1300 York Avenue, New York, New York

Abstract 215
1. Introduction 216
2. Immune Ignorance and Tolerance 217
3. Melanoma and Vitiligo 219
4. Active Immunization with Differentiation Antigens as Altered Self ... 222
5. Passive Immunization with Antibodies Against Differentiation Antigens ... 226
6. Adoptive Transfer of CD8[+] T Cells Specific for Differentiation Antigens
   in Adoptive Immunotherapy 228
7. Blockade of CTLA-4 228
8. Overcoming Effects of Suppressor Populations of T Cells 229
9. Dendritic Cells as Adjuvants 230
10. Mouse Model of Spontaneous Melanoma-Associated Vitiligo 230
11. Clinical Trials in Melanoma 231
12. Conclusions 233
    References 234

Abstract

A relationship between melanoma and vitiligo, a skin disorder characterized by the loss of melanocytes, has been postulated for many decades. In some cases, vitiligo is almost certainly a manifestation of autoimmune-mediated destruction of melanocytes. Melanocytes and melanoma cells share melanocyte differentiation antigens. Based on a number of observations, de novo vitiligo developing in patients with melanoma has been regarded as a sign of good prognosis. The immune system tolerates or ignores differentiation antigens because these antigens are self-derived. Therefore, immune tolerance or ignorance must be overcome to prime naïve T and B cells to induce cancer immunity and autoimmunity against melanocyte differentiation antigens.

Mouse models of concurrent melanoma and autoimmune vitiligo have revealed strategies to overcome immune ignorance or tolerance to melanocyte differentiation antigens: immunization with self-antigens as altered self (e.g., orthologues or mutated versions), expression in viral vectors, passive immunization with antibodies or T cells, incorporating potent adjuvants into active immunization, and blockade or removal of a downregulatory mechanism. Extensive investigations into the mechanisms that lead to tumor immunity and autoimmunity elicited by certain differentiation antigens have further revealed a variety of distinct cellular and molecular requirements, which are redundant and alternative.

1. Introduction

The foundation of cancer immunity is the recognition of antigen by the host's immune system. Appealing targets are unique/mutated self-molecules (e.g., point mutations, translocations). Counter-intuitively, self-antigens have been found so far to be the most common antigens recognized by the immune system of the host with cancer. Self-antigens include differentiation antigens (expressed by cancer cells and their normal cell counterparts), overexpressed antigens (present in a variety of normal tissues, but overexpressed by cancer), and germ cell/cancer-testes antigens (expressed by germ cells and cancers, but not adult somatic tissues).

Studies in mice using syngeneic transplanted tumors have shown that unique antigens are the most potent tumor-rejection antigens (Prehn and Main, 1957). However, weaker antigens that are shared by tumors and normal tissues are revealed in these experiments (Prehn and Main, 1957). Furthermore, unique antigens are best characterized for carcinogen-induced tumors in mice involving intensive exposure to mutagens, which probably have little relevance to most human cancers. On the other hand, weaker shared antigens are particularly relevant for spontaneously arising tumors, which are presumably most pertinent to human cancers (Prehn and Main, 1957; Turk *et al.*, 2004). For these reasons, developing immunotherapy strategies against unique antigens has been hindered by the substantial difficulties in identification and creation of vaccines for individual patients, often limited supply or unavailability of autologous tumor for vaccine preparation, and by their less persuasive role in spontaneous tumors (Hewitt *et al.*, 1976; Turk *et al.*, 2004).

Self-antigens should be invisible to the immune system. However, a substantial body of work from the past 20 years has shown that: (1) self-antigens are recognized by the immune system of autologous cancer patients (Old, 1981; Vijayasaradhi *et al.*, 1990); (2) active and passive immunizations against self-antigens have antitumor and therapeutic effects in laboratory models (Hara *et al.*, 1995; Naftzger *et al.*, 1996); (3) passive immunization against self-antigens is effective in cancer patients (Dudley *et al.*, 2002; Houghton *et al.*, 1985; McLaughlin *et al.*, 1998; Vadhan-Raj *et al.*, 1988); and (4) tolerance exists to cancer self-antigens (Weber *et al.*, 1998). These findings have put self-antigens at center stage for the development of immune therapies for cancer, including active, adoptive cellular, and monoclonal antibody (mAb) therapies. For clinical studies, differentiation and overexpressed antigens have been the overwhelmingly prevalent targets (e.g., mAb against differentiation antigens CD20, CD33, CD52, and epithelial cell adhesion molecule (EpCAM), and overexpressed antigens Her2 and epidermal growth factor (EGF) receptors), although germ cell/cancer-testes antigens are also gaining attention.

2. Immune Ignorance and Tolerance

T cells are positively selected for survival during development in the thymus via signals elicited by complexes of self-peptides with MHC molecules (Nikolic-Zugic and Bevan, 1990). Positive selection is the process by which thymocytes with low affinity for a self-MHC/peptide complex expressed on epithelial cells of the thymic cortex are saved from apoptosis by a signal provided by T-cell receptor (TCR) ligation. On the other hand, to avoid autoimmunity, T cells with strong reactivity against self-peptide/MHC complexes are negatively selected by deletion through interaction between these thymocytes and thymic dendritic cells (DCs) (Brocker *et al.*, 1997), but more weakly self-reactive T cells survive to populate the repertoire. In fact, the repertoire of T cells is positively selected for low-level self-reactivity. Similarly, strongly self-reactive B cells are deleted in bone marrow. Nonetheless, T and B cells recognizing self-antigens, including tissue-restricted antigens, populate a variety of tissues, such as secondary lymphoid organs and the blood. Self-reactive T cells with high-affinity TCR recognition that happen to escape into the periphery may become activated, but are then deleted by apoptosis. In contrast, self-reactive T cells with low/intermediate affinity TCR that are presented antigenic self-peptides in the absence of costimulatory signals either ignore antigens or undergo anergy. Self-reactive B cells are likewise ignorant or tolerized in the periphery. Self-antigens are often ignored by the immune system, especially those with qualitatively poor agonistic properties or that are sequestered in privileged tissues or expressed at extremely low levels (Mapara and Sykes, 2004).

This pool of low avidity self-reactive T cells discriminates nonself-antigens of pathogens by strong agonist cross-reactivity to foreign antigens in the context of adjuvant/proinflammatory signals. However, once activated, these low avidity T cells have the ability to reject tumors (Bullock *et al.*, 2001; Dyall *et al.*,

1998). A corollary to these observations is that, despite abundant self-reactivity in the peripheral immune system, priming of immune cells against self-antigens is restricted by insufficient signals. These observations explain the paradox that T cells against self-antigens on cancer are present in the repertoire but do not respond to tumors. A variety of strategies for active immunization have been successfully used to overcome ignorance or tolerance to self-antigens on melanoma (Table 1).

Postthymic mechanisms further contribute to maintaining tolerance to self-antigens. Continuous presentation of self-antigens by antigen-presenting cells (APCs) in the absence of APC maturation and activation maintains tolerance, fosters T-cell anergy or apoptosis, and potentially maintains regulatory T cells (Treg) postthymically (Albert et al., 2001; Banchereau and Steinman, 1998; Belz et al., 2002; Chen et al., 2004; Davey et al., 2002; Ehl et al., 1998; Gilliet and Liu, 2002; Groux et al., 2004; Guery and Adorini 1995; Hawiger, 2001; Steinman and Nussenzweig, 2002; Steinman et al., 2000, 2003). Treg cells, seemingly omnipresent in immunology research nowadays, are major regulators of postthymic tolerance, playing a central function in downregulation of immunity and prevention of autoimmunity. Natural (thymus-derived) Treg cells, crucial for maintaining tolerance to self-antigens, are CD4/CD25, Foxp3, glucocorticoid-induced tumor necrosis factor (TNF) receptor (GITR), and cytotoxic T-lymphocyte antigen-4 (CTLA-4) positive, although none of

Table 1 Strategies to Overcome Immunologic Ignorance or Tolerance to Self-Antigens

Strategy	Examples
Immunization against self-antigens using altered self	Expression in xenogeneic cells
	Xenogeneic orthologous antigen
	Syngeneic antigen with foreign sequences
	Heteroclitic epitopes/super-agonist altered peptide ligands
Recombinant viral vectors	Vaccinia and other poxviruses
	Adeno- and adeno-associated viruses
	Alphaviruses
Adjuvants	Cytokines: ex. IL-2, IL-7, IL-12, IL-15, GM-CSF
	Costimulators: ex. B7–1, B7–2, OX40 ligand
	Toll-like receptor ligands and other activation receptors on APCs: ex. CpG motif in bacterial DNA
	Dendritic cells
Removal of tolerance mechanisms	Blockade of CTLA-4
	Depletion of regulatory populations of T cells
	Inhibition/depletion myeloid suppressor cells
Passive immunization	Monoclonal antibodies
	Adoptive transfer of T cells

these markers is absolutely specific for functional Treg cells (Fontenot et al., 2003; Hori et al., 2003; Muriglan et al., 2004; Sakaguchi et al., 1995; Scotto et al., 2004; Shimizu et al., 1999). Natural Treg cells mediate suppression by cell-contact mechanisms, at least in *in vitro* assays. They are anergic and inhibit T-cell responses through suppression of IL-2 production or by competition for IL-2, among other mechanisms.

The notion of effective antigen presentation gets to the heart of adjuvant effects—to overcome insufficient activation of innate APCs due to inadequate signals for costimulation and survival. Thus, one of the effects of successful adjuvants is to provoke or provide these signals. The tolerogenic function of immature DCs is at least in part due to limited expression of costimulatory (CD80 and CD86) and survival-promoting (e.g., OX40 and 4-1BB ligands) molecules. CD80 and CD86 bind to CD28, which is constitutively expressed by T cells; upon activation, CTLA-4, a high-affinity inhibitory receptor for CD80, downregulates T cells. Blockade of CTLA-4 has significant antitumor activity in patients with metastatic melanoma, with responses corresponding to the autoimmune side effects (Hodi et al., 2003; Phan et al., 2003; Robinson et al., 2004; Sanderson et al., 2005). Furthermore, other inhibitory signals for T cells, such as PD-1L1, PD-L2, B7x, and others, seem to abound in peripheral tissues. Thus, in addition to active immunization to direct the immune system, modulation of mechanisms that downregulate immune responses will be required. Ultimately, it is most likely that the combination of active or passive immunization for specificity combined with immune modulation will be required for successful, rational immunotherapy of cancer.

3. Melanoma and Vitiligo

Melanoma arises from the malignant transformation of melanocytes. Most melanomas arise in the skin, with a few percent arising in the eye (choroid and ciliary body), and rare melanomas arising from mucous membranes, leptomeninges, and other noncutaneous sites. Primary melanoma in the skin usually arises from melanocytes sitting on the basement membrane of the epidermis, although occasional melanomas may arise from dermal or junctional (dermal/epidermal junction) nevi. Because melanocytes in most mouse strains reside in the epithelia surrounding hair follicles, melanoma in mice should arise from hair follicles and not surface epithelia. Infiltration of T cells among primary melanoma lesional cells is an independent prognostic factor for improved survival and decreased risk of metastases. Presumably related to a host response, regression is frequently found in primary melanomas, characterized often as pink or white areas with infiltration of inflammatory cells, particularly macrophage-like cells laden with pigment (melanophages).

Occasional primary melanomas completely regress, with disease manifesting as metastases usually in lymph nodes. Outcome in these patients is unaffected by complete regression of the primary melanoma. Rather, the clinical course is dominated by the metastatic melanoma cells, since survival is the same as for patients with regional metastases and intact primary tumors. These observations suggest a complicated relationship between the host immune system and primary versus metastatic melanoma, suggesting that immune responses able to destroy primary melanoma cells are ineffective against metastatic tumors.

Numerous melanoma antigens that are recognized by the immune system of melanoma patients have been characterized, more than for any other cancer type. Melanoma antigens include: mutated antigens (e.g., mutations in β-catenin, cyclin dependent kinase 4 (CDK4), CDC27), germ cell/cancer-testis antigens (e.g., MAGE, BAGE, GAGE, NY-ESO-1), and differentiation antigens (e.g., tyrosinase, tyrosinase-related protein 1 (TYRP1)/gp75, dopachrome tautomerase (DCT)/TRP-2, gp100/pmel-17, Melan-A/MART-1). Differentiation antigens are expressed by melanoma and melanocytes and are frequently recognized by the immune system of patients with melanoma (Houghton et al., 2001).

Vitiligo is an acquired disorder characterized by circumscribed hypopigmented macules on the skin that result from the loss of melanocytes. A major function of melanocytes, which are derived from neural crest cells and distributed to the basal cell layer of the epidermis, is the synthesis, storage, and transfer of melanin pigments packaged in melanosomes to surrounding keratinocytes, to protect the host from inflammatory and mutagenic effects of ultraviolet radiation. Vitiligo is found at a prevalence of 1% of the world population, regardless of gender, ethnicity, or color of the skin (Das et al., 2001). Although the precise etiology remains to be established, several lines of evidence have suggested that autoimmune mechanisms are involved in the pathogenesis of vitiligo. First, vitiligo is frequently associated with known autoimmune disorders, such as autoimmune thyroiditis, pernicious anemia, type I diabetes mellitus, and myasthenia gravis, while immunosuppressive regimens can produce repigmentation in patients with vitiligo (Grimes et al., 2002). Second, autoantibodies against melanocyte differentiation antigens (tyrosinase, TYRP1/TRP-1/gp75, DCT/TRP-2, and gp100/pmel-17), and melanin-concentrating hormone receptor 1 are present in the sera of a significantly higher proportion of patients with vitiligo than that of healthy individuals. The presence and level of the autoantibodies are correlated with the activity of vitiligo (Kemp et al., 1998a,b; 2002; Song et al., 1994). Furthermore, sera of patients with vitiligo can lyse cultured human melanocytes in vitro by both complement-mediated cytotoxicity and antibody-dependent cellular cytotoxicity (ADCC) (Gilhar et al., 1995). On the other hand, cytotoxic CD8$^+$

T lymphocytes that recognize peptides from tyrosinase, gp100/pmel-17, and Melan-A/Mart-1 are also found in patients with vitiligo and the presence of these cells is closely related to disease activity (Lang et al., 2001; Ogg et al., 1998; Palermo et al., 2001). In vitro studies showed that $CD8^+$ T cells derived from vitiligo lesions are specific for differentiation antigens, with cytolytic activity against cultured human melanocytes (Ogg et al., 1998).

Further evidence for a role for autoimmunity in the pathogenesis of vitiligo comes from the occurrence of concurrent hypopigmentation in patients with melanoma. Patients with melanoma are known to occasionally develop de novo hypopigmentation synchronous with or following a diagnosis of melanoma. Melanoma-associated vitiligo occurs as hypopigmentation either surrounding melanoma (Sutton's phenomenon) or distant from melanoma, which is pathologically indistinguishable from Sutton's nevus or common vitiligo, respectively (Bystryn et al., 1987; Nordlund et al., 1983). This association has been called melanoma-associated vitiligo or melanoma-associated leukoderma and has been linked to improved prognosis (Bystryn et al., 1987; Duhra and Ilchyshyn, 1991; Nordlund et al., 1983). Furthermore, the development of vitiligo during or following chemotherapy, immunotherapy, or biochemotherapy treatment of melanoma is associated with a higher likelihood of response to treatment, and de novo appearance of vitiligo has been observed at a much higher frequency in responding patients than in nonresponders. These observations suggest that death of melanoma cells during therapy cross-primes immune responses to normal melanocytes, but these observations do not distinguish whether the autoimmunity against the melanocyte antigen actually directly contributes to response or improved prognosis.

Reports have investigated the mechanism of concurrent vitiligo and tumor immunity in melanoma. Becker et al. (1999) demonstrated the presence of clonally expanded T cells with identical TCR β-variable regions in a melanoma tumor and the surrounding vitiliginous halo. In another study, Le Gal et al. (2001) showed that vitiligo-infiltrating lymphocytes in patients with melanoma are $CD8^+$ T cells predominantly expressing skin-homing receptor, cutaneous lymphocyte-associated antigen. They have a clonal or oligoclonal TCR profile and recognize differentiation antigens (Le Gal et al., 2001). Remarkably, a patient with metastatic melanoma treated with $CD8^+$ T-cell clones developed inflammatory lesions around pigmented areas of skin after infusion of T cells, developing vitiligo associated with complete absence of melanocytes at biopsy (Yee et al., 2000). Infiltrating T cells from skin and tumor revealed tetramer-positive MelanA/MART-1 reactive T cells with identical CDR3 sequences as the infused T cells. These last observations provide strong evidence that cytotoxic $CD8^+$ T cells against melanocyte differentiation antigens can mediate vitiligo. Thus, the occurrence of vitiligo in patients with melanoma may result from an immune response directed against differentiation antigens shared by melanoma and melanocytes, leading to destruction of normal melanocytes and melanoma cells. Several groups, including our own, have established different mouse models of concurrent tumor immunity and autoimmune vitiligo. These models show that there are multiple pathways to tumor immunity and autoimmunity, which are induced by overcoming ignorance or tolerance to differentiation antigens.

4. Active Immunization with Differentiation Antigens as Altered Self

The poorly immunogenic B16 melanoma is a highly aggressive tumor derived from syngeneic C57BL/6 mice that expresses no MHC class II and very low levels of MHC class I. Like most human melanomas and normal melanocytes, B16 and other mouse melanoma express differentiation antigens, including tyrosinase, TYRP1, DCT, and gp100. Most experimental models of melanoma and vitiligo have been based on experiments using this tumor. In mouse skin, DCT^+ stem cells of the melanocyte lineage exist in the bulge area of hair follicles. Differentiating mouse melanocytes are distributed from progenitors in the bulge to the epithelium surrounding the hair bulb to produce melanin pigments during the anagen (active) phase of hair growth (Nishimura et al., 2002). Mouse epidermis does not usually contain melanocytes because, unlike human keratinocytes, mouse keratinocytes do not produce the stem cell factor/kit ligand that is required to induce migration of kit-expressing melanocytes throughout the basal cell layer of the epidermis (Kunisada et al., 1998). Transgenic expression of the stem cell factor/kit ligand by keratinocytes under a keratin promoter leads to population of the mouse basal epidermis by melanocytes (Kunisada et al., 1998). Mouse autoimmune vitiligo is, therefore, usually manifested as patchy white areas consisting of hypopigmented hairs.

C57BL/6 mice did not generate any detectable autoantibodies or $CD8^+$ T-cell responses to TYRP1 when immunized with either irradiated B16 melanoma cells (up to 5×10^7 cells) or purified mouse TYRP1 protein or peptides in the presence of various adjuvants. On the other hand, immunization with lysates of Sf9 insect cells expressing mouse TYRP1 by a baculovirus vector could elicit production of autoantibodies but not $CD8^+$ T-cell responses to TYRP1, providing the first evidence that ignorance or tolerance to melanosomal self-antigens can be overcome (Naftzger et al., 1996). Immunized mice showed protection against challenge with a lethal dose of B16 melanoma and the development of autoimmune vitiligo. Tumor protection could be transferred to naïve mice with serum from immunized mice. Although the Sf9 insect cells produced an immature form of TYRP1 that contained nonprocessed high mannose carbohydrate chains, indicating lack of processing beyond the endoplasmic reticulum upon translation, immunized mice produced IgG antibodies recognizing mature full-length TYRP1 (Naftzger et al., 1996). These results suggest that a differentiation glycoprotein presented to the host as an immature processed form or as an aggregated form in Sf9 cells can overcome ignorance or tolerance. In addition, it is likely that the Sf9 lysates provide adjuvant effects for activation of APCs that contribute to immunogenicity.

4.1. Active Immunization with Xenogeneic DNA

Immunization with xenogeneic orthologous proteins is another strategy to elicit immunity to self-antigens, a time-honored method to induce autoimmunity in mouse models. Immunization with bacterial plasmid carrying full-length DNA that encodes orthologous proteins has been shown by our group to overcome immune tolerance to the mouse differentiation antigens TYRP1, DCT, tyrosinase, and gp100 in C57BL/6 mice (Bowne et al., 1999; Goldberg et al., 2005; Hawkins et al., 2000; Weber et al., 1998).

Dendritic cells must undergo maturation in order to trigger adaptive immune responses. Dendritic cells are activated by surface receptors, including: (1) activating Fc receptors (FcR), (2) toll-like receptors (TLRs) by distinct molecules of infectious pathogens (bacteria, viruses, and parasites), and (3) CD40 receptors by agonist signals from CD40 ligand. Activation signals lead to upregulation of MHC, antigen processing, costimulatory molecules, cytokine/chemokine receptors, and cytokine/chemokine secretion. Plasmacytoid DCs are the major source of type I IFNs, but also make IL-12 (although less than myeloid DCs), thus promoting T-cell activation (Colonna et al., 2004). In mice, both myeloid and plasmacytoid DCs express TLR7 and TLR9, while in humans these receptors are expressed mainly by plasmacytoid DCs. TLR9 is relevant because it signals activation of DCs by binding unmethylated CpG nucleotides present at high levels in prokaryotic and viral DNA. CpGs provide adjuvant effects for plasmid DNA vaccines (Chu et al., 1997, 2000; Hemmi et al., 2000; Klinman et al., 1996, 2000; Salio et al., 2004; Sato et al., 1996; Schneeberger et al., 2004; Sparwasser et al., 2000; Sun et al., 1998; Weiner et al., 1997). TLR9, with other TLRs that sense intracellular bacteria and viruses, is located within endosomes normally sequestered from the host cell's nucleic acids. Thus, activation by CpG-containing polynucleotides requires cell uptake.

In experiments using high-pressure particle bombardment delivered by gene gun for cellular uptake of CpG-containing DNA, we tested DNA vaccines made from bacterial plasmid containing immunostimulatory CpG sequences. Xenogeneic DNA vaccines with human orthologues encoding each of these melanocyte differentiation antigens were delivered to the mouse skin via gene gun. In the skin, Langerhans cells and interstitial DCs presumably take up the antigen of interest, either directly or through uptake from products made by surrounding cells. Xenogeneic immunization overcame immune ignorance or tolerance, resulting in protection against a challenge with B16 melanoma as well as the development of autoimmune vitiligo. However, the cellular and molecular requirements differed, depending on the antigen.

C57BL/6 mice immunized with human TYRP1 DNA developed autoantibodies against mouse TYRP1 with concurrent tumor immunity and autoimmunity, while MHC II$^{-/-}$ mice did not. Depletion experiments further demonstrated that CD4$^+$ T cells and natural killer (NK) cells were required to reject B16 melanoma. FcR$\gamma^{-/-}$ mice, which lack the FcγR types I and III, also showed no protection against tumor challenge. On the other hand, activating FcγR was not required to develop vitiligo (Weber et al., 1998). Notably, in most cases, tumor immunity and autoimmunity were independent of CD8$^+$ T cells. These results indicated that immunization against TYRP1 produced immunity mediated by IgG antibody responses that depend on CD4$^+$ T-cell help in an IFN-γ-dependent manner. Further, these autoantibodies elicit tumor immunity mediated by activating FcγRs, probably present on tissue macrophages, as well as autoimmunity that is independent of FcγR. Insights into mechanisms were further revealed by studies with mAb against TYRP1, discussed below under Section 5 (Passive Immunization with Antibodies Against Differentiation Antigens).

In contrast to TYRP1 studies, immunization with human DCT and human gp100 DNA induced cellular immunity mediated by CD8$^+$ T cells. Tumor immunity and autoimmunity were induced by immunization with human DCT DNA, and although CD8$^+$ T cells were required at both the immunization and the effector phases, CD4$^+$ T cells were necessary only at the immunization phase to provide T cell help. Interestingly, only autoimmunity, but not tumor immunity, required perforin, whereas both tumor immunity and autoimmunity proceeded in the absence of Fas (Bowne et al., 1999). In addition, immunization with human DCT DNA did not induce either tumor immunity or autoimmunity in IFN-$\gamma^{-/-}$ mice; however, tumor immunity was restored by repletion with recombinant mouse IFN-γ (Wolchok, 2001). Finally, human gp100-induced tumor immunity and autoimmunity required CD8$^+$ T cells, but not CD4$^+$ T cells, although CD4$^+$ T cells augmented immunity (Hawkins et al., 2000).

4.2. Active Immunization with Syngeneic DNA Linked to Foreign Sequences

Enhanced green fluorescent protein (EGFP) from jellyfish is a widely used intracellular reporter molecule to assess gene transfer and expression; it is also known to induce strong humoral and cellular immune responses (Stripecke et al., 1999). C57BL/6 mice immunized with cDNA encoding a fusion protein between EGFP and mouse DCT via gene gun showed protection against challenge with B16 melanoma and developed autoimmune vitiligo, while both tumor immunity and autoimmunity were abrogated in either MHC II$^{-/-}$ or I$^{-/-}$ mice. Immunization induced CD8$^+$ T cells but not autoantibodies against mouse DCT, although autoantibodies against EGFP could be detected in immunized sera (Steitz et al., 2002). These results are in agreement with regard to mechanism for mice immunized with xenogeneic human DCT DNA (Bowne et al., 1999). Thus, ignorance or tolerance was broken by immunization with cDNA coding a differentiation antigen linked to xenogeneic helper sequences.

4.3. Active Immunization with Recombinant Viruses Expressing Differentiation Antigens

Recombinant viruses encoding tumor antigens effectively deliver antigens of interest to appropriate antigen processing compartments in APCs of the host to elicit humoral and cellular immune responses, involving both CD4$^+$ and CD8$^+$ T cells. Vaccinia virus, the agent used for smallpox immunization, is a member of the orthopoxvirus genus and has a broad host range. The poxvirus genome consists of a linear double-stranded DNA and can accept large inserts of foreign DNA (Rocha et al., 2004). In C57BL/6 mice immunized with recombinant vaccinia viruses expressing mouse tyrosinase, TYRP1, DCT, gp100, and Melan-A/MART-1, remarkably only mice inoculated with a vaccinia virus expressing mouse TYRP1 showed tumor protection and autoimmune vitiligo (Overwijk et al., 1999). High titers of mouse TYRP1-specific antibodies were detected in immunized C57BL/6 mice and MHC I$^{-/-}$ mice, but not MHC II$^{-/-}$ mice, while mouse TYRP1-specific CD8$^+$ T cells could not be found. MHC II$^{-/-}$ mice as well as C57BL/6 mice depleted of CD4$^+$ cells develop neither vitiligo nor tumor protection. On the other hand, MHC I$^{-/-}$ mice still developed vitiligo, although at a lower rate than control mice, and showed tumor protection, indicating that tumor immunity and autoimmunity induced by a vaccinia virus expressing mouse TYRP1 were dependent on antibodies and CD4$^+$ T cells (Overwijk et al., 1999).

Adenoviruses are nonenveloped viruses containing a linear double-stranded DNA genome that does not integrate into the host cell genome. Adenoviruses infect both dividing and resting cells. Immunization with a recombinant adenovirus expressing human DCT resulted in much greater protective immunity than did vaccination with a recombinant adenovirus expressing mouse DCT. Furthermore, only mice immunized with human DCT, but not mouse DCT, developed vitiligo, suggesting that autoimmunity may depend on the potency of the vaccine. Immunization with an adenovirus expressing human DCT induced both autoantibodies and $CD8^+$ T-cell responses against mouse DCT. Tumor immunity and autoimmunity in immunized mice were abrogated only when both $CD4^+$ and $CD8^+$ T cells were depleted, while B cells were not required (Lane et al., 2004). Interestingly, only intradermally immunized mice developed vitiligo, while intramuscular immunization did not elicit autoimmunity, although both groups of mice showed comparable tumor protection. Furthermore, mice intramuscularly immunized with an adenovirus expressing human DCT developed vitiligo by local inflammation of the skin, such as intradermal injection of control vector or complete Freund's adjuvant (Lane et al., 2004). These results may suggest that local nonspecific inflammatory responses triggered the recruitment of cytotoxic T lymphocytes (CTL) specific to mouse DCT to the skin, similar to trauma- or sunburn-induced vitiligo in humans.

Studies have shown that propagation-incompetent alphavirus vectors, called virus-like replicon particles (VRPs), encoding tyrosinase induced both antibody and T-cell responses to mouse tyrosinase (Goldberg et al., 2005). Notably, VRPs encoding mouse tyrosinase generated stronger T-cell responses and antibody responses in a higher proportion of mice than VRPs encoding human tyrosinase.

5. Passive Immunization with Antibodies Against Differentiation Antigens

The mouse IgG_{2a} monoclonal antibody TA99 specifically recognizes both the human and mouse TYRP1 glycoproteins (Vijayasaradhi et al., 1990). Hara et al. (1995) showed that systemic treatment with TA99 induced protection against a lethal challenge with B16 melanoma and elicited autoimmune vitiligo, providing the initial experimental evidence that passively transferred immunity against melanocyte antigens can produce vitiligo. The threshold dose of TA99 required for hypopigmentation was fivefold greater than that required for tumor rejection. This difference in susceptibility suggests that one manner of uncoupling autoimmunity and tumor immunity may be related to quantitative differences in thresholds. For instance, antibodies can access solid tumors more easily due to leaky vasculature, while access to melanocytes, which sit on the basement membrane at the basal layer of the epidermis and in the epithelia of hair follicles, may be more difficult.

Interestingly, depletion of specific cell populations revealed that antibody-dependent tumor rejection was dependent on NK cells and partially on $CD4^+$ T cells, but not $CD8^+$ T cells, while hypopigmentation occurred in the absence of these cell populations (Hara et al., 1995). These observations were the first to experimentally show that tumor immunity and autoimmunity are linked and to demonstrate that they can have distinct requirements.

5.1. The Cellular and Molecular Requirements for TA99-Induced Tumor Protection

The Fc region of TA99 is required for tumor rejection, initially suggested by the observation that F(ab′)$_2$ fragments of TA99 had no detectable antitumor activity (Takechi *et al.*, 1996). Using mice that lack the activating FcγR types I and III (FcRγ$^{-/-}$) or the inhibitory FcγR type II (FcγRII$^{-/-}$), the effect of passive immunization of TA99 on B16 melanoma was tested following a lethal dose administered by intravenous challenge. The protective effect of TA99 was completely eliminated in FcRγ$^{-/-}$ mice (Clynes *et al.*, 1998), while FcγRII$^{-/-}$ mice immunized with TA99 showed significantly higher protection against a challenge with B16 melanoma than control mice (Clynes *et al.*, 2000). NK cells have been regarded as a principal cell population involved in ADCC, but direct cell-lytic activity of NK cells probably does not contribute to TA99-induced tumor rejection. Because NK cells express only the type III FcγR, but not type II FcγR, increased tumor rejection seen in FcγRII$^{-/-}$ mice cannot be attributed to NK cells. Furthermore, the antitumor effect of TA99 was intact in severe combined immune deficient (SCID)/Beige mice, which lack NK cells with cytolytic capacity as well as mature T and B cells (Takechi *et al.*, 1996). Instead, macrophages, which express FcγRs II and III, almost certainly function as the dominant effector cell population in this protection, perhaps by mediating an ADCC or phagocytic response or through production of cytotoxic molecules, such as nitric oxide and peroxynitrite (Clynes *et al.*, 1998, 2000).

5.2. The Cellular and Molecular Requirements for TA99-Induced Vitiligo

Passive immunization with the mouse IgG$_{2a}$ monoclonal antibody TA99 induced vitiligo in C57BL/6 mice irrespective of NK, CD4$^+$ T, or CD8$^+$ T cells (Hara *et al.*, 1995). Activating FcR containing common γ chain are known to be necessary in many mouse models of autoimmune diseases, such as autoimmune hemolytic anemia, glomerulonephritis, and collagen-induced arthritis (Ravetch and Clynes, 1998). In contrast, autoimmune vitiligo induced by TA99 proceeded in the absence of FcR γ chain (Clynes *et al.*, 1998). Although mice deficient in complement (C3$^{-/-}$) also developed vitiligo suggesting complement-independence, TA99 could not induce vitiligo in double-deficient FcRγ$^{-/-}$,C3$^{-/-}$ mice lacking both functional activating FcRs and a functional complement pathway. When lethally irradiated, double-deficient mice were reconstituted with bone marrow from FcRγ$^{-/-}$ mice or C3$^{-/-}$ mice, both groups of mice developed vitiligo after TA99 immunization (Trcka *et al.*, 2002). These results indicated that complement and FcγR mediate autoimmune vitiligo by redundant mechanisms. More specifically, adoptive transfer of FcRγ$^{+/-}$ bone marrow-derived macrophages from C3$^{-/-}$ background mice could reconstitute the autoimmune response in double-deficient FcRγ$^{-/-}$, C3$^{-/-}$ mice. Collectively, FcγR-bearing macrophages mediate TA99-inducing vitiligo, and, in the absence of functional macrophages, complement plays an alternative role in mediating vitiligo in this model (Trcka et al., 2002).

6. Adoptive Transfer of CD8$^+$ T Cells Specific for Differentiation Antigens in Adoptive Immunotherapy

The pmel-1 strain of C57BL/6 mice is TCR transgenic mice expressing the Vα1Vβ13 TCR that recognizes an H-2D^b-restricted mouse gp100$_{25-33}$ epitope. Despite the fact that more than 90% of CD8 T cells in pmel-1 mice are specific for mouse gp100, pmel-1 mice do not reject B16 melanoma, indicating that CD8$^+$ T cells in pmel-1 mice are functionally ignorant or tolerant. Adoptive transfer of pmel-1 splenocytes did not confer tumor protection upon C57BL/6 mice (Overwijk et al., 2003). In contrast, C57BL/6 mice adoptively transferred with pmel-1 splenocytes followed by immunization with a recombinant fowlpox virus encoding human gp100$_{25-33}$, combined with concurrent administration of IL-2, showed strong tumor rejection of established tumors and autoimmune vitiligo. This result shows that previously ignorant or tolerant self-reactive T cells were activated by a xenogeneic peptide ligand and IL-2 to lyse B16 melanoma and normal melanocytes. Furthermore, even mice bearing large (>50 mm^2), established B16 melanoma tumors could be effectively treated by this combination treatment (Overwijk et al., 2003).

7. Blockade of CTLA-4

To induce effective activation of naïve T cells, both interaction between TCR and antigen/MHC complex (signal 1) and engagement of CD28 on the surface of T cells with CD80 and CD86 expressed on APCs (signal 2) are required. Cytotoxic T-lymphocyte antigen-4 is a CD28 homologue expressed on activated T cells. Cytotoxic T-lymphocyte antigen-4 binds to CD80 and CD86 with higher affinity than CD28 and antagonizes ongoing T-cell activation (Salomon and Bluestone, 2001). CD4$^+$CD25$^+$ regulatory T cells constitutively express CTLA-4. Downregulation of T cells by CTLA-4 following activation, arguably combined with effects on Treg cells, has been suggested to underlie the role of CTLA-4 in downregulating immune responses (Takahashi et al., 2000). Combination treatment consisting of administration of anti-CTLA-4 blockade mAb and vaccination with irradiated granulocyte/macrophage colony-stimulating factor (GM-CSF)-expressing B16 melanoma cells, which is known to induce specific tumor immunity to B16 melanoma (Dranoff et al., 1993), induced concurrent tumor protection and autoimmune vitiligo. Both tumor immunity and autoimmunity induced by this combination treatment were dependent on $CD8^+$ T cells, but not $CD4^+$ T cells or B cells (van Elsas et al., 1999). Fas–FasL interaction and perforin were also required at the effector phase. These data show that blockade of CTLA-4 led to activation of ignorant or tolerized CTL specific to differentiation antigens to attack both B16 melanoma and normal melanocytes. $CD8^+$ T cells recognizing a peptide from mouse DCT were expanded in treated mice (van Elsas et al., 2001).

Blockade of CTLA-4 by mAb can augment $CD8^+$ T-cell responses against DCT and gp100 and enhance rejection of B16 melanoma (Gregor et al., 2004; Sutmuller et al., 2001; van Elsas et al., 2001). Of note, the ability of CTLA-4 blockade to enhance vaccine-induced T-cell responses was only observed when blockade occurred after initial priming, with booster vaccinations. These results suggest that costimulation during boosting is particularly critical in expanding autoreactive T cells against melanoma differentiation antigens following priming immunizations.

8. Overcoming Effects of Suppressor Populations of T Cells

$CD4^+$ Treg cells have been implicated as central players in downmodulating T-cell dependent immunity at the level of tumor. Several studies have shown that depleting $CD4^+$ or $CD25^+$ cells enhances rejection of tumors (Golgher et al., 2002; Nagai et al., 2000, 2004; Onizuka et al., 1999; Shimizu et al., 1999; Sutmuller et al., 2001). Interleukin-12 is a heterodimeric cytokine consisting of p40 and p35 subunits, mainly produced by APCs, and induces a Th1-type immune reaction by activating NK cells, NKT cells, and CTL to produce IFN-γ. B16 melanoma cells were transfected with plasmid vectors expressing cDNA encoding IL-12p40 and IL-12p35, and stable transfectants producing bioactive IL-12p70 were cloned. IL-12-producing B16 melanoma cells showed retarded tumor growth in C57BL/6 mice compared with control vector-transfected B16. Depletion of $CD4^+$ T cells resulted in complete regression of IL-12-producing B16 melanoma in most challenged mice with concurrent vitiligo, while depletion of $CD8^+$ T cells or NK cells accelerated the tumor growth (Nagai et al., 2000). These results suggested that tolerance to differentiation antigens was abrogated by depletion of suppressor populations in $CD4^+$ T cells.

The GITR molecule is expressed at high levels by Treg cells (Nocentini et al., 1997; Shimizu et al., 2002). Agonist mAb against GITR disable suppressive properties of Treg cells as well as provide costimulation for activated T cells, and treatment of mice with agonist mAb enhances tumor immunity (Shimizu et al., 2002).

Concomitant tumor immunity describes the responses to a progressive tumor that rejects the same tumor at a remote site in the host. Using a model of concomitant tumor immunity with B16 melanoma, we showed that immunity was $CD8^+$-dependent and predominantly directed against shared melanoma antigens, specifically differentiation antigens including DCT and gp100 (Turk *et al.*, 2004). Immunity was enhanced by carefully timed pretreatment with low-dose cyclophosphamide (an alkylating agent that has been postulated to selectively destroy or disable Treg cells), depletion of $CD4^+$ cells, or treatment with the agonist anti-GITR mAb DTA-1. All these observations supported a role for Treg cells in downmodulating concomitant immunity against B16. In order to establish that Treg cells were in fact involved, $Foxp3^+CD25^+CD4^+$ T cells were adoptively transferred from naïve mice into immune deficient mice along with $CD8^+$ T cells previously activated against B16. These experiments directly demonstrated that naturally occurring Treg cells efficiently suppress concomitant tumor immunity using adoptive transfer experiments.

9. Dendritic Cells as Adjuvants

Dendritic cells are the most potent APCs, and antigen presentation by fully matured DCs can break tolerance to self-antigens. Almost all organs contain a small population of immature DCs serving as sentinels through their high endocytic and phagocytic capacity. Once DCs capture pathogenic antigens in concert with stimulatory signals by pattern-recognition receptors, they mature and migrate toward secondary lymphoid organs where DCs present or cross-present peptide/MHC complexes to naïve T cells. Because mature DCs express high levels of both MHC class I and II as well as costimulatory molecules, they are capable of activating both naïve $CD4^+$ T cells and naïve $CD8^+$ T cells (Fong and Engleman, 2000). Schreurs *et al.* (2000) generated mature DC *in vitro* by culturing bone marrow cells with GM-CSF and IL-4 and loaded native peptides from mouse DCT on DCs. Immunization with native peptide-loaded DCs induced protective immunity against a challenge with B16 melanoma, and notably this treatment induced only sporadic development of autoimmune vitiligo, although no studies investigated the mechanisms that disconnected tumor immunity from autoimmunity (Schreurs *et al.*, 2000). Importantly, the peptides that bound to MHC class I with higher affinity elicited higher levels of protective immunity against B16 melanoma. On the other hand, immunization with either native peptides in incomplete Freund's adjuvant or plasmid DNA encoding mouse DCT did not elicit protective immunity against B16 melanoma (Schreurs *et al.*, 2000).

10. Mouse Model of Spontaneous Melanoma-Associated Vitiligo

MT/*ret* transgenic mice expressing the human *ret* oncogene fused to the metallothionein-I promoter-enhancer have congenital melanosis throughout the skin and develop benign melanocytic lesions several months after birth, followed by development of melanoma that metastasizes to lymph nodes, lung, and brain (Kato et al., 1998). Addition of zinc to the water given to MT/*ret* mice from birth resulted in both earlier and more rapidly progressing invasive melanoma lesions. Additionally, one half of the mice developed vitiligo that occurred as hypopigmentation both surrounding tumors and distant from tumors. Interestingly, MT/*ret* mice with vitiligo had significantly fewer melanoma nodules compared with mice of the same age without vitiligo, and mice with vitiligo more frequently had $CD8^+$ T cells that recognize peptides derived from DCT and gp100 than mice without vitiligo. Furthermore, MT/*ret* mice with vitiligo were more resistant to a challenge with cells from a syngeneic melanoma cell line (Melan-ret) than mice without vitiligo, which was dependent on $CD8^+$ T cells (Lengagne et al., 2004). These results support the observation that spontaneous appearance of vitiligo is associated with an improved prognosis in patients with metastatic melanoma.

11. Clinical Trials in Melanoma

Based on animal studies, numerous clinical trials with immunotherapy have treated patients with melanoma, especially metastatic cases, partly because melanoma is quite resistant to conventional chemotherapy and radiation therapy. Because differentiation antigens are the most frequently targeted antigens in the studies, patients with melanoma who showed clinical responses to immunotherapy have occasionally developed autoimmune responses to normal melanocytes, including vitiligo. IL-2 is produced by helper T cells to activate CTL and NK cells. It is the only immunotherapy agent approved by the US Food and Drug Administration for the treatment of patients with stage IV melanoma. Metaanalyses of clinical data of treatment with IL-2 have shown that the overall objective response rate of high-dose bolus IL-2 regimen is 15%, with 8% being complete (Atkins et al., 1999; Phan et al., 2001). Among patients with metastatic melanoma who received IL-2 therapy, 48% of responders developed vitiligo, while 82% of nonresponders had no vitiligo, indicating a strong relationship between clinical responses and development of vitiligo ($p \leq 10^{-6}$) (Phan et al., 2001; Rosenberg and White, 1996).

11.1. Adoptive Transfer of Tumor Infiltrating Lymphocytes

T-cell populations derived from so-called tumor infiltrating lymphocytes (TILs) in patients with melanoma contain T cells recognizing melanoma differentiation antigens. Tumor infiltrating lymphocytes are typically tolerized, but the immunological capacity of TILs can be restored by *in vitro* culture with IL-2 (Ridolfi et al., 2003). Despite the transfer of large numbers of highly active T-cell clones to differentiation antigens, rapid clearance in the number of transferred T cells *in vivo* has prevented a long-lasting CTL effect. Dudley *et al.* (2002) demonstrated that adoptively transferred tumor-reactive lymphocytes from TILs, after expansion, could be used to repopulate the immune repertoire following nonmyeloablative chemotherapy, in some cases leading to repopulation of most of the T-cell repertoire by expansion of infused cells (Dudley *et al.*, 2002). After treatment with nonmyeloablative chemotherapy consisting of cyclophosphamide and fludarabine, each patient was infused with *in vitro* expanded autologous lymphocytes, containing both $CD4^+$ and $CD8^+$ T cells, followed by high-dose IL-2 therapy. In a preliminary report, 6 out of 13 patients achieved a partial response and 4 other patients showed mixed responses. Among patients who demonstrated objective cancer regression, five patients developed autoimmune-mediated destruction of melanocytes, including four patients with vitiligo and one patient with anterior uveitis (Dudley *et al.*, 2002). Remarkably, despite antimelanoma reactive T cells comprising a large majority of T cells in several patients, only partial regressions were observed, suggesting mechanisms in or around the tumor to disable potentially reactive T cells. Follow-up observations have suggested that transfer of tumor-reactive $CD8^+$ T cells with $CD4^+$ T cells after treatment by nonmyeloablative chemotherapy to create recovering T-cell homeostasis leads to long-lasting clonal expansion of transferred $CD8^+$ T cells.

11.2. Blockade of CTLA-4

Syngeneic peptides from differentiation antigens are poorly immunogenic because of their low/intermediate TCR and/or MHC affinity. Heteroclitic peptides whose anchor residues are optimized to achieve higher affinity can prime CTL that cross-react with the original peptides (Dyall *et al.*, 1998). Vaccination with heteroclitic peptides from differentiation antigens can induce specific $CD8^+$ T-cell responses in a number of clinical trials (Rosenberg *et al.*, 1998, 2003). Combination treatment of anti-CTLA-4 mAb combined with immunization using two MHC class I-restricted heteroclitic peptides from gp100 [$gp100_{209-217}$(210M), $gp100_{280-288}$(288V)] with incomplete Freund's adjuvant lead to objective responses in 3 out of 14 patients, with 2 additional patients showing mixed responses. Notably, six patients developed substantial autoimmune toxicities, including dermatitis, colitis, hypophysitis, and hepatitis, and two patients developed vitiligo. This clinical trial indicated that anti-CTLA-4 mAb overcame ignorance or tolerance to various self-antigens, including melanocyte differentiation antigens (Phan *et al.*, 2003).

11.3. Vaccination with Autologous DCs

Establishment of *in vitro* culture methods for generating DCs from precursor cells has enabled the use of DCs as adjuvants for immunotherapy. Culturing with GM-CSF and IL-4 induces peripheral blood monocytes to differentiate into DCs, while DCs can also be generated from CD34$^+$ cells mobilized in peripheral blood by granulocyte colony-stimulating factor (G-CSF) in the presence of GM-CSF and TNFα. Both DCs are known to effectively present or cross-present antigenic peptides to naïve T cells, leading to activation of antigen-specific cytotoxic and helper T cells. There are different strategies to load antigens onto DCs: pulsing with tumor-derived peptides or autologous tumor lysates, transfection with cDNA or RNA encoding tumor antigens, and transduction with recombinant viruses expressing tumor antigens (Nestle, 2000). The first report by Nestle *et al.* (1998) has been followed by many other phase I/II clinical trials of DC vaccines in patients with metastatic melanoma, with some observations of concomitant vitiligo (Banchereau *et al.*, 2001; Di Nicola *et al.*, 2004; Mackensen *et al.*, 2000; Smithers *et al.*, 2003).

12. Conclusions

Mouse models of concurrent melanoma and vitiligo have established the proof of principle that autoimmunity can generate vitiligo. These experimental systems have provided opportunities to investigate the cellular and molecular

Table 2 Mechanisms of Uncoupling Cancer Immunity and Autoimmunity

Targeted antigen	Mechanism	Divergence between tumor immunity and autoimmunity
TYRP1 (xenogeneic DNA, mAb)	Overlapping and redundant pathways	*Tumor immunity*: dependent on FcγR-expressing macrophages *Autoimmunity*: dependent on FcγR-expressing macrophages and/or complement
DCT (xenogeneic DNA)	Distinct molecular requirements	*Tumor immunity*: independent of perforin or Fas *Autoimmunity*: dependent on perforin, independent of Fas
TYRP1 (mAb), DCT (expression in viral vector)	Potency of vaccine	Higher threshold for autoimmunity than for tumor immunity
DCT (expression in viral vector)	Route of immunization	Induction of autoimmunity by intradermal, but not intramuscular immunization

requirements of tumor immunity and autoimmunity elicited against self-antigens. There are multiple distinct pathways that can potentially lead to tumor immunity and autoimmunity, and some experimental systems have succeeded in uncoupling tumor immunity from autoimmunity (Table 2). For example, immunization against TYRP1 elicits antibody responses, but only tumor immunity requires activating FcγR, whereas autoimmunity proceeds in the absence of these receptors. On the other hand, immunization against DCT induces $CD8^+$-dependent immunity, with only perforin required in autoimmunity, but not tumor immunity. In addition, development of concomitant vitiligo may depend on the potency of the vaccine and on the route of immunization. Although unwanted, in some cases vitiligo can be an acceptable side effect during immunotherapy for a high-risk melanoma, especially because autoimmunity seems to have a higher threshold than tumor immunity. On the other hand, immune reactivity to tumors that arise from critical tissues might lead to unacceptable autoimmune sequelae. To establish strategies that block autoimmunity but allow tumor immunity to proceed is, therefore, one of the challenges for the future.

References

Albert, M. L., Jegathesan, M., and Darnell, R. B. (2001). Dendritic cell maturation is required for the cross-tolerization of CD8+ T cells. *Nat. Immunol.* **2**, 1010–1017.

Atkins, M. B., Lotze, M. T., Dutcher, J. P., Fisher, R. I., Weiss, G., Margolin, K., Abrams, J., Sznol, M., Parkinson, D., Hawkins, M., Paradise, C., Kunkel, L., *et al.* (1999). High-dose recombinant interleukin 2 therapy for patients with metastatic melanoma: Analysis of 270 patients treated between 1985 and 1993. *J Clin. Oncol.* **17**, 2105–2116.

Banchereau, J., Palucka, A. K., Dhodapkar, M., Burkeholder, S., Taquet, N., Rolland, A., Taquet, S., Coquery, S., Wittkowski, K. M., Bhardwaj, N., Pineiro, L., Steinman, R., *et al.* (2001). Immune and clinical responses in patients with metastatic melanoma to CD34(+) progenitor-derived dendritic cell vaccine. *Cancer Res.* **61**, 6451–6458.

Banchereau, J., and Steinman, R. M. (1998). Dendritic cells and the control of immunity. *Nature* **392**, 245–252.

Becker, J. C., Guldberg, P., Zeuthen, J., Brocker, E. B., and Straten, P. T. (1999). Accumulation of identical T cells in melanoma and vitiligo-like leukoderma. *J. Invest. Dermatol.* **113**, 1033–1038.

Belz, G. T., Behrens, G. M. N., Smith, C. M., Miller, J. F. A. P., Jones, C., Lejon, K., Fathman, C. G., Mueller, S. N., Shortman, K., Carbone, F. R., and Heath, W. R. (2002). The CD8{alpha}+ dendritic cell is responsible for inducing peripheral self-tolerance to tissue-associated antigens. *J. Exp. Med.* **196**, 1099–1104.

Bowne, W. B., Srinivasan, R., Wolchok, J. D., Hawkins, W. G., Blachere, N. E., Dyall, R., Lewis, J. J., and Houghton, A. N. (1999). Coupling and uncoupling of tumor immunity and autoimmunity. *J. Exp. Med.* **190**, 1717–1722.

Brocker, T., Riedinger, M., and Karjalainen, K. (1997). Targeted expression of major histocompatibility complex (MHC) class II molecules demonstrates that dendritic cells can induce negative but not positive selection of thymocytes *in vivo*. *J. Exp. Med.* **185**, 541–550.

Bullock, T. N., Mullins, D. W., Colella, T. A., and Engelhard, V. H. (2001). Manipulation of avidity to improve effectiveness of adoptively transferred CD8(+) T cells for melanoma immunotherapy in human MHC class I-transgenic mice. *J. Immunol.* **167,** 5824–5831.

Bystryn, J. C., Rigel, D., Friedman, R. J., and Kopf, A. (1987). Prognostic significance of hypopigmentation in malignant melanoma. *Arch. Dermatol.* **123,** 1053–1055.

Chen, T. C., Cobbold, S. P., Fairchild, P. J., and Waldmann, H. (2004). Generation of anergic and regulatory T cells following prolonged exposure to a harmless antigen. *J. Immunol.* **172,** 5900–5907.

Chu, R. S., Targoni, O. S., Krieg, A. M., Lehmann, P. V., and Harding, C. V. (1997). CpG oligodeoxynucleotides act as adjuvants that switch on T helper 1 (TH1) immunity. *J. Exp. Med.* **186,** 1623–1631.

Chu, W., Gong, X., Li, Z., Takabayashi, K., Ouyang, H., Chen, Y., Lois, A., Chen, D. J., Li, G. C., Karin, M., and Raz, E. (2000). DNA-PKcs is required for activation of innate immunity by immunostimulatory DNA. *Cell* **103,** 909–918.

Clynes, R., Takechi, Y., Moroi, Y., Houghton, A., and Ravetch, J. V. (1998). Fc receptors are required in passive and active immunity to melanoma. *Proc. Natl. Acad. Sci. USA* **95,** 652–656.

Clynes, R. A., Towers, T. L., Presta, L. G., and Ravetch, J. V. (2000). Inhibitory Fc receptors modulate *in vivo* cytotoxicity against tumor targets. *Nat. Med.* **6,** 443–446.

Colonna, M., Trinchieri, G., and Liu, Y. J. (2004). Plasmacytoid dendritic cells in immunity. *Nat. Immunol.* **5,** 1219–1226.

Das, P. K., van den Wijngaard, R. M., Wankowicz-Kalinska, A., and Le Poole, I. C. (2001). A symbiotic concept of autoimmunity and tumour immunity: Lessons from vitiligo. *Trends Immunol.* **22,** 130–136.

Davey, G. M., Kurts, C., Miller, J. F. A. P., Bouillet, P., Strasser, A., Brooks, A. G., Carbone, F. R., and Heath, W. R. (2002). Peripheral deletion of autoreactive CD8 T cells by cross presentation of self-antigen occurs by a Bcl-2-inhibitable pathway mediated by Bim. *J. Exp. Med.* **196,** 947–955.

Di Nicola, M., Carlo-Stella, C., Mortarini, R., Baldassari, P., Guidetti, A., Gallino, G. F., Del Vecchio, M., Ravagnani, F., Magni, M., Chaplin, P., Cascinelli, N., *et al.* (2004). Boosting T cell-mediated immunity to tyrosinase by vaccinia virus-transduced, CD34(+)-derived dendritic cell vaccination: A phase I trial in metastatic melanoma. *Clin. Cancer Res.* **10,** 5381–5390.

Dranoff, G., Jaffee, E., Lazenby, A., Golumbek, P., Levitsky, H., Brose, K., Jackson, V., Hamada, H., Pardoll, D., and Mulligan, R. C. (1993). Vaccination with irradiated tumor cells engineered to secrete murine granulocyte-macrophage colony-stimulating factor stimulates potent, specific, and long-lasting anti-tumor immunity. *Proc. Natl. Acad. Sci. USA* **90,** 3539–3543.

Dudley, M. E., Wunderlich, J. R., Robbins, P. F., Yang, J. C., Hwu, P., Schwartzentruber, D. J., Topalian, S. L., Sherry, R., Restifo, N. P., Hubicki, A. M., Robinson, M. R., Raffeld, M., *et al.* (2002). Cancer regression and autoimmunity in patients after clonal repopulation with antitumor lymphocytes. *Science* **298,** 850–854.

Duhra, P., and Ilchyshyn, A. (1991). Prolonged survival in metastatic malignant melanoma associated with vitiligo. *Clin. Exp. Dermatol.* **16,** 303–305.

Dyall, R., Bowne, W. B., Weber, L. W., LeMaoult, J., Szabo, P., Moroi, Y., Piskun, G., Lewis, J. J., Houghton, A. N., and Nikolic-Zugic, J. (1998). Heteroclitic immunization induces tumor immunity. *J. Exp. Med.* **188,** 1553–1561.

Ehl, S., Aichele, P., Ramseier, H., Barchet, W., Hombach, J., Pircher, H., Hengartner, H., and Zinkernagel, R. M. (1998). Antigen persistence and time of T-cell tolerization determine the efficacy of tolerization protocols for prevention of skin graft rejection. *Nat. Med.* **4,** 1015–1019.

Fong, L., and Engleman, E. G. (2000). Dendritic cells in cancer immunotherapy. *Annu. Rev. Immunol.* **18,** 245–273.

Fontenot, J. D., Gavin, M. A., and Rudensky, A. Y. (2003). Foxp3 programs the development and function of CD4+CD25+ regulatory T cells. *Nat. Immunol.* **4,** 330–336.
Gilhar, A., Zelickson, B., Ulman, Y., and Etzioni, A. (1995). In vivo destruction of melanocytes by the IgG fraction of serum from patients with vitiligo. *J. Invest. Dermatol.* **105,** 683–686.
Gilliet, M., and Liu, Y.-J. (2002). Generation of human CD8 T regulatory cells by CD40 ligand-activated plasmacytoid dendritic cells. *J. Exp. Med.* **195,** 695–704.
Goldberg, S. M., Bartido, S. M., Gardner, J. P., Guevara-Patiño, J. A., Montgomery, S. C., Perales, M. A., Maughan, M. F., Dempsey, J., Donovan, G. P., Olson, W. C., Houghton, A. N., and Wolchok, J. D. (2005). Comparison of two cancer vaccines targeting tyrosinase, plasmid DNA and recombinant alphavirus replicon particles. *Clin. Cancer Res.* **11,** 8114–8121.
Golgher, D., Jones, E., Powrie, F., Elliott, T., and Gallimore, A. (2002). Depletion of CD25+ regulatory cells uncovers immune responses to shared murine tumor rejection antigens. *Eur. J. Immunol.* **32,** 3267–3275.
Gregor, P. D., Wolchok, J. D., Ferrone, C. R., Buchinshky, H., Guevara-Patino, J. A., Perales, M. A., Mortazavi, F., Bacich, D., Heston, W., Latouche, J. B., Sadelain, M., Allison, J. P., *et al.* (2004). CTLA-4 blockade in combination with xenogeneic DNA vaccines enhances T-cell responses, tumor immunity and autoimmunity to self antigens in animal and cellular model systems. *Vaccine* **22,** 1700–1708.
Grimes, P. E., Soriano, T., and Dytoc, M. T. (2002). Topical tacrolimus for repigmentation of vitiligo. *J. Am. Acad. Dermatol.* **47,** 789–791.
Groux, H., Fournier, N., and Cottrez, F. (2004). Role of dendritic cells in the generation of regulatory T cells. *Semin. Immunol.* **16,** 99–106.
Guery, J.-C., and Adorini, L. (1995). Dendritic cells are the most efficient in presenting endogenous naturally processed self-epitopes to class II-restricted T cells. *J. Immunol.* **154,** 536–544.
Hara, I., Takechi, Y., and Houghton, A. N. (1995). Implicating a role for immune recognition of self in tumor rejection: Passive immunization against the brown locus protein. *J. Exp. Med.* **182,** 1609–1614.
Hawiger, D. (2001). Dendritic cells induce peripheral T cell unresponsiveness under steady state conditions *in vivo. J. Exp. Med.* **194,** 769–779.
Hawkins, W. G., Gold, J. S., Dyall, R., Wolchok, J. D., Hoos, A., Bowne, W. B., Srinivasan, R., Houghton, A. N., and Lewis, J. J. (2000). Immunization with DNA coding for gp100 results in CD4 T-cell independent antitumor immunity. *Surgery* **128,** 273–280.
Hemmi, H., Takeuchi, O., Kawai, T., Kaisho, T., Sato, S., Sanjo, H., Matsumoto, M., Hoshino, K., Wagner, H., Takeda, K., and Akira, S. (2000). A Toll-like receptor recognizes bacterial DNA. *Nature* **408,** 740–745.
Hewitt, H. B., Blake, E. R., and Walder, A. S. (1976). A critique of the evidence for active host defense against cancer, based on personal studies of 27 murine tumours of spontaneous origin. *Br. J. Cancer* **33,** 241–259.
Hodi, F. S., Mihm, M. C., Soiffer, R. J., Haluska, F. G., Butler, M., Seiden, M. V., Davis, T., Henry-Spires, R., MacRae, S., Willman, A., Padera, R., Jaklitsch, M. T., *et al.* (2003). Biologic activity of cytotoxic T lymphocyte-associated antigen 4 antibody blockade in previously vaccinated metastatic melanoma and ovarian carcinoma patients. *Proc. Natl. Acad. Sci. USA* **100,** 4712–4717.
Hori, S., Nomura, T., and Sakaguchi, S. (2003). Control of regulatory T cell development by the transcription factor Foxp3. *Science* **299,** 1057–1061.
Houghton, A. N., Gold, J. S., and Blachere, N. E. (2001). Immunity against cancer: Lessons learned from melanoma. *Curr. Opin. Immunol.* **13,** 134–140.
Houghton, A. N., Mintzer, D., Cordon-Cardo, C., Welt, S., Fliegel, B., Vadhan, S., Carswell, E., Melamed, M. R., Oettgen, H. F., and Old, L. J. (1985). Mouse monoclonal IgG3 antibody

detecting GD3 ganglioside: A phase I trial in patients with malignant melanoma. *Proc. Natl. Acad. Sci. USA* **82**, 1242–1246.

Kato, M., Takahashi, M., Akhand, A. A., Liu, W., Dai, Y., Shimizu, S., Iwamoto, T., Suzuki, H., and Nakashima, I. (1998). Transgenic mouse model for skin malignant melanoma. *Oncogene* **17**, 1885–1888.

Kemp, E. H., Gawkrodger, D. J., Watson, P. F., and Weetman, A. P. (1998a). Autoantibodies to human melanocyte-specific protein pmel17 in the sera of vitiligo patients: A sensitive and quantitative radioimmunoassay (RIA). *Clin. Exp. Immunol.* **114**, 333–338.

Kemp, E. H., Waterman, E. A., Gawkrodger, D. J., Watson, P. F., and Weetman, A. P. (1998b). Autoantibodies to tyrosinase-related protein-1 detected in the sera of vitiligo patients using a quantitative radiobinding assay. *Br. J. Dermatol.* **139**, 798–805.

Kemp, E. H., Waterman, E. A., Hawes, B. E., O'Neill, K., Gottumukkala, R. V., Gawkrodger, D. J., Weetman, A. P., and Watson, P. F. (2002). The melanin-concentrating hormone receptor 1, a novel target of autoantibody responses in vitiligo. *J. Clin. Invest.* **109**, 923–930.

Klinman, D. M., Ishii, K. J., and Verthelyi, D. (2000). CpG DNA augments the immunogenicity of plasmid DNA vaccines. *Curr. Top. Microbiol. Immunol.* **247**, 131–142.

Klinman, D. M., Yi, A. K., Beaucage, S. L., Conover, J., and Krieg, A. M. (1996). CpG motifs present in bacteria DNA rapidly induce lymphocytes to secrete interleukin 6, interleukin 12, and interferon gamma. *Proc. Natl. Acad. Sci. USA* **93**, 2879–2883.

Kunisada, T., Lu, S. Z., Yoshida, H., Nishikawa, S., Mizoguchi, M., Hayashi, S., Tyrrell, L., Williams, D. A., Wang, X., and Longley, B. J. (1998). Murine cutaneous mastocytosis and epidermal melanocytosis induced by keratinocyte expression of transgenic stem cell factor. *J. Exp. Med.* **187**, 1565–1573.

Lane, C., Leitch, J., Tan, X., Hadjati, J., Bramson, J. L., and Wan, Y. (2004). Vaccination-induced autoimmune vitiligo is a consequence of secondary trauma to the skin. *Cancer Res.* **64**, 1509–1514.

Lang, K. S., Caroli, C. C., Muhm, A., Wernet, D., Moris, A., Schittek, B., Knauss-Scherwitz, E., Stevanovic, S., Rammensee, H. G., and Garbe, C. (2001). HLA-A2 restricted, melanocyte-specific CD8+ T lymphocytes detected in vitiligo patients are related to disease activity and are predominantly directed against MelanA/MART1. *J. Invest. Dermatol.* **116**, 891–897.

Le Gal, F. A., Avril, M. F., Bosq, J., Lefebvre, P., Deschemin, J. C., Andrieu, M., Dore, M. X., and Guillet, J. G. (2001). Direct evidence to support the role of antigen-specific CD8(+) T cells in melanoma-associated vitiligo. *J. Invest. Dermatol.* **117**, 1464–1470.

Lengagne, R., Le Gal, F. A., Garcette, M., Fiette, L., Ave, P., Kato, M., Briand, J. P., Massot, C., Nakashima, I., Renia, L., Guillet, J. G., and Prevost-Blondel, A. (2004). Spontaneous vitiligo in an animal model for human melanoma: Role of tumor-specific CD8+ T cells. *Cancer Res.* **64**, 1496–1501.

Mackensen, A., Herbst, B., Chen, J. L., Kohler, G., Noppen, C., Herr, W., Spagnoli, G. C., Cerundolo, V., and Lindemann, A. (2000). Phase I study in melanoma patients of a vaccine with peptide-pulsed dendritic cells generated *in vitro* from CD34(+) hematopoietic progenitor cells. *Int. J. Cancer* **86**, 385–392.

Mapara, M. Y., and Sykes, M. (2004). Tolerance and cancer: Mechanisms of tumor evasion and strategies for breaking tolerance. *J. Clin. Oncol.* **22**, 1136–1151.

McLaughlin, P., Grillo-Lopez, A. J., Link, B. K., Levy, R., Czuczman, M. S., Williams, M. E., Heyman, M. R., Bence-Bruckler, I., White, C. A., Cabanillas, F., Jain, V., Ho, A. D., *et al.* (1998). Rituximab chimeric anti-CD20 monoclonal antibody therapy for relapsed indolent lymphoma: Half of patients respond to a four-dose treatment program. *J. Clin. Oncol.* **16**, 2825–2833.

Muriglan, S. J., Ramirez-Montagut, T., Alpdogan, O., Van Huystee, T. W., Eng, J. M., Hubbard, V. M., Kochman, A. A., Tjoe, K. H., Riccardi, C., Pandolfi, P. P., Sakaguchi, S., Houghton, A. N., et al. (2004). GITR activation induces an opposite effect on alloreactive CD4(+) and CD8(+) T cells in graft-versus-host disease. *J. Exp. Med.* **200,** 149–157.

Naftzger, C., Takechi, Y., Kohda, H., Hara, I., Vijayasaradhi, S., and Houghton, A. N. (1996). Immune response to a differentiation antigen induced by altered antigen: A study of tumor rejection and autoimmunity. *Proc. Natl. Acad. Sci. USA* **93,** 14809–14814.

Nagai, H., Hara, I., Horikawa, T., Oka, M., Kamidono, S., and Ichihashi, M. (2000). Elimination of CD4(+) T cells enhances anti-tumor effect of locally secreted interleukin-12 on B16 mouse melanoma and induces vitiligo-like coat color alteration. *J. Invest. Dermatol.* **115,** 1059–1064.

Nagai, H., Horikawa, T., Hara, I., Fukunaga, A., Oniki, S., Oka, M., Nishigori, C., and Ichihashi, M. (2004). In vivo elimination of CD25 regulatory T cells leads to tumor rejection of B16F10 melanoma, when combined with interleukin-12 gene transfer. *Exp. Dermatol.* **13,** 613–620.

Nestle, F. O. (2000). Dendritic cell vaccination for cancer therapy. *Oncogene* **19,** 6673–6679.

Nestle, F. O., Alijagic, S., Gilliet, M., Sun, Y., Grabbe, S., Dummer, R., Burg, G., and Schadendorf, D. (1998). Vaccination of melanoma patients with peptide- or tumor lysate-pulsed dendritic cells. *Nat. Med.* **4,** 328–332.

Nikolic-Zugic, J., and Bevan, M. J. (1990). Role of self-peptides in positively selecting the T-cell repertoire. *Nature* **344,** 65–67.

Nishimura, E. K., Jordan, S. A., Oshima, H., Yoshida, H., Osawa, M., Moriyama, M., Jackson, I. J., Barrandon, Y., Miyachi, Y., and Nishikawa, S. (2002). Dominant role of the niche in melanocyte stem-cell fate determination. *Nature* **416,** 854–860.

Nocentini, G., Giunchi, L., Ronchetti, S., Krausz, L. T., Bartoli, A., Moraca, R., Migliorati, G., and Riccardi, C. (1997). A new member of the tumor necrosis factor/nerve growth factor receptor family inhibits T cell receptor-induced apoptosis. *Proc. Natl. Acad. Sci. USA* **94,** 6216–6221.

Nordlund, J. J., Kirkwood, J. M., Forget, B. M., Milton, G., Albert, D. M., and Lerner, A. B. (1983). Vitiligo in patients with metastatic melanoma: A good prognostic sign. *J. Am. Acad. Dermatol.* **9,** 689–696.

Ogg, G. S., Rod Dunbar, P., Romero, P., Chen, J. L., and Cerundolo, V. (1998). High frequency of skin-homing melanocyte-specific cytotoxic T lymphocytes in autoimmune vitiligo. *J. Exp. Med.* **188,** 1203–1208.

Old, L. J. (1981). Cancer immunology: The search for specificity—G. H. A. Clowes memorial lecture. *Cancer Res.* **41,** 361–375.

Onizuka, S., Tawara, I., Shimizu, J., Sakaguchi, S., Fujita, T., and Nakayama, E. (1999). Tumor rejection by in vivo administration of anti-CD25 (interleukin-2 receptor alpha) monoclonal antibody. *Cancer Res.* **59,** 3128–3133.

Overwijk, W. W., Lee, D. S., Surman, D. R., Irvine, K. R., Touloukian, C. E., Chan, C. C., Carroll, M. W., Moss, B., Rosenberg, S. A., and Restifo, N. P. (1999). Vaccination with a recombinant vaccinia virus encoding a "self" antigen induces autoimmune vitiligo and tumor cell destruction in mice: Requirement for CD4(+) T lymphocytes. *Proc. Natl. Acad. Sci. USA* **96,** 2982–2987.

Overwijk, W. W., Theoret, M. R., Finkelstein, S. E., Surman, D. R., de Jong, L. A., Vyth-Dreese, F. A., Dellemijn, T. A., Antony, P. A., Spiess, P. J., Palmer, D. C., Heimann, D. M., Klebanoff, C. A., et al. (2003). Tumor regression and autoimmunity after reversal of a functionally tolerant state of self-reactive CD8+ T cells. *J. Exp. Med.* **198,** 569–580.

Palermo, B., Campanelli, R., Garbelli, S., Mantovani, S., Lantelme, E., Brazzelli, V., Ardigo, M., Borroni, G., Martinetti, M., Badulli, C., Necker, A., and Giachino, C. (2001). Specific cytotoxic T lymphocyte responses against Melan-A/MART1, tyrosinase and gp100 in vitiligo by the use of major histocompatibility complex/peptide tetramers: The role of cellular immunity in the etiopathogenesis of vitiligo. *J. Invest. Dermatol.* **117,** 326–332.

Phan, G. Q., Attia, P., Steinberg, S. M., White, D. E., and Rosenberg, S. A. (2001). Factors associated with response to high-dose interleukin-2 in patients with metastatic melanoma. *J. Clin. Oncol.* **19,** 3477–3482.

Phan, G. Q., Yang, J. C., Sherry, R. M., Hwu, P., Topalian, S. L., Schwartzentruber, D. J., Restifo, N. P., Haworth, L. R., Seipp, C. A., Freezer, L. J., Morton, K. E., Mavroukakis, S. A., *et al.* (2003). Cancer regression and autoimmunity induced by cytotoxic T lymphocyte-associated antigen 4 blockade in patients with metastatic melanoma. *Proc. Natl. Acad. Sci. USA* **100,** 8372–8377.

Prehn, R. T., and Main, J. M. (1957). Immunity to methylcholanthrene-induced sarcomas. *J. Natl. Cancer Inst.* **18,** 769–778.

Ravetch, J. V., and Clynes, R. A. (1998). Divergent roles for Fc receptors and complement *in vivo. Annu. Rev. Immunol.* **16,** 421–432.

Ridolfi, L., Ridolfi, R., Riccobon, A., De Paola, F., Petrini, M., Stefanelli, M., Flamini, E., Ravaioli, A., Verdecchia, G. M., Trevisan, G., and Amadori, D. (2003). Adjuvant immunotherapy with tumor infiltrating lymphocytes and interleukin-2 in patients with resected stage III and IV melanoma. *J. Immunother.* **26,** 156–162.

Robinson, M. R., Chan, C. C., Yang, J. C., Rubin, B. I., Gracia, G. J., Sen, H. N., Csaky, K. G., and Rosenberg, S. A. (2004). Cytotoxic T lymphocyte-associated antigen 4 blockade in patients with metastatic melanoma: A new cause of uveitis. *J. Immunother.* **27,** 478–479.

Rocha, C. D., Caetano, B. C., Machado, A. V., and Bruna-Romero, O. (2004). Recombinant viruses as tools to induce protective cellular immunity against infectious diseases. *Int. Microbiol.* **7,** 83–94.

Rosenberg, S. A., and White, D. E. (1996). Vitiligo in patients with melanoma: Normal tissue antigens can be targets for cancer immunotherapy. *J. Immunother. Emphasis Tumor Immunol.* **19,** 81–84.

Rosenberg, S. A., Yang, J. C., Schwartzentruber, D. J., Hwu, P., Marincola, F. M., Topalian, S. L., Restifo, N. P., Dudley, M. E., Schwarz, S. L., Spiess, P. J., Wunderlich, J. R., Parkhurst, M. R., *et al.* (1998). Immunologic and therapeutic evaluation of a synthetic peptide vaccine for the treatment of patients with metastatic melanoma. *Nat. Med.* **4,** 321–327.

Rosenberg, S. A., Yang, J. C., Schwartzentruber, D. J., Hwu, P., Topalian, S. L., Sherry, R. M., Restifo, N. P., Wunderlich, J. R., Seipp, C. A., Rogers-Freezer, L., Morton, K. E., Mavroukakis, S. A., *et al.* (2003). Recombinant fowlpox viruses encoding the anchor-modified gp100 melanoma antigen can generate antitumor immune responses in patients with metastatic melanoma. *Clin. Cancer Res.* **9,** 2973–2980.

Sakaguchi, S., Sakaguchi, N., Asano, M., Itoh, M., and Toda, M. (1995). Immunologic self-tolerance maintained by activated T cells expressing IL-2 receptor alpha-chains (CD25). Breakdown of a single mechanism of self-tolerance causes various autoimmune diseases. *J. Immunol.* **155,** 1151–1164.

Salio, M., Palmowski, M. J., Atzberger, A., Hermans, I. F., and Cerundolo, V. (2004). CpG-matured murine plasmacytoid dendritic cells are capable of *in vivo* priming of functional CD8 T cell responses to endogenous but not exogenous antigens. *J. Exp. Med.* **199,** 567–579.

Salomon, B., and Bluestone, J. A. (2001). Complexities of CD28/B7: CTLA-4 costimulatory pathways in autoimmunity and transplantation. *Annu. Rev. Immunol.* **19,** 225–252.

Sanderson, K., Scotland, R., Lee, P., Liu, D., Groshen, S., Snively, J., Sian, S., Nichol, G., Davis, T., Keler, T., Yellin, M., and Weber, J. (2005). Autoimmunity in a phase I trial of a fully human anti-cytotoxic T-lymphocyte antigen-4 monoclonal antibody with multiple melanoma peptides and

Montanide ISA 51 for patients with resected stages III and IV melanoma. *J. Clin. Oncol.* **23**, 741–750.

Sato, Y., Roman, M., Tighe, H., Lee, D., Corr, M., Nguyen, M.-D., Silverman, G. J., Lotz, M., Carson, D. A., and Raz, E. (1996). Immunostimulatory DNA sequences necessary for effective intradermal gene immunization. *Science* **273**, 352–354.

Schneeberger, A., Wagner, C., Zemann, A., Luhrs, P., Kutil, R., Goos, M., Stingl, G., and Wagner, S. N. (2004). CpG motifs are efficient adjuvants for DNA cancer vaccines. *J. Invest. Dermatol.* **123**, 371–379.

Schreurs, M. W., Eggert, A. A., de Boer, A. J., Vissers, J. L., van Hall, T., Offringa, R., Figdor, C. G., and Adema, G. J. (2000). Dendritic cells break tolerance and induce protective immunity against a melanocyte differentiation antigen in an autologous melanoma model. *Cancer Res.* **60**, 6995–7001.

Scotto, L., Naiyer, A. J., Galluzzo, S., Rossi, P., Manavalan, J. S., Kim-Schulze, S., Fang, J., Favera, R. D., Cortesini, R., and Suciu-Foca, N. (2004). Overlap between molecular markers expressed by naturally occurring CD4+CD25+ regulatory T cells and antigen specific CD4+CD25+ and CD8+CD28- T suppressor cells. *Hum. Immunol.* **65**, 1297–1306.

Shimizu, J., Yamazaki, S., and Sakaguchi, S. (1999). Induction of tumor immunity by removing CD25+CD4+ T cells: A common basis between tumor immunity and autoimmunity. *J. Immunol.* **163**, 5211–5218.

Shimizu, J., Yamazaki, S., Takahashi, T., Ishida, Y., and Sakaguchi, S. (2002). Stimulation of CD25 (+)CD4(+) regulatory T cells through GITR breaks immunological self-tolerance. *Nat. Immunol.* **3**, 135–142.

Smithers, M., O'Connell, K., MacFadyen, S., Chambers, M., Greenwood, K., Boyce, A., Abdul-Jabbar, I., Barker, K., Grimmett, K., Walpole, E., and Thomas, R. (2003). Clinical response after intradermal immature dendritic cell vaccination in metastatic melanoma is associated with immune response to particulate antigen. *Cancer Immunol. Immunother.* **52**, 41–52.

Song, Y.-H., Connor, E., Li, Y., Zorovich, B., Balducci, P., and Maclaren, N. (1994). The role of tyrosinase in autoimmune vitiligo. *Lancet* **344**, 1049–1052.

Sparwasser, T., Vabulas, R. M., Villmow, B., Lipford, G. B., and Wagner, H. (2000). Bacterial CpG-DNA activates dendritic cells *in vivo*: T helper cell-independent cytotoxic T cell responses to soluble proteins. *Eur. J. Immunol.* **30**, 3591–3597.

Steinman, R. M., Hawiger, D., and Nussenzweig, M. C. (2003). Tolerogenic dendritic cells. *Annu. Rev. Immunol.* **21**, 685–711.

Steinman, R. M., and Nussenzweig, M. C. (2002). Inaugural Article: Avoiding horror autotoxicus: The importance of dendritic cells in peripheral T cell tolerance. *Proc. Natl. Acad. Sci. USA* **99**, 351–358.

Steinman, R. M., Turley, S., Mellman, I., and Inaba, K. (2000). The induction of tolerance by dendritic cells that have captured apoptotic cells. *J. Exp. Med.* **191**, 411–416.

Steitz, J., Bruck, J., Gambotto, A., Knop, J., and Tuting, T. (2002). Genetic immunization with a melanocytic self-antigen linked to foreign helper sequences breaks tolerance and induces autoimmunity and tumor immunity. *Gene Ther.* **9**, 208–213.

Stripecke, R., Carmen Villacres, M., Skelton, D., Satake, N., Halene, S., and Kohn, D. (1999). Immune response to green fluorescent protein: Implications for gene therapy. *Gene Ther.* **6**, 1305–1312.

Sun, S., Zhang, X., Tough, D. F., and Sprent, J. (1998). Type I interferon-mediated stimulation of T cells by CpG DNA. *J. Exp. Med.* **188**, 2335–2342.

Sutmuller, R. P., van Duivenvoorde, L. M., van Elsas, A., Schumacher, T. N., Wildenberg, M. E., Allison, J. P., Toes, R. E., Offringa, R., and Melief, C. J. (2001). Synergism of cytotoxic T lymphocyte-associated antigen 4 blockade and depletion of cd25(+) regulatory T cells in antitumor therapy reveals alternative pathways for suppression of autoreactive cytotoxic T lymphocyte responses. *J. Exp. Med.* **194,** 823–832.

Takahashi, T., Tagami, T., Yamazaki, S., Uede, T., Shimizu, J., Sakaguchi, N., Mak, T. W., and Sakaguchi, S. (2000). Immunologic self-tolerance maintained by CD25(+)CD4(+) regulatory T cells constitutively expressing cytotoxic T lymphocyte-associated antigen 4. *J. Exp. Med.* **192,** 303–310.

Takechi, Y., Hara, I., Naftzger, C., Xu, Y., and Houghton, A. N. (1996). A melanosomal membrane protein is a cell surface target for melanoma therapy. *Clin. Cancer Res.* **2,** 1837–1842.

Trcka, J., Moroi, Y., Clynes, R. A., Goldberg, S. M., Bergtold, A., Perales, M. A., Ma, M., Ferrone, C. R., Carroll, M. C., Ravetch, J. V., and Houghton, A. N. (2002). Redundant and alternative roles for activating Fc receptors and complement in an antibody-dependent model of autoimmune vitiligo. *Immunity* **16,** 861–868.

Turk, M. J., Guevara-Patino, J. A., Rizzuto, G. A., Engelhorn, M. E., Sakaguchi, S., and Houghton, A. N. (2004). Concomitant tumor immunity to a poorly immunogenic melanoma is prevented by regulatory T cells. *J. Exp. Med.* **200,** 771–782.

Vadhan-Raj, S., Cordon-Cardo, C., Carswell, E., Mintzer, D., Dantis, L., Duteau, C., Templeton, M. A., Oettgen, H. F., Old, L. J., and Houghton, A. N. (1988). Phase I trial of a mouse monoclonal antibody against GD3 ganglioside in patients with melanoma: Induction of inflammatory responses at tumor sites. *J. Clin. Oncol.* **6,** 1636–1648.

van Elsas, A., Hurwitz, A. A., and Allison, J. P. (1999). Combination immunotherapy of B16 melanoma using anti-cytotoxic T lymphocyte-associated antigen 4 (CTLA-4) and granulocyte/macrophage colony-stimulating factor (GM-CSF)-producing vaccines induces rejection of subcutaneous and metastatic tumors accompanied by autoimmune depigmentation. *J. Exp. Med.* **190,** 355–366.

van Elsas, A., Sutmuller, R. P., Hurwitz, A. A., Ziskin, J., Villasenor, J., Medema, J. P., Overwijk, W. W., Restifo, N. P., Melief, C. J., Offringa, R., and Allison, J. P. (2001). Elucidating the autoimmune and antitumor effector mechanisms of a treatment based on cytotoxic T lymphocyte antigen-4 blockade in combination with a B16 melanoma vaccine. Comparison of prophylaxis and therapy. *J. Exp. Med.* **194,** 481–490.

Vijayasaradhi, S., Bouchard, B., and Houghton, A. N. (1990). The melanoma antigen gp75 is the human homologue of the mouse b (brown) locus gene product. *J. Exp. Med.* **171,** 1375–1380.

Weber, L. W., Bowne, W. B., Wolchok, J. D., Srinivasan, R., Qin, J., Moroi, Y., Clynes, R., Song, P., Lewis, J. J., and Houghton, A. N. (1998). Tumor immunity and autoimmunity induced by immunization with homologous DNA. *J. Clin. Invest.* **102,** 1258–1264.

Weiner, G. J., Liu, H. M., Wooldridge, J. E., Dahle, C. E., and Krieg, A. M. (1997). Immunostimulatory oligodeoxynucleotides containing the CpG motif are effective as immune adjuvants in tumor antigen immunization. *Proc. Natl. Acad. Sci. USA* **94,** 10833–10837.

Wolchok, J., Srinivasan, R., Perales, M.-A., Houghton, A. N., Bowne, W., and Blachere, N. (2001). Alternative roles for IFN-gamma in the immune response to DNA vaccines encoding related melanosomal antigens. *Cancer Immun.* **1,** 9–19.

Yee, C., Thompson, J. A., Roche, P., Byrd, D. R., Lee, P. P., Piepkorn, M., Kenyon, K., Davis, M. M., Riddell, S. R., and Greenberg, P. D. (2000). Melanocyte destruction after antigen-specific immunotherapy of melanoma: Direct evidence of T cell-mediated vitiligo. *J. Exp. Med.* **192,** 1637–1644.

Immunity to Melanoma Antigens: From Self-Tolerance to Immunotherapy

Craig L. Slingluff, Jr., Kimberly A. Chianese-Bullock, Timothy N.J. Bullock, William W. Grosh, David W. Mullins, Lisa Nichols, Walter Olson, Gina Petroni, Mark Smolkin, and Victor H. Engelhard

Departments of Surgery and Microbiology, Public Health Sciences, Medicine, Pathology, Human Immune Therapy Center, Beirne Carter Center for Immunology Research, University of Virginia, Charlottesville, Virginia

Abstract 243
1. Introduction 244
2. Molecular Definition of Tumor Antigens Recognized by CD8 T Cells 245
3. Why Study Peptide Vaccines? 246
4. Clinical Studies with Peptide Vaccines 248
5. Vaccination with Single Melanoma Peptide and Nonspecific Helper Peptide in Adjuvant 248
6. Evaluation of Immune Responses in the Sentinel Immunized Node 250
7. Vaccination with Peptides in Adjuvant Is More Immunogenic than a Dendritic Cell Vaccine Using Monocyte Derived Immature DC Pulsed with Peptides 250
8. Low-Dose IL-2 Administered Early with Multipeptide Vaccine Does Not Augment Immunogenicity 251
9. Expanding the Repertoire of Melanoma Reactivity Using Multipeptide Vaccines 252
10. *Ex Vivo* Analyses of T-Cell Responses to Class I MHC Restricted Peptides ... 259
11. Modulation of Responses by Combination of CD4 and CD8 T-Cell Vaccination, and Modulation of Regulatory Function 260
12. Cancer Vaccine Development Requires Elucidation of Biology of the Host–Tumor Relationship in Human and Murine Systems, *In Vivo* and *In Vitro* 265
13. A Murine Model to Evaluate Immunity to the MDP-Derived Peptide Ag from Tyrosinase 266
14. Nature of Self-Tolerance to mTyR$_{369}$ and Its Effect on Tumor Control 267
15. MDP-Specific Immune Responses in Tolerant Mice Enable Control of Tumor Outgrowth 273
16. Peptide-Pulsed Exogenous DC as a Vehicle to Influence the Quality of the Tumor-Specific Immune Response 275
17. Summary of Preclinical and Clinical Studies and Future Directions 282
References 284

Abstract

The development of effective immune therapy for cancer is a central goal of immunologists in the 21st century. Our laboratories have been deeply involved in characterization of the immune response to melanoma and translation of laboratory discoveries into clinical trials. We have identified a cohort of peptide antigens presented by Major Histocompatibility Complex (MHC) molecules on *melanoma cells and widely recognized by T cells from melanoma patients. These have been incorporated into peptide-based vaccines that induce $CD8^+$ and $CD4^+$ T-cell responses in 80–100% of patients. Major objective clinical tumor regressions have been observed in some patients, and overall survival in vaccinated patients exceeds expected stage-specific survival. New clinical trials will determine the value of combination of melanoma helper peptides (MHP) into multipeptide vaccines targeting CD8 cells. New trials will also evaluate new approaches to modulating the host–tumor relationship and will develop new combination therapies. Parallel investigations in murine models are elucidating the immunobiology of the melanoma–host relationship and addressing issues that are not feasible to approach in human trials. Based on the fact that the largest cohort of melanoma antigens are derived from normal proteins concerned with pigment production, we have evaluated the mechanisms of self-tolerance to tyrosinase (Tyr) and have determined how T cells in an environment of self-tolerance are impacted by immunization. Using peptide-pulsed dendritic cells as immunogens, we have also used the mouse model to establish strategies for quantitative and qualitative enhancement of antitumor immunity. This information creates opportunities for a new generation of therapeutic interventions using cancer vaccines.*

1. Introduction

Cellular immune responses to melanoma occur spontaneously and are evident by the presence of melanoma-antigen specific T cells infiltrating tumors, regional lymph nodes (LN), and peripheral blood of most patients (Slingluff *et al.*, 1988, 1989). The ability of melanoma-reactive CD8 T cells to mediate tumor regression after *in vitro* expansion and adoptive transfer is evidence that they recognize Ags relevant to tumor control (Rosenberg *et al.*, 1988). The definition of such Ags provides the basis for a therapeutic vaccine and for stimulation of more effective CD8 T cells for adoptive immunotherapy. The largest category of peptide Ags that are both widely displayed on melanomas in association with class I MHC molecules and recognized by CD8 T cells from multiple patients originate from proteins associated with pigment production in normal melanocytes. These melanocyte differentiation proteins (MDP) include tyrosinase (Tyr), gp100, MART-1/Melan-A, tyrosinase-related protein-1 (TRP-1) and TRP-2. Peptides from many of these Ags are presented by multiple class I or class II MHC molecules, emphasizing their generality. Positive clinical responses have been associated with MDP-directed immunotherapies (Jager *et al.*, 2000; Kawakami *et al.*, 1995; Nestle *et al.*, 1998b; Pass *et al.*, 1998; Rosenberg *et al.*, 1998; Slingluff *et al.*, 2003) emphasizing the importance of these proteins as immune targets and strongly suggesting their importance in the development of vaccines for tumor control in a spectrum of patients.

Importantly, melanoma regression occurring spontaneously or in association with several forms of immunotherapy has been associated with autoimmune skin depigmentation and melanocyte destruction (vitiligo) in patients (Brystryn *et al.*, 1987; Nordlund *et al.*, 1983; Rosenberg and White 1996; Yee *et al.*, 2000) and murine models (Overwijk *et al.*, 1999; Steitz *et al.*, 2000; van Elsas *et al.*, 1999). Over the last 15 years, our laboratories have been concerned with the identification of these antigens incorporating them into vaccines for immunotherapy of melanoma patients, and utilizing murine models to understand the factors influencing their immunogenicity.

2. Molecular Definition of Tumor Antigens Recognized by CD8 T Cells

The peptides incorporated into many of the vaccines we have studied were directly identified by mass spectrometry in combination with cytotoxic T lymphocyte (CTL) lines derived from melanoma patients. The peptides identified in our early work were all derived from the MDPs gp100 or Tyr and restricted by Human Leukocyte Antigen (HLA)-A1, HLA-A2, or HLA-A3 (Cox *et al.*, 1994; Kittlesen *et al.*, 1998; Skipper *et al.*, 1996a,b). All were displayed on melanomas isolated from multiple patients, indicating their generality as targets. They were also recognized by T cells from multiple patients, indicating the existence of an intrinsic immune response that could potentially be augmented by vaccination. Additionally, two of these four peptides contained posttranslational modifications that were only discernable by using the mass spectrometry approach but which dramatically influenced T cell recognition. One of these involved deamidation of asparagine 371 in the $Tyr_{369-377}$ peptide to an aspartic acid residue (Skipper *et al.*, 1996a). This is now known to occur during the removal of N-linked carbohydrates by peptide *N*-glycanase during antigen processing (Altrich-VanLith *et al.*, 2006), and a similar modification has been identified in epitopes derived from other glycoproteins (Ferris *et al.*, 1999; Mosse *et al.*, 2001; Selby *et al.*, 1999; Skipper *et al.*, 1996a). A second modification involved the attachment of a free cysteine residue to a cysteine in the $Tyr_{243-251}$ peptide via a disulfide bond (Kittlesen *et al.*, 1998). While this cysteinylation modification has been found in other epitopes (Meadows *et al.*, 1997; Pierce *et al.*, 1999), the Tyr peptide itself contained two cysteine residues allowing for displacement of the free cysteine by disulfide exchange. We established that CTL specific for this melanoma peptide recognized a modified peptide in which Cys244 was substituted with serine residue (Kittlesen *et al.*, 1998). These results establish the value of antigen identification using this direct approach.

More recently, we have identified two other peptides on melanoma cells that are not derived from MDP. One of these, RLSNRLLLR, is derived from a novel cancer-testis antigen, called TAG, that is expressed in approximately 90% of melanomas (Hogan *et al.*, 2004). We have also established the naturally processed forms for several antigens identified by other groups, and have also determined that several of these are presented by multiple class I MHC molecules (summarized in Table 1). We have also begun to explore the use of mass spectrometry to identify peptides that represent attractive candidates for vaccine development based on their differential expression in tumor cells. Since disregulated phosphorylation of cell signaling molecules is a hallmark of cellular transformation, phosphorylated peptides from these proteins may be excellent immune rejection antigens. Using mass spectrometry, we have established that phosphorylated peptides are naturally processed and presented by class I MHC molecules, and that CD8 T cells that specifically recognize them can be elicited by vaccination (Zarling et al., 2000). More recently, we have established that the repertoire of these peptides varies with tumor type and have identified a small cohort of phosphorylated peptides that are being characterized for their value in cancer vaccines (Zarling et al., 2006).

3. Why Study Peptide Vaccines?

We have chosen to focus on vaccines using synthetic MHC-associated peptides for multiple reasons. The use of defined peptides, as opposed to full-length proteins, ensures that the vaccine represents the actual antigens processed and presented by melanoma cells by avoiding uncertainties of antigen processing efficiency and selectivity. While the relevance of individual peptides is limited both by MHC restriction and the heterogeneity of antigen expression among tumor cells, defined synthetic peptides are easily combinable into multipeptide vaccines that mitigate both of these concerns. While current peptide vaccines exclude antigens that are unique to individual patients, they also avoid administration of large numbers of self-proteins whose influence on the immune response is uncertain. Peptides are also easily modifiable by chemical means, permitting creation of synthetic peptides that are more immunogenic and less susceptible to degradation *in vivo* than native peptides. From a practical standpoint, high-grade synthetic peptides are relatively cheap and easy to produce, and vaccines that employ them are easier to evaluate than those based on whole cells or viruses because of lower regulatory hurdles. Thus, peptide vaccines are feasible to study without corporate support. Finally, vaccines for cancer patients seek to stimulate a therapeutic immune response, as opposed to the protective immunity that has been the primary goal of vaccination for infectious disease. Virtually all vaccines for cancer patients are also exploring new technologies. Simply put, we know relatively little about how best to vaccinate cancer patients. The use of defined antigens allows direct evaluation of preexisting and vaccine-induced responses. Clinical investigations with peptide vaccines offer a special opportunity to evaluate the immune

Table 1 Characterization of Naturally Processed MHC Class I Associated Peptides on Melanomas

Epitope	Sequence[a]	MHC restriction	Reference
Antigens Discovered At UVa			
gp100$_{280-288}$	YLEPGPVTA	HLA-A2	(Cox et al., 1994)
Tyr$_{369-377D}$	YMDGTMSQV[b]	HLA-A2	(Skipper et al., 1996a)
gp100$_{17-25}$	ALLAVGATK	HLA-A3, HLA-A11, HLA-A31, HLA-A68	(Hogan et al., 2005; Skipper et al., 1996b)
Tyr$_{243-251}$	KCDICTDEY	HLA-A1	(Kittlesen et al., 1998)
TAG-1,2	RLSNRLLLR	HLA-A3	(Hogan et al., 2004)
Unknown	SQNFPGSQK	HLA-A3	(Hogan et al., 2003)
Naturally processed peptide established using mass spectrometry			
gp100$_{154-162}$	KTWGQYWQV (Bakker et al., 1995)	HLA-A2	(Skipper et al., 1999)
gp100$_{209-217}$	ITDQVPFSV (Kawakami et al., 1995)	HLA-A2	(Skipper et al., 1999)
gp100$_{476-485}$	VLYRYGSFSV (Kawakami et al., 1995)	HLA-A2	(Skipper et al., 1999)
MART-1/MelanA$_{27-35}$	AAGIGILTV (Kawakami et al., 1994)	HLA-A2	(Skipper et al., 1999)
Naturally processed form established to associate with MHC supertype members			
gp100	ALNFPGSQK (Kawakami et al., 1998)	HLA-A3, HLA-A11	(Hogan et al., 2005)
gp100	LIYRRRLMK (Kawakami et al., 1998)	HLA-A3	(Hogan et al., 2005)
NY-ESO-1	AAQERRVPR (Wang et al., 1998)	HLA-A3	(Hogan et al., 2005)
NY-ESO-1	ASGPGGGAPR (Wang et al., 1998)	HLA-A3, HLA-A31	(Hogan et al., 2005)
NY-ESO-1	LLGPGRPYR (Wang et al., 1998)	HLA-A3, HLA-A31	(Hogan et al., 2005)

[a] Peptides originally discovered by other investigators are listed with the appropriate citation.
[b] Posttranslational modification N→D due to N-linked glycosylation.

response at a molecular level and to characterize the host–tumor relationship while optimizing cancer immunotherapy.

4. Clinical Studies with Peptide Vaccines

As peptide antigens for cancer-reactive T cells were first identified in the early 1990s, there was no meaningful experience with use of these peptide epitopes in cancer vaccines. The goal of our clinical studies has been to optimize peptide vaccines for melanoma by sequential studies that are adequately powered to provide definitive answers to critical questions toward this goal. Our vaccine program is an ongoing series of phase I and phase II clinical trials, dedicated largely to developing effective ways to vaccinate with peptides. Most of the trials have been randomized trials, allowing evaluation of two or more approaches in parallel. Each has contributed to our stepwise process of vaccine optimization.

5. Vaccination with Single Melanoma Peptide and Nonspecific Helper Peptide in Adjuvant

Our first phase I melanoma vaccine trial evaluated administration of the HLA-A*0201-restricted peptide gp100$_{280-288}$ (Table 1) in adjuvant with or without a tetanus toxoid peptide restricted by multiple HLA-DR alleles. This tetanus peptide was administered to stimulate helper T cells. It was modified from the reported sequence of tetanus toxoid by the addition of an alanine residue to the N-terminus, thus avoiding spontaneous conversion of the N-terminal glutamine residue to pyroglutamate (Slingluff *et al.*, 2001). Twenty-two patients were randomized to receive the gp100 peptide alone, the gp100 peptide and the tetanus helper peptide, or a fusion peptide encoding both the gp100 peptide sequence and the tetanus helper sequence. Patients were also randomized to receive the vaccine in one of two different adjuvants: Montanide ISA-51 (Seppic, Inc.) or QS-21 (Aquila Pharmaceuticals).

5.1. Immunization with gp100$_{280-288}$ and Tetanus Peptides Induces CD8 and CD4 Immune Responses in the Blood

ELIspot and IFN-γ secretion assays, performed on peripheral blood lymphocytes (PBL) stimulated with peptide *ex vivo*, detected peptide-reactive T cell responses in only 3 of 21 patients (Slingluff *et al.*, 2001). We evaluated the response to the tetanus helper peptide by measuring proliferative responses to that peptide *in vitro*, in a 5-day tritiated thymidine incorporation assay. The maximal increases in reactivity to the tetanus helper peptide were observed for the patients who were vaccinated with the gp100 peptide and the tetanus helper peptide (as free peptides) in Montanide ISA-51 adjuvant. These were predominantly Th1 responses, based on the generation of IFN-γ but not IL4 or IL10 in response to peptide. These and subsequent data supported continuing use of this tetanus helper peptide as a free peptide added to vaccine regimens with Montanide ISA-51.

5.2. Survival Results

The patients on this trial had resected stage IIB-IV melanoma. The multicenter clinical trials of high-dose IFN-α can be used as a comparator for an estimate of the expected survival in this population. The patients on Eastern Cooperative Oncology Group (ECOG) 1690 included stage III patients (75%) and stage IIB patients (25%) as reported (Kirkwood et al., 2000). Thus, the patients on our small trial would be expected to have the same or poorer prognosis than patients on the observation arm on the ECOG 1690 and ECOG 1684 trials. However, the survival and progression-free survival for patients on this trial, in fact, are comparable to what was reported for patients who received high-dose IFN (HDI) on each of the ECOG trials, with 74% survival at 4.5 years in our published results (data not shown; compared to 62% and 55% 3 year survival on HDI arms of ECOG 1690 and ECOG 1684, respectively (Kirkwood et al., 1996, 2000). Longer follow-up of our patients reveals an 8-year overall survival rate for this high-risk patient population of approximately 53% (Fig. 1). The actuarial survival data for this first generation peptide vaccine trial Mel16, thus, are encouraging, though it is impossible to compare these groups in a rigorous manner for significance.

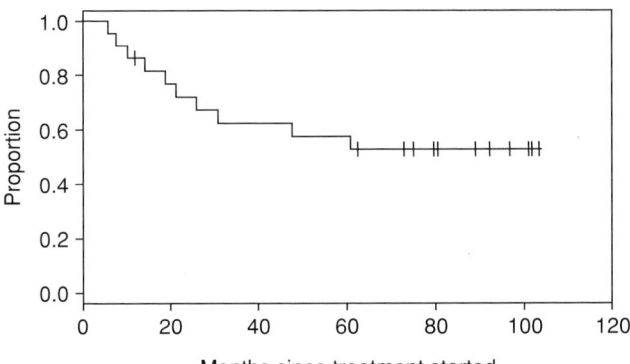

Figure 1 Overall survival of patients on Mel16 trial. Follow-up information at or beyond 5 years is available for almost all living patients.

6. Evaluation of Immune Responses in the Sentinel Immunized Node

Because the CD8 T cell response in the trial described above was difficult to detect in the PBL but clinical outcome was good, we developed another approach to immune monitoring by evaluation of the CD8 T cell response in a lymph node draining a replicate vaccination site after three immunizations. We developed this approach with the expectation that this node should be the site of primary immune response and therefore may serve as an excellent immunologic compartment in which to measure immunogenicity of the vaccine. We were concerned that immune responses measured in circulating PBL are a less direct measure, as they may be affected by dilution, by systemic tumor factors, and by trafficking from the blood to tumor sites.

This node was harvested using standard techniques for sentinel node biopsy, thus, it is called the sentinel-immunized node (SIN). The first trial using this approach was a randomized phase II trial evaluating vaccination with a mixture of 4 melanoma peptides and the tetanus helper peptide, either pulsed on autologous dendritic cells or administered directly in emulsion with Montanide ISA-51 adjuvant and granulocyte-macrophage colony stimulating factor (GM-CSF). For those patients vaccinated with peptides in adjuvant with GM-CSF, CD8 T cell responses were detectable in 80% of patients in the SIN, but in only 42% of patients in their peripheral blood (Slingluff et al., 2003). This suggests that evaluation of the SIN is a more sensitive assessment of vaccine immunogenicity. CD8 T cells expanded from the SIN were also capable of lysing melanoma cells that naturally express the source melanoma proteins, thus, the T cells generated have adequate affinity to cause tumor cell lysis (Yamshchikov et al., 2001). We have continued to incorporate this approach in many of our trials both for its value in measuring immunogenicity and for its potential for elucidating the biology of T cell trafficking into and out of secondary lymphoid organs.

7. Vaccination with Peptides in Adjuvant Is More Immunogenic than a Dendritic Cell Vaccine Using Monocyte Derived Immature DC Pulsed with Peptides

The trial mentioned earlier, and several others, incorporated 4 melanoma peptides including two HLA-A*0201-restricted peptides ($gp100_{280-288}$ and $Tyr_{369-377D}$), the HLA-A3-restricted peptide $gp100_{17-25}$, and the HLA-A1-restricted peptide $Tyr_{240-251S}$ (Table 1). This vaccine preparation is abbreviated 4MP. These peptides have been coadministered with the tetanus helper peptide described earlier. In the first of these trials, Mel31, immune responses were substantially greater in number and magnitude when the 4MP and tetanus peptides were administered as an emulsion with Montanide ISA-51 and GM-CSF than when administered as peptide-pulsed dendritic cells (DC) (Slingluff *et al.*, 2003). The DC used in that trial expressed phenotypic markers of immature DC, but did induce allogeneic MLR *in vitro*. Patients on that study also received low-dose IL-2 in conjunction with the vaccines. Objective clinical responses were observed in 2 of 13 patients vaccinated in this manner, and in 1 patient vaccinated with peptides pulsed on DC. We remain uncertain about how to proceed with future dendritic cell vaccines because of the complexity of regulation of monocyte-derived human DC. The high immune response rate in the patients vaccinated with the peptides in emulsion with GM-CSF and Montanide ISA-51 supported continued investigation of this approach to peptide vaccination.

8. Low-Dose IL-2 Administered Early with Multipeptide Vaccine Does Not Augment Immunogenicity

The trial described in an earlier section used low-dose IL-2 empirically, with encouraging immunologic and clinical outcomes. However, there was some toxicity attributable to the IL-2. The next trial was designed to assess whether low-dose IL-2 augments the CD8 T cell response to vaccination with 4MP and to assess its toxicity more definitively. Patients received 4MP in GM-CSF and Montanide ISA-51 weekly for 6 weeks, with harvest of a sentinel immunized node 1 week after the third vaccine. Patients were randomized to receive low-dose IL-2 (3 Mu/m^2/day $\times$ 42 days) either beginning 1 week after the first vaccine, or beginning after harvest of the SIN. Thus, for patients with "upfront" IL-2, immune responses in the SIN reflected the results of vaccination with IL-2, whereas in patients with "delayed" IL-2, the SIN reflects results of vaccination without effects of IL-2.

8.1. Immunologic Results

The primary endpoint for this trial design was the T cell response in the SIN. The trial was powered to detect a doubling of immunogenicity with the addition of IL-2 ("upfront" IL-2 arm versus "delayed" IL-2 arm, as measured in the SIN). The study showed paradoxically that the CTL response was reduced by approximately 50% in the "upfront" IL-2 group (Slingluff *et al.*, 2003). This difference was statistically significant. A similar negative effect was observed in the PBL after three vaccines. Thus, the low-dose IL-2 regimen used in this trial appears to decrease T cell responses to peptide vaccines, when administered on the schedule used in the "upfront" arm of the trial.

We have since begun to evaluate effects of this low-dose IL-2 regimen to understand how it may have inhibited T-cell responses. Approximately 1 week after starting this low-dose IL-2, there was a peak in systemic serum IL-5 associated with other changes suggestive of a Th2 shift in circulating T cell responses (Cragun *et al.*, 2005; Woodson *et al.*, 2004). The data suggest that early administration of IL-2 creates a Th2 dominant immunologic environment at a time when induction of CD8 T cell responses is desired. This may have decreased the CD8 T-cell response. Study of the effects of this regimen on regulatory T cells is planned. Interestingly, this low-dose IL-2 regimen was associated with induction of transient autoimmune toxicities (Chianese-Bullock *et al.*, 2005b). Thus, despite the negative results in this trial, this regimen does have immunologic effects that may be useful in immune therapy.

8.2. Clinical Outcome Data

Updates in clinical outcome data show that the 5-year survival rate for patients on this trial receiving vaccine and delayed IL-2 is 74% and for patients receiving vaccine and upfront IL-2 is only 47% (Fig. 2A). These values are based on very mature follow-up data. This study enrolled only 40 patients, so it was not powered to identify differences in clinical outcome for the two arms of the trial. Nonetheless, the p value for this survival curve difference approaches significance, at 0.12. Also, the disease-free survival curves show a trend toward better outcome for patients in which IL-2 administration was delayed (Fig. 2B). Regardless, the overall survival and disease-free survival rates for patients receiving these vaccines in adjuvant is higher than expected, with overall 5-year survival of approximately 60%, and 5-year disease-free survival of approximately 40% (not shown). These findings are very provocative for two reasons. First, the clinical outcome is better for the patient group with higher T-cell responses. Second, these data suggest that the timing of IL-2 administration may have significant effects on immune responses to vaccination and on clinical outcome of combination immunotherapy. These data provide justification for a larger randomized trial to test for definitive survival benefit with vaccination and low-dose IL-2 in the adjuvant setting, which is being planned now.

9. Expanding the Repertoire of Melanoma Reactivity Using Multipeptide Vaccines

One limitation of vaccines based on a small number of peptides is the heterogeneity of tumor antigen expression in human cancers. First-generation peptide vaccines have commonly used a single peptide antigen restricted by a single

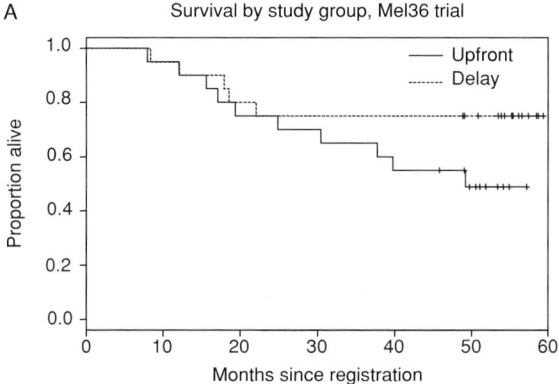

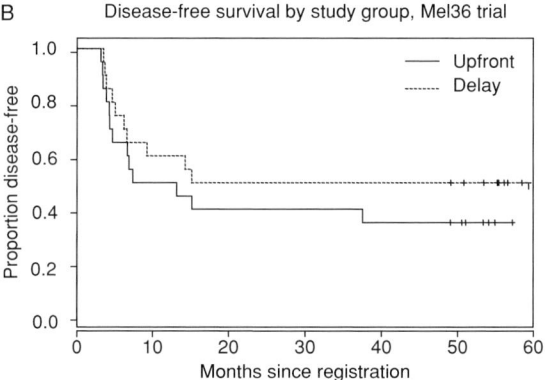

Figure 2 Overall survival and the disease-free survival of patients on Mel36 trial. Patients received the 4MP peptide vaccine and low-dose IL-2 on the "upfront" schedule (Upfront) and for patients receiving the 4MP peptide vaccine and low-dose IL-2 on the "delayed" schedule (Delay). Follow-up information at 45–60 months is available for all living patients.

HLA class I molecule. However, metastatic tumors contain a heterogeneous population of cells with respect to protein expression. Based on the emergence of metastases that have lost expression of target antigens (Riker et al., 1999; Thurner et al., 1999), vaccines that incorporate single melanoma derived epitopes may be inadequate in generating a complete immune response against the tumor. Furthermore, there is heterogeneity in the T-cell repertoire of patients reactive to melanoma antigens. We hypothesized that vaccines incorporating larger numbers of peptide antigens (1) would induce T-cell responses in a larger percentage of patients and (2) would lead to T-cell responses directed against multiple antigens, with a greater probability of tumor eradication. These hypotheses were prompted also by the observation in patient VMM5 of a process we describe as immune adaptation, where a spontaneous shift of T-cell repertoire was adaptive for an immune escape phenotype.

9.1. Long-Term Survivor of Metastatic Melanoma Developed Spontaneous Shift of Repertoire of CD8 T Cell for Melanoma Antigens

We evaluated CD8 T-cell responses to HLA-A2-restricted peptide antigens, in tumor-involved and tumor-free nodes. Of particular interest is a shift observed in the CD8 T-cell repertoire coincident with the development of antigen loss by the tumor. The HLA-A°0201$^+$ patient VMM5 was originally diagnosed with melanoma on his back, and recurred twice in LN over approximately 12 years, then remained disease-free with surgical therapy only until he died 5 years later at the age of 91 of unrelated causes. This surprising clinical outcome prompted detailed investigation of the host–tumor relationship. The first tumor presented at least six peptide epitopes restricted by HLA-A2, including MART-1/MelanA$_{27-35}$ and Tyr$_{369-377D}$ (Skipper et al., 1996a, 1999; Slingluff et al., 1993). T cells infiltrating the first recurrent tumor had dominant reactivity to the MART-1 peptide but did not recognize the Tyr peptide. However, melanoma cells in the second recurrent tumor failed to present the MART-1$_{27-35}$ peptide but continued to present Tyr$_{369-377D}$. Interestingly, there was a coinciding change in the reactivity of T cells both in the recurrent tumor and in the peripheral blood, such that the dominant T-cell reactivity at the time of the second recurrence was to the Tyr$_{369-377D}$ peptide. This finding (Yamshchikov et al., 2005) suggests that immune reactivity to subdominant epitopes may develop in patients and function as a defense against immune escape due to antigen loss by tumor cells. This provides rationale for vaccinating against panels of antigens including those that may not be immunodominant.

9.2. Twelve-Peptide Vaccine Improves Breadth and Magnitude of T-Cell Response Compared to Four-Peptide Vaccine

Over 50 peptide epitopes for melanoma-reactive CD8 T cell have been defined, but only a few have been studied in human clinical trials (Jaeger et al., 1996; Marchand et al., 1995; Nestle et al., 1998a; Rosenberg et al., 1998; Scheibenbogen et al., 2000; Weber et al., 1999). Also, most studies have focused on HLA-A2 restricted peptides, particularly those that are available through the Clinical Trials Evaluation Program (CTEP), which are now in multicenter trials through ECOG. Thus, trials limited to HLA-A2 restricted peptides exclude over 50% of patients, and are limited in their antigenic breadth. To address these issues, we developed a vaccine using 12 peptides derived from both MDP and cancer-testis antigens, with four restricted by each of three different MHC molecules (12MP) (Table 2). This mixture included 5 peptides not, to our knowledge, previously evaluated in humans.

9.2.1. Vaccination with Peptide Mixtures: Overall Results

We completed enrollment of 51 patients on this trial, with 50 patients evaluable for immune responses by ELIspot assay after one *in vitro* stimulation. Overall, 10 of the 12 peptides were found to be immunogenic. Only $Tyr_{146-156}$ and $MAGE-A1_{161-169}$ have not been associated with T-cell responses yet, but were evaluable in only 6 HLA-A1$^+$ patients. A larger experience with both peptides is necessary to estimate the rate of immunogenicity more precisely. Furthermore, T-cell responses to these peptides may be augmented by coadministration of helper peptides from corresponding Tyr and MAGE-A1, which are included in the helper peptide mixture in the current ongoing studies (see later section). T cells generated from vaccinated patients were able to lyse melanoma cell targets naturally expressing the peptide antigens, in a specific manner (Chianese-Bullock *et al.*, 2005a).

In patients vaccinated with 4MP, responses were detected only to the peptides included in that vaccine even though the lymphocytes were stimulated *in vitro* with all of the 12 peptides prior to the assay. This typically led to responses to only one peptide per patient on that arm. For patients vaccinated with 12MP, responses were commonly observed to multiple peptides for each relevant HLA restriction element. Overall, for patients vaccinated with 12MP, 100% had an immune response to at least one peptide in the blood or SIN, and 83% responded to at least one peptide in the blood alone (Table 2). The rates of detectable immune responses were lower in patients vaccinated with 4MP ($p < 0.05$ for the response in PBL or SIN). Furthermore, the cumulative T cell response magnitude for *all* 12 peptides was approximately 2–2.5-fold higher for patients vaccinated with 12MP than those vaccinated with 4MP ($p = 0.03$ for the SIN, Fig. 3).

9.2.2. Peptides Not Previously Evaluated in Humans Found to be Immunogenic

Four of the 5 peptides not previously tested in humans were immunogenic, including $MAGE-A10_{254-262}$, $gp100_{614-622}$, $MAGE-A1_{96-104}$, and $NY-ESO-1_{53-62}$ (Slingluff *et al.*, 2004). Furthermore, at least three of these induced T cells have adequate avidity to recognize their cognate peptide antigens when

Table 2 Immune Responses to Peptides in 12MP Vaccine Preparation

Epitope	Sequence	MHC	Reference	N^a	Patients with immune response by IVS ELIspot[b]		
					PBL	SIN	Overall
Tyr$_{240-251}$S	**_DAEKSDICTDEY_**	A1	(Kittlesen et al., 1998)	16	69%	86%	81%
Tyr$_{146-156}$	SSDYVIPIGTY		(Kawakami et al., 1998; Kittlesen et al., 1998)	6	0%	0%	0%
MAGE-A1$_{161-169}$	EADPTGHSY		(Traversari et al., 1992)	6	0%	0%	0%
MAGE-A3$_{168-176}$	EVDPIGHLY		(Celis et al., 1994; Gaugler et al., 1994)	6	67%	33%	83%
Tyr$_{369-377}$D	**_YMDGTMSQV_**	A2	(Skipper et al., 1996a)	27	44%	44%	56%
gp100$_{209-217}$M	IMDQVPFSV		(Kawakami et al., 1995)	12	75%	100%	100%
gp100$_{280-288}$	YLEPGPVTA		(Cox et al., 1994)	27	0%	8%	7%
MAGE-A10$_{254-262}$	GLYDGMEHL		(Huang et al., 1999)	12	75%	67%	83%
_gp100_$_{17-25}$	**_ALLAVGATK_**	A3	(Skipper et al., 1996b)	20	75%	84%	90%
gp100$_{614-622}$	LIYRRRLMK		(Kawakami et al., 1998)	13	62%	31%	62%
MAGE-A1$_{96-104}$	SLFRAVITK		(Chaux et al., 1999a)	13	62%	75%	77%
NY-ESO-1$_{53-62}$	ASGPGGGAPR		(Wang et al., 1998)	13	46%	38%	46%
4MP overall[b]		all		26	69%	72%	77%
12MP overall[b]		all		24	83%	92%	100%

Index peptides are shown in bold italics. These three, and a fourth peptide shown in italics were included in 4MP.
[a]Number of evaluable patients with each HLA type.
[b]For peptides included in both 4MP and 12MP preparations, data from both arms are shown.

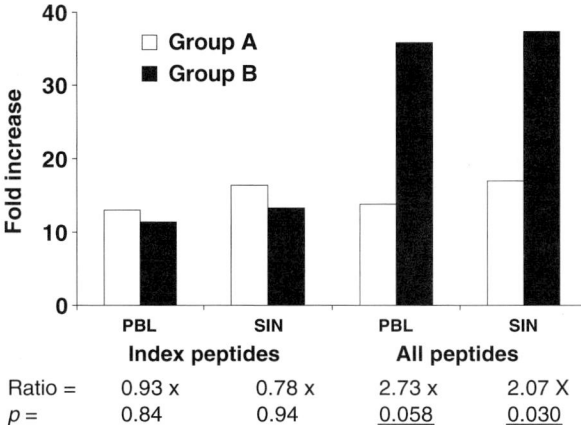

Figure 3 The magnitude of the T-cell response to index peptides or to all peptides in the vaccine preparation was determined as a maximum fold-increase over baseline, and these values were summed for each patient. These values were averaged across the study populations for Group A (vaccinated with 4MP mixture) or for Group B (vaccinated with 12MP mixture). The magnitude of the T-cell response to vaccination is reported here for responses to index peptides only, and to all peptides, overall. The ratio of the T-cell response magnitude for Group B relative to Group A is reported below the x-axis, and the p-value for differences between study groups is shown.

naturally processed and presented on melanoma cells (Chianese-Bullock et al., 2005a).

9.2.3. Competition for Binding to Class I MHC Molecules Does Not Diminish CD8 T-Cell Responses to Lower Affinity Peptides

One concern with using the 12MP vaccine was that peptides would compete for binding to MHC molecules such that peptides with high affinity would prevent binding of those with lower affinity. To evaluate this possible inhibition of immunogenicity, the Mel39 trial was designed to compare responses to one index peptide for each HLA molecule (HLA-A1, -A2, and -A3) in both study arms. The index peptides were $Tyr_{240-251S}$ (HLA-A1), $Tyr_{369-377D}$ (HLA-A2), and $gp100_{17-25}$ (HLA-A3) (Table 2). The cumulative data reveal no difference in the frequency of T-cell responses to the index peptides in the blood or the SIN, or overall (p values (Chi-sq) in PBL = 0.75, SIN = 0.79, overall = 0.71) (Slingluff et al., 2004). Furthermore, the magnitudes of the T-cell response to index peptides in the PBL or SIN were comparable for both groups (Fig. 3). Thus, these data taken together support the conclusion that competition for MHC binding does not diminish immunogenicity of multiple peptides administered in the manner used in this study.

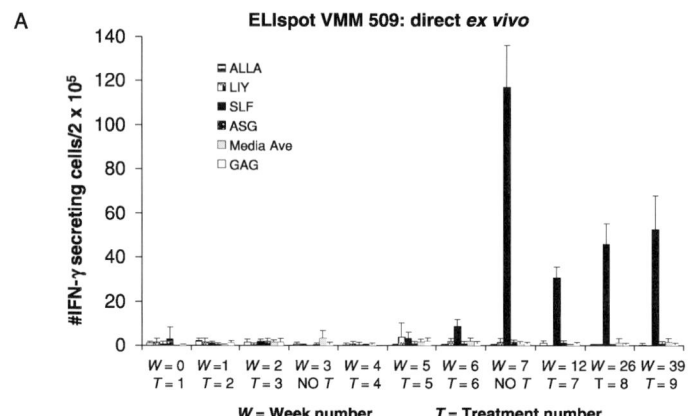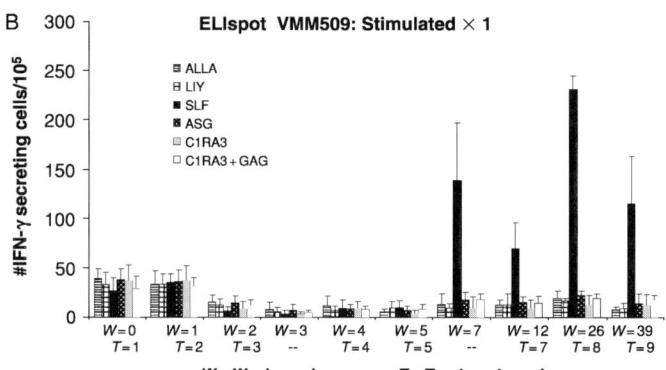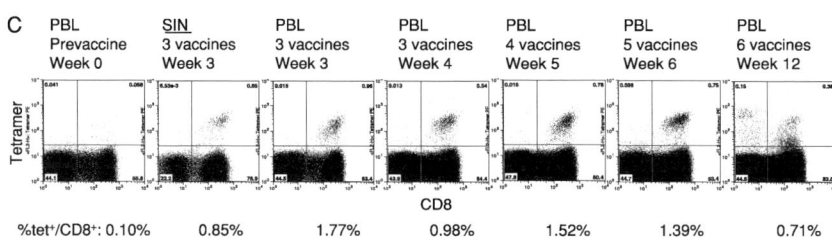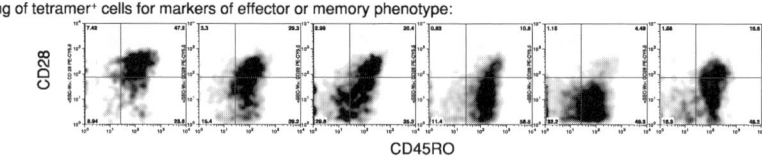

10. *Ex Vivo* Analyses of T-Cell Responses to Class I MHC Restricted Peptides

To date, our analyses of CD8 T-cell responses have primarily used ELIspot assays after one *in vitro* sensitization (IVS ELIspot). However, in our newer studies, we are evaluating T-cell responses without an *in vitro* sensitization by ELIspot and tetramer analyses cryopreserved lymphocytes. Direct ELIspot assays performed *ex vivo* detect vaccine-induced T cells, after vaccination with 12MP. An example is shown for an HLA-A3$^+$ patient, which demonstrates responses to the MAGE-A1$_{96-104}$ peptide after 5 weekly vaccines that increased with subsequent vaccinations (Fig. 4A). The later samples had 30–116 responding T cells per 200,000 PBL. Assuming that approximately 10% of PBL are CD8 cells, this assay shows the induction of functional antigen-specific T cells representing 0.15–0.58% of circulating CD8 T cells. Comparison to the IVS ELIspot assay performed after one sensitization reveals a comparable pattern of response (Fig. 4B).

Tetramers were obtained in the past, from the NIAID-sponsored core facility in Atlanta, and results are published (Slingluff, Jr. *et al.*, 2003). Currently, we obtain tetramers from Beckman-Coulter. We have validated tetramers for 7 of the 12 peptides [Tyr$_{240-251}$S (using Tyr$_{242-251}$), Tyr$_{369-377}$D, gp100$_{209-217}$M (using gp100 $_{209-217}$), gp100$_{280-288}$, MAGE-A10$_{254-262}$, gp100$_{17-25}$, and gp100$_{614-622}$]. Validation was performed with peptide-reactive T-cell lines obtained from patients with preexisting or vaccine-stimulated reactivity to the relevant peptide. Validation of the MAGE-A3$_{168-176}$/HLA-A1 tetramer is pending. For the

Figure 4 Characteristics of vaccine reactive T cells. (A–B) ELIspot data from an example patient vaccinated with the 12MP and tetanus peptides, in an emulsion of Montanide ISA-51 adjuvant and GM-CSF. PBL sample dates are labeled on the *x*-axis based on vaccine treatment number (*T*) and week since study initiation (*W*). Prevaccine blood was drawn on the same date of the first vaccine, but prior to vaccine administration, and is labeled $W = 0$, $T = 1$. The PBL were assayed against the 4 HLA-A3-restricted melanoma peptides in the 12MP mixture and are abbreviated with the single letter abbreviations for the first several amino acids: gp100$_{17-25}$ (ALLA), gp100$_{614-622}$ (LIY), MAGE-A1$_{96-104}$ (SLF), NY-ESO-1$_{53-62}$ (ASG). (A) Data from ELIspot assay performed directly *ex vivo* on cryopreserved lymphocytes. Cryopreserved PBL were incubated in assay wells with one of the test peptides alone, or (as negative controls) with media alone or with an irrelevant HIV-gag peptide (GAG). (B) Data from ELIspot assay performed after one *in vitro* sensitization with the 12MP mixture. After 14 days, the expanded PBMC were incubated in assay wells with C1R-A3 antigen-presenting cells pulsed with one of the test peptides, or (as negative controls) C1R-A3 cells alone (C1RA3), or C1R-A3 cells pulsed with the irrelevant HIV-gag peptide (GAG). (C) For another patient, tetramer data are shown for HLA-A3/ALLAVGATK (gp100 $_{17-25}$) in an HLA-A3$^+$ patient on the Mel39 trial. Tetramer$^+$ cells accounted for almost 2% of circulating CD8 cells. Under each data plot for tetramer$^+$ CD8$^+$ cells, data are shown for the proportion of Tetramer$^+$ cells that stain with CD28 and/or CD45RO.

remaining peptides in the 12-peptide mixture (Tyr$_{146-156}$, MAGE-A1$_{161-169}$, MAGE-A1$_{96-104}$, NY-ESO-1$_{53-62}$) validation failed, tetramers could not be made, or validation has not been addressed because T cells are not available.

Using tetramers we have observed increases in peptide reactive T cells with vaccination, with up to 2% of circulating CD8 T cells recognizing individual peptides. In Fig. 4C tetramer data are shown for HLA-A3/ALLAVGATK (gp100$_{17-25}$) in an HLA-A3$^+$ patient on the Mel39 trial. There is a substantial decrease in CD28 staining during repeated weekly vaccines, then an increase in CD28 staining 6 weeks after the last vaccine. The cells are predominantly CD45RO$^+$; so the changes in CD28 staining may suggest an initial increase in the proportion of effector-T cells, and then a reversion to more of an effector memory phenotype as the numbers of tetramer-positive cells decreases 6 weeks after the last vaccine. These are anecdotal data but show the ability to detect T-cell responses directly *ex vivo*. They also show that it is feasible to begin to characterize the T-cell response to vaccination, and how these data may explain observed changes in the magnitude of the response.

11. Modulation of Responses by Combination of CD4 and CD8 T-Cell Vaccination, and Modulation of Regulatory Function

The work presented above demonstrates the ability to induce specific CD8 T-cell responses with peptide vaccines in patients with melanoma. However, the magnitude of the T-cell responses remains low in most patients, and clinical responses have been observed in only 3–6% of patients in most series. Thus, it is critical now to identify strategies to improve the magnitude of the responses and to improve clinical response rates. Our current approach toward vaccination in the adjuvant setting is to evaluate vaccination to recruit melanoma-specific CD4 T cells with multipeptide vaccination and to combine that with strategies to modulate regulatory mechanisms, in addition to continued multipeptide vaccination to activate CD8 cells.

A limited view of helper T cells as simply a source of IL-2 has yielded to a greater understanding of the more fundamental and comprehensive role of CD4 cells in initiation and maintenance of CD8 T-cell responses to tumors (Kayaga *et al.*, 1999; Pardoll and Topalian, 1998). Furthermore, adoptive therapy with CD4 T cells has been shown to induce tumor protection in some model systems (Kahn *et al.*, 1991). Thus, the protective immunity induced by tumor cell vaccines appears to be mediated both by CD8 and CD4 T cells.

Despite the acknowledged importance of stimulating helper T cells as a component of active immunotherapy, the effect of a helper cell stimulus on CTL responses has not been addressed definitively. In one vaccine study,

CD8 T-cell responses to class I MHC-associated Tyr peptides appeared to be increased by coadministration of keyhole limpet hemocyanin (KLH) (Scheibenbogen et al., 2003). Our approach in past studies incorporates a tetanus helper peptide also with the intention of providing nonspecific helper-T cell stimulation at the site of vaccination. However, vaccination with cytotoxic T-cell epitopes may be more successful when the vaccine includes helper epitopes from the same protein(s) rather than with nonspecific helper epitopes. A small number of trials have been performed to test this concept in the setting of a single class I restricted peptide and a single class II restricted peptide (Knutson et al., 2001; Phan et al., 2003; Wong et al., 2004). Overall, there has been a paucity of human experience with tumor-associated helper peptides in cancer patients, and much of the work has been limited to pilot studies and to a very limited number of peptides. Definitive evaluation is warranted of whether vaccination with melanoma-associated helper peptides can induce antigen-reactive $CD4^+$ T-cell responses and whether vaccination with melanoma-associated helper peptides can increase $CD8^+$ responses, compared to vaccination with a nonspecific helper peptide. We have initiated three clinical trials to test these hypotheses.

11.1. Immunogenicity and Possible Clinical Benefit of Vaccination with a Mixture of 6 Melanoma Helper Peptides

Peptides presented by class II MHC molecules for recognition by CD4 cells have been identified less readily than those associated with class I MHC molecules. We have collaborated with the laboratory of Dr Walter Storkus, at the Pittsburgh Cancer Institute, to identify several peptides from MART-1/Melan-A, Tyr, and gp100 presented by HLA-DR molecules (Kierstead et al., 2001; Zarour et al., 2000). Additional epitopes have been identified from cancer-testis antigens. A summary of class II MHC associated peptide epitopes that have been defined has been published in a recent review (Novellino et al., 2005). We are currently performing a phase I/II trial (Mel41) of vaccination with a mixture of 6 melanoma helper peptides (6MHP) (Table 3). In this study, patients are vaccinated with 200–800 μg of each peptide and GM-CSF and Montanide ISA-51 adjuvant in each of two vaccine sites on days 1, 8, and 15. One week after the third vaccine, a SIN is harvested from the groin, representing a draining node from the replicate vaccine site in that thigh. Three additional vaccines are given weekly at the primary vaccination site. The trial design included a phase I dose escalation component and a subsequent randomized phase II component at three dose levels. The phase I component has been completed, with at least 3 patients accrued sequentially to each of three dose levels (200, 400, and 800 μg/dose of each peptide), and safety is supported at each dose level.

Table 3 Class II MHC Restricted Melanoma Peptides Used in 6MHP Vaccine

Epitope	Peptide sequence	MHC	Reference
Tyr$_{56-70}$	AQNILLSNAPLGPQFP[a]	DR4	(Topalian et al., 1996)
Tyr$_{388-406}$	FLLHHAFVDSIFEQWLQRHRP	DR15	(Kobayashi et al., 1998)
Melan-A/MART-1$_{51-73}$	RNGYRALMDKSLHVGTQCALTRR	DR4	(Zarour et al., 2000)
MAGE-A3$_{281-295}$	TSYVKVLHHMVKISG	DR11	(Manici et al., 1999)
MAGE-A1,2,3,6$_{121-134}$	LLKYRAREPVTKAE	DR13	(Chaux et al., 1999b)
Gp100$_{44-59}$	WNRQLYPEWTEAQRLD	DR4/DR1	(Halder et al., 1997; Li et al., 1998)

[a]This peptide has been modified by addition of an N-terminal alanine residue to prevent cyclization of glutamine.

11.1.1. Preliminary Immunologic Findings

Preliminary immunologic data were obtained from five patients from this trial. Mononuclear cells from the SIN of these five patients were evaluated in triplicate for proliferative responses to each of the 6MHP and the tetanus helper peptide. Supernatants were also collected from these cultures and were evaluated for Th1 and Th2 cytokines. As controls, SIN samples from five patients on the Mel31 trial (vaccinated with 4 class I MHC-restricted melanoma peptides and the tetanus peptide in the same adjuvant) were evaluated for proliferative responses to the 6MHP and to the tetanus helper peptide. Responses (stimulation indices >4) were detected in four of five patients on the Mel41 trial (patients 582, 537, 504, and 425), with reactivity to 1, 4, 6, and 3 different peptides, respectively (Fig. 5A). In contrast, no reactivity was observed to any of the MHP in patients from Mel31. However, tetanus peptide reactivity was seen in all five patients vaccinated with that peptide but only at low level in one of five patients on Mel41 (Fig. 5B). The patients responding to the 6MHP peptides often expressed HLA-DR molecules different from those for which the corresponding peptides have been reported to be restricted. This supports the hypothesis that they are promiscuous in binding to varied HLA-DR molecules.

Supernatants from these proliferation assays were assayed by multiplex bead assay for the Th1 cytokines IFN-γ, TNF-α, and IL-2, and for the Th2 cytokines IL-5, IL-4, and IL-10. The principal findings in this pilot analysis were that the

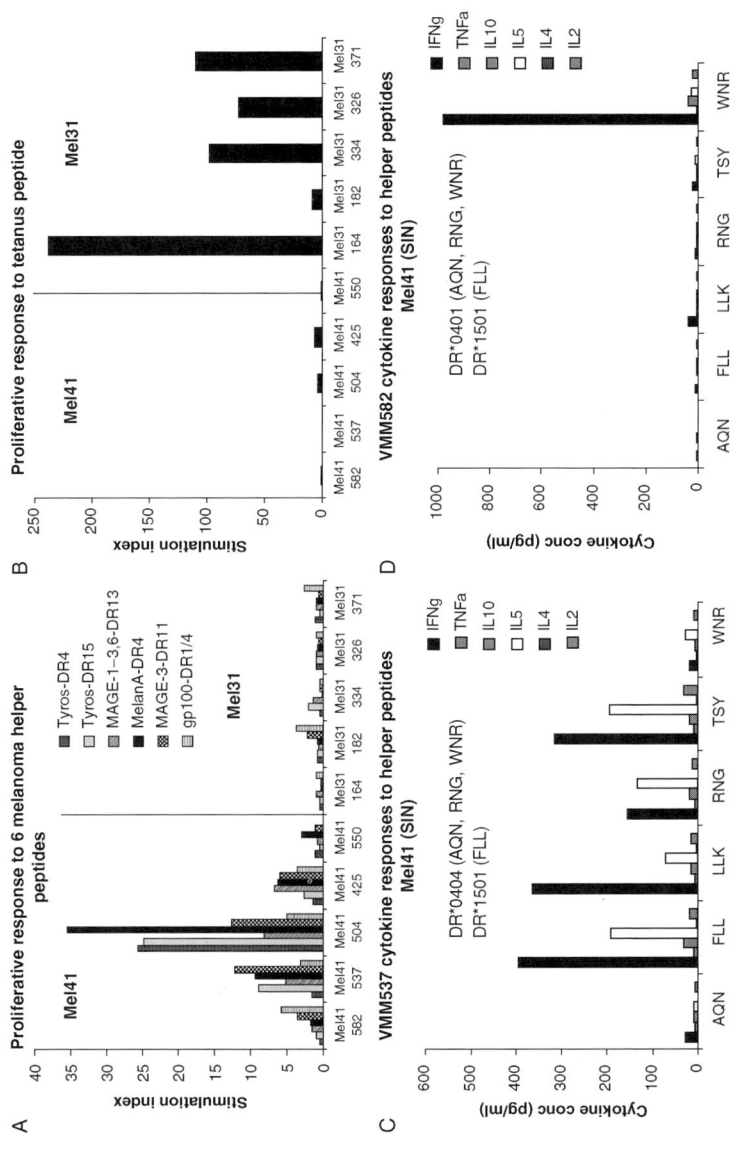

Figure 5 Proliferative and cytokine responses to helper peptides in sentinel immunized nodes. (A–B) Proliferative responses to the 6MHP (A) and to the tetanus helper peptide (B) were measured in a 5-day tritiated thymidine uptake assay on cell suspensions obtained from sentinel immunized nodes for patients on the Mel31 and Mel41 trials. Results are reported as stimulation indices (SI > 4 considered positive). (C–D) Cytokine levels were measured in culture supernatants. Note that the peptides to which reactivity was measured are abbreviated by the first three amino acids of the sequence. These are listed in the same order as the peptides listed in Fig. 5A, though in Fig. 5A the peptides are identified by their source protein. The full sequences are listed and defined in Table 3.

263

dominant cytokines detected were IFN-γ and IL-5, suggesting a balanced Th1/Th2 response. In most cases, the amount of IFN-γ detected was slightly higher than that of IL-5. Representative cytokine data are presented for patient VMM537 (Fig. 5C). For patient 582, the proliferative and cytokine responses were limited to a single peptide, and the response was almost exclusively a Th1 response (Fig. 5D). These preliminary data support the immunogenicity of all six helper peptides, the induction of Th1/Th2 balanced or Th1 dominant responses, and promiscuity of the helper peptides for varied HLA-DR molecules.

11.1.2. Preliminary Clinical Outcomes

Patients have been eligible for this Mel41 study if they have stage IIIB, IIIC, or IV melanoma, whether resected or measurable. Thus far, of 12 patients with measurable disease in whom clinical response may be assessed, 2 patients have experienced objective partial clinical responses (17%). At this point, these data suggest possible clinical benefit by vaccination with the mixture of MHP.

11.2. Trial Design for Evaluation of MHP in Combination Vaccines for Patients with Advanced Melanoma (E1602)

The University of Virginia is leading the ECOG trial E1602, for patients with advanced measurable metastatic melanoma, who are randomized to one of four arms: (1) 12MP alone, (2) 12MP and tetanus helper peptide, (3) 12MP and 6MHP, and (4) 6MHP alone. That trial opened in 2005 and is accruing patients. Immunologic and clinical response data will be collected for all study arms, and data will be collected for T-cell responses in blood, SIN, and tumor deposits. Importantly, work by Walter Storkus' group demonstrates that patients with renal cell cancer mount a Th2 dominant response to tumor antigen when they have advanced measurable disease, whereas patients with resected disease mount a Th1 dominant response (Tatsumi et al., 2002). Thus, it is critical also to evaluate the role of helper peptides separately in patients without measurable disease as well as in those with measurable disease.

11.3. Trial Design for Evaluation of MHP and Combination with Cyclophosphamide for Melanoma Patients in the Adjuvant Setting (Mel44)

For patients without measurable disease but at high risk for recurrence of melanoma (resected stages IIB-IV melanoma), we have initiated an ongoing clinical trial, UVA-Mel44, which is designed to evaluate the safety and immunogenicity of administration of peptide mixtures containing melanoma-derived class I and class II MHC-restricted peptides, and the effects of pretreatment with cyclophosphamide. It is being conducted at the University of Virginia, MD Anderson Cancer Center, and Fox Chase Cancer Center.

11.3.1. Vaccination with Helper Peptide Mixtures

Patients are randomized among four study arms by vaccination with the tetanus helper peptide (Group A, Group B) or with the 6MHP (Group C, Group D). Patients in all arms are vaccinated with the 12MP preparation (Table 2). This protocol will permit evaluation of whether addition of MDP and cancer-testis antigen derived class II MHC-restricted peptides and activation of T_h responses augment the magnitude and persistence of CD8 T cell responses to the class I MHC-restricted peptides in the vaccine. It is also a large enough study (168 patients) that some data on clinical outcome will be evaluable.

11.3.2. Effects of Cyclophosphamide Pretreatment

This trial was also designed to evaluate the safety and immunologic effects of administration of cyclophosphamide prior to initiation of the vaccine series. Thus, patients are randomized, also, either to receive (Groups B and D) or not (Groups A and C) a single dose of cyclophosphamide (300 mg/m^2) before the first vaccine. The literature, and unpublished experience, contains conflicting data on the effects of pretreatment with cyclophosphamide. In this fairly large study, we will be able to assess the effects on both CD8 and CD4 T-cell responses to defined peptide antigens, so it should be possible to make definitive conclusions about its effects. We also will evaluate effects on serum cytokine levels and on T-cell subsets, especially regulatory T cells. We expect this to be the beginning of a more comprehensive analysis of combination therapies for melanoma using vaccines and chemotherapy, targeted molecular therapies, or radiation, in the years ahead.

12. Cancer Vaccine Development Requires Elucidation of Biology of the Host–Tumor Relationship in Human and Murine Systems, In Vivo and In Vitro

Our early work on identification of MHC-associated peptide epitopes for melanoma-reactive T cells, and parallel work in other laboratories worldwide, led to characterization of some of the relevant antigens for immune rejection of melanoma and other cancers. However, it was probably naïve for us to think that vaccination with one or several peptides alone could lead to clinical cures in most patients. The fact that melanoma metastasizes and progresses in patients with clinically normal immune systems suggest that those tumors have developed mechanisms for immune escape. This is strongly supported by murine studies (Shankaran et al., 2001) and by clinical observation in humans (Yamshchikov et al., 2005). We are convinced that the concept of immune therapy, and the approach of peptide vaccines in particular, has merit for the prevention of death due to melanoma. However, there is clearly a lot of work to be done in elucidating the immunobiology of the host–tumor relationship in the cancer-bearing host. Clinical trials of peptide vaccines are uniquely valuable for their use of specific molecular targets of the T-cell response, and the ability to dissect elements of the immune response to those antigens.

Importantly, peptide vaccine strategies in murine models are also critically important for characterizing immunobiological principles that may have relevance in humans and that may be evaluable in a subsequent clinical trial. It is impossible to perform in humans some of the critically important studies, and murine models provide valuable opportunities for progress toward successful immunotherapy of melanoma and other cancers. Our research groups are increasingly integrating their clinical and laboratory findings for the purposes of continued progress in understanding the host–tumor relationship and development of optimal immune therapies for melanoma.

13. A Murine Model to Evaluate Immunity to the MDP-Derived Peptide Ag from Tyrosinase

MDPs are among the most widely expressed melanoma antigens. However, one concern with using them in melanoma vaccines is that their success may be impeded by self-tolerance. To date there has been no detailed study of how tolerance to any Ag expressed in melanocytes is established, maintained, or broken, despite the clinical relevance of this information. A second concern is the lack of knowledge concerning effective immunotherapies based on the use of peptide antigens. Again, it is difficult to evaluate alternative strategies rapidly in the setting of human clinical trials. For these reasons, we have developed a murine model to explore the relationship between self-tolerance, skin depigmentation, and immunotherapy for melanoma. Our model uses C57Bl/6 (B6) mice that express a recombinant class I MHC molecule termed "AAD," which consists of the peptide-binding region of human HLA-A*0201 linked to the CD8-binding domain of murine H-2D^d. AAD-restricted CD8 T-cell responses are similar in strength to those restricted by murine class I molecules (Newberg et al., 1996), and the AAD-restricted peptide epitopes recognized by these mice are the same as recognized by HLA-A*0201$^+$ humans (Engelhard et al., 1991; Man et al., 1995; Shirai et al., 1995; Vitiello et al., 1991; Wentworth et al., 1996a,b). B6 mice are Tyr$^+$, and the murine homolog of the HLA-A*0201-restricted Tyr$_{369-377D}$ epitope, termed $\underline{m}$Tyr$_{369}$, differs only by a substitution of F for Y at P1. This change does not significantly influence binding affinity for HLA-A*0201, enabling us to use the AAD transgenic mouse to measure responses against either peptide. We also backcrossed a mutation comprising a complete deletion of the Tyr gene (Rinchik et al., 1993) into the B6-AAD lineage, enabling us to assess self-tolerance to Tyr, and specifically to mTyr$_{369}$. Subsequently, we isolated mTyr$_{369}^{+}$ AAD-specific CD8 T-cell clones from AAD^{+} albino mice, and have developed transgenic mice expressing one of these receptors, designated FH. Finally, we have transfected B16-F1 melanoma cells, which also are mTyr^{+}, with the AAD molecule enabling us to assess the relationship of immune reactivity to mTyr to control of that tumor.

14. Nature of Self-Tolerance to mTyR$_{369}$ and Its Effect on Tumor Control

14.1. Deletion of mTyr$_{369}$-Specific CD8 Cells is Induced by Ag Encounter in Peripheral LN but Not Thymus

We evaluated immune responses to mTyr$_{369}$ after immunization of mice with either a recombinant vaccinia virus encoding full-length mTyr (mTyr-vac) (Colella et al., 2000) or bone marrow-derived DC (BMDC) that had been cultured in GM-CSF and IL4, matured in the presence of either TNFα (Bullock et al., 2000) or CD40L (Bullock et al., 2001) and then pulsed with synthetic peptides. We harvested spleen or peripheral LN at the peak of the response and determined the number of mTyr$_{369}$-specific CD8 T cells by intracellular IFN-γ accumulation (IFN-γ-ICS) and by staining with mTyr$_{369}^{+}$ HLA-A*0201 tetramers. This *ex vivo* approach avoids prolonged *in vitro* T-cell culture, which we have shown to modify their characteristics (Bullock et al., 2001). Immune responses to mTyr$_{369}$ in AAD^{+} albinos were robust, while responses in AAD^{+}Tyr^{+} mice were very low, indicating that self-tolerance to this antigen is based at least in part on diminished T-cell reactivity.

Tyr is expressed exclusively in melanocytes in the basal layer of the epidermis, hair follicles, and retinal pigment epithelium (Gimenez et al., 2003; Han et al., 2002; Kunisada et al., 1998; Porter et al., 1999; Slominski et al., 1994; Tief et al., 1996), although high-cycle PCR analysis has suggested that low level expression is widespread in many tissues (Battyani et al., 1993) including the thymus (Battyani et al., 1993; Derbinski et al., 2001). Nonetheless, thymic tissue from AAD^{+}Tyr^{+} donors implanted into neonatally thymectomized AAD^{+} albino hosts did not diminish responses to mTyr$_{369}$, and responses to mTyr$_{369}$ in thymectomized AAD^{+}Tyr^{+} hosts implanted with thymic tissue from AAD^{+} albino donors remained undetectable (Nichols et al., 2006), suggesting that tolerance to mTyr$_{369}$ did not result from exposure of developing T cells to this Ag on thymic epithelial cells. In addition, there is no alteration in either the number or differentiation state of $\underline{m}Tyr_{369}$-specific FH TCR transgenic (tgTCR) cells in the thymuses of AAD^+Tyr^+ and AAD^+ albino mice. This confirms that tolerance to $\underline{m}Tyr_{369}$ is not due to immature T-cell encounter with this Ag in the thymus, and suggests that it is due to mature T-cell encounter with Ag in the periphery.

The development of CD8 T-cell tolerance toward Ags expressed selectively in several peripheral nonlymphoid tissues has been studied using mice expressing tgTCR (Kurts et al., 1997; Limmer et al., 1998, 2000; Mayerova et al., 2004; Morgan et al., 1999; Ohlen et al., 2001, 2002; Tanchot et al., 1998; Vezys et al., 2000). These studies have established that in some cases, CD8 T cells exposed to Ag in this way sometimes express a subset of activation markers, followed by limited proliferation and deletion without acquisition of effector function. However, CD8 cells could persist in an unactivated (ignorant) state if the level was sufficiently low (Kurts et al., 1999), or persist in an anergic state (Limmer et al., 1998, 2000; Ohlen et al., 2001, 2002; Tanchot et al., 1998). We evaluated the nature of peripheral self-tolerance to $\underline{m}Tyr_{369}$ by adoptive transfer of CFSE-labeled Thy 1.2^+FH^+ CD8 cells from AAD^+ albino donors into Tyr^+ or albino Thy 1.1^+AAD^+ recipients. After 3 days, cells reisolated from the peripheral LN of albino hosts were still at rest, while those from Tyr^+ hosts had undergone several cell divisions (Fig. 6). T cells activated by endogenous Tyr underwent apoptotic death, and the number of cells remaining after 14d was at the lower limit of detection (Nichols et al., 2006). This establishes that self-tolerance to Tyr is based in part on T cell activation-induced deletion and is the first description of peripheral deletion as a mechanism for tolerance to an Ag expressed in melanocytes.

14.2. Endogenous Tyr Presentation by Radioresistant Antigen Presenting Cells

It has been established that CD8 deletional tolerance to Ag expressed in the pancreatic islets is due to cross-presentation of Ag by DC localized to pancreatic LN (Kurts et al., 1997; Morgan et al., 1999) but has not been evaluated in other models. We investigated the nature of the $\underline{m}Tyr_{369}$-expressing cells that mediate deletional self-tolerance in peripheral LN. T-cell activation was not observed in the spleen, suggesting that it was mediated by skin-draining dendritic cells that cross-presented endogenous Tyr. Based on the hypothesis that these cells should be DC derived from radiosensitive precursors, we created chimeras in which bone marrow from AAD^{neg} donors was introduced into lethally irradiated AAD^+Tyr^+ recipients, as well as the converse $AAD^+ \rightarrow AAD^{neg}Tyr^+$ chimeras. Surprisingly, we found that proliferation and

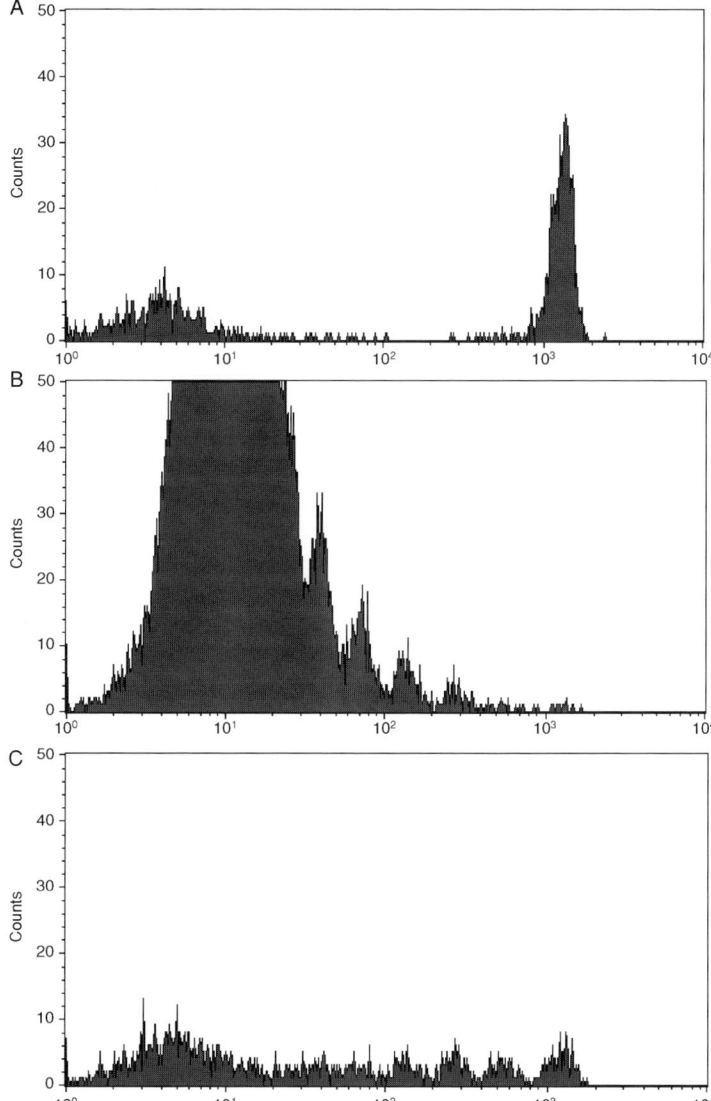

Figure 6 FH tgTCR$^+$ T cells are activated but fail to accumulate after adoptive transfer into AAD$^+$Tyr$^+$ recipients. FH tgTCR$^+$ from albino Thy 1.2 donors were CFSE-labeled and transferred into AAD$^+$ recipients. Cells were gated on tgTCR (Va8 and Vb11) and CD8 indicated Thy 1.1 recipients. In some cases, recipients were immunized with mTyr-vac. Peripheral LN were harvested and analyzed by flow cytometry 3 days later.

Table 4 Peripheral Deletion of mTyr369-Specific CD8 T Cells is Mediated by a Radioresistant Cell in Peripheral LN

Bone marrow donor	Bone marrow recipient	Response of adoptively transferred mTyr$_{369}$-specific T cells in peripheral LN
AAD$^+$	AAD^{neg} albino	No activation
AAD^{neg}	AAD$^+$ albino	No activation
none	AAD$^+$ Tyr$^+$	Proliferation and deletion
AAD^{neg}	AAD$^+$ Tyr$^+$	Proliferation and deletion
AAD$^+$	AAD^{neg} Tyr$^+$	No activation

FH T cells were labeled with CFSE and adoptively transferred into the indicated bone marrow chimera. Peripheral LN were harvested 72 h later. CFSE dilution was evaluated by flow cytometry.

deletion of adoptively transferred FH T cells remained intact in the AAD^{neg}→AAD$^+$Tyr$^+$ chimeras but did not occur in the AAD$^+$→AAD^{neg}Tyr$^+$ chimeras (Table 4). The latter result is particularly unexpected, inasmuch as more than 90% of the peripheral CD11b$^+$ and CD11c$^+$ cells were AAD$^+$ after reconstitution (Nichols et al., 2006). As with control mice, T-cell activation under these circumstances led to proliferation followed by deletion. These results indicate that presentation of endogenous mTyr$_{369}$ leading to activation-induced deletion of T cells is mediated by radioresistant cells. It is extremely unlikely that the responsible cells are melanocytes, since they are sessile and have not been found in any lymphoid compartment. Conversely, epidermal Langerhans cells (LC) develop from skin-resident precursors that are resistant to gamma irradiation (Allan et al., 2003; Merad et al., 2002, 2004), and we have identified a population of AAD^{hi} cells with an LC-like phenotype in the peripheral LN but not spleen of AAD^{neg}→AAD$^+$Tyr$^+$ chimeras (Nichols et al., 2006). In addition, LC are located in the epidermis and hair follicles in proximity to melanocytes and carry melanin granules into the peripheral LN of hyperpigmented mice (Hemmi et al., 2001). Taken together, these results strongly suggest that self-tolerance to Tyr, and perhaps to other MDP, is based on cross-presentation by LC. Previous studies have failed to find a role for LC in promoting immunity to cutaneous viruses (Allan et al., 2003; Zhao et al., 2003), although they do play a role in the development of graft-versus-host disease (Merad et al., 2004). It has been suggested that a transgenic Ag expressed in keratinocytes of the skin is cross-presented both by LC and another uncharacterized antigen presenting cells (APC) (Mayerova et al., 2004). However, Ag presentation by LC alone leads to T-cell activation. Using the same maneuver, however, we have demonstrated that presentation of mTyr$_{369}$ by a radio-resistant DC subset in peripheral LN leads to tolerance.

Thus, our work provides the first indication that LC can mediate self-tolerance as well as immunity.

14.3. A Residual Repertoire of Tyr-Specific T Cells in Tyr$^+$ Mice

Despite our inability to detect responses to mTyr$_{369}$ in AAD$^+$Tyr$^+$ mice, they responded relatively well to the closely related human Tyr$_{369-377D}$ epitope (Bullock et al., 2000; Colella et al., 2000), and T-cell lines established on Tyr$_{369-377D}$ cross-reacted on mTyr$_{369}$ (Bullock et al., 2001; Colella et al., 2000). When AAD$^+$ albino mice were immunized with Tyr$_{369-377D}$, and their bulk T cells analyzed *ex vivo* at the peak of a primary response for intracellular IFN-γ accumulation in response to either Tyr$_{369-377D}$ or mTyr$_{369}$, the peptide dose response curves were superimposable and all T cells responded to both epitopes (Bullock and Engelhard, 2006; Engelhard et al., 2002). Thus, in the absence of self-tolerance, few T cells in AAD$^+$ albino mice distinguish between these peptides. However, in AAD$^+$Tyr$^+$ mice immunized with Tyr$_{369-377D}$, only about half of these T cells could cross-react on mTyr$_{369}$ at the maximum peptide dose, and these cells also required 2–3 logs more mTyr$_{369}$ than Tyr$_{369-377D}$ for equivalent recognition (Bullock and Engelhard, 2006). These results indicate that a significant fraction of the mTyr$_{369}$ repertoire has been deleted or anergized in AAD$^+$Tyr$^+$ mice, but by analogy with human melanoma patients, self-tolerance is incomplete. The mTyr$_{369}$-specific T cells remaining have a low avidity for this peptide. The inability of mTyr$_{369}$ to induce discernable proliferation in Tyr$^+$ mice, while it does induce IFN-γ secretion from cells activated with Tyr$_{369-377D}$, is reminiscent of the hierarchical responses to altered peptide ligands (Hemmer et al., 1998), and suggests that many of the mTyr$_{369}$-specific T cells remaining in AAD$^+$Tyr$^+$ mice recognize mTyr$_{369}$ as a weak or partial agonist, while recognizing Tyr$_{369-377D}$ as a full agonist.

14.4. Controlled Entry of Activated Tyr-Specific CD8 T Cells Into Skin

Although we have successfully stimulated the residual mTyr$_{369}$ specific T cells in AAD$^+$Tyr$^+$ mice to delay melanoma outgrowth (see the following sections), we have been unable to induce vitiligo by multiple immunizations of AAD$^+$Tyr$^+$ mice with Tyr$_{369-377D}$-pulsed DC or human or murine Tyr-vac, with or without anti-CTLA4 as an immune enhancement (Colella et al., 2000, unpublished). In contrast to active immunization, adoptive transfer of activated mTyr$_{369}$ specific T-cell lines and clones, as well as naïve splenocytes from AAD$^+$ albino mice, into adult AAD$^+$Tyr$^+$ recipients, regularly causes the development of localized vitiligo within 3 weeks (Colella et al., 2000; Engelhard et al., 2000; Mullins et al., 2001). Importantly, vitiligo induction after adoptive transfer required coadministration of IL-2 and sublethal (700R) irradiation. Irradiation induces release of IL-1, TNFα and IL-6 (Ganss et al., 2002) and upregulates VCAM1 and E-selectin on endothelial cells (Quarmby et al., 1999, 2000), potentially promoting T-cell extravasation into the skin. Indeed, we found that irradiation results in a general increase of CD8 T cells in the skin within 24 h (Fig. 7). After adoptive transfer of CFSE-labeled T-cell lines, we also observed that about 60% of the skin-associated CD8 T cells were mTyr$_{369}$-specific in AAD$^+$Tyr$^+$ recipients, while less than 2% were specific in AAD$^+$ albino mice or using labeled T cells of an irrelevant specificity. These results suggest that another mechanism to maintain self-tolerance to mTyr$_{369}$ and other MDP is limited accessibility of activated T cells to the skin due to the absence of local inflammation or potentially, because of inappropriate expression of homing receptors on the T cells (see later). This mechanism is unlikely to compromise immunity to metastatic melanoma, but may limit immunity to early stage disease. It may also explain the irregular occurrence and localized distribution of vitiligo in melanoma patients.

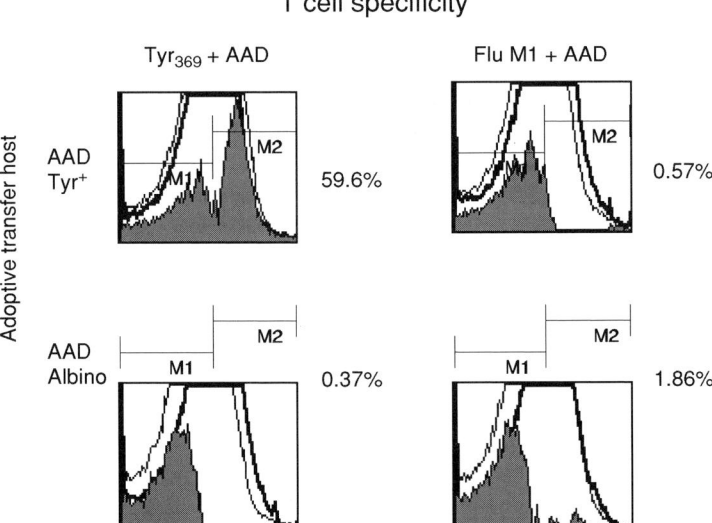

Figure 7 Selective accumulation of mTyr$_{369}$ specific T cells in skin of irradiated AAD$^+$Tyr$^+$ mice. 5×10^7 CFSE labeled T cells were injected IP into 700R irradiated or unirradiated mice. 24 h later, 1 cm^2 skin sections were harvested and dissociated in 0.5% collagenase. Single cell suspensions were analyzed for CFSE and CD8$^+$. Solid histograms represent the net number of CD8$^+$ cells in irradiated skin after subtraction of the control histogram. M1 and M2 gates define CFSE − and + populations representing endogenous and adoptively transferred CD8 T cells, respectively. Percentages are the fraction of the CD8 population that is CFSE$^+$.

14.5. Self-Tolerance to Tyr Impairs Control of B16-AAD Tumor Outgrowth

To gain insight into the impact of tolerance to Tyr on the ability to control melanoma tumors, we evaluated the outgrowth of B16 melanomas transfected with the AAD molecule in Tyr^+ and albino mice. B16-AAD endogenously processes and presents mTyr$_{369}$ (Colella et al., 2000; Engelhard et al., 2000; Mullins et al., 2001). In keeping with the low level response to mTyr$_{369}$ in AAD^+Tyr^+ mice, B16-AAD subcutaneous tumors and lung metastases grew as rapidly in these animals mice as did untransfected B16 itself (Mullins et al., 2001). Outgrowth of B16-AAD was delayed in AAD^+ albino mice, while outgrowth of B16 in these animals was no different from that of their Tyr^+ counterparts. This established that self-tolerance to Tyr substantially compromised the ability of mice to control B16-AAD. Furthermore, the only Tyr-derived epitopes relevant for tumor control in naïve albino mice are presented by AAD, and not by endogenous $H-2^b$ molecules.

15. MDP-Specific Immune Responses in Tolerant Mice Enable Control of Tumor Outgrowth

15.1. Tumor Control in mTyr$_{369}$-Tolerant Mice After Immunization with Tyr Peptides

The work summarized above suggests that tolerance to mTyr$_{369}$ in naïve T cells is based on both activation-induced deletion and ignorance within different segments of a broad-based T-cell repertoire. An important question is whether elements of this repertoire can be activated to control tumors effectively. For other MDP-derived Ags, immunotherapy strategies involving melanocyte destruction (Daniels et al., 2004), inflammatory processes in the skin (Daniels et al., 2004; Steitz et al., 2000), activation of CD4 T cells (Antony et al., 2005; Steitz et al., 2005), and IL-2 (Overwijk et al., 2003) have each been shown to tip the balance from self-tolerance to autoimmunity. However, it is not clear if these maneuvers rescue activated T cells destined for deletional self-tolerance (Ehl et al., 1998), or enhance the activation of low-affinity T cells (Goverman, 1999), or both. Immunization of AAD^+ albino mice with CD40L-matured DC that had been pulsed with the human Tyr$_{369-377D}$ peptide completely prevented the outgrowth of B16-AAD as a subcutaneous tumor (Mullins et al., 2001). Importantly, immunization of AAD^+Tyr^+ mice with these same DC delayed the outgrowth of B16-AAD as a subcutaneous tumor (Mullins et al., 2001), and substantially reduced the number of experimental lung metastases (Engelhard et al., 2002). The level of control was comparable to that seen in naïve AAD^+ albino mice (Mullins et al., 2001). A weaker but significant effect was seen after immunization of AAD$^+$Tyr$^+$ mice with murine mTyr$_{369}$-pulsed DC. Thus, by using human Tyr$_{369-377D}$ peptide for activation, mTyr$_{369}$-reactive T cells in tolerant mice can be as effective in controlling tumor outgrowth as those from nontolerant animals.

Given the diminished reactivity and low avidity of residual mTyr$_{369}$-specific T cells in AAD$^+$Tyr$^+$ mice, an important question arising is how immunization leads to the development of a cohort of memory T cells that are effective against a mTyr$_{369}^+$ tumor. We addressed this by examining the functional avidity of primary and recall effector cells *ex vivo* (measured as the concentration of peptide pulsed onto stimulator cells that elicited half-maximal IFN-γ-ICS) after immunization of either AAD$^+$ albino or AAD$^+$Tyr$^+$ mice. In albino mice, the functional avidity of recall effector cells for the immunogen, Tyr$_{369-377D}$, as well as mTyr$_{369}$, increases by 10–20-fold over that of primary effectors (Bullock and Engelhard, 2006; Bullock *et al.*, 2003). In Tyr$^+$ mice, there is a similar increase in functional avidity for Tyr$_{369-377D}$, but the functional avidity for mTyr$_{369}$ increases by almost 100-fold (Bullock and Engelhard, 2006). This avidity change results in substantial recognition of B16 tumor as well. It is not yet clear if the general increase in avidity driven by immunization reflects selection of higher avidity T cells within the repertoire or a change in the properties of memory T cells relative to naïve T cells with the same TCR (Bullock *et al.*, 2003). However, the disproportionate gain in avidity for self-antigen in the context of self-tolerance suggests that immunization may rescue T cells with high avidity for mTyr$_{369}$ from deletional self-tolerance.

15.2. Immune Responses to Other MDP Peptides and Tumor Control

The murine MDP gp100 also contains sequences that are highly homologous to known HLA-A*0201-restricted human gp100 epitopes (Colella *et al.*, 2000; Engelhard *et al.*, 2002). We were particularly interested in gp100$_{209-217}$ because the sequence is identical in both species and it is processed and presented on B16-AAD melanoma (Colella *et al.*, 2000; Engelhard *et al.*, 2000; Mullins *et al.*, 2001). gp100$_{209-217}$ was not immunogenic when pulsed onto CD40L-activated DC (Bullock *et al.*, 2000), consistent with the possibility that self-tolerance limits responsiveness. However, gp100$_{209-217M}$, which contains a substitution that decreases its rate of dissociation from HLA-A*0201 by a factor of 10, was immunogenic. In contrast to mTyr$_{369}$, T-cell lines established and maintained on the altered peptide gp100$_{209-217M}$ showed diminished cross-reactivity with gp100$_{209}$ (Bullock *et al.*, 2000), and this was even more evident when lower peptide doses were used to increase avidity (Bullock *et al.*, 2001). Thus, these two peptides are antigenically distinguishable by T cells, despite the fact that the difference between them is an anchor residue that is not directly exposed in the peptide-MHC complex. This also suggested that the augmented immunogenicity of gp100$_{209-217M}$ might be due to its recognition as a stronger agonist than the unmodified self-Ag, as we had previously observed with Tyr$_{369-377D}$. Importantly, the ability of T-cell lines initially activated using gp100$_{209-217M}$ to control the outgrowth of B16-AAD after adoptive transfer was correlated with their avidity for gp100$_{209-217}$ and not that for gp100$_{209-217M}$. Nonetheless, in the context of a single immunization, gp100$_{209-217M}$ stimulated more effective immunity against B16-AAD than did gp100$_{209-217}$ (Mullins et al., 2001). Collectively, these results confirm that the enhanced immunogenicity of modified peptides may be particularly useful to overcome self-tolerance, but suggest that their antigenic distinctiveness may diminish their utility in continually augmenting responses against the original Ag, particularly in the context of repetitive immunization.

16. Peptide-Pulsed Exogenous DC as a Vehicle to Influence the Quality of the Tumor-Specific Immune Response

Because DC comprise several different subsets and their maturation state is regulated by a variety of stimuli, there is no general agreement on what constitutes a "best" preparation of DC for tumor immunotherapy, nor is it possible to rigorously compare human and murine DC preparations. Nonetheless, we have used the murine tumor model to explore two issues that offer insight into the use of DC in human clinical trials. First, DC are unique antigen delivery vehicles because they distribute selectively into different lymphoid compartments when injected into the body by different routes (Eggert et al., 1999; Lappin et al., 1999; Morse et al., 1999; Mullins et al., 2003; Okada et al., 2001). Second, the use of DC pulsed with synthetic peptide antigens enables manipulation of the immunogen in two ways: varying the number of cells injected and varying the density of antigen presented on each cell. Using BMDC that had been cultured in GM-CSF+IL4 and then matured in the presence of either TNFα (Bullock et al., 2000) or CD40L (Bullock et al., 2001), we have explored how these different factors influence the quality of the immune response and tumor immunity in mice.

16.1. Route of Immunization Determines Location of T-cell Activation and Antitumor Efficacy

Subcutaneous (SC) injection of CD40L-activated BMDC resulted in a rapid and selective influx of cells into the draining peripheral LN (Mullins and Engelhard, 2006a). About 3000 DC accumulated in the axillary LN, regardless of the number injected. Additional DC accumulated in the spleen over the next several hours in proportion to the number injected, presumably representing a "spillover" of cells into the circulation. However, no accumulation of DC in any other LN was seen at any point. Intravenously (IV) injected DC migrated to spleen, and failed to access any peripheral or mesenteric LN (Mullins et al., 2003), with the exception of the paratracheal LN of the mediastinum (Sheasley-O'Neill et al., 2006). Primary CD8 T-cell responses were confined to these DC-infiltrated compartments. Similarly, T-cell activation after intraperitoneal (IP) injection of DC is confined to mesenteric and mediastinal LN (Sheasley-O'Neill et al., 2006). This contrasts strongly with the systemic primary immune responses induced by vaccinia virus introduced via either SC or IV routes (Mullins et al., 2003). Interestingly, T-cell activation by BMDC in different lymphoid compartments also led to the acquisition of different homing-associated integrins on T cells, and their differential accumulation in peripheral tissues (Sheasley-O'Neill et al., 2006). Bone marrow-derived DC do not induce some of these integrins in vitro, and our results suggest that they collaborate with elements of different LN microenvironments to do so in vivo. The selective accumulation of activated T cells in peripheral tissues is surprising, since peptide-pulsed DC are not expected to create an inflammatory focus as would an active infection. Activation of Ag-specific T cells in peripheral LN also gave rise to a population of memory T cells that infiltrated peripheral LN in noncontiguous drainages. However, T cells activated in the spleen were incapable of accessing peripheral LN (Mullins et al., 2003). Although adhesion molecules and chemokine receptors that enable homing of central memory cells to peripheral or intestinal LN have been defined (Mora et al., 2005; Rott et al., 1996), regulation of T-cell migration to spleen is not understood (Kraal et al., 1995; Nolte et al., 2002). Thus, BMDC localize in different lymphoid compartments depending on injection route, resulting in localized primary CD8 T-cell responses and differential distributions of both effector and memory T cells. The use of BMDC has also uncovered a previously unknown population of spleen-homing or spleen resident memory T cells.

To determine whether control of tumor correlated with location of memory T cells, mice immunized with mTyr$_{369}$-pulsed CD40L-activated DC were challenged with B16-AAD melanoma, delivered by either SC or IV injection to induce, respectively, solid tumors or lung lesions. SC delivery of immunizing DC, which induced Ag-specific memory T cells in both peripheral LN and spleen, enabled control of both subcutaneous solid tumors and lung lesions (Mullins et al., 2003) (Fig. 8). We further defined the requirement for peripheral LN by selectively ablating them in AAD$^+$ albino mice treated in utero with LTβR-Ig (Mullins et al., 2003; Rennert et al., 2001). These mice also controlled lung lesions but failed to control subcutaneous B16-AAD. Similarly,

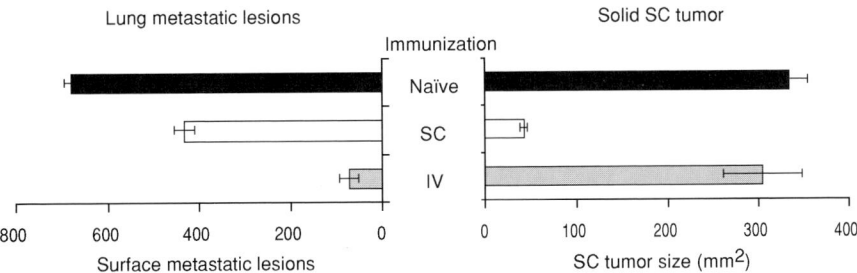

Figure 8 Control of melanoma outgrowth correlates with route of DC immunization. AAD$^+$ mice were injected, either SC in the scapular area or IV in the lateral tail vein, with 1×10^5 CD40L-activated autologous DC that were pulsed for 3 h at 37°C with 1 μg/ml of Tyr$_{369-377D}$. Three weeks later, immunized and naïve mice were challenged with 4×10^5 B16-AAD cells injected SC or IV. Tumor outgrowth was assessed 21 days later.

IV-immunized mice, in which tumor-reactive memory T cells were confined to spleen and absent in peripheral LN, significantly controlled lung lesions but failed to control subcutaneous solid tumors (Fig. 8). The ability to control lung lesions was absent in immunized Hox11 knockout mice, which lack spleens but have normal LN.

Collectively these data suggest that the distribution of CD8 memory cells induced by DC influences the ability to control outgrowth of a subsequently injected tumor. We have recently demonstrated that Ags from B16 melanoma, including mTyr$_{369}$, are cross-presented in only those lymphoid compartments draining the tumor (Hargadon et al., 2006). This suggests that the number of preexisting memory T cells in tumor-draining LN is one critical determinant of control. A second determinant may be the acquisition, by effectors activated in these compartments, of selective homing properties that enable them to infiltrate the tumor growing in different sites in the body. These results suggest that DC immunization route should be considered as one basis for improving tumor immunotherapy in human clinical trials.

16.2. Overcoming the Limited Antitumor Immune Response in Individual LN

The limited capacity for activated DC (~3000) of axillary LN draining an injection site has important consequences—this number of DC limits the size of primary and recall immune responses and the ability to control subcutaneous tumors (Mullins and Engelhard, 2006a; Mullins et al., 2003). In contrast, the size of these responses in spleen and control of lung tumors is correlated with the number of DC injected either SC or IV over the entire

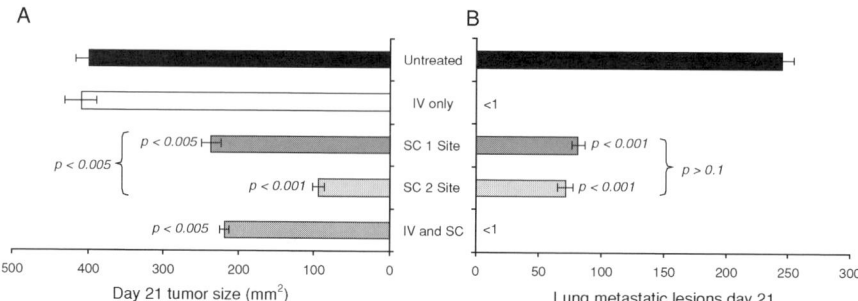

Figure 9 Multisite immunization enhances antitumor efficacy of peptide-pulsed DC immunization. AAD$^+$ mice were injected with 10^5 CD40L-activated DC that were pulsed for 3 h at 37°C with 1 μM Tyr$_{369}$Y. In some groups, DC were equally divided between 2 SC sites or between SC and IV delivery. Twenty-one days later, mice were challenged with 4×10^5 B16-AAD tumor cells, either SC (A) or IV (B). Tumor outgrowth was assessed 21 days after tumor induction.

range of 10^3–10^6 cells. We have evaluated several strategies to overcome the limitation on immunity imposed by DC infiltration into LN. First, because primary responses initiated by DC in individual LN result in memory T cells that redistribute to noncontiguous drainages, we tested whether distributing DC into two noncontiguous LN, leading to discrete primary responses in each, would also increase the size of the recall response in every peripheral LN and thus improve antitumor efficacy. Indeed, delivery of DC into two noncontiguous LN beds lead to substantially larger recall responses in a third noncontiguous drainage and significantly decreased outgrowth of subcutaneous as opposed to lung-localized, B16-AAD melanoma (Fig. 9). This observation also emphasizes the fact that the number of antigen-specific T cells activated in an individual LN is significantly less than the total number of such cells in the whole animal, and emphasizes the possibility to activate a larger fraction of the total through distributed immunization.

We also exploited the observation that an initial influx of activated DC can condition an LN to accept a much larger population of subsequently-injected DC (Martín-Fontecha et al., 2003). We observed a significant increase in the infiltration of labeled Ag-bearing DC into the draining LN after pretreatment with unpulsed DC (Mullins and Engelhard, 2006a), and this was accompanied by both increased primary immune response magnitude and subsequent tumor control. Taken together with the limited number of T cells that can be activated in individual LN mentioned above, this result suggests that the larger number of DC present in the node may recruit a larger number of naïve T cells into the same node. Finally, we asked whether immunization using DC pulsed with two different peptides could improve control of melanoma outgrowth, compared with single epitope immunization. Indeed, immunization with Tyr$_{369-377D}$ and gp100$_{209}$ copulsed DC increased the total number of melanoma Ag-specific CD8 T cells in the primary response and a correlative improvement in tumor control (Mullins and Engelhard, 2006a). Use of two epitopes on the immunizing DC did not compromise the magnitude of Ag-specific response to either epitope. It remains to be determined whether this effectiveness is related simply to an overall increase in the number of tumor-specific effector cells, irrespective of epitope specificity, or whether specificity for multiple epitopes provides more effective control of Ag loss variants. Collectively, however, these results emphasize that the limited distribution of exogenous DC upon immunization will activate only a fraction of the Ag-specific T cells present in the immune system as a whole. It is likely that the same limitations apply using peptide-in-adjuvant vaccine formulations that create a depot effect. They will also limit the memory T cells that become activated upon repetitive vaccination to the fraction in the node draining the injection site. Effective recruitment of the larger repertoire of Ag-specific T cells available within the body as a whole represents an important and overlooked opportunity to improve the immune response to tumors.

16.3. Altering Peptide Density on APC: Influence on T-Cell Avidity, Response Magnitude, and Tumor Control

It is well-established that the use of lower amounts of peptide Ag *in vitro* enables the outgrowth of CD8 T-cell lines with higher avidities, and these lines are more effective in mediating antiviral and antitumor immunity (Alexander-Miller *et al.*, 1996a; Derby *et al.*, 2001; Zeh, III *et al.*, 1999). This is in keeping with the idea that lowering the Ag density leads to the preferential activation of T cells with higher affinity TCR, and thus avidity, skewing the repertoire of the responding population in the process. However, using tTCR$^+$ cells, cell lines with high or low-functional avidity have been isolated by culture in the presence of low or high concentration of peptide, respectively (Cawthon *et al.*, 2001), suggesting the existence of mechanisms to regulate avidity independent of repertoire selection. Regardless of the mechanism, we established T-cell lines with progressively higher functional avidities from AAD$^+$Tyr$^+$ mice by culture with spleen cells that had been pulsed with progressive lower amounts of human Tyr$_{369-377D}$. High avidity was associated with increased cross-reactive recognition of mTyr$_{369}$ (Bullock *et al.*, 2001). The highest avidity lines recognized these two peptides equally, despite the fact that mTyr$_{369}$ is a self-Ag, and their avidities for mTyr$_{369}$ were comparable to those of the highest avidity T-cell lines we have isolated from AAD$^+$ albino mice (Bullock *et al.*, 2001; Colella *et al.*, 2000). This suggests either that we are selecting out a minor subset of T cells that persist *in vivo* despite tolerance, or that *in vitro* culture conditions enable a modification of avidity and cross-reactivity. Most importantly, the higher avidity T cells demonstrated progressively better ability to control B16-AAD outgrowth in a therapeutic setting (Bullock *et al.*, 2001).

Based on the ability to select for high avidity CD8 T cells with better recognition of melanoma cells using low densities of mTyr$_{369}$ *in vitro*, we tested whether the avidity of CD8 T-cell responses *in vivo* could be similarly improved by manipulating the density of peptide Ag displayed on the surface of the immunizing DC. Increasing the density of Tyr$_{369-377D}$ displayed on DC over a broad range increased the number of Ag-specific T cells measured *ex vivo* at the peak of both primary (Bullock *et al.*, 2000) and recall responses (Bullock *et al.*, 2003). However, we found that all primary effector T-cell populations had identical functional and structural (determined as the concentration of Tyr$_{369-377D}$ tetramers necessary for half-maximal staining of T cells) avidities, regardless of the peptide density on the DC used to elicit them (Bullock *et al.*, 2003). These data suggested that the peptide density-based selection of primary CD8 effector T cells with different avidities does not occur. The reasons for this surprising result are not clear. However, it should be kept in mind that the density of antigen on a cross-presenting APC may bear little relationship to that expressed on a tumor or a virally-infected cell, and there may be advantages in activating a population of T cells with a broad distribution of avidities (resulting in the same average avidity on the whole), regardless of the antigen density displayed on the DC itself. Whether this is true and how it is achieved mechanistically remains to be determined.

In contrast to the results with primary effector cells, mice primed with DC presenting a lower density of Tyr$_{369-377D}$ did give rise to recall effectors with relatively higher functional and structural avidities after challenge with a recombinant vaccinia virus expressing human Tyr (hTyr-vac) (Bullock *et al.*, 2003). While the avidities of memory cells could not be determined directly because of their low frequency, this result suggests that cells entering the memory pool have undergone peptide-density based selection. We also examined whether memory cells could undergo peptide-density based selection for avidity during activation of the recall response. Mice that had been primed with hTyr-vac were challenged with DC that presented high or low epitope densities. Recall CD8 T cells generated with high-peptide density had lower functional and structural avidities than those generated with low-peptide density, demonstrating that peptide-density based selection occurs during the expansion of recall T cells (Bullock *et al.*, 2003). The magnitudes of these responses were less influenced by peptide Ag density than those of the primary responses. Importantly, a greater proportion of the high avidity recall

T cells expanded by challenge with low-peptide density recognized melanoma cells. Because several studies (Bachmann *et al.*, 1999; Curtsinger *et al.*, 1998; Pihlgren *et al.*, 1996), including our own (Bullock *et al.*, 2003), have demonstrated an overall increase in the avidity of recall effectors compared to primary effectors, it is not clear whether these avidity differences are due to a maturation process in individual T cells or selection of different TCR within the repertoire.

As mentioned earlier, the overall magnitude of the immune response generally increased as the density of presented Ag was increased. However, at the highest densities used, the primary response diminished substantially. This has been observed with several peptide Ags and is not limited to self-Ags (Bullock *et al.*, 2000; Mullins and Engelhard, 2006b). High concentrations of peptide Ag have been shown to induce apoptosis of high avidity CD8 effector cells *in vitro* (Alexander-Miller *et al.*, 1996b). In a vaccinia virus model, excessive Ag expression was associated with the accumulation of tetramer$^+$ cells that did not produce IFN-γ (Kaech *et al.*, 2002), while in another system, immunization with peptide in adjuvant was associated with "functional deletion" (Toes *et al.*, 1996). However, this was reversed when the peptide was administered on DC (Toes *et al.*, 1998), suggesting that the effect was due to binding of free peptide to nonprofessional APC. In a third system, peptide-pulsed splenic DC induced anergy that was reversed by IL12 (Grohmann *et al.*, 1997). The mechanism responsible in our system is not clear, since our DC are washed to remove unbound peptide before immunization, and they secrete IL12 after maturation with CD40L (Bullock *et al.*, 2001).

To determine whether peptide Ag density on immunizing DC affected the ability to control tumors growing in different sites, we evaluated B16-AAD outgrowth following IV or SC immunization using DC pulsed with a range of Tyr$_{369-377D}$ concentrations. SC delivery of peptide-pulsed DC led to dose dependent CD8 responses in both draining LN and spleen, but the pulsing concentration that stimulated an optimal response in peripheral LN was 3 logs lower than in the spleen (Mullins and Engelhard, 2006b). The dose-dependent magnitude of the CD8 response in peripheral LN and spleen correlated directly with control of subcutaneous tumor and lung lesions, respectively. The dose dependence of CD8 responses in spleen induced by IV immunization was the same as that induced by SC immunization, and no response in peripheral LN was observed at any dose (Mullins and Engelhard, 2006b). Again, control of lung tumor paralleled the response magnitude, and no control of subcutaneous tumor was observed at any dose. We hypothesized that the difference in optimal epitope density between peripheral LN and spleen might arise from differences in DC migration time to these organs, coupled with the progressive shedding of pulsed peptide: SC-injected DC saturate draining LN within 30 min, whereas SC- or IV-injected DC take 4 h to reach a maximal number in spleen (Mullins and Engelhard, 2006a). However, the same dose–response curve was observed when DC were directly injected into the spleen (Mullins and Engelhard, 2006b). Thus, there is a clear optimum peptide density for the induction of maximal immune responses, and this is influenced by the characteristics of lymphoid compartments that differ between peripheral LN and spleen. Epitope density is not usually considered a variable in DC-based clinical trials. Indeed, the peptide concentrations used by some investigators (Jonuleit et al., 2001; Panelli et al., 2000) may lead to a supra-optimal peptide display and diminished responses. Collectively, our results suggest that peptide-density based selection of memory T cells and recall effectors could be a successful strategy for enhancing immunotherapy, although application of this approach is relatively complex.

17. Summary of Preclinical and Clinical Studies and Future Directions

When our group began to focus on tumor immunology and immunotherapy of melanoma, molecular definition of T-cell epitopes had not yet been initiated. By exploiting the new technology of tandem mass spectrometry of our colleague Donald Hunt, we have participated in the identification and characterization of the antigenic targets of CD4 and CD8 T cells. This work continues in our group, and we are convinced that there are additional important antigens that remain to be discovered and characterized. We are excited about the prospect of incorporating in the next generation of peptide vaccines some of the new antigens identified here and at other institutions and are particularly enthusiastic about characterizing MHC-associated phosphor-peptides that may be relevant immunologic targets on cancer cells with upregulation of critical cell growth or metastasis pathways.

Despite our continued work on antigen identification, we share the growing perception that identification of antigens is insufficient for optimizing cancer vaccines. Our future directions over the next decade will include at least 4 additional major themes: (1) tumor-associated immune dysfunction and immune escape, (2) tolerance and autoimmunity, (3) immunobiologic principles governing activation and targeting of T-cell responses to cancer antigens, and (4) combination therapies that augment antigen-specific immune activation.

Over the last several years, knowledge concerning the immune response to melanoma has exploded, and with it the opportunities to develop new immunotherapeutic approaches to treat it. This work has also led to important new questions about the relationship between self-tolerance and tumor-specific immunity, as well as how best to stimulate T-cell responses that will be durable and therapeutic. These issues are difficult to address in a comprehensive fashion in the course of clinical trials, necessitating the development of highly relevant preclinical models. These studies ideally result in new hypotheses to test in the clinical setting. Similarly, as clinical trials are performed, careful immunologic correlates suggest new questions to pursue in the preclinical setting.

Our work and that of other laboratories has identified Tyr and the Tyr_{369} epitope as significant targets for melanoma-specific immune responses and immunotherapy. By focusing preclinical work on immune responses to this antigen, we have identified several unique aspects of tolerance and autoimmunity to this MDP-derived Ag that have not been previously described in any other model of which we are aware. In particular, the regional control of immunity and the site-specific limitations on T-cell response provide impetus to develop human clinical trials to exploit these new findings.

In our clinical trials, we have developed peptide mixtures and delivery systems and schedules that induce immune responses in 80–100% of patients, and that are associated with clinical outcomes that exceed expectations. However, there is substantial work to do in augmenting the magnitude, breadth, and persistence of the T-cell responses and in characterizing the host- and tumor-related factors that limit optimal immune response generation. As we move into the next phase of studies, both our laboratory and clinical investigations will partner to address these questions.

Particularly, troubling is the fact that T cells infiltrating tumor deposits are often tolerized, inactivated, or negatively regulated. Similar effects may be observed on tumor-infiltrating dendritic cells (Mellor and Munn, 2004). These effects combine with other forms of immune escape as challenges to our success in immune therapy. On the other hand, if the immune system had no effect on melanoma progression, such immune escape would not be necessary. Thus, the high prevalence of immune escape phenotypes among metastatic melanomas is evidence that melanoma cells without immune escape phenotypes are selectively destroyed by the native antitumor immune response. The clinical experience with melanoma vaccines mirrors this biologic reality. In a minority of patients, objective clinical responses have been observed with cancer vaccines, and some of them have been durable. However, the overall clinical response rate with melanoma vaccines has been low (Das et al., 2001; Dunbar et al., 1999; Jager et al., 2001; Meidenbauer et al., 2003; Nestle et al., 1998b; Palermo et al., 2001; Rosenberg et al., 1998; Yamshchikov et al., 2001). While it is tempting to view these low clinical response rates to cancer vaccines as failure, it is illustrative to consider the myriad forms of medical and surgical therapies that "failed" to a similar degree in their early development but have now become standard and successful approaches in contemporary medical practice. These include liver transplantation, heart surgery, chemotherapy for Hodgkin's disease, and monoclonal antibody therapy for cancer. All of these became successful by a combination of an increased depth of scientific knowledge and improved technology. The challenges for the next generation of studies in cancer vaccine development are to increase knowledge of the host–tumor relationship and to develop new technology that increases the effectiveness of cancer vaccines. Clinical and laboratory (preclinical and postclinical) investigations with peptide vaccines offer particular opportunities for advancing knowledge that is relevant not only to the specific use of melanoma vaccines in humans, but also in understanding the development of the immune response at a fundamental level.

Acknowledgments

This work was supported by PHS grants AI20963, CA78400, and AI059996 (to VHE) and CA78519, CA57653, and CA89937 to CLS. The work was also supported in part by Schering-Plough Research Institute; Argonex, Inc.; Chiron Corporation; the Human Immune Therapy Center at the University of Virginia (funded by the Cancer Research Institute), the Cancer Center Support Grant (NIH P30CA44579) at the University of Virginia, and the General Clinical Research Center at the University of Virginia (RR00847).

References

Alexander-Miller, M. A., Leggatt, G. R., and Berzofsky, J. A. (1996a). Selective expansion of high- or low-avidity cytotoxic T lymphocytes and efficacy for adoptive immunotherapy. *Proc. Natl. Acad. Sci. USA* **93,** 4102–4107.

Alexander-Miller, M. A., Leggatt, G. R., Sarin, A., and Berzofsky, J. A. (1996b). Role of antigen, CD8, and cytotoxic T lymphocyte (CTL) avidity in high dose antigen induction of apoptosis of effector CTL. *J. Exp. Med.* **184,** 485–492.

Allan, R. S., Smith, C. M., Belz, G. T., van Lint, A. L., Wakim, L. M., Heath, W. R., and Carbone, F. R. (2003). Epidermal viral immunity induced by CD8alpha+ dendritic cells but not by Langerhans cells. *Science* **301,** 1925–1928.

Altrich-VanLith, M. L., Polefrone, J. M., Ostankovitch, M., Shabanowitz, J., Hunt, D. F., and Engelhard, V. H. (2006). Deamidation and Amino Terminal Processing of a T cell Epitope from Tyrosinase Requires ER to Cytosol Translocation, Peptide-N-glycanase, and ERAP1.

Antony, P. A., Piccirillo, C. A., Akpinarli, A., Finkelstein, S. E., Speiss, P. J., Surman, D. R., Palmer, D. C., Chan, C. C., Klebanoff, C. A., Overwijk, W. W., Rosenberg, S. A., and Restifo, N. P. (2005). CD8+ T cell immunity against a tumor/self-antigen is augmented by CD4+ T helper cells and hindered by naturally occurring T regulatory cells. *J. Immunol.* **174,** 2591–2601.

Bachmann, M. F., Gallimore, A., Linkert, S., Cerundolo, V., Lanzavecchia, A., Kopf, M., and Viola, A. (1999). Developmental regulation of Lck targeting to the CD8 coreceptor controls signaling in naive and memory T cells. *J. Exp. Med.* **189,** 1521–1530.

Bakker, A. B., Schreurs, M. W., Tafazzul, G., de Boer, A. J., Kawakami, Y., Adema, G. J., and Figdor, C. G. (1995). Identification of a novel peptide derived from the melanocyte-specific gp100 antigen as the dominant epitope recognized by an HLA-A2.1-restricted anti-melanoma CTL line. *Int. J. Cancer* **62,** 97–102.

Battyani, Z., Xerri, L., Hassoun, J., Bonerandi, J. J., and Grob, J. J. (1993). Tyrosinase gene expression in human tissues. *Pigment Cell Res.* **6,** 400–405.

Brystryn, J.-C., Rigel, D., Friedman, R. J., and Kopf, A. (1987). Prognostic significance of hypopigmentation in malignant melanoma. *Arch. Dermatol.* **123,** 1053–1055.

Bullock, T. N., Mullins, D. W., Colella, T. A., and Engelhard, V. H. (2001). Manipulation of avidity to improve effectiveness of adoptively transferred $CD8^+$ T cells for melanoma immunotherapy in human MHC class I-transgenic mice. *J. Immunol.* **167,** 5824–5831.

Bullock, T. N., Mullins, D. W., and Engelhard, V. H. (2003). Antigen density presented by dendritic cells *in vivo* differentially affects the number and avidity of primary, memory, and recall CD8+ T cells. *J. Immunol.* **170,** 1822–1829.

Bullock, T. N. J., Colella, T. A., and Engelhard, V. H. (2000). The density of peptides displayed by dendritic cells affects immune responses to human tyrosinase and gp100 in HLA-A2 transgenic mice. *J. Immunol.* **164,** 2354–2361.

Bullock, T. N. J., and Engelhard, V. H. (2006). Differential avidity maturation after immunization of self-tolerant mice .

Cawthon, A. G., Lu, H., and Alexander-Miller, M. A. (2001). Peptide requirement for CTL activation reflects the sensitivity to CD3 engagement: Correlation with CD8ab versus CD8aa expression. *J. Immunol.* **167,** 2577–2584.

Celis, E., Tsai, V., Crimi, C., DeMars, R., Wentworth, P. A., Chesnut, R. W., Grey, H. M., Sette, A., and Serra, H. M. (1994). Induction of anti-tumor cytotoxic T lymphocytes in normal humans using primary cultures and synthetic peptide epitopes. *Proc. Natl. Acad. Sci. USA* **91,** 2105–2109.

Chaux, P., Luiten, R., Demotte, N., Vantomme, V., Stroobant, V., Traversari, C., Russo, V., Schultz, E., Cornelis, G. R., Boon, T., and van der Bruggen, P. (1999a). Identification of five MAGE-A1 epitopes recognized by cytolytic T lymphocytes obtained by *in vitro* stimulation with dendritic cells transduced with MAGE-A1. *J. Immunol.* **163,** 2928–2936.

Chaux, P., Vantomme, V., Stroobant, V., Thielemans, K., Corthals, J., Luiten, R., Eggermont, A. M. M., Boon, T., and van der Bruggen, P. (1999b). Identification of MAGE-3 epitopes presented by HLA-DR molecules to CD4+ T lymphocytes. *J. Exp. Med.* **189,** 767–777.

Chianese-Bullock, K. A., Pressley, J., Garbee, C., Hibbitts, S., Murphy, C., Yamshchikov, G., Petroni, G. R., Bissonette, E. A., Neese, P. Y., Grosh, W. W., Merrill, P., Fink, R., Woodson, E. M., Wiernasz, C. J., Patterson, J. W., and Slingluff, C. L., Jr. (2005a). MAGE-A1-, MAGE-A10-, and gp100-derived peptides are immunogenic when combined with granulocyte-macrophage colony-stimulating factor and montanide ISA-51 adjuvant and administered as part of a multipeptide vaccine for melanoma. *J. Immunol.* **174,** 3080–3086.

Chianese-Bullock, K. A., Woodson, E. M., Tao, H., Boerner, S. A., Smolkin, M., Grosh, W. W., Neese, P. Y., Merrill, P., Petroni, G. R., and Slingluff, C. L., Jr. (2005b). Autoimmune toxicities associated with the administration of antitumor vaccines and low-dose interleukin-2. *J. Immunother.* **28,** 412–419.

Colella, T. A., Bullock, T. N. J., Russell, L. B., Mullins, D. W., Overwijk, W., Luckey, C. J., Pierce, R. A., Restifo, N. P., and Engelhard, V. H. (2000). Self-tolerance to the murine homologue of a tyrosinase-derived melanoma antigen: Implications for tumor immunotherapy. *J. Exp. Med.* **191,** 1221–1231.

Cox, A. L., Skipper, J., Chen, Y., Henderson, R. A., Darrow, T. L., Shabanowitz, J., Engelhard, V. H., Hunt, D. F., and Slingluff, C. L., Jr. (1994). Identification of a peptide recognized by five melanoma-specific human cytotoxic T cell lines. *Science* **264,** 716–719.

Cragun, W. C., Yamshchikov, G. V., Bissonette, E. A., Smolkin, M. E., Eastham, S., Petroni, G. R., Schrecengost, R. S., Woodson, E. M., and Slingluff, C. L., Jr. (2005). Low-dose IL-2 induces cytokine cascade, eosinophilia, and a transient Th2 shift in melanoma patients. *Cancer Immunol. Immunother.* **54,** 1095–1105.

Curtsinger, J. M., Lins, D. C., and Mescher, M. F. (1998). CD8+ memory T cells (CD44high, Ly-6C+) are more sensitive than naive cells to (CD44low, Ly-6C-) to TCR/CD8 signaling in response to antigen. *J. Immunol.* **160,** 3236–3243.

Daniels, G. A., Sanchez-Perez, L., Diaz, R. M., Kottke, T., Thompson, J., Lai, M., Gough, M., Karim, M., Bushell, A., Chong, H., Melcher, A., Harrington, K., and Vile, R. G. (2004). A simple method to cure established tumors by inflammatory killing of normal cells. *Nat. Biotechnol.* **22,** 1125–1132.

Das, P. K., van den Wijngaard, R. M., Wankowicz-Kalinska, A., and Le Poole, I. C. (2001). A symbiotic concept of autoimmunity and tumour immunity: Lessons from vitiligo. *Trends Immunol.* **22,** 130–136.

Derbinski, J., Schulte, A., Kyewski, B., and Klein, L. (2001). Promiscuous gene expression in medullary thymic epithelial cells mirrors the peripheral self. *Nat. Immunol.* **2,** 1032–1039.

Derby, M. A., Alexander-Miller, M. A., Tse, R., and Berzofsky, J. A. (2001). High-avidity CTL exploit two complementary mechanisms to provide better protection against viral infection than low-avidity CTL. *J. Immunol.* **166,** 1690–1697.

Dunbar, P. R., Chen, J. L., Chao, D., Rust, N., Teisserenc, H., Ogg, G. S., Romero, P., Weynants, P., and Cerundolo, V. (1999). Cutting edge: Rapid cloning of tumor-specific CTL suitable for adoptive immunotherapy of melanoma. *J. Immunol.* **162,** 6959–6962.

Eggert, A. A., Schreurs, M. W., Boerman, O. C., Oyen, W. J., de Boer, A. J., Punt, C. J., Figdor, C. G., and Adema, G. J. (1999). Biodistribution and vaccine efficiency of murine dendritic cells are dependent on the route of administration. *Cancer Res.* **59,** 3340–3345.

Ehl, S., Hombach, J., Aichele, P., Rulicke, T., Odermatt, B., Hengarter, H., Zinkernagel, R., and Pircher, H. (1998). Viral and bacterial infections interfere with peripheral tolerance induction and activate CD8+ T cells. *J. Exp. Med.* **187,** 763–774.

Engelhard, V. H., Bullock, T. N., Colella, T. A., and Mullins, D. W. (2000). Direct identification of human tumor-associated peptide antigens and a preclinical model to evaluate their use. *Cancer J. Sci. Am.* **6**(Suppl. 3), S272–S280.

Engelhard, V. H., Bullock, T. N., Colella, T. A., Sheasley, S. L., and Mullins, D. W. (2002). Antigens derived from melanocyte differentiation proteins: Self-tolerance, autoimmunity, and use for cancer immunotherapy. *Immunol. Rev.* **188,** 136–146.

Engelhard, V. H., Lacy, E., and Ridge, J. P. (1991). Influenza A specific, HLA-A2.1 restricted cytotoxic T lymphocytes from HLA-A2.1 transgenic mice recognize fragments of the M1 protein. *J. Immunol.* **146,** 1226–1232.

Ferris, R. L., Hall, C., Sipsas, N. V., Safrit, J. T., Trocha, A., Koup, R. A., Johnson, R. P., and Siliciano, R. F. (1999). Processing of HIV-1 envelope glycoprotein for class I-restricted recognition: Dependence on TAP1/2 and mechanisms for cytosolic localization. *J. Immunol.* **162,** 1324–1332.

Ganss, R., Ryschich, E., Klar, E., Arnold, B., and Hammerling, G. J. (2002). Combination of T-cell therapy and trigger of inflammation induces remodeling of the vasculature and tumor eradication. *Cancer Res.* **62,** 1462–1470.

Gaugler, B., Van den Eynde, B., van der Bruggen, P., Romero, P., Gaforio, J. J., De Plaen, E., Lethe, B., Brasseur, F., and Boon, T. (1994). Human gene MAGE-3 codes for an antigen recognized on a melanoma by autologous cytolytic T lymphocytes. *J. Exp. Med.* **179,** 921–930.

Gimenez, E., Lavado, A., Giraldo, P., and Montoliu, L. (2003). Tyrosinase gene expression is not detected in mouse brain outside the retinal pigment epithelium cells. *Eur. J. Neurosci.* **18,** 2673–2676.

Goverman, J. (1999). Tolerance and autoimmunity in TCR transgenic mice specific for myelin basic protein. *Immunol. Rev.* **169,** 147–159.

Grohmann, U., Bianchi, R., Ayroldi, E., Belladonna, M. L., Surace, D., Fioretti, M. C., and Puccetti, P. (1997). A tumor-associated and self-antigen peptide presented by dendritic cells may induce T cell anergy *in vivo*, but IL-12 can preent or revert the anergic state. *J. Immunol.* **158,** 3593–3602.

Halder, T., Pawelec, G., Kirkin, A. F., Zeuthen, J., Meyer, H. E., Kun, L., and Kalbacher, H. (1997). Isolation of novel HLA-DR restricted potential tumor-associated antigens from the melanoma cell line FM3. *Cancer Res.* **57,** 3238–3244.

Han, R., Baden, H. P., Brissette, J. L., and Weiner, L. (2002). Redefining the skin's pigmentary system with a novel tyrosinase assay. *Pigment Cell Res.* **15,** 290–297.

Hargadon, K. M., Sheasley-O'Neill, S. L., Nichols, L. A., Bullock, T. N. J., and Engelhard, V. H. (2006). Incomplete differentiation of tumor-specific $CD8^+$ T cells in the face of tumor cell metastasis to draining lymph nodes.

Hemmer, B., Stefanova, I., Vergelli, M., Germain, R. N., and Martin, R. (1998). Relationships among TCR ligand potency, thresholds for effector function elicitation, and the quality of early signaling events in human T cells. *J. Immunol.* **160,** 5807–5814.

Hemmi, H., Yoshino, M., Yamazaki, H., Naito, M., Iyoda, T., Omatsu, Y., Shimoyama, S., Letterio, J. J., Nakabayashi, T., Tagaya, H., Yamane, T., Ogawa, M., *et al.* (2001). Skin antigens in the steady state are trafficked to regional lymph nodes by transforming growth factor-beta1-dependent cells. *Int. Immunol.* **13,** 695–704.

Hogan, K. T., Coppola, M. A., Gatlin, C. L., Thompson, L. W., Shabanowitz, J., Hunt, D. F., Engelhard, V. H., Ross, M. M., and Slingluff, C. L., Jr. (2004). Identification of novel and widely expressed cancer/testis gene isoforms that elicit spontaneous cytotoxic T-lymphocyte reactivity to melanoma. *Cancer Res.* **64,** 1157–1163.

Hogan, K. T., Coppola, M. A., Gatlin, C. L., Thompson, L. W., Shabanowitz, J., Hunt, D. F., Engelhard, V. H., Slingluff, C. L., Jr., and Ross, M. M. (2003). Identification of a shared epitope recognized by melanoma-specific, HLA-A3-restricted cytotoxic T lymphocytes. *Immunol. Lett.* **90,** 131–135.

Hogan, K. T., Sutton, J. N., Chu, K. U., Busby, J. A., Shabanowitz, J., Hunt, D. F., and Slingluff, C. L., Jr. (2005). Use of selected reaction monitoring mass spectrometry for the detection of specific MHC class I peptide antigens on A3 supertype family members. *Cancer Immunol. Immunother.* **54,** 359–371.

Huang, L. Q., Brasseur, F., Serrano, A., De Plaen, E., van der Bruggen, P., Boon, T., and Van Pel, A. (1999). Cytolytic T lymphocytes recognize an antigen encoded by MAGE-A10 on a human melanoma. *J. Immunol.* **162,** 6849–6854.

Jaeger, E., Bernhard, H., Romero, P., Ringhoffer, M., Arand, M., Karbach, J., Ilsemann, C., Hagedorn, M., and Knuth, A. (1996). Generation of cytotoxic T-cell responses with synthetic melanoma-associated peptides *in vivo*: Implications for tumor vaccines with melanoma-associated antigens. *Int. J. Cancer* **66,** 162–169.

Jager, D., Jager, E., and Knuth, A. (2001). Vaccination for malignant melanoma: Recent developments. *Oncology* **60,** 1–7.

Jager, E., Maeurer, M., Hohn, H., Karbach, J., Jager, D., Zidianakis, Z., Bakhshandeh-Bath, A., Orth, J., Neukirch, C., Necker, A., Reichert, T. E., and Knuth, A. (2000). Clonal expansion of Melan A-specific cytotoxic T lymphocytes in a melanoma patient responding to continued immunization with melanoma-associated peptides. *Int. J. Cancer* **86,** 538–547.

Jonuleit, H., Giesecke-Tuettenberg, A., Tuting, T., Thurner-Schuler, B., Stuge, T. B., Paragnik, L., Kandemir, A., Lee, P. P., Schuler, G., Knop, J., and Enk, A. H. (2001). A comparison of two types of dendritic cell as adjuvants for the induction of melanoma-specific T-cell responses in humans following intranodal injection. *Int. J. Cancer* **93,** 243–251.

Kaech, S. M., Wherry, E. J., and Ahmed, R. (2002). Effector and memory T-cell differentiation: Implications for vaccine development. *Nature Rev. Immunol.* **2,** 251–262.

Kahn, M., Sugawara, H., McGowan, P., Okuno, K., Nagoya, S., Hellstrom, K. E., and Greenberg, P. (1991). CD4+ T cell clones specific for the human p97 melanoma-associated antigen can eradicate pulmonary metastases from a murine tumor expressing the p97 antigen. *J. Immunol.* **146,** 3235–3241.

Kawakami, Y., Eliyahu, S., Jennings, C., Sakaguchi, K., Kang, X., Southwood, S., Robbins, P. F., Sette, A., Appella, E., and Rosenberg, S. A. (1995). Recognition of multiple epitopes in the human melanoma antigen gp100 by tumor-infiltrating T lymphocytes associated with *in vivo* tumor regression. *J. Immunol.* **154,** 3961–3968.

Kawakami, Y., Eliyahu, S., Sakaguchi, K., Robbins, P. F., Rivoltini, L., Yannelli, J. R., Appella, E., and Rosenberg, S. A. (1994). Identification of the immunodominant peptides of the MART-1 human melanoma antigen recognized by the majority of HLA-A2-restricted tumor infiltrating lymphocytes. *J. Exp. Med.* **180,** 347–352.

Kawakami, Y., Robbins, P. F., Wang, X., Tupesis, J. P., Parkhurst, M. R., Kang, X., Sakaguchi, K., Appella, E., and Rosenberg, S. A. (1998). Identification of new melanoma epitopes on melanosomal proteins recognized by tumor infiltrating T lymphocytes restricted by HLA-A1, -A2, and -A3 alleles. *J. Immunol.* **161,** 6985–6992.

Kayaga, J., Souberbielle, B. E., Sheikh, N., Morrow, W. J., Scott-Taylor, T., Vile, R., Chong, H., and Dalgleish, A. G. (1999). Anti-tumour activity against B16-F10 melanoma with a GM-CSF secreting allogeneic tumour cell vaccine. *Gene Ther.* **6,** 1475–1481.

Kierstead, L. S., Ranieri, E., Olson, W., Brusic, V., Sidney, J., Sette, A., Kasamon, Y. L., Slingluff, C. L. J., Kirkwood, J. M., and Storkus, W. J. (2001). gp100/pmel17 and tyrosinase encode multiple epitopes recognized by Th1-type CD4+ T cells. *Br. J. Cancer* **85,** 1738–1745.

Kirkwood, J. M., Ibrahim, J. G., Sondak, V. K., Richards, J., Flaherty, L. E., Ernstoff, M. S., Smith, T. J., Rao, U., Steele, M., and Blum, R. H. (2000). High- and low-dose interferon alfa-2b in high-risk melanoma: First analysis of intergroup trial E1690/S9111/C9190. *J. Clin. Oncol.* **18,** 2444–2458.

Kirkwood, J. M., Strawderman, M. H., Ernstoff, M. S., Smith, T. J., Borden, E. C., and Blum, R. H. (1996). Interferon alfa-2b adjuvant therapy of high-risk resected cutaneous melanoma: The Eastern Cooperative Oncology Group Trial EST 1684 (see comments). *J. Clin. Oncol.* **14,** 7–17.

Kittlesen, D. J., Thompson, L. W., Gulden, P. H., Skipper, J. C., Colella, T. A., Shabanowitz, J. A., Hunt, D. F., Engelhard, V. H., and Slingluff, C. L., Jr. (1998). Human melanoma patients recognize an HLA-A1-restricted CTL epitope from tyrosinase containing two cysteine residues: Implications for tumor vaccine development. *J. Immunol.* **160,** 2099–2106.

Knutson, K. L., Schiffman, K., and Disis, M. L. (2001). Immunization with a HER-2/neu helper peptide vaccine generates HER-2/neu CD8 T-cell immunity in cancer patients. *J. Clin. Invest.* **107,** 477–484.

Kobayashi, H., Kokubo, T., Sato, K., Kimura, S., Asano, K., Takahashi, H., Iizuka, H., Miyokawa, N., and Katagiri, M. (1998). CD4+ T cells from peripheral blood of a melanoma patient recognize peptides derived from nonmutated tyrosinase. *Cancer Res.* **58,** 296–301.

Kraal, G., Schornagel, K., Streeter, P. R., Holzmann, B., and Butcher, E. C. (1995). Expression of the mucosal vascular addressin, MAdCAM-1, on sinus-lining cells in the spleen. *Am. J Pathol.* **147,** 763–771.

Kunisada, T., Lu, S. Z., Yoshida, H., Nishikawa, S., Nishikawa, S., Mizoguchi, M., Hayashi, S., Tyrrell, L., Williams, D. A., Wang, X., and Longley, B. J. (1998). Murine cutaneous mastocytosis and epidermal melanocytosis induced by keratinocyte expression of transgenic stem cell factor. *J. Exp. Med.* **187,** 1565–1573.

Kurts, C., Kosaka, H., Carbone, F. R., Miller, J. F. A. P., and Heath, W. R. (1997). Class I-restricted cross-presentation of exogenous self-antigens leads to deletion of autoreactive $CD8^+$ T Cells. *J. Exp. Med.* **186,** 239–245.

Kurts, C., Sutherland, R. M., Davey, G., Li, M., Lew, A. M., Blanas, E., Carbone, F. R., Miller, J. F., and Heath, W. R. (1999). CD8 T cell ignorance or tolerance to islet antigens depends on antigen dose. *Proc. Natl. Acad. Sci. USA* **96,** 12703–12707.

Lappin, M. B., Weiss, J. M., Delattre, V., Mai, B., Dittmar, H., Maier, C., Manke, K., Grabbe, S., Martin, S., and Simon, J. C. (1999). Analysis of mouse dendritic cell migration *in vivo* upon subcutaneous and intravenous injection. *Immunology* **98,** 181–188.

Li, K., Adibzadeh, M., Halder, T., Kalbacher, H., Heinzel, S., Muller, C., Zeuthen, J., and Pawelec, G. (1998). Tumour-specific MHC-class-II-restricted responses after *in vitro* sensitization to synthetic peptides corresponding to gp100 and Annexin II eluted from melanoma cells. *Cancer Immunol. Immunother.* **47,** 32–38.

Limmer, A., Ohl, J., Kurts, C., Ljunggren, H. G., Reiss, Y., Groettrup, M., Momburg, F., Arnold, B., and Knolle, P. A. (2000). Efficient presentation of exogenous antigen by liver endothelial cells to CD8+ T cells results in antigen-specific T-cell tolerance. *Nat. Med.* **6,** 1348–1354.

Limmer, A., Sacher, T., Alferink, J., Kretschmar, M., Schonrich, G., Nichterlein, T., Arnold, B., and Hammerling, G. J. (1998). Failure to induce organ-specific autoimmunity by breaking of tolerance: Importance of the microenvironment. *Eur. J. Immunol.* **28,** 2395–2406.

Man, S., Newberg, M. H., Crotzer, V. L., Luckey, C. J., Williams, N. S., Chen, Y., Huczko, E. L., Ridge, J. P., and Engelhard, V. H. (1995). Definition of a human T cell epitope from influenza A non-structural protein 1 using HLA-A2.1 transgenic mice. *Int. Immunol.* **7,** 597–605.

Manici, S., Sturniolo, T., Imro, M. A., Hammer, J., Sinigaglia, F., Noppen, C., Spagnoli, G., Mazzi, B., Bellone, M., Dellabona, P., and Protti, M. P. (1999). Melanoma cells present a MAGE-3 epitope to CD4(+) cytotoxic T cells in association with histocompatibility leukocyte antigen DR11. *J. Exp. Med.* **189,** 871–876.

Marchand, M., Weynants, P., Rankin, E., Arienti, F., Belli, F., Parmiani, G., Cascinelli, N., Bourlond, A., Vanwijck, R., Humblet, Y., Canon, J. L., Laurent, C., et al. (1995). Tumor regression responses in melanoma patients treated with a peptide encoded by gene MAGE-3. *Int. J. Cancer* **63,** 883–885.

Martín-Fontecha, A., Sebastiani, S., Hopken, U. E., Uguccioni, M., Lipp, M., Lanzavecchia, A., and Sallusto, F. (2003). Regulation of dendritic cell migration to the draining lymph node: Impact on T lymphocyte traffic and priming. *J. Exp. Med.* **198,** 615–621.

Mayerova, D., Parke, E. A., Bursch, L. S., Odumade, O. A., and Hogquist, K. A. (2004). Langerhans cells activate naive self-antigen-specific CD8 T cells in the steady state. *Immunity* **21,** 391–400.

Meadows, L. R., Wang, W., den Haan, J. M., Blokland, E., Reinhardus, C., Drijfhout, J. W., Shabanowitz, J., Pierce, R., Agulnik, A., Bishop, C. E., Hunt, D. F., Goulmy, E., and Engelhard, V. H. (1997). The HLA-A°0201-restricted HY antigen contains a posttranslationally modified cysteine that significantly affects T cell recognition. *Immunity* **6,** 273–281.

Meidenbauer, N., Marienhagen, J., Laumer, M., Vogl, S., Heymann, J., Andreesen, R., and Mackensen, A. (2003). Survival and tumor localization of adoptively transferred Melan-A-specific T cells in melanoma patients. *J. Immunol.* **170,** 2161–2169.

Mellor, A. L., and Munn, D. H. (2004). IDO expression by dendritic cells: Tolerance and tryptophan catabolism. [Review, 151 refs]. *Nat. Rev. Immunol.* **4,** 762–774.

Merad, M., Hoffmann, P., Ranheim, E., Slaymaker, S., Manz, M. G., Lira, S. A., Charo, I., Cook, D. N., Weissman, I. L., Strober, S., and Engleman, E. G. (2004). Depletion of host Langerhans cells before transplantation of donor alloreactive T cells prevents skin graft-versus-host disease. *Nat. Med.* **10**, 510–517.

Merad, M., Manz, M. G., Karsunky, H., Wagers, A., Peters, W., Charo, I., Weissman, I. L., Cyster, J. G., and Engleman, E. G. (2002). Langerhans cells renew in the skin throughout life under steady-state conditions. *Nat. Immunol.* **3**, 1135–1141.

Mora, J. R., Cheng, G., Picarella, D., Briskin, M., Buchanan, N., and von Andrian, U. H. (2005). Reciprocal and dynamic control of CD8 T cell homing by dendritic cells from skin- and gut-associated lymphoid tissues. *J. Exp. Med.* **201**, 303–316.

Morgan, D. J., Kreuwel, H. T., and Sherman, L. A. (1999). Antigen concentration and precursor frequency determine the rate of CD8+ T cell tolerance to peripherally expressed antigens. *J. Immunol.* **163**, 723–727.

Morse, M. A., Coleman, R. E., Akabani, G., Niehaus, N., Coleman, D., and Lyerly, H. K. (1999). Migration of human dendritic cells after injection in patients with metastatic malignancies. *Cancer Res.* **59**, 56–58.

Mosse, C. A., Hsu, W., and Engelhard, V. H. (2001). Tyrosinase degradation via two pathways during reverse translocation to the cytosol. *Biochem. Biophys. Res. Commun.* **285**, 313–319.

Mullins, D. W., Bullock, T. N., Colella, T. A., Robila, V. V., and Engelhard, V. H. (2001). Immune responses to the HLA-A°0201-restricted epitopes of tyrosinase and glycoprotein 100 enable control of melanoma outgrowth in HLA-A°0201- transgenic mice. *J. Immunol.* **167**, 4853–4860.

Mullins, D. W., and Engelhard, V. H. (2006a). Limited infiltration of exogenous dendritic cells and naïve T cells restricts immune responses in peripheral lymph nodes.

Mullins, D. W., and Engelhard, V. H. (2006b). The immunogenicity of exogenous dendritic cells differs in lymph nodes and spleen.

Mullins, D. W., Sheasley, S. L., Ream, R. M., Bullock, T. N., Fu, Y. X., and Engelhard, V. H. (2003). Route of immunization with peptide-pulsed dendritic cells controls the distribution of memory and effector T cells in lymphoid tissues and determines the pattern of regional tumor control. *J. Exp. Med.* **198**, 1023–1034.

Nestle, F. O., Alijagic, S., Gilliet, M., Sun, Y., Grabbe, S., Dummer, R., Burg, G., and Schadendorf, D. (1998b). Vaccination of melanoma patients with peptide- or tumor lysate-pulsed dendritic cells. *Nat. Med.* **4**, 328–332.

Nestle, F. O., Alijagic, S., Gilliet, M., Sun, Y., Grabbe, S., Dummer, R., Burg, G., and Schadendorf, D. (1998a). Vaccination of melanoma patients with peptide- or tumor lysate-pulsed dendritic cells. *Nat. Med.* **4**, 328–332.

Newberg, M. H., Smith, D. H., Haertel, S. B., Vining, D. R., Lacy, E., and Engelhard, V. H. (1996). Importance of MHC class I a2 and a3 domains in the recognition of self and non-self MHC molecules. *J. Immunol.* **156**, 2473–2480.

Nichols, L. A., Colella, T. A., Chen, Y., and Engelhard, V. H. (2006). Self-tolerance to tyrosinase, an antigen expressed in melanocytes and melanoma is via deletion mediated by a radioresistant antigen presenting cell in the periphery.

Nolte, M. A., Hamann, A., Kraal, G., and Mebius, R. E. (2002). The strict regulation of lymphocyte migration to splenic white pulp does not involve common homing receptors. *Immunology* **106**, 299–307.

Nordlund, J. J., Kirkwood, J. M., Forget, B. M., Milton, G., Albert, D. M., and Lerner, A. B. (1983). Vitiligo in patients with metastatic melanoma: A good prognostic sign. *J. Am. Acad. Dermatol.* **9**, 689–696.

Novellino, L., Castelli, C., and Parmiani, G. (2005). A listing of human tumor antigens recognized by T cells: March 2004 update. [Review, 220 refs]. *Cancer Immunol. Immunother.* **54**, 187–207.

Ohlen, C., Kalos, M., Cheng, L. E., Shur, A. C., Hong, D. J., Carson, B. D., Kokot, N. C., Lerner, C. G., Sather, B. D., Huseby, E. S., and Greenberg, P. D. (2002). CD8(+) T cell tolerance to a tumor-associated antigen is maintained at the level of expansion rather than effector function. *J. Exp. Med.* **195,** 1407–1418.

Ohlen, C., Kalos, M., Hong, D. J., Shur, A. C., and Greenberg, P. D. (2001). Expression of a tolerizing tumor antigen in peripheral tissue does not preclude recovery of high-affinity CD8+ T cells or CTL immunotherapy of tumors expressing the antigen. *J. Immunol.* **166,** 2863–2870.

Okada, N., Tsujino, M., Hagiwara, Y., Tada, A., Tamura, Y., Mori, K., Saito, T., Nakagawa, S., Mayumi, T., Fujita, T., and Yamamoto, A. (2001). Administration route-dependent vaccine efficiency of murine dendritic cells pulsed with antigens. *Br. J. Cancer* **84,** 1564–1570.

Overwijk, W. W., Lee, D. S., Surman, D. R., Irvine, K. R., Touloukian, C. E., Chan, C. C., Carroll, M. W., Moss, R., Rosenberg, S. A., and Restifo, N. P. (1999). Vaccination with a recombinant vaccinia virus encoding a "self" antigen induces autoimmune vitiligo and tumor cell destruction in mice: Requirement for CD4(+) T lymphocytes. *Proc. Natl. Acad. Sci. USA* **96,** 2982–2987.

Overwijk, W. W., Theoret, M. R., Finkelstein, S. E., Surman, D. R., de Jong, L. A., Vyth-Dreese, F. A., Dellemijn, T. A., Antony, P. A., Spiess, P. J., Palmer, D. C., Heimann, D. M., Klebanoff, C. A., *et al.* (2003). Tumor regression and autoimmunity after reversal of a functionally tolerant state of self-reactive CD8+ T cells. *J. Exp. Med.* **198,** 569–580.

Palermo, B., Campanelli, R., Garbelli, S., Mantovani, S., Lantelme, E., Brazzelli, V., Ardigo, M., Borroni, G., Martinetti, M., Badulli, C., Necker, A., and Giachino, C. (2001). Specific cytotoxic T lymphocyte responses against Melan-A/MART1, tyrosinase and gp100 in vitiligo by the use of major histocompatibility complex/peptide tetramers: The role of cellular immunity in the etiopathogenesis of vitiligo. *J. Invest. Dermatol.* **117,** 326–332.

Panelli, M. C., Wunderlich, J., Jeffries, J., Wang, E., Mixon, A., Rosenberg, S. A., and Marincola, F. M. (2000). Phase 1 study in patients with metastatic melanoma of immunization with dendritic cells presenting epitopes derived from the melanoma-associated antigens MART-1 and gp100. *J. Immunother.* **23,** 487–498.

Pardoll, D. M., and Topalian, S. L. (1998). The role of CD4+ T cell responses in antitumor immunity. *Curr. Opin. Immunol.* **10,** 588–594.

Pass, H. A., Schwarz, S. L., Wunderlich, J. R., and Rosenberg, S. A. (1998). Immunization of patients with melanoma peptide vaccines: Immunologic assessment using the ELISPOT assay (see comments). *Cancer J. Sci. Am.* **4,** 316–323.

Phan, G. Q., Touloukian, C. E., Yang, J. C., Restifo, N. P., Sherry, R. M., Hwu, P., Topalian, S. L., Schwartzentruber, D. J., Seipp, C. A., Freezer, L. J., Morton, K. E., Mavroukakis, S. A., *et al.* (2003). Immunization of patients with metastatic melanoma using both class I- and class II-restricted peptides from melanoma-associated antigens. *J. Immunother.* **26,** 349–356.

Pierce, R. A., Field, E. D., den Haan, J. M., Caldwell, J. A., White, F. M., Marto, J. A., Wang, W., Frost, L. M., Blokland, E., Reinhardus, C., Shabanowitz, J., Hunt, D. F., *et al.* (1999). Cutting edge: The HLA-A°0101-restricted HY minor histocompatibility antigen originates from DFFRY and contains a cysteinylated cysteine residue as identified by a novel mass spectrometric technique. *J. Immunol.* **163,** 6360–6364.

Pihlgren, M., Dubois, P. M., Tomkowiak, M., Sjogren, T., and Marvel, J. (1996). Resting memory CD8+ T cells are hyperreactive to antigenic challenge *in vitro*. *J. Exp. Med.* **184,** 2141–2151.

Porter, S. D., Hu, J., and Gilks, C. B. (1999). Distal upstream tyrosinase S/MAR-containing sequence has regulatory properties specific to subsets of melanocytes. *Dev. Genet.* **25,** 40–48.

Quarmby, S., Hunter, R. D., and Kumar, S. (2000). Irradiation induced expression of CD31, ICAM-1 and VCAM-1 in human microvascular endothelial cells. *Anticancer Res.* **20,** 3375–3381.

Quarmby, S., Kumar, P., and Kumar, S. (1999). Radiation-induced normal tissue injury: Role of adhesion molecules in leukocyte-endothelial cell interactions. *Int. J. Cancer* **82,** 385–395.

Rennert, P. D., Hochman, P. S., Flavell, R. A., Chaplin, D. D., Jayaraman, S., Browning, J. L., and Fu, Y. X. (2001). Essential role of lymph nodes in contact hypersensitivity revealed in lymphotoxin-alpha-deficient mice. *J. Exp. Med.* **193,** 1227–1238.

Riker, A., Cormier, J., Panelli, M., Kammula, U., Wang, E., Abati, A., Fetsch, P., Lee, K. H., Steinberg, S., Rosenberg, S., and Marincola, F. (1999). Immune selection after antigen-specific immunotherapy of melanoma. *Surgery* **126,** 112–120.

Rinchik, E. M., Stoye, J. P., Frankel, W. N., Coffin, J., Kwon, B. S., and Russell, L. B. (1993). Molecular analysis of viable spontaneous and radiation-induced albino (c)-locus mutations in the mouse. *Mut. Res.* **286,** 199–207.

Rosenberg, S. A., Packard, B. S., Aebersold, P. M., Solomon, D., Topalian, S. L., Toy, S. T., Simon, P., Lotze, M. T., Yang, J. C., and Seipp, C. A. (1988). Use of tumor-infiltrating lymphocytes and interleukin-2 in the immunotherapy of patients with metastatic melanoma. A preliminary report. *N. Engl. J. Med.* **319,** 1676–1680.

Rosenberg, S. A., and White, D. E. (1996). Vitiligo in patients with melanoma—normal tissue antigens can be targets for cancer immunotherapy. *J. Immunother. Emphasis Tumor Biol.* **19,** 81–84.

Rosenberg, S. A., Yang, J. C., Schwartzentruber, D. J., Hwu, P., Marincola, F. M., Topalian, S. L., Restifo, N. P., Dudley, M. E., Schwarz, S. L., Spiess, P. J., Wunderlich, J. R., Parkhurst, M. R., *et al.* (1998). Immunologic and therapeutic evaluation of a synthetic peptide vaccine for the treatment of patients with metastatic melanoma. *Nat. Med.* **4,** 321–327.

Rott, L. S., Briskin, M. J., Andrew, D. P., Berg, E. L., and Butcher, E. C. (1996). A fundamental subdivision of circulating lymphocytes defined by adhesion to mucosal addressin cell adhesion molecule-1. Comparison with vascular cell adhesion molecule-1 and correlation with beta 7 integrins and memory differentiation. *J. Immunol.* **156,** 3727–3736.

Scheibenbogen, C., Schadendorf, D., Bechrakis, N. E., Nagorsen, D., Hofmann, U., Servetopoulou, F., Letsch, A., Philipp, A., Foerster, M. H., Schmittel, A., Thiel, E., and Keilholz, U. (2003). Effects of granulocyte-macrophage colony-stimulating factor and foreign helper protein as immunologic adjuvants on the T-cell response to vaccination with tyrosinase peptides. *Int. J. Cancer* **104,** 188–194.

Scheibenbogen, C., Schmittel, A., Keilholz, U., Allgauer, T., Hofmann, U., Max, R., Thiel, E., and Schadendorf, D. (2000). Phase 2 trial of vaccination with tyrosinase peptides and granulocyte-macrophage colony-stimulating factor in patients with metastatic melanoma. *J. Immunother.* **23,** 275–281.

Selby, M., Erickson, A., Dong, C., Cooper, S., Parham, P., Houghton, M., and Walker, C. M. (1999). Hepatitis C virus envelope glycoprotein E1 originates in the endoplasmic reticulum and requires cytoplasmic processing for presentation by class I MHC molecules. *J. Immunol.* **162,** 669–676.

Shankaran, V., Ikeda, H., Bruce, A. T., White, J. M., Swanson, P. E., Old, L. J., and Schreiber, R. D. (2001). IFNgamma and lymphocytes prevent primary tumour development and shape tumour immunogenicity. *Nature* **410,** 1107–1111.

Sheasley-O'Neill, S. L., Dispenza, M. C., Brinkmann, V., and Engelhard, V. H. (2006). CD8 T cell homing receptor expression and localization to lymphoid and non-lymphoid tissues depends upon the compartment in which activation by exogenous DC occurs.

Shirai, M., Arichi, T., Nishioka, M., Nomura, T., Ikeda, K., Kawanishi, K., Engelhard, V. H., Feinstone, S. M., and Berzofsky, J. A. (1995). CTL responses of HLA-A2.1-transgenic mice specific for hepatitis C viral peptides predict epitopes for CTL of humans carrying HLA-A2.1. *J. Immunol.* **154,** 2733–2742.

Skipper, J. C., Gulden, P. H., Hendrickson, R. C., Harthun, N., Caldwell, J. A., Shabanowitz, J., Engelhard, V. H., Hunt, D. F., and Slingluff, C. L., Jr. (1999). Mass-spectrometric evaluation of

HLA-A°0201-associated peptides identifies dominant naturally processed forms of CTL epitopes from MART-1 and gp100. *Int. J. Cancer* **82**, 669–677.

Skipper, J. C., Hendrickson, R. C., Gulden, P. H., Brichard, V., Van Pel, A., Chen, Y., Shabanowitz, J., Wolfel, T., Slingluff, C. L. J., Boon, T., Hunt, D. F., and Engelhard, V. H. (1996a). An HLA-A2-restricted tyrosinase antigen on melanoma cells results from posttranslational modification and suggests a novel pathway for processing of membrane proteins. *J. Exp. Med.* **183**, 527–534.

Skipper, J. C., Kittlesen, D. J., Hendrickson, R. C., Deacon, D. D., Harthun, N. L., Wagner, S. N., Hunt, D. F., Engelhard, V. H., and Slingluff, C. L., Jr. (1996b). Shared epitopes for HLA-A3-restricted melanoma-reactive human CTL include a naturally processed epitope from Pmel-17/gp100. *J. Immunol.* **157**, 5027–5033.

Slingluff, C. L., Petroni, G., Bullock, K. A., Bissonette, E., Hibbitts, S., Murphy, C., Anderson, N., Grosh, W. W., Neese, P. Y., and Fink, R. (2004). Immunological results of a phase II randomized trial of multipeptide vaccines for melanoma, pp. abstract number 7503.

Slingluff, C. L., Jr., Petroni, G. R., Yamshchikov, G. V., Barnd, D. L., Eastham, S., Galavotti, H., Patterson, J. W., Deacon, D. H., Hibbitts, S., Teates, D., Neese, P. Y., Grosh, W. W., *et al.* (2003). Clinical and immunologic results of a randomized phase II trial of vaccination using four melanoma peptides either administered in granulocyte-macrophage colony-stimulating factor in adjuvant or pulsed on dendritic cells (see comment). *J. Clin. Oncol.* **21**, 4016–4026.

Slingluff, C. L. J., Cox, A. L., Henderson, R. A., Hunt, D. F., and Engelhard, V. H. (1993). Recognition of human melanoma cells by HLA-A2.1-restricted cytotoxic T lymphocytes is mediated by at least six shared peptide epitopes. *J. Immunol.* **150**, 2955–2963.

Slingluff, C. L. J., Darrow, T., Vervaert, C., Quinn-Allen, M. A., and Seigler, H. F. (1988). Human cytotoxic T cells specific for autologous melanoma cells: Successful generation from lymph node cells in seven consecutive cases. *J. Natl. Cancer Inst.* **80**, 1016–1026.

Slingluff, C. L. J., Darrow, T. L., and Seigler, H. F. (1989). Melanoma-specific cytotoxic T cells generated from peripheral blood lymphocytes. Implications of a renewable source of precursors for adoptive cellular immunotherapy (see comments). *Ann. Surg.* **210**, 194–202.

Slingluff, C. L. J., Yamshchikov, G., Neese, P., Galavotti, H., Eastham, S., Engelhard, V. H., Kittlesen, D., Deacon, D., Hibbitts, S., Grosh, W. W., Petroni, G., Cohen, R., *et al.* (2001). Phase I trial of a melanoma vaccine with gp100 (280–288) peptide and tetanus helper peptide in adjuvant: Immunologic and clinical outcomes. *Clin. Cancer Res.* **7**, 3012–3024.

Slominski, A., Paus, R., Plonka, P., Chakraborty, A., Maurer, M., Pruski, D., and Lukiewicz, S. (1994). Melanogenesis during the anagen-catagen-telogen transformation of the murine hair cycle. *J. Invest Dermatol.* **102**, 862–869.

Steitz, J., Bruck, J., Lenz, J., Buchs, S., and Tuting, T. (2005). Peripheral CD8+ T cell tolerance against melanocytic self-antigens in the skin is regulated in two steps by CD4+ T cells and local inflammation: Implications for the pathophysiology of vitiligo. *J. Invest Dermatol.* **124**, 144–150.

Steitz, J., Bruck, J., Steinbrink, K., Enk, A., Knop, J., and Tuting, T. (2000). Genetic immunization of mice with human tyrosinase-related protein 2: Implications for the immunotherapy of melanoma. *Int. J. Cancer* **86**, 89–94.

Tanchot, C., Guillaume, S., Delon, J., Bourgeois, C., Franzke, A., Sarukhan, A., Trautmann, A., and Rocha, B. (1998). Modifications of CD8+ T cell function during *in vivo* memory or tolerance induction. *Immunity* **8**, 581–590.

Tatsumi, T., Kierstead, L. S., Ranieri, E., Gesualdo, L., Schena, F. P., Finke, J. H., Bukowski, R. M., Mueller-Berghaus, J., Kirkwood, J. M., Kwok, W. W., and Storkus, W. J. (2002). Disease-associated bias in T helper type 1 (Th1)/Th2 CD4(+) T cell responses against MAGE-6 in HLA-DRB10401(+) patients with renal cell carcinoma or melanoma. *J. Exp. Med.* **196**, 619–628.

Thurner, B., Haendle, I., Roder, C., Dieckmann, D., Keikavoussi, P., Jonuleit, H., Bender, A., Maczek, C., Schreiner, D., von Den Driesch, P., Brocker, E. B., Steinman, R. M., et al. (1999). Vaccination with mage-3A1 peptide-pulsed mature, monocyte-derived dendritic cells expands specific cytotoxic T cells and induces regression of some metastases in advanced stage IV melanoma. *J. Exp. Med.* **190,** 1669–1678.

Tief, K., Hahne, M., Schmidt, A., and Beerman, F. (1996). Tyrosinase, the key enzyme in melanin synthesis, is expressed in murine brain. *Eur. J. Biochem.* **241,** 12–16.

Toes, R. E., Blom, R. J., Offringa, R., Kast, W. M., and Melief, C. J. (1996). Enhanced tumor outgrowth after peptide vaccination. Functional deletion of tumor-specific CTL induced by peptide vaccination can lead to the inability to reject tumors. *J. Immunol.* **156,** 3911–3918.

Toes, R. E., van der Voort, E. I., Schoenberger, S. P., Drijfhout, J. W., van Bloois, L., Storm, G., Kast, W. M., Offringa, R., and Melief, C. J. (1998). Enhancement of tumor outgrowth through CTL tolerization after peptide vaccination is avoided by peptide presentation on dendritic cells. *J. Immunol.* **160,** 4449–4456.

Topalian, S. L., Gonzales, M. I., Parkhurst, M., Li, Y. F., Southwood, S., Sette, A., Rosenberg, S. A., and Robbins, P. F. (1996). Melanoma-specific CD4+ T cells recognize nonmutated HLA-DR-restricted tyrosinase epitopes. *J. Exp. Med.* **183,** 1965–1971.

Traversari, C., van der Bruggen, P., Luescher, I. F., Lurquin, C., Chomez, P., Van Pel, A., De Plaen, E., Amar-Costesec, A., and Boon, T. (1992). A nonapeptide encoded by human gene MAGE-1 is recognized on HLA-A1 by cytolytic T lymphocytes directed against tumor antigen MZ2-E. *J. Exp. Med.* **176,** 1453–1457.

van Elsas, A., Hurwitz, A. A., and Allison, J. P. (1999). Combination immunotherapy of B16 melanoma using anti-cytotoxic T lymphocyte-associated antigen 4 (CTLA-4) and granulocyte/macrophage colony-stimulating factor (GM-CSF)-producing vaccines induces rejection of subcutaneous and metastatic tumors accompanied by autoimmune depigmentation. *Proc. Natl. Acad. Sci. USA* **96,** 2982.

Vezys, V., Olson, S., and Lefrancois, L. (2000). Expression of intestine-specific antigen reveals novel pathways of CD8 T cell tolerance induction. *Immunity* **12,** 505–514.

Vitiello, A., Marchesini, D., Furze, J., Sherman, L. A., and Chestnut, R. W. (1991). Analysis of the HLA-restricted influenza-specific cytotoxic T lymphocyte response in transgenic mice carrying a chimeric human-mouse class I major histocompatibility complex. *J. Exp. Med.* **173,** 1007–1015.

Wang, R. F., Johnston, S. L., Zeng, G., Topalian, S. L., Schwartzentruber, D. J., and Rosenberg, S. A. (1998). A breast and melanoma-shared tumor antigen: T cell responses to antigenic peptides translated from different open reading frames. *J. Immunol.* **161,** 3598–3606.

Weber, J. S., Hua, F. L., Spears, L., Marty, V., Kuniyoshi, C., and Celis, E. (1999). A phase I trial of an HLA-A1 restricted MAGE-3 epitope peptide with incomplete Freund's adjuvant in patients with resected high-risk melanoma. *J. Immunother.* **22,** 431–440.

Wentworth, P. A., Sette, A., Celis, E., Sidney, J., Southwood, S., Crimi, C., Stitely, S., Keogh, E., Wong, N. C., Livingston, B., Alazard, D., Vitiello, A., et al. (1996a). Identification of A2-restricted hepatitis C virus-specific cytotoxic T lymphocyte epitopes from conserved regions of the viral genome. *Int. Immunol.* **8,** 651–659.

Wentworth, P. A., Vitiello, A., Sidney, J., Keogh, E., Chesnut, R. W., Grey, H., and Sette, A. (1996b). Differences and similarities in the A2.1-restricted cytotoxic T cell repertoire in humans and human leukocyte antigen-transgenic mice. *Eur. J. Immunol.* **26,** 97–101.

Wong, R., Lau, R., Chang, J., Kuus-Reichel, T., Brichard, V., Bruck, C., and Weber, J. (2004). Immune responses to a class II helper peptide epitope in patients with stage III/IV resected melanoma. *Clin. Cancer Res.* **10,** 5004–5013.

Woodson, E. M., Chianese-Bullock, K. A., Wiernasz, C. J., Bissonette, E. A., Grosh, W. W., Neese, P. Y., Merrill, P. K., Barnd, D. L., Petroni, G. R., and Slingluff, C. L., Jr. (2004). Assessment of the toxicities of systemic low-dose interleukin-2 administered in conjunction with a melanoma peptide vaccine. *J. Immunother.* **27,** 380–388.

Yamshchikov, G. V., Barnd, D. L., Eastham, S., Galavotti, H., Patterson, J. W., Deacon, D. H., Teates, D., Neese, P., Grosh, W. W., Petroni, G. R., Engelhard, V. H., and Slingluff, C. L., Jr. (2001). Evaluation of peptide vaccine immunogenicity in draining lymph nodes and blood of melanoma patients. *Int. J. Cancer* **92,** 703–711.

Yamshchikov, G. V., Mullins, D. W., Chang, C. C., Ogino, T., Thompson, L., Pressley, J., Galavotti, H., Aquila, W., Deacon, D., Ross, W. G., Patterson, J. W., Engelhard, V. H., *et al.* (2005). Sequential immune escape and shifting of T cell responses in a long-term survivor of melanoma. *J. Immunol.* **174,** 6863–6871.

Yee, C., Thompson, J. A., Roche, P., Byrd, D. R., Lee, P. P., Piepkorn, M., Kenyon, K., Davis, M. M., Riddell, S. R., and Greenberg, P. D. (2000). Melanocyte destruction after antigen-specific immunotherapy of melanoma: Direct evidence of T cell-mediated vitiligo. *J. Exp. Med.* **192,** 1637–1644.

Zarling, A. L., Ficarro, S. B., White, F. M., Shabanowitz, J., Hunt, D. F., and Engelhard, V. H. (2000). Phosphorylated peptides are naturally processed and presented by major histocompatibility complex class I molecules *in vivo. J. Exp. Med.* **192,** 1755–1762.

Zarling, A. L., Polefrone, J. M., Hopkins, L. M., Evans, A. M., Shabanowitz, J., Lewis, S. T., Hunt, D. F., and Engelhard, V. H. (2006). Phosphoproteomic evaluation of the class I MHC peptide repertoire on cancer cells.

Zarour, H. M., Kirkwood, J. M., Kierstead, L. S., Herr, W., Brusic, V., Slingluff, C. L. J., Sidney, J., Sette, A., and Storkus, W. J. (2000). Melan-A/MART-1(51–73) represents an immunogenic HLA-DR4-restricted epitope recognized by melanoma-reactive CD4(+) T cells. *Proc. Natl. Acad. Sci. USA* **97,** 400–405.

Zeh, H. J., III, Perry-Lalley, D., Dudley, M. E., Rosenberg, S. A., and Yang, J. C. (1999). High avidity CTLs for two self-antigens demonstrate superior *in vitro* and *in vivo* antitumor efficacy. *J. Immunol.* **162,** 989–994.

Zhao, X., Deak, E., Soderberg, K., Linehan, M., Spezzano, D., Zhu, J., Knipe, D. M., and Iwasaki, A. (2003). Vaginal submucosal dendritic cells, but not Langerhans cells, induce protective Th1 responses to herpes simplex virus-2. *J. Exp. Med.* **197,** 153–162.

Checkpoint Blockade in Cancer Immunotherapy

Alan J. Korman,* Karl S. Peggs,[†] and James P. Allison[†]

*Medarex Inc., Milpitas, California
[†]Howard Hughes Medical Institute, Memorial Sloan-Kettering Cancer Center, New York, New York

  Abstract.. 297
1. Introduction 297
2. The Extended CD28:B7 Immunoglobulin Superfamily............................... 300
3. Preclinical Models of Checkpoint Blockade as Tumor Immunotherapy......... 310
4. Clinical Trials of CTLA-4 Blockade: Overview 317
5. Other Potential Coinhibitory Targets for Checkpoint Blockade 323
6. Conclusions... 328
   References.. 329

Abstract

The progression of a productive immune response requires that a number of immunological checkpoints be passed. Passage may require the presence of excitatory costimulatory signals or the avoidance of negative or coinhibitory signals, which act to dampen or terminate immune activity. The immunoglobulin superfamily occupies a central importance in this coordination of immune responses, and the CD28/cytotoxic T-lymphocyte antigen-4 (CTLA-4):B7.1/B7.2 receptor/ligand grouping represents the archetypal example of these immune regulators. In part the role of these checkpoints is to guard against the possibility of unwanted and harmful self-directed activities. While this is a necessary function, aiding in the prevention of autoimmunity, it may act as a barrier to successful immunotherapies aimed at targeting malignant self-cells that largely display the same array of surface molecules as the cells from which they derive. Therapies aimed at overcoming these mechanisms of peripheral tolerance, in particular by blocking the inhibitory checkpoints, offer the potential to generate antitumor activity, either as monotherapies or in synergism with other therapies that directly or indirectly enhance presentation of tumor epitopes to the immune system. Such immunological molecular adjuvants are showing promise in early clinical trials. This review focuses on the results of the archetypal example of checkpoint blockade, anti-CTLA-4, in preclinical tumor models and clinical trials, while also highlighting other possible targets for immunological checkpoint blockade.

1. Introduction

Progress in antitumor immunotherapy has been aided by advances in the understanding of antigen presentation and the rules governing polarization of subsequent immune responses toward $CD4^+$ or $CD8^+$ compartments and

Th1/Th2 or Tc1/Tc2 phenotypes. A number of approaches aimed at enhancing tumor-specific activities have provided important proofs of principle in both murine models and early clinical trials in humans. However, while many methodologies aimed at enhancing these earliest of events in the immune response (such as peptide or protein vaccines, dendritic cell vaccines loaded with peptides or modified to express tumor antigens, DNA vaccines with or without modifications to enhance $CD8^+$ T-cell responses, and cytokine-secreting cellular vaccines derived from primary tumor) have provided encouraging results in specific preclinical models, or have been demonstrated to enable the generation of measurable antitumor activity based on sensitive laboratory read-outs of immunological reactivity, the generation of prolonged, objectively quantifiable and clinically meaningful responses in patients has proven more difficult than initially envisaged. Of course, part of the difficulty arises from the fact that the tumors are host-derived and express mostly the same array of self-antigens as the cell types from which they arise. Many of the molecules identified as potentially therapeutic targets in human cancers are self or "altered self" antigens, either aberrantly expressed or overexpressed on malignant cells. Overcoming multiple mechanisms of peripheral tolerance to these tumor-associated targets may prove crucial for effective recruitment of the immune effectors required for successful immune-based therapies. Just as our knowledge of the sentinel role of dendritic cells (T-cell extrinsic elements) in directing the outcome of early events in immune responses has expanded, we have also become increasingly aware of the roles of both T-cell intrinsic cell-autonomous regulatory elements, and of T-cell intrinsic non cell-autonomous mediators (regulatory T cells) in the induction of peripheral tolerance. And as we have learned more about the rules governing the progression of productive immune responses, we have discovered an extended network of immunological checkpoints that need to be passed in order for these responses to proceed. Attention to these immunological bottlenecks may prove critical for us to fully harness the therapeutic potential of immunotherapy.

Given the latent destructive capacity inherent in the mammalian adaptive immune system, it is perhaps no surprise that multiple immunological checkpoints are in place to prevent inappropriate activation events such as those targeted toward self-antigens. However, the true complexity of these pathways has only relatively recently become apparent, and continues to be unraveled with the discovery of new molecules whose physiological significance remains uncertain. At a basic level these checkpoints may be viewed as those that are required to provide additional excitatory costimulatory activity for progression of immune priming or activation, initiation of cell division, or development of particular effector phenotypes following T-cell receptor (TCR) ligation, and those that provide "coinhibitory" influences and which may be more important both for the prevention of the initiation of inappropriately directed responses and for limiting the size, duration, or premature focusing of immune responses once initiated. As a group these molecules allow fine-tuning of the response to TCR ligation by cognate antigen. Each feeds into overlapping or identical downstream signaling pathways and by virtue of the contribution of multiple costimulatory signals with overlapping but nonredundant function acts as a rheostat for T-cell activation, survival, and function.

The initial foundation of self-tolerance is a fundamental function of the central tolerance established through positive and negative selection in the thymus. Self-proteins are processed and presented in association with self-major histocompatability complex (MHC) molecules on the surface of thymic antigen presenting cells (APCs). The subsequent outcome of interactions with T cells depends on the avidity between TCRs and self-peptide-MHC complexes. Interactions of very low-avidity result in T-cell deletion by apoptotic death by neglect, while high-avidity interactions result in similar termination of T cells by apoptotic negative selection. Intermediate-avidity binding provides positive selection with further T-cell differentiation and establishment of a T-cell repertoire characterized by a population of relatively weakly autoreactive T cells. Subthreshold recognition of self-antigens may thus be a prerequisite for the generation and survival of regulatory T cells and both naïve and memory T cells. This ontogeny has important implications for tumor immunotherapy in a system now established to include rheostatic mechanisms for resetting the threshold for T-cell activation events. If T cells capable of responding to tumor epitopes are present in the host, therapeutic manipulation of activation thresholds could recruit these cells, or enhance their functional capabilities sufficiently to effect meaningful antitumor activity. Evidence suggesting the existence of such tumor-reactive T cells can be derived from correlative studies in a number of human cancers demonstrating prolonged survival and/or reduced metastases in those patients who have greater levels of intratumor infiltration with T cells (Marrogi et al., 1997; Naito et al., 1998; Nakano et al., 2001; Vesalainen et al., 1994; Zhang et al., 2003a).

It is also apparent that the evolution of the malignant phenotype of tumor cells could be characterized by adaptations involving these regulatory molecules, which could enhance evasion of the immune responses that target aberrant cell outgrowth. For example, reduced expression of costimulatory ligands could render the malignant cells "invisible" to the immune system, while overexpression of coinhibitory ligands could effectively dampen or terminate active antitumor immunity (Iwai et al., 2002; Townsend and Allison, 1993). Subjugation of regulatory T-cell populations could also affect a similar outcome (Curiel et al., 2004; Liyanage et al., 2002; Viguier et al., 2004; Woo et al., 2001, 2002). Examples of all of these mechanisms have now been described in a variety of murine tumor models and human cancers, providing further impetus for attempts to manipulate these pathways for therapeutic benefit. Blockade of any of the inhibitory checkpoints could potentially enhance any preexistent antitumor immunity, and synergize with other therapies that either directly or indirectly augment such activities.

One further general point needs to be addressed when considering the potential of immune checkpoint blockade as a therapeutic modality. These checkpoints have a vital physiological role in limiting the potential damage that can be caused by an auto-reactive T-cell repertoire. Blockade might theoretically result in uncontrolled auto-reactivity and significant toxicity. Adverse immune events have been noted in some of the early clinical trials of cytotoxic T-lymphocyte antigen-4 (CTLA-4) blockade (Attia *et al.*, 2005; Phan *et al.*, 2003b; Ribas *et al.*, 2005b; Sanderson *et al.*, 2005). A question of vital importance is whether such adverse events are an inherent part of effective checkpoint blockade, or whether they can be dissociated by manipulation of dose scheduling, targeting immunological rather than clinical endpoints as a primary objective, or by combinatorial approaches involving strategies that will enhance presentation of tumor-selective antigens to the immune system over-and-above those of normal tissues. This review focuses on CTLA-4 blockade in tumor immunotherapy as the prototypical example of checkpoint blockade in order to address these issues, and highlight other potential targets warranting further exploration.

2. The Extended CD28:B7 Immunoglobulin Superfamily

Since the initial description of the costimulatory receptor ligand pair of CD28: B7, an extended family of structurally and functionally related molecules have been described, which due to their commonality with the immunoglobulin variable-like (IgV) and constant (IgC) domains of the immunoglobulins have become known collectively as the CD28:B7 immunoglobulin superfamily. The CD28 family is composed of CD28, CTLA-4, inducible T-cell costimulator (ICOS), programmed death-1 (PD-1), and B- and T-lymphocyte attenuator (BTLA). CD28 and ICOS typify costimulatory family members, whereas CTLA-4, PD-1, and BTLA appear to be coinhibitory. Both PD-1 and BTLA possess immunoreceptor tyrosine-inhibitory plus/minus tyrosine-switch motifs (ITIMs and ITSMs) and, like CTLA-4, are able to recruit phosphatases such as Src-homology protein tyrosine phosphatase-2 (SHP-2). Each immunoglobulin superfamily member, except BTLA, is characterized by a single extracellular IgV domain followed by a short cytoplasmic tail (although the major human form of B7-H3 uniquely contains two extracellular tandem IgV-IgC domains (Sun *et al.*, 2002)). The crystal structure of BTLA, in contrast, suggests it to be a member of the I-set of Ig domains (Compaan et al., 2005). CD28, CTLA-4, and ICOS have an unpaired cysteine that allows them to homodimerize on the cell surface, while neither PD-1 nor BTLA has an unpaired cysteine and both likely exist as monomers on the cell surface (Compaan et al., 2005; Zhang et al., 2004). The seven known members of the B7 family (B7.1, B7.2, ICOS-L, PD-L1, PD-L2, B7-H3, and B7x/B7-H4) are characterized by extracellular IgV-like and IgC-like domains and short intracellular cytoplasmic domains (19–62 amino acids). The intracellular domains contain serine and threonine residues, which may have significance as potential phosphorylation sites given the evidence that B7-family members can signal into the cell on which they are expressed. They are predicted to form homodimers at the cell surface (as shown for B7.1), although B7.2 likely exists as a monomer (Schwartz et al., 2001; Zhang et al., 2003b). The ligand for BTLA has been identified as the tumor-necrosis factor (TNF) receptor family member herpesvirus entry mediator (HVEM) (Sedy et al., 2005), providing a previously unknown structural interaction allowing reverse signaling from a TNF receptor family member toward lymphocytes that may be a barrier to T-cell activation. This, and the I-set structure, suggests that BTLA may be evolutionarily the most distantly related of the CD28 family.

2.1. CD28/CTLA-4:B7.1/B7.2: The Archetypal Immune Regulators

2.1.1. CD28: The Original Second Signal

The ability of CD28-dependent signaling to rescue T-cell clones from TCR-mediated anergy was recognized in the early 1990s (Harding et al., 1992), and the critical role of engagement by either of the structurally-homologous B7.1 (CD80) and B7.2 (CD86) ligand pair for costimulatory activity also established (Hathcock et al., 1994; Linsley et al., 1991). Blocking antibodies to B7.1 or B7.2 diminished, and a combination of both or a CTLA-4-Ig fusion protein effectively eliminated T-cell responses to a variety of *in vitro* and *in vivo* stimuli (Lenschow and Bluestone, 1993). Meanwhile, $CD28^{-/-}$ knockout mice showed severe diminution of most T-cell responses (although the ability to reject some viruses was retained, and subsequent studies suggested that the duration of TCR stimulation may determine the costimulatory requirement of certain T-cell responses) (Kundig et al., 1996; Shahinian et al., 1993), and B7.1/B7.2 double knockout mice demonstrated a virtual absence of T-cell responses (Borriello et al., 1997). Dendritic cells (DCs) expressed the highest levels of these costimulatory ligands, particularly after activating stimuli, and also demonstrated an enhanced ability to sample, process, and present exogenous antigen back to the adaptive immune system via the intermediary of MHC molecules. They became drawn as the sentinels of the immune system.

CD28 is constitutively expressed by most mouse T cells, 90% of human $CD4^+$ T cells and 50% of human $CD8^+$ T cells. The restricted localization of B7.1 and B7.2 expression to lymphoid and antigen-presenting cells (such as DCs, macrophages, and activated B cells) provides a compartmentalization that may function as a means by which early events in T-cell activation are directed to maintain peripheral tolerance by restricting T-cell activation to areas of inflammation or injury. B7.2 is expressed at a low level in nonactivated DCs and can be rapidly upregulated by a variety of activating stimuli (infection, tissue injury, inflammatory cytokines, and interaction of DCs with activated T cells). B7.1 is virtually absent from nonactivated DCs, is upregulated by similar stimuli but is expressed on the cell surface later than the peak of B7.2 expression.

There are no clearly defined differences in the downstream biochemical effects of ligation of CD28 by B7.1 or B7.2 respectively, and mice that are deficient for either B7.1 or B7.2 show that they have partially overlapping functions. The functional differences that can be observed may be more a result of the differences in expression kinetics of the two ligands than of any unique biochemical properties of the signals they induce. Provision of signaling via both TCR and CD28 results in dramatic changes in numerous aspects of T-cell function, the most immediate of which include rearrangement of plasma-membrane and cytoskeletal components, reorientation of the microtubule organizing center (MTOC), accelerated intracellular vesicular trafficking, and both general and locus-specific chromatin changes that are concomitant with nuclear localization and the activation of transcription factors (reviewed in Acuto and Michel, 2003). While the majority of these changes can be directed by strong and long-lasting supra-physiological stimulation via the TCR alone, the TCR ligation conditions that occur *in vivo* under normal circumstances are likely to generate only short-lasting and incomplete activation events that are insufficient to cause cell proliferation and differentiation, and which more likely result in the induction of anergy or cell death. In addition, some biological outcomes of TCR ligation do appear to have a mandatory requirement for CD28 signaling. Isolated CD28 ligation results in transient expression of a restricted number of the same genes induced by TCR ligation with no discernable dedicated signaling element, but engagement in concert with TCR ligation strongly amplifies weak TCR signals and modifies the gene regulation induced by TCR stimulation (Diehn *et al.*, 2002; Riley *et al.*, 2002). Thus, ligation of CD28 decreases the number of ligated TCRs that are required for a given biological response (Viola and Lanzavecchia,

1996), resulting in an apparent dependency on a qualitative second signal when TCR occupancy is low.

The recognition that B7 expression could enhance T-cell responses led to studies in murine models confirming that transfection-induced expression of B7.1/B7.2 on many immunogenic tumors resulted in T-cell mediated rejection in both a prophylactic and treatment setting (Chen *et al.*, 1992, 1994; Townsend and Allison, 1993). The efficacy of antitumor activity depended on inherent tumor immunogenicity (Chen *et al.*, 1994). Primary rejection of tumor cells was frequently documented to result in long-term protection against a secondary challenge, even with the B7⁻ parental tumor, as well as eradication of preestablished micro-metastases. Protection was demonstrated to be due to $CD8^+$ T cells by depletion studies, and it was initially envisaged that $CD8^+$ cytotoxic T cells (CTL) were being primed directly by transfected tumor cells. Bone marrow chimera experiments in which the haplotype of the reconstituted APC population was distinct from that of the tumor, however, demonstrated that while B7-transfected tumor could directly serve as APC for the priming of naïve CTL *in vivo*, the efficiency of this process was far less than that of CTL priming by the host's APC, requiring multiple immunizations to establish detectable responses as compared to the single immunization required for responses restricted to the haplotype of the bone marrow (Huang *et al.*, 1996). These findings suggested that B7 expression might enhance an initial wave of direct tumor lysis, but that it was the efficient cross-presentation of tumor debris via DCs that resulted in the majority of the enhanced immunogenicity seen with $B7^+$ tumors, consistent with the earlier finding that generation of effective systemic immunity was dependent on inherent tumor immunogenicity and that immunity to the parental tumor could be established. Nonimmunogenic tumors might be targeted by the initial wave of direct B7-directed killing of transfected cells but would not then generate potent systemic immunity.

2.1.2. CTLA-4 as a T Cell Intrinsic Cell-Autonomous Negative Regulator

CTLA-4 was recognized as a closely related homologue of CD28 capable of binding both of the B7.1/B7.2 ligand pair well before its true function became apparent. Following its establishment as a key negative regulator of immune responses these four molecules became acknowledged as perhaps the most important cofactors functioning at the tip of an immunological cascade. Together they act as the arbiters of initial immunological "stop–go" decisions, and emerged as the archetypal example of interdependent antagonistic costimulatory/inhibitory pathways. It has subsequently become apparent that their role may not be as straight forward as the simple licensing of "stop–go" signaling, but that they may be more subtly involved in the shaping of the immune repertoire and that their interdependence, coupled with the tight control of the temporal and spatial kinetics of their expression, might enable a mechanism to escape the restraints imposed by system based purely on Boolean logic. CTLA-4 has significantly higher affinities for both B7 ligands than does CD28. The interaction of CTLA-4 with B7.1 is of higher affinity than that with B7.2, whereas CD28 is predicted to bind to B7.2 more effectively than B7.1 (Collins *et al.*, 2002). Ligand binding is important for the accumulation of both CD28 and CTLA-4 at the synapse. While CD28 is recruited to the synapse in the absence of B7.1 and B7.2 binding, it is not effectively stabilized there, and its localization can be disrupted by CTLA-4. The latter is more critically dependent on ligand binding for concentration at the synapse (Pentcheva-Hoang *et al.*, 2004). The structure of cocrystals of CTLA-4 and B7.1 suggests that these molecules may form extended lattice-like networks, enabled by the distal positioning of CTLA-4 binding sites from the B7.1 dimer interface (Stamper *et al.*, 2001; van der Merwe and Davis, 2003). This contrasts with a likely monovalent interaction between CD28 and B7.2 (Collins *et al.*, 2002). The function of CTLA-4 as a negative regulator of CD28-dependent T-cell responses is perhaps most strikingly demonstrated by the phenotype of CTLA-4 knockout mice, which succumb to a rapidly lethal polyclonal CD4-dependent lympho-proliferation within 3–4 weeks of birth (Chambers *et al.*, 1997; Tivol *et al.*, 1995; Waterhouse *et al.*, 1995).

It is likely that the temporal and spatial separation of expression of CD28 and CTLA-4 are critical for regulation of immune responses. CTLA-4 expression is difficult to detect on resting T cells, but it is recognized to influence some of the earliest events in T-cell activation (Blair *et al.*, 1998; Brunner *et al.*, 1999). It undergoes complex intracellular trafficking mediated by its binding to the clathrin-adaptor molecules AP-1 and AP-2 (Chuang *et al.*, 1997; Shiratori *et al.*, 1997; Zhang and Allison, 1997), and is mobilized from intracellular vesicles in the proximity of the MTOC to the synaptic site of TCR engagement rapidly after TCR engagement (Egen and Allison, 2002). Strong TCR agonists are more efficient at inducing translocation of CTLA-4 to the immunological synapse, suggesting that TCR signal strength itself may inversely influence subsequent signaling elements. In contrast to CD28, CTLA-4 has a short cell-surface half-life in activated T cells, and surface expression is thus tightly linked to gene transcription and/or translation. In the unphosphorylated state, an intracellular localization motif mediates rapid binding to AP-2, endocytosis, and lysosomal targeting (Shiratori *et al.*, 1997). Its ability to form a lattice structure of alternating CTLA-4 and B7.1 homodimers coupled to the 500–2500-fold higher affinities for both ligands than those of CD28 (Greene *et al.*, 1996) provides one possible physical mechanism for its role as a negative regulator of CD28 signaling. It may exclude CD28 from the immunological synapse and out-compete it for the shared ligands. Transfection of T cells with CTLA-4 expressing mutations or truncations provide confirmatory evidence for the hypothesis that the CTLA-4 cytoplasmic tail is not always necessary for inhibitory function and that competition for shared ligands may be an important mechanism of inhibition (Carreno et al., 2000; Nakaseko et al., 1999). Expression of a mutant CTLA-4 molecule without a functional intracellular domain blocked the massive lethal lymphoproliferation that characterizes CTLA-4$^{-/-}$ mice completely (Takahashi et al., 2005), or partially (Chikuma et al., 2005; Masteller et al., 2000) depending on the surface expression level, presumably as a consequence of competition for CD28/B7 ligation or indoleamine 2,3-dioxygenase (IDO) induction (Fallarino et al., 2003). However, although such competition may be most effective when B7 levels are limiting, direct signaling through the tail appears to be necessary if B7 levels are high (Carreno et al., 2000). In addition, an alternatively spliced ligand independent form of CTLA-4 (liCTLA-4) lacking the B7.1/B7.2 ligand-binding domain has been reported to be expressed on resting T cells, particularly on $CD4^+CD45Rb^{lo}$ cells, to be rapidly downregulated following T-cell activation, and to inhibit both T-cell proliferation and cytokine production (Vijayakrishnan et al., 2004). It has been speculated that this isoform controls survival and/or homeostasis of naïve T-cell subsets. Taken together, the results suggest that inhibitory signals are transduced via both ligand-independent and B7 ligation-dependent mechanisms to maximize negative signaling. One important aspect of the mechanism of inhibition is that a direct physical competition with CD28 for ligand binding may be negated by antibodies that block the ligand interaction, resulting in a more effective blockade than agents that specifically target the CTLA-4 signaling pathway. While the precise mechanisms by which CTLA-4 inhibits T-cell responses remain unclear, the importance of the codependence of its activity on CD28-mediated signaling is emphasized by gene expression analyses demonstrating that CTLA-4 engagement selectively blocked augmentation of gene regulations by CD28-mediated costimulation but did not ablate gene regulation induced by TCR triggering alone (Riley et al., 2002).

Two distinct, but not mutually exclusive, models that attempt to integrate the effects of CTLA-4 engagement within the framework of TCR and CD28 signaling and subsequent biological responses have been proposed. They have been termed the threshold and attenuation models (Chambers et al., 2001). In the threshold model CTLA-4 increases the TCR and/or CD28 signal strength required for activation of a naïve T cell, and effectively prevents those cells receiving low amounts of stimulation from proceeding to a state of full activation. This could be affected by competition with CD28 for B7.1/B7.2 on APCs under conditions when CD28-B7.1/B7.2 signaling is limiting for

T-cell activation. The lymphoproliferation in CTLA-4$^{-/-}$ mice is dependent on both CD28 costimulation and TCR signals generated from low-affinity peptide-MHC interactions. The absence of B7.1 and B7.2 signals ablates the autoimmune phenotype in triple-mutant mice deficient in B7.1, B7.2, and CTLA-4 (Mandelbrot et al., 1999). CTLA-4 could set the threshold for activation above that delivered by the weak TCR signals that will be an inevitable function of thymic positive selection. When CD28-B7.1/B7.2 signaling is not limiting, CTLA-4 could restrict cell division following T-cell activation (Brunner et al., 1999; Doyle et al., 2001; Krummel and Allison, 1996), and hence attenuate rather than prevent T-cell responses. If this inhibition of expansive capacity were differentially regulated as a function of TCR signal strength (Chambers et al., 1999; Egen and Allison, 2002), the antigen-driven selection of T cells bearing high-affinity TCRs that occurs during T-cell responses might be decreased allowing the maintenance of a broader diversity of clonal responses early during antigen encounter. Attenuation of T-cell expansion could also influence the induction of T-cell anergy, as T cells can be rendered anergic if they fail to progress through enough rounds of division (Vanasek et al., 2001).

TCR transgenic T cells from CTLA-4-deficient mice allowed the study of the role of CTLA-4 in the regulation of peptide specific responses. These studies indicated that the inhibitory effect of CTLA-4 was more pronounced during secondary rather than primary responses, and indicated a role in both CD4$^+$ and CD8$^+$ T-cell responses (Chambers et al., 1998, 1999; Luhder et al., 2000). Together the data are consistent with a model in which chronic T-cell stimulation results in persistently higher levels of CTLA-4 expression. Thus, CTLA-4 blockade offered a further potential mechanism by which to try to enhance the antitumor responses of preexistent chronically stimulated tumor-reactive T cells by a combination of reducing the threshold for activation of weakly reacting clones and removal of the attenuation of subsequent T-cell proliferation, the effect of which might be accentuated by prior upregulation of CTLA-4 in the higher affinity population (Fig. 1). Blockade might result in the promotion of higher affinity clones that would otherwise be more restricted by CTLA-4 signaling.

2.1.3. CTLA-4 as a Non Cell-Autonomous Regulator: Regulatory T Cells and Dendritic Cells

The function of CTLA-4 has so far been discussed with respect to a cell-autonomous mode of action that is T-cell intrinsic (i.e., a direct action mediated via a receptor located on the helper or effector T cell). Adoptive transfer experiments demonstrate that CTLA-4-deficient T cells show enhanced responsiveness to antigenic stimulation compared to wild-type cells,

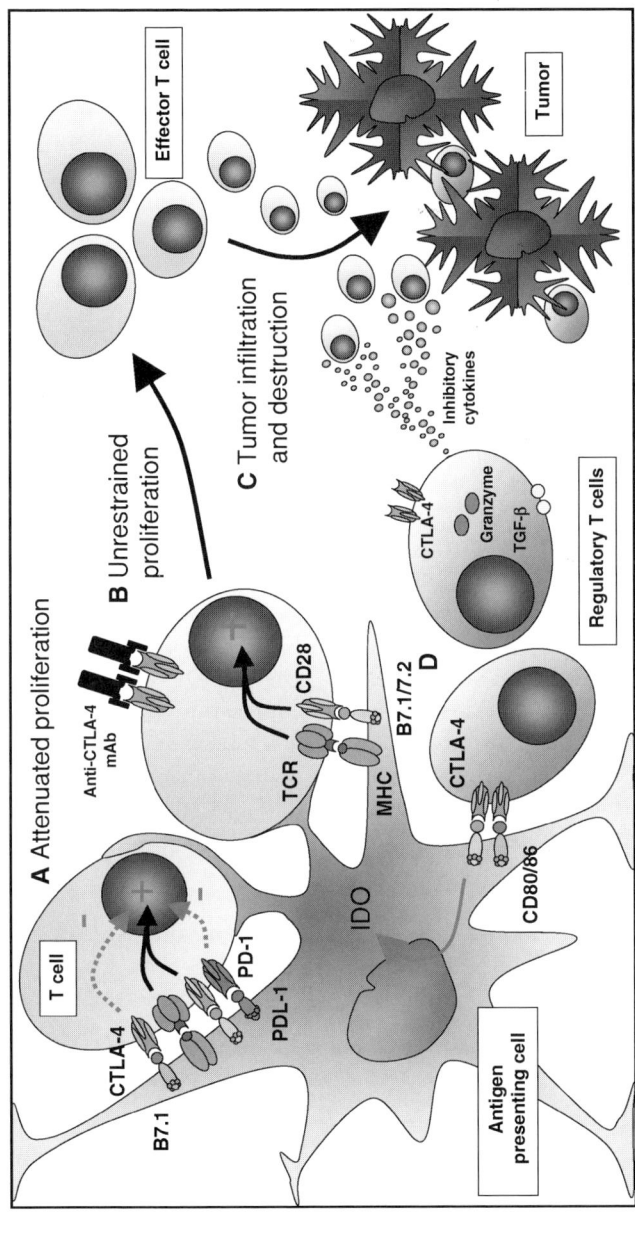

Figure 1 CTLA-4 blockade in cancer immunotherapy. Dendritic cells can sample tumor antigens and present them to T cells. (A) Although activation of dendritic cells may result in upregulation of B7.1/B7.2, the potentially responsive T cells expressing reactive TCR may be inhibited from effector function by inhibitory signaling via CTLA-4 and PD-1. (B) Blockade of CTLA-4 signaling may allow unopposed CD28 costimulation, resulting in recruitment of these T cells as antitumor effectors, either directly or as helpers of CD8-mediated T cells responses. (C) Activated cytotoxic T cells can then affect antitumor responses. (D) CTLA-4 expressing regulatory T cell populations may still be locally active in suppressing antitumor responses. Their activity could also be directly downregulated by CTLA-4 blockade, although the relative importance of CTLA-4 expression to their function remains controversial. (**See Plate 9 in color insert at the end of the book.**)

confirming the importance of a cell-autonomous mechanism of CTLA-4-mediated inhibition (Greenwald et al., 2001). However, negative regulatory mechanisms within the immune cascade include those that invoke additional subsets of cells, including regulatory T cells (in which CTLA-4 could potentially fulfill a T-cell intrinsic, non cell-autonomous regulatory role) and dendritic cells (T-cell extrinsic regulators). The role of immunoglobulin coinhibitory family members in the function of both continues to be elucidated. Both are important targets in their own right for manipulation in the field of immunotherapy. Data has demonstrated the presence of infiltrating $CD4^+CD25^+Foxp3^+$ regulatory T cells in human ovarian, breast, pancreatic, and lung carcinoma, and metastatic melanoma (Curiel et al., 2004; Liyanage et al., 2002; Viguier et al., 2004; Woo et al., 2001). A number of T-cell subtypes with regulatory or suppressive activity are now recognized. They fall broadly into one of two categories: those which are continuously produced by the thymus, express CD4, CD25, and GITR, and appear crucially dependent on the expression of the X-linked forkhead/winged helix transcription factor, Foxp3, for their development [so-called "naturally occurring" regulatory T (Treg) cells]; and those which arise as a result of "tolerogenic" encounters in the periphery [interleukin (IL)-10-producing, Foxp3-negative Tr1 cells (Groux et al., 1997; Levings et al., 2001a) and TGFβ-producing Th3 cells (Weiner, 2001) being the best characterized of these "inducible" or "adaptive" regulatory T cells]. In addition, $CD4^+CD25^-Foxp3^+$ T cells with regulatory capabilities have also been described (Zhou et al., 2005). $CD4^+CD25^+$ regulatory T cells are selected by high-affinity interactions in the thymus (Caton et al., 2004; Jordan et al., 2001), although the factors dictating the choice between Treg development and T cell negative selection remain unclear. Interactions between CD28 and B7.1/B7.2 are implicated in the selection process as it is defective in mice lacking these molecules, helping to explain the unexpected finding of increased severity and accelerated onset of diabetes that develops in $CD28^{-/-}$ and $B7.1/B7.2^{-/-}$ NOD mice (Salomon et al., 2000). The finding that the $CD4^+CD25^+$ Treg subset constitutively expresses CTLA-4 at high levels (Salomon et al., 2000) led to the suggestion that it may be important in the function of these cells and that "blockade" with monoclonal antibodies may suppress the function of or mediate the depletion of these cells. An alternative explanation for the high levels of CTLA-4 that does not require the invocation of additional mechanisms of function is that its role in $CD4^+CD25^+$ Treg is the same as in other T cells. That is, it works in a cell-autonomous fashion to restrict proliferation of a population of T cells with higher affinities for self than those of nonregulatory populations, and that the higher levels of CTLA-4 are a manifestation of chronic stimulation by self-antigen *in vivo*.

Precise details of the mechanisms involved in effecting suppression in different immune responses are not yet entirely clear. $CD4^+CD25^+$ Treg are able to suppress the proliferation of other T cells in an antigen-nonspecific manner, although Treg activation is antigen specific. Activity *in vitro* appears to be cytokine-independent and to involve direct interactions between T cells (Gondek *et al.*, 2005; Thornton and Shevach, 2000), while in many *in vivo* experimental systems suppression requires TGF-β or IL-10 (Fahlen *et al.*, 2005). CTLA-4 has been implicated in $CD4^+CD25^+$ Treg function in some, but not all, studies. Inhibition of the CTLA-4 pathway by using antibodies or CTLA-4 deficient regulatory cells reduces suppressor function in some experimental systems (Read *et al.*, 2000; Takahashi *et al.*, 2000). Normal mice treated with high doses of anti-CTLA-4 or a mixture of anti-CTLA-4 and anti-CD25 develop autoimmune gastritis, and the administration of anti-CTLA-4 reverses the Treg-mediated inhibition of $CD25^-$ T cell induced colitis *in vivo* (Read *et al.*, 2000). It is of course difficult to exclude the possibility of a T cell intrinsic cell-autonomous mechanism of action in these studies via the direct blockade of inhibitory signals via CTLA-4 on effector populations. The finding that bone marrow chimeras generated from $CTLA-4^{-/-}$ and wild-type $CTLA-4^{+/+}$ donors are protected from the lethal lymphoproliferative disorder that characterizes the $CTLA-4^{-/-}$ mice (Bachmann *et al.*, 1999) has also been used to suggest an important non cell-autonomous role for CTLA-4 in negative regulation of T-cell responses. Wild-type CTLA-4 expressing regulatory T cells are obvious candidate populations to mediate these effects. In two alternate, but not mutually exclusive, models, CTLA-4 could be required for the normal development or maintenance of a regulatory population, or could be key to the inhibitory function of these cells. In this respect, the finding that CTLA-4 binding to B7.1/B7.2 appears to result in backward or "outside-in" signaling, resulting in induction of IDO in dendritic cells, which in turn leads to immune suppression as a consequence of tryptophan depletion and production of pro-apoptotic metabolites, may have relevance (Fallarino *et al.*, 2003).

Further evidence supports the possibility of a similar direct effect on T cells (a truly T-cell intrinsic, non cell-autonomous activity). B7.2, but not B7.1, is constitutively expressed on some resting T cells, and both can be upregulated. $CD4^+CD25^-$ effector T cells from $B7.1/B7.2^{-/-}$ mice are resistant to suppression by $CD4^+CD25^+$ Treg compared to wild-type $CD4^+CD25^-$ effector T cells *in vitro*, and these cells provoke a lethal wasting disease in lymphopaenic mice despite the presence of regulatory T cells (Paust *et al.*, 2004). Susceptibility of B7.1/B7.2-deficient cells to suppression could be restored by lentiviral-based expression of full-length B7.1 or B7.2, but not of truncated molecules lacking the transmembrane/cytoplasmic domain, despite restoration of CD28-dependent costimulatory activity by these truncation mutants. In addition,

T cells that constitutively overexpress B7.2 exhibit reduced alloreactivity and graft-versus-host disease mortality in murine transplantation models (Taylor et al., 2004). Conversely, T cells from B7.1/B7.2$^{-/-}$ mice effect accelerated alloresponses and increased graft-versus-host disease-related mortality. The downregulation of responsiveness mediated via B7.1/B7.2 appeared to be dependent on interaction with T cell-associated CTLA-4. Collectively these data suggest that bi-directional signaling may also be important in T-cell regulation by B7.1/B7.2-CTLA-4 interactions.

Anti-CTLA-4 does not, however, successfully reverse *in vitro* suppression in all studies (Chai et al., 2002; Thornton and Shevach, 1998). Studies with human cultured cells have suggested that CTLA-4 blockade has only a moderate or no effect on the suppressive function of $CD4^+CD25^+$ regulatory T cells (Annunziato et al., 2002; Levings et al., 2001b). In addition, CTLA-4 expression does not appear to be critical for the development of $CD4^+CD25^+$ T cells within the thymus of CTLA-4$^{-/-}$ mice (Kataoka et al., 2005), and $CD4^+CD25^+CD62L^+$ T cells from CTLA-4-deficient mice with the CTLA-4Ig transgene express levels of Foxp3 that are similarly high to those of wild-type Treg by Western blot analysis, suggesting that they are of the same lineage (Tang et al., 2004). Both of these CTLA-4$^{-/-}$ Treg populations exhibit regulatory function in *in vitro* assays that is equivalent to that of wild-type Treg cells, although the mechanism of suppression may differ as there is some evidence of compensatory changes in CTLA-4$^{-/-}$ Treg that enable them to suppress in a partially TGF-β-dependent fashion in *in vitro* assays, unlike their wild-type counterparts (Tang et al., 2004). Thus, data suggest that the role of CTLA-4 in both the development and function of $CD4^+CD25^+$ Treg is, at least, partially redundant.

3. Preclinical Models of Checkpoint Blockade as Tumor Immunotherapy

The demonstration that blockade of CTLA-4/B7 interactions with anti-CTLA-4 monotherapy was able to induce rejection of several types of established transplantable tumors in mice, including colon carcinoma, fibrosarcoma, prostatic carcinoma, lymphoma, and renal carcinoma was an important proof of principle establishing checkpoint blockade as a potentially viable therapeutic modality (Kwon et al., 1997; Leach et al., 1996; Shrikant et al., 1999; Sotomayor et al., 1999; Yang et al., 1997). Antitumor activity appears dependent on inherent tumor immunogenicity and response longevity, in terms of ability to reject subsequent tumor challenge, is variable. The failure of anti-CTLA-4 monotherapy in the less immunogenic tumors (e.g., B16 melanoma) led to the exploration of its combination with vaccination approaches. Irradiated tumor vaccines that are engineered to produce granulocyte-macrophage colony stimulating factor (GMCSF) are highly effective as prophylaxis in tumor challenge experiments but poorly effective in treatment models. Combination with CTLA-4 blockade in the B16 melanoma model results in synergism of activity, which can cause tumor rejection if initiated 4 days after tumor implantation, and significant retardation in tumor growth if delayed by up to 1 week (van Elsas et al., 1999). A similar effect was observed for the poorly immunogenic SM1 mammary carcinoma line (Hurwitz et al., 1998) and in a transgenic model of prostate carcinoma (Hurwitz et al., 2000). Analogous synergism is observed with DNA rather than cellular vaccines. Xenogeneic or heteroclitic DNA vaccines have shown some promise in preclinical murine models, and combination with CTLA-4 blockade enhanced T-cell responses to melanoma differentiation antigens (tyrosinase-related protein 2 and gp100) and enhanced B16 tumor rejection (Gregor et al., 2004). The effect was stronger when anti-CTLA-4 was administered with booster vaccinations with the suggestion that the sequence and schedule of administration of CTLA-4 blockade may be an important variable to consider in clinical studies. CTLA-4 blockade also increased the T-cell responses to prostate-specific membrane antigen (PSMA) when given with the booster rather than the priming vaccinations.

In the B16 melanoma vaccination/CTLA-4 blockade models, rejection is accompanied by depigmentation, reminiscent of that seen in patients with melanoma who respond to immunotherapy, and suggesting that the immune targets for these responses may be normally expressed differentiation antigens. Depigmentation is uncommon following vaccination alone, suggesting that CTLA-4 blockade is important in breaking peripheral tolerance in this system. Importantly it is not seen with anti-CTLA-4 monotherapy. An additional manipulation that may enhance therapeutic efficacy in murine models is depletion of $CD25^+$ Treg cells. Depletion prior to combination therapy results in induction of increased numbers of TRP-$2^{180-188}$-specific T cells and an enhanced ability to reject larger tumor burdens (Sutmuller et al., 2001). Efficacy of the antitumor therapy correlated with the extent of autoimmune skin depigmentation as well as with the frequency of TRP-$2^{180-188}$-specific cytotoxic T cells detected in the periphery.

Combination of CTLA-4 blockade with a number of other therapeutic modalities has confirmed the versatility of a therapy which can enhance immune responses induced by a variety of interventions. Multiple mechanisms may account for this effect, such as reducing tumor burden, increasing the available pool of tumor antigen, or upregulating costimulatory molecules. Ionizing radiation is an important component in the management of breast cancer, but although the primary tumor can be successfully treated by surgery and radiotherapy, metastatic breast cancer remains a therapeutic challenge. CTLA-4 blockade has no effect on primary tumor growth or survival in the poorly immunogenic metastatic mouse mammary carcinoma 4T1 model when used as a monotherapy (Demaria et al., 2005). Radiotherapy delays the growth of the primary tumor, but in the absence of CTLA-4 blockade survival is not improved compared to control mice. In contrast, mice treated with radiotherapy and CTLA-4 blockade demonstrate a statistically significant survival advantage, correlating with an inhibition of the formation of metastatic lesions within the lung. This activity required $CD8^+$ T cells, while $CD4^+$ T cells were dispensable (Demaria et al., 2005) as in earlier studies of CTLA-4 blockade as a therapeutic rather than prophylactic modality (van Elsas et al., 1999). Chemotherapy is another mainstay for the treatment of many human malignancies with which CTLA-4 blockade may synergize. Anti-CTLA-4 monotherapy is ineffective in retarding tumor growth in the murine MOPC-315 tumor system, but demonstrates significant therapeutic benefits when combined with a subtherapeutic dose of the chemotherapeutic agent melphalan (Mokyr et al., 1998).

Finally, combination of anti-CTLA-4 with both peptide vaccination and CpG, which acts as an immunological adjuvant by activating the innate immunity via Toll-like receptor (TLR)-9 signaling, has also been shown to enhance antitumor immunity in the B16 melanoma model (Davila et al., 2003). The antitumor effect of this combination immunotherapy required both $CD4^+$ and $CD8^+$ T lymphocytes.

3.1. CTLA-4 Blockade in Tumor Immunotherapy: A Cell-Autonomous or Noncell-Autonomous Mode of Action?

There are no data that definitively address the issue of the role of CTLA-4 blockade on Treg cells as opposed to helper/effector cells during antitumor therapy. Studies documenting the possibility of Treg depletion have given contradictory results. Depletion was not seen in the lymph nodes of BALB/c mice following administration of blocking antibody despite the induction of autoimmunity (Takahashi et al., 2000) and did not occur following therapy in nonhuman primates (Keler et al., 2003). However, blood samples from human subjects receiving anti-CTLA antibody indicate that there may be a reduction in the percentage of $CD4^+CD25^+$ T cells that has been suggested to imply a depletion of the Treg compartment (Attia et al., 2005). Depletion of $CD25^+$ cells prior to tumor challenge significantly increases the effectiveness of combination therapy with CTLA-4 blockade and cellular vaccines (Sutmuller et al.,

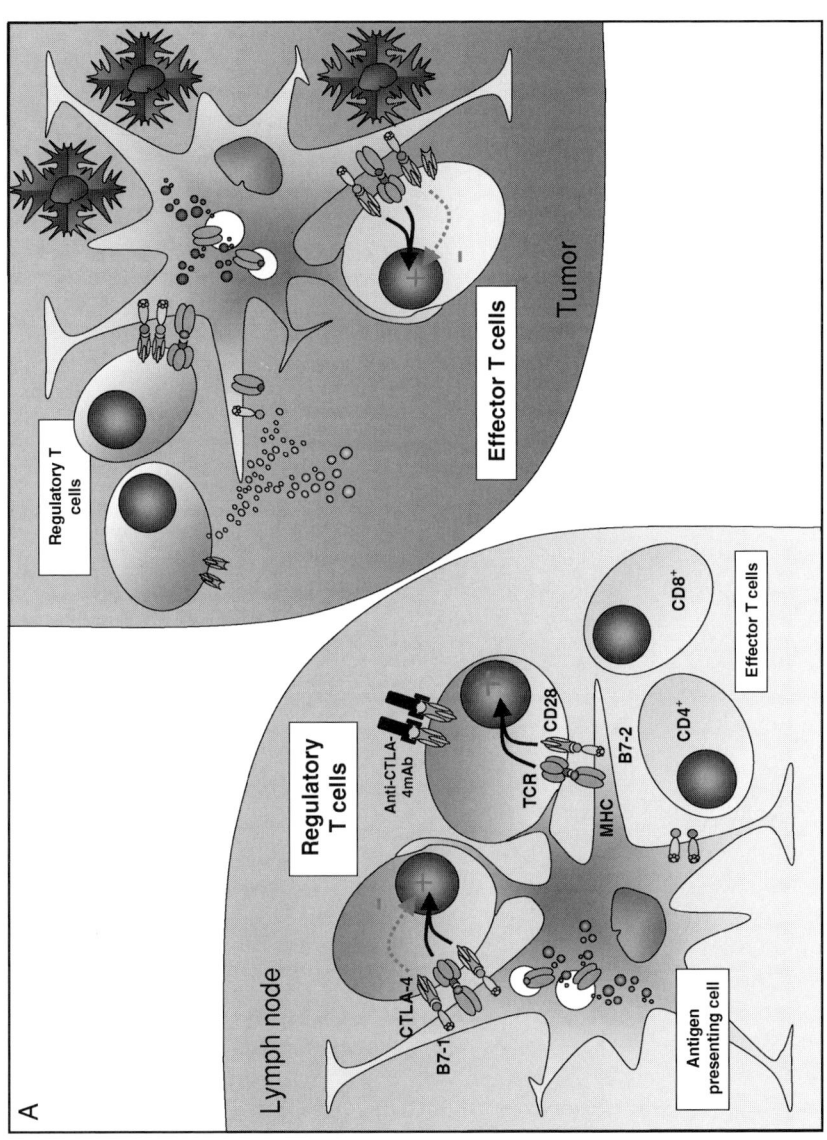

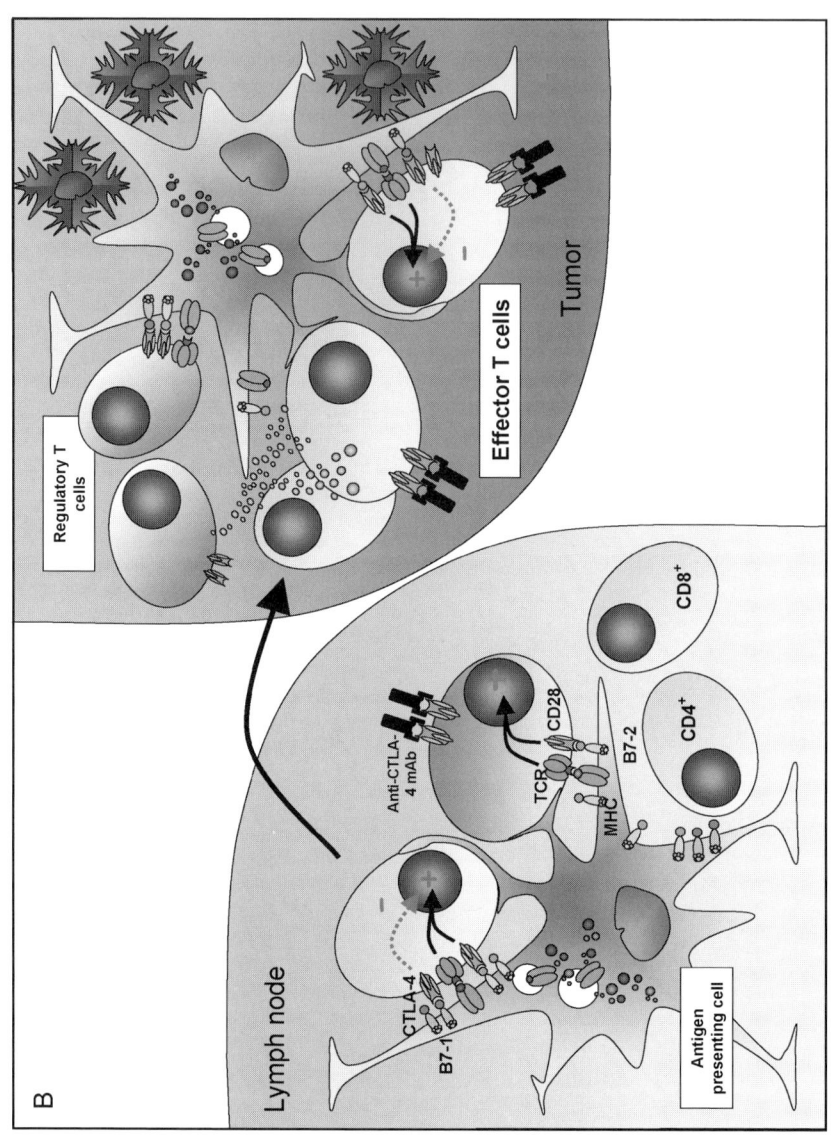

2001). If the efficacy of CTLA-4 blockade was dependent on inhibition of $CD4^+CD25^+$ Treg activity, one might predict that depletion of $CD4^+CD25^+$ Treg prior to blockade would abrogate its activity to some degree. The synergism in the effects of CTLA-4 blockade and depletion of $CD4^+CD25^+$ Treg cells suggests that $CD25^+$ regulatory T cells and CTLA-4 signaling represent two alternative pathways for suppression of autoreactive T-cell immunity, although it does not formally exclude a direct effect on Treg function, particularly if this were effected through the $CD4^+CD25^-Foxp3^+$ population, which is not depleted by CD25-depleting antibodies.

Studies in our laboratory favor a T cell intrinsic cell-autonomous mode of action of anti-CTLA-4 on both the effector and regulatory compartments (Quezada et al., manuscript submitted). Anti-CTLA-4 increased proliferation of the purified $CD4^+CD25^-$ effector population and was unable to inhibit the suppressive capacity of $CD4^+CD25^+$ regulatory T cells at a 1:1 suppressor: effector ratio in standard in vitro suppressor assays. In addition, chronic anti-CTLA-4 therapy in vivo (over a period of 2 weeks) induced expansion of intranodal Treg rather than depletion, suggesting a direct cell-autonomous effect of blockade of CTLA-4-mediated inhibitory signaling on the Treg. In a mouse model of the poorly immunogenic B16 melanoma tumor, tumor growth induced the expansion and accumulation of Treg in the lymph nodes in absence of any therapy. Anti-CTLA-4 monotherapy resulted in a further accumulation of Treg within the lymph nodes, presumably driven by self-antigen (Fig. 2A), but did not result in increased intratumoral T-cell infiltration. Administration of a GM-CSF-expressing B16 cellular vaccine facilitated efficient priming of tumor-specific effector T cells. As a monotherapy this enhanced tumor infiltration by $CD8^+$ T cells. However, intratumoral proliferation was still presumably under

Figure 2 CTLA-4 blockade and cellular vaccines in poorly immunogenic tumors: the effect of CTLA-4 blockade and vaccination with a GM-CSF expressing cellular vaccine for poorly immunogenic tumors may depend on the local antigenic milieu and priming history of the T cells. In the nonvaccinated host (A) a direct effect on Treg may predominate due to higher TCR affinities, lower requirements for costimulation and predominance of self-antigen presentation, resulting in a relative expansion of Treg compared to other T-cell populations. The tumor infiltrate is characterized by a relatively high proportion of Treg and very low levels of $CD8^+$ T cells. CTLA-4 blockade under these conditions still favors Treg over effector T cells. In the vaccinated host (B) the preferential presentation of tumor-associated antigens in association with high levels of costimulatory molecules allows expansion of effector T-cell populations that can traffic to the tumor, although these cells will now upregulate CTLA-4 expression. Vaccination may be insufficient on its own to eradicate tumor due to the presence of both cell-autonomous and non cell-autonomous inhibitory circuits. The addition of CTLA-4 blockade now tips the balance in favor of the effector population, perhaps aided by the numerical superiority of these cells over tumor-resident Treg resulting in tumor eradication. (**See Plate 10 in color insert at the end of the book.**)

the restraints imposed by CTLA-4 mediated signaling and tumor growth was not arrested. Combination with CTLA-4 blockade resulted in maximal effects on nonregulatory T cell numbers by allowing unrestrained proliferation driven by tumor antigens, resulting in the inversion of the ratio of effectors to regulators (Fig. 2B). The data suggest that with combination therapy the priming induced by the cellular vaccine results in a massive increase in the effector compartment within the tumor and once the inhibitory cellular restraints imposed by CTLA-4 signaling are removed the inhibitory activities of the Treg are overwhelmed, resulting in tumor rejection. In the absence of the cellular vaccine, insufficient effector T-cells infiltrate the tumor and the outcome of CTLA-4 blockade still favors Treg over the effector populations resulting in continued tumor growth. Hence, the overall outcome will depend on the priming history of the T-cell populations and the local antigenic milieu. It remains difficult to completely exclude an additional non cell-autonomous effect mediated via inhibition of Treg function and further studies addressing these issues are clearly warranted.

3.2. Adverse Immune Manifestations of CTLA-4 Blockade in Preclinical Models

The ability of anti-CTLA-4 to exacerbate autoimmunity in experimental models is well established (Hurwitz *et al.*, 1997). In general, autoimmunity has been amplified when mice are vaccinated with self-antigens in combination with CTLA-4 blockade (Karandikar *et al.*, 1996; Luhder *et al.*, 1998; Perrin *et al.*, 1996; Wang *et al.*, 2001). While preclinical studies of antitumor immunity demonstrated the potential for CTLA-4 blockade in tumor immunotherapy, they also illustrated the possibility of induction of autoimmunity. However, toxicities were limited to predicted "target" tissues sharing the same epitopic topiary as the cellular vaccines (depigmentation in the melanoma model (van Elsas *et al.*, 1999), prostatitis in the prostate cancer model (Hurwitz *et al.*, 2000)). More serious systemic toxicities were not documented, perhaps in part due to the shorter duration of therapy, and shorter half life of the original hamster antimouse antibody (clone 9H10) used in these studies as compared to that of the fully human antibody used for subsequent clinical studies. Nonhuman primates treated with CTLA-4 blockade and a human melanoma whole cell vaccine showed enhanced development of antibodies to some self-antigens, in particular to those present in lysates prepared from their melanocyte rich iris tissue (Keler *et al.*, 2003). Continued administration of anti-CTLA-4 in high doses for up to 6 months, however, did not result in any clinically or pathologically detectable end organ damage, even in those animals with detectable humoral anti-self responses.

4. Clinical Trials of CTLA-4 Blockade: Overview

Inhibition of the activity of CTLA-4 has begun to be tested in humans through the use of human antibodies developed using mice that are transgenic for human immunoglobulin loci. MDX-010 is a human IgG1 antibody that binds human and rhesus CTLA-4 and inhibits the binding of CTLA-4 to B7.1 and B7.2. In preclinical studies in cynomolgus monkeys, the antibody was shown to augment antibody responses to a Hepatitis B surface antigen vaccine and a human melanoma cell line, SK-MEL (Keler et al., 2003). These studies also revealed that multiple dosing at 10 mg/kg resulted in no serious adverse events. CP-675, 206, another human antibody to human CTLA-4 in development, is an IgG2 isotype and blocks B7 ligand binding (Ribas et al., 2005a). MDX-010 has a reported half life of 12–14 days (Davis et al., 2002), while CP-675, 206 has been reported as 22.1 days (Ribas et al., 2005a). This difference may be due to the different isotypes of the antibodies. These antibodies have entered human clinical trials and have been tested in multiple therapeutic regimens.

CTLA-4 blockade has been predominantly tested in metastatic melanoma and in renal cancer, those cancers in which immunological responses are thought to be most relevant. In these settings, treatment by anti-CTLA-4 antibodies is capable of inducing objective tumor responses as monotherapy. These responses can be durable in nature with several ongoing after several years. The response rate to monotherapy is variable (from 5 to 13%). Dosing has ranged from single doses of 0.01–15 mg/kg and repeated dosing from 3 to 15 mg/kg at various frequencies of administration. Redosing or maintenance dosing in those patients showing clinical benefit have also been explored. It remains unclear what the optimal scheduling is for CTLA-4 blockade either in monotherapy or concurrently with vaccines. Other cancers in which CTLA-4 blockade has been tested include prostate, ovarian, breast, and colon carcinomas.

In studies in which CTLA-4 blockade is combined with gp100 melanoma peptides, objective durable responses have also been noted (Attia et al., 2005; Phan et al., 2003b). These have involved multiple subcutaneous skin lesions, as well as multiple visceral sites in the lung as well as brain metastases. CTLA-4 blockade did not result in increased numbers of antigen specific T cells when the antipeptide responses were measured in peripheral blood relative to historical controls. The lack of augmented antigen specific responses using CTLA-4 blockade has also been observed using other peptides as well (Sanderson et al., 2005). Vaccination with peptide vaccines may indirectly result in the activation and increase in numbers of tumor-specific T cells with specificity distinct from the tumor antigen immunogen as shown by the work of Lurquin et al. (2005).

It is likely that monotherapy is able to activate preexisting antitumor responses. However, it is also possible that *de novo* antitumor responses are also generated. T-cell subset analysis in patients treated with MDX-010 revealed that HLA-DR$^+$ T cells were increased as well as frequent increases in CD45RO T cells (Attia *et al.*, 2005; Maker *et al.*, 2005a; Phan *et al.*, 2003b). These cells may include those effector T cells or their precursors that are responsible for the antitumor effects as well as the adverse events observed with anti-CTLA-4 treatment. In addition, CTLA-4 blockade is unlikely to function through effects on Treg cells, since patients treated with anti-CTLA-4 do not show demonstrable changes in Treg activity (Maker *et al.*, 2005a).

4.1. Clinical Trials of CTLA-4 Blockade: Adverse Events

Treatment with anti-CTLA-4 antibodies is frequently accompanied by a wide variety of adverse events. The most common events involve the skin (rash and pruritis) and the gastrointestinal tract (diarrhea and colitis). In a small number of patients, these side effects can be of a serious nature (Grade III/IV). In a collection of 198 patients with metastatic melanoma and renal cancer that were treated with MDX-010 in a variety of regimens, Grade III/IV colitis was observed in 21% of the patients (Beck *et al.*, 2005). These adverse events are due to inflammatory T-cell infiltrates where studied. Infiltrates of CD4 and CD8 T cells can be observed in skin and colon biopsies. Other serious adverse events include hypophysitis, uveitis, and hepatitis (Blansfield *et al.*, 2005; Phan *et al.*, 2003b; Ribas *et al.*, 2005a; Robinson *et al.*, 2004); it is presumed that these events are also the consequence of inflammatory T-cell infiltration. Colectomy has been necessary in some cases of colitis and two deaths were observed in a combination trial with DTIC, although these may be ascribed to causes other than anti-CTLA-4 (Fischkoff *et al.*, 2005; Korman *et al.*, 2005). The adverse events can appear at various times after anti-CTLA-4 treatment. Management of these adverse events includes cessation of drug and treatment with high-dose steroids. Steroid use can temper the inflammation in most cases and paradoxically antitumor responses have been observed to be maintained after steroid use (Attia *et al.*, 2005). While glucocorticoids have multiple activities and are thought to impair T-cell responses, their use may not impair activated T-cells responses as shown in a murine model in which dexamethasone treatment did not alter the effectiveness of adoptive cell therapy (Hinrichs *et al.*, 2005). Tumor-necrosis factor blockade has also been used in the management of colitis in a small number of patients (Beck *et al.*, 2005). In some trials, no treatment of the adverse events was attempted and resolution of many of the side effects occurred over time after cessation of antibody treatment (Ribas et al., 2005b).

One of the observations from these studies is that serious adverse events (Grade III/IV) may be correlated with effective antitumor responses (Attia et al., 2005; Beck et al., 2005; Phan et al., 2003b). For example, in patients with enterocolitis, Beck et al. (2005) report that 45% and 46% of patients with metastatic melanoma and renal cell cancer, respectively showed objective tumor responses. This suggests that a component of T-cell activation is directed at tumor antigens as well as putative self-antigens and that CTLA-4 blockade may overcome tolerance to self-antigens. However, in no instance has specificity of the T cells mediating the adverse events been determined. It is most likely that nonantigen specific expansion/infiltration of T cells catalyzes these adverse events. In this respect, these side events are suggestive of the phenotype of the CTLA-4 knockout mouse. While the adverse event profile of CTLA-4 blockade has frequently been referred to as autoimmune in nature, it should be noted that the phenomenon of uncontrolled T-cell proliferation in the murine system has not been shown to be directed at specific self-antigens.

4.2. Clinical Trials of CTLA-4 Blockade: Specific Trials

4.2.1. Monotherapy for Malignant Melanoma

MDX-010 was initially given to 17 patients in a phase I clinical trial at a single dose of 3 mg/kg. At this dose level the drug was well tolerated and side effects of rash were noted. There were two partial responses. Many of the patients in this trial received vaccines at various times prior to treatment with MDX-010. It was observed that prior treatment with GM-CSF modified vaccines engendered a greater frequency of immune cell infiltrates into the tumors and tumor necrosis, although objective responses were not noted in these patients (Hodi et al., 2003).

Dose escalation studies have been carried out for CP-675, 206 as a single agent in 39 patients that included 34 patients with melanoma using from doses of 0.01–15 mg/kg (Ribas et al., 2005a). Dose limiting toxicities were observed at 15 mg/kg and a maximum tolerated dose was considered to be 10 mg/kg. Two complete and 2 partial responses were noted out of 34 melanoma patients (response rate of 12%) with responses continuing from 24+ to 35+ months. Further studies with CP-675, 206 have explored multiple dosing regimens at high-antibody levels in malignant melanoma (16 patients at 10 mg/kg and 10 patients at 15 mg/kg every 3 months) (Reuben et al., 2005). Five objective responses were noted. In addition, monthly dosing of CP-675, 206 from 3 to 10 mg/kg has been examined in 14 patients (Ribas et al., 2005a). Adverse events included Grade III diarrhea and were similar to those adverse events previously observed. One patient had an ongoing response while receiving 10 doses at 10 mg/kg with the sole adverse event of autoimmune thyroiditis. These studies suggest that prolonged CTLA-4 blockade may be tolerated in some individuals.

4.2.2. Monotherapy for Renal Cell Carcinoma

MDX-010 has been administered to renal cancer patients at a dose of 3 mg/kg every 3 weeks ($n = 38$ or 3 mg/kg followed by 1 mg/mg every 3 weeks ($n = 21$) (Yang et al., 2005). In the 3 mg/kg cohort, 5 responses of partial duration were noted with 3 ongoing (8+, 10+, and 12+); 1 partial response was noted in the 3/1 cohort. All the responders were among the group with serious adverse events. A similar profile of adverse events was described (enteritis, colitis, hypophysitis, and rash) that are similar to that observed in malignant melanoma. The type of adverse events does not appear to correlate with the type of cancer. The contribution of prior IL-2 treatment in these patients remains to be analyzed since the majority of these patients were previously treated IL-2 nonresponders.

4.3. CTLA-4 Blockade and Vaccines

After initial single dose trials of MDX-010, multiple dosing trials were initiated together with peptide vaccines in patients with Stage 4 nonresectable metastatic melanoma (Attia et al., 2005; Phan et al., 2003b). This vaccine consists of two modified peptides from the melanocyte antigen gp100 that are restricted by HLA-A2 administered with the adjuvant Montanide. A total of 56 patients were treated: one cohort of 29 patients were treated with 3 mg/kg of MDX-010 every 3 weeks together with peptide vaccinations (for 1–12 cycles) and a second cohort of 27 were treated with an initial dose of 3 mg/kg and peptide vaccination followed by 1 mg/kg of MDX-010 and peptide vaccinations every 3 weeks (2–12 cycles completed). Four patients out of 29 (14%) patients in the high-dose group had objective clinical responses with 2 complete and 1 partial response (continuing for 2–3 years). The response rate in the second cohort was 3/27 (11%) with 2 partial responses continuing greater than 2 years. There appeared to be no significant differences either in efficacy between the two cohorts or the frequency of induction of adverse events. Treatment with MDX-010 was associated with significant immune related adverse events and these adverse events were associated with antitumor activity. Of 14 patients with grade III/IV toxicities, 5 tumor responses were noted, while 2 responses were noted among 42 patients without grade III/IV toxicity.

It is unclear from the above studies whether there is an effect of the vaccine and/or adjuvant in the clinical responses. Vaccination with gp100 peptides had previously been shown to induce antigen specific T-cell responses but few significant antitumor responses (Phan *et al.*, 2003a). The gp100 vaccine together with MDX-010 generates no greater T-cell responses than that previously described for the peptides alone; however, these responses are monitored in peripheral blood and may not reflect the number or activity of antigen specific T-cells at effector sites. Thus it is possible that the effects observed are a consequence of MDX-010 alone. A phase III trial comparing response rates among groups treated with vaccine/adjuvant alone, MDX-010 alone, and MDX-010 together with vaccine/adjuvant will address this question directly.

CTLA-4 blockade may reactivate antitumor responses as seen in patients in which administration of anti-CTLA-4 has been given after prior vaccination with various types of vaccines. In one study of nine previously vaccinated patients with advanced cancer there was clear evidence of antitumor activity. In patients who had been previously vaccinated with autologous GM-CSF-secreting tumor cell vaccines, anti-CTLA-4 induced extensive tumor necrosis along with lymphocytic and granulocytic infiltration of tumors in each of three patients with metastatic melanoma and CA-125 levels were stabilized or decreased in two of two patients with metatastic ovarian carcinoma (Hodi *et al.*, 2003). In another example, a complete response (CR) was obtained after treatment with anti-CTLA-4 antibody after tumor progression occurred despite multiple DC/Mart-1 peptide vaccinations (Ribas *et al.*, 2004) . In addition, T cell reactivity to additional tumor antigens as well as infectious agents were augmented in this patient following CTLA-4 blockade. These observations, albeit limited in number, suggest that anti-CTLA-4 was able to reactivate latent antitumor responses and prolong objective antitumor responses.

4.4. Anti-CTLA-4 and Chemotherapy

MDX-010 has been combined with the chemotherapeutic, dacarbazine (DTIC) in patients with unresectable metastatic melanoma (Fischkoff *et al.*, 2005). MDX-010 (3 mg/kg) was administered monthly for 4 cycles together with DTIC (250 mg/m2 for 5 consecutive days for up to 6 cycles); in addition, there was a second arm where MDX-010 (3 mg/kg for 4 cycles) alone was administered. In the combination arm 6/35 responses were noted for a response rate of 17.1%. This included 2 complete responses (ongoing at 17+ and 20+ months) and 4 partial responses (one ongoing at 21+ months). Two partial responses were noted in the 35 patients in the monotherapy arm (both ongoing at 16 and 18 months). In addition, a significant increase in overall survival (14.2 months for MDX-010 and DTIC and 11.2 months for MDX-010) as well as

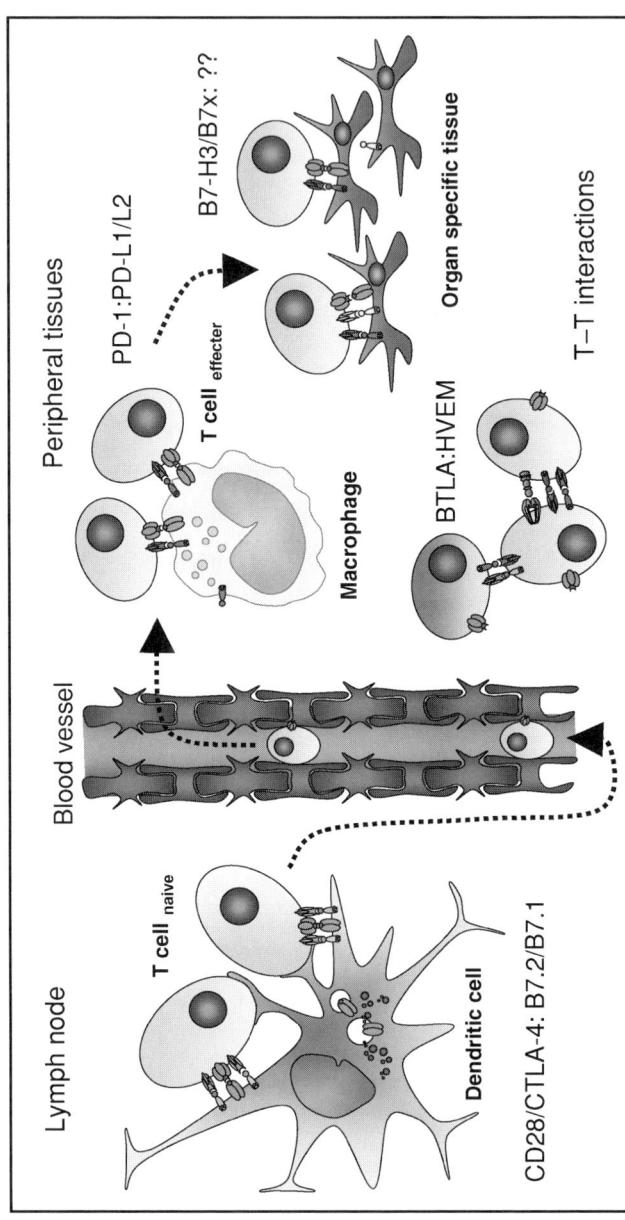

Figure 3 Immunological inhibitory checkpoints: potential therapeutic targets. All of the members of the immunoglobulin superfamily that act as inhibitory checkpoints are potential targets for manipulation in immunotherapies. CD28/CTLA-4:B7.1/B7.2 are centrally important for the initial activation of naïve T cells and regulation of the clonal composition of the responding repertoire following migration of activated dendritic cells to lymphoid organs. As activated effectors traffic back into peripheral tissues they come under the influence of PD1:PD-L1/L2 mediated signaling, both as a result of interactions with tissue macrophages and with ligands expressed on malignant cells. B7-H3 and B7x could be poised to act as the final arbiters of the fate of T effector interactions with nonlymphoid target tissues, and could potentially protect any tumor cells expressing them from cytotoxic T cell mediated killing. The potential for cross-talk between T-cell populations via many of these pathways is complex, particularly as activated T cells can upregulate receptors and/or

progression-free survival was observed in the MDX-010 groups relative to historical values for DTIC (Fischkoff et al., 2005). Adverse events, such as colitis, were also observed in this trial including two deaths.

4.5. Anti-CTLA-4 and IL-2

High-dose bolus IL-2 is an approved treatment for metastatic melanoma that results in response rates of ~15% of which a high percentage can be durable (Atkins et al., 1999; Rosenberg, 2000). Thirty-six patients have been treated with a combination of MDX-010 and high-dose bolus IL-2 in a dose escalation trial of MDX-010 (Maker et al., 2005b). Twelve patients were treated with MDX-010 at 0.1, 0.3, 1, and 2 mg/kg (3 patients per group) while 24 patients were treated at 3 mg/kg of MDX-010. The response rate in all groups was 22.2% (3 complete and 5 partial responses) with ongoing responses in 6 patients of 13–19+ month duration. Given the response rate to MDX-010 together with gp100 peptides described above, it appears that the combination resulted in an additive effect. Five of 36 patients experienced Grade III/IV adverse events, but the association of inflammatory adverse events with outcome was not observed in this study. This may be explained by responses that are due to IL-2 treatment alone, which is not expected to result in an adverse event profile like that for anti-CTLA-4. An alternative explanation is that IL-2 promotes the activity of regulatory T cells, which may limit the inflammatory reactions of those T cells that are otherwise activated by anti-CTLA-4; however, this must be accomplished while retaining the activity of those T-effector cells that mediate antitumor activity.

5. Other Potential Coinhibitory Targets for Checkpoint Blockade

Given its earlier identification compared to other members of the immunoglobulin superfamily and its position at the tip of the regulatory cascade, CTLA-4 blockade was a natural first choice for investigation as a therapeutic intervention in immune-based therapies. However, the identification of other inhibitory checkpoints has highlighted other potential targets for therapeutic blockade (Fig. 3). These include PD-1 and its ligands PD-L1 and PD-L2, and possibly B7-H3, B7x/B7-H4, and BTLA.

PD-1 is more broadly expressed than CD28/CTLA-4. It is expressed on activated, but not resting, $CD4^+$ and $CD8^+$ T cells, B cells, monocytes,

---

ligands, which can potentially signal bidirectionally. Blockade of BTLA may remove inhibitory restraints imposed by HVEM-expressing cells, but effects on T–T interactions mediated by blockade of CTLA-4, PD-1/PD-L1, or B7-H3 are also possible. (**See Plate 11 in color insert at the end of the book.**)

and at low levels on NKT cells. It shares the same pattern as CTLA-4 of dual ligands (PD-L1 (B7-H1) and PD-L2 (B7-DC)). PD-1 displays a higher affinity for PD-L2 than for PD-L1 (Youngnak et al., 2003). The ligands exhibit distinct expression profiles (reviewed in Greenwald et al., 2005). PD-L1 is expressed on resting and upregulated on activated B, T, myeloid, and dendritic cells, and on $CD4^+CD25^+$ Treg cells. It is also expressed on nonhematopoietic cells including microvascular endothelial cells and in nonlymphoid organs including heart, lung, pancreas, muscle, and placenta. This distribution suggests that interactions of ligands and receptors may be important in regulating effector T-cell responses in the peripheral tissues by "professional" APCs, such as DCs, macrophages, and also endothelial cells. PD-L2 is induced by cytokines on macrophages and DCs. The widespread expression of PD-L1 and expression of PD-1 on T cells, B cells, and macrophages presents ample opportunities for bidirectional signaling, further complicated by evidence of "outside-in" signaling (Dong et al., 2003; Nguyen et al., 2002; Radhakrishnan et al., 2004).

In a situation somewhat reminiscent of the early studies of CTLA-4 function, controversy exists over the function of PD-1. Studies using antibodies specific for PD-1 or the natural ligands demonstrate that engagement of PD-1 is able to inhibit T-cell proliferation under suboptimal CD3 stimulation (Carter et al., 2002; Freeman et al., 2000; Latchman et al., 2001). At high-antigen concentrations the TCR/CD28 signal predominates over PD-L1 or PD-L2 transduced signals, although cytokine production may be diminished. Colocalization of PD-1 with TCR/CD28 is necessary for this inhibitory activity. The phenotype of $PD-1^{-/-}$ mice also provides evidence for an inhibitory role of the receptor (Nishimura et al., 1999, 2001). These mice develop an autoimmune phenotype, delayed in onset compared to $CTLA-4^{-/-}$ mice, and characterized by high titers of autoantibodies in keeping with a negative regulatory effect on T and/or B cells. The phenotype manifested depends on the genetic background of the mouse. PD-1 deficiency on the C57BL/6 background results in development of a late-onset progressive arthritis and lupus-like glomerulonephritis (Nishimura et al., 1999), while on the BALB/c background it results in development of a lethal dilated cardiomyopathy that shows incomplete penetrance, with concomitant evidence of autoantibodies to troponin-1 (Nishimura et al., 2001). $PD-L1^{-/-}$ mice accumulate $CD8^+$ T cells in the liver that do not mediate spontaneous hepatic disease but which can enhance autoimmune hepatitis when experimentally challenged (Dong et al., 2004). Numerous models of autoimmune disease, and transplantation and graft-versus-host disease provide additional evidence that inhibition of PD-1/PD-L1 signaling results in enhanced severity and/or accelerated onset of disease, or that signaling induced by PD-L1Ig can synergize with conventional immunosuppressive drugs to enhance graft survival. However, other evidence points to a possible costimulatory role of PD-1 engagement (Dong et al., 1999; Tamura et al., 2001; Tseng et al., 2001; Wang et al., 2003), and PD-L2$^{-/-}$ DCs have a reduced capacity to stimulate CD4$^+$ T cells (Shin et al., 2003). Site-directed mutagenesis studies in both PD-L1 and PD-L2 demonstrate mutations that can abrogate binding to PD-1 but which retain or enhance costimulatory activity (Wang et al., 2003). The possibility that an undiscovered second stimulatory receptor exists that interacts with the PD-L1/L2 ligands would add further symmetry to the similarities with the CD28/CTLA-4:CD80/86 pathway, and remains an intriguing possibility. Finally, the likelihood that this pathway has functional importance in the induction or function of regulatory T cell or DC populations appears increasingly probable (Aramaki et al., 2004; Baecher-Allan et al., 2001).

The expression of PD-L1 and PD-L2 by a range of murine and human tumors has led to the hypothesis that this may be a mechanism by which they evade immune surveillance. PD-L1 is expressed on many human carcinomas (mammary, cervical, lung, ovarian, colonic, renal), as well as melanoma, glioblastoma, some primary T-cell lymphomas, and most thymic epithelial tumors including thymomas and thymic carcinoma (Blank et al., 2004; Brown et al., 2003; Dong et al., 2002; Thompson et al., 2004). In renal cancer, PD-L1 expression on tumors and on infiltrating T cells is associated with poor prognosis (Thompson et al., 2004). By contrast, PD-L2 is highly expressed on Hodgkin's lymphoma cell lines and is the best genomic discriminator between primary mediastinal B-cell lymphoma and other less favorable diffuse large B-cell lymphomas (Rosenwald et al., 2003). PD-L1 and PD-L2 expression has been observed alone and together in esophageal cancer and poor survival is associated with either PD-L1 or PD-L2 expression (Ohigashi et al., 2005).

Transfection of murine tumors with PD-L1 rendered them less susceptible to the specific T-cell antigen receptor-mediated lysis by cytotoxic T cells *in vitro*, and markedly enhanced tumor growth and invasiveness *in vivo* (Iwai et al., 2002). Both effects could be reversed by blockade by anti-PD-L1 antibody (Iwai et al., 2002; Strome et al., 2003). Transfection with PD-L1 was able to negate the enhanced immunogenicity conferred by transfection of P815 mastocytoma cells with CD80 (Dong et al., 2002). The 4T1 mammary cell carcinoma is PD-L1 negative in culture but expresses PD-L1 *in vivo* (or can be induced to express PD-L1 in culture by γ-IFN) (Hirano et al., 2005). This tumor is refractory to tumor rejection mediated by an agonistic anti-41BB antibody, an activating receptor that is a member of the TNF family of receptors. While anti-41BB shows a modest decrease in tumor growth, treatment with anti-41BB together with anti-PD-L1 results in dramatic tumor rejection. Murine myeloma cell lines naturally express PD-L1, and their growth *in vivo* was also inhibited significantly, but transiently, by the administration of anti-PD-L1 antibody, although a direct effect of the antibody on the growth of the tumor (by other mechanisms such as ADCC) was not excluded. Their growth was suppressed completely in syngeneic PD-1-deficient mice (Iwai et al., 2002). In addition, PD-1$^{-/-}$ CD8$^+$ TCR transgenic T cells caused tumor rejection in an adoptive transfer model in which wild-type and CTLA-4 $^{-/-}$ T cells failed to mediate rejection (Blank et al., 2004). These results are consistent with a model in which CTLA-4 is more vital for regulation of CD4$^+$ T-cell responses, particularly early at the APC interface, whereas PD-1 has a relatively minor role at this stage (when CD28 costimulation can overcome its inhibitory effects (Carter et al., 2002)) but a more critical role in suppressing the execution of T-cell effector function against cells that do not express CD80/86 (Fig. 3). Intriguingly, PD-L2 expression on J558 plasmacytoma cells actually enhanced CD8-mediated immunity, tumor rejection, and establishment of immunological memory to subsequent rechallenge (Liu et al., 2003). The effect was evident for PD-1$^{-/-}$ as well as wild-type-T cells, suggesting that it may be mediated by interaction with a receptor other than PD-1.

Very few studies have examined the ability of anti-PD-1 antibodies to promote antitumor responses directly. Two metastatic models have been shown to be sensitive to PD-1 blockade (Iwai et al., 2005). Utilizing CT26, a colon carcinoma that metastasizes to the lung after intravenous injection, tumor growth was inhibited by 50% after treatment with anti-PD-1 antibody. This study also reported that B16 melanoma metastasis to the liver after intrasplenic injection of tumor cells, in which PD-L1 expression was found to be upregulated in vivo, could be inhibited by anti-PD1 treatment. In studies using the immunogenic fibrosarcoma line, Sa1N, PD-1 blockade was able to prevent the outgrowth of tumor in unstaged tumors and showed a partial effect on staged tumors. Sa1N cells were unable to express PD-L1. This suggests that host PD-L1 expression in dendritic cells and/or APCs play a role in limiting antitumor responses (unpublished data).

Other possible targets for checkpoint blockade are currently somewhat more speculative. B7-H3 (B7-RP2) and B7x (B7-H4, B7-S1) are the most recently described B7 family members, which currently remain orphan ligands. They display greater similarity to each other than other family members. Both B7-H3 and B7x/B7-H4 appear to bind to a receptor(s) expressed on activated but not naïve T cells, but the identity of the receptor(s) remains unclear. The broad tissue distribution and inducible nature of both ligands has led to the suggestion that they downregulate immune responses in the periphery and play a role in regulating T-cell tolerance. In addition, the presence in tumor cells suggests a possible role in immune evasion as suggested for PD-L1, and another potential target for immune manipulation in tumor therapy.

B7-H3 is not constitutively expressed but can be induced, on T and B cells, NK cells, and monocytes. It is expressed on immature and mature myeloid DC. It has very general mRNA expression in nonlymphoid tissues (e.g., heart, kidney, testes, and nasal epithelium). It has been reported to possess both stimulatory and inhibitory functions. These contradictory findings are yet to be fully reconciled but might be explained by the existence of two receptors with opposing function, or the effects of signaling mediated by different cell types. The phenotype of B7-H3-deficient mice supports an inhibitory role, with enhanced severity of pathology under Th1-polarizing conditions in airway inflammation experiments coupled with increased T-cell responses and accelerated development of experimental autoimmune encephalomyelitis (Suh et al., 2003). However, expression of B7-H3 by transfection of the mouse P815 tumor line enhanced its immunogenicity, leading to the regression of tumors and amplification of tumor-specific $CD8^+$ CTL responses (Luo et al., 2004). In addition, intratumoral injection of an expression plasmid encoding B7-H3 led to complete regression of 50% EL4 tumors. Mice whose tumors completely regressed resisted a challenge with parental tumor cells, indicating systemic immunity had been generated. This immunity was mediated by $CD8^+$ T and NK cells. These tumor models suggest a positive costimulatory function for B7-H3, implying that blocking antibodies may actually reduce rather than enhance antitumor activity.

B7x/B7-H4 appears to be a further negative regulator of T-cell responses, and to inhibit proliferation and cytokine production in both $CD4^+$ and $CD8^+$ T cells (Prasad et al., 2003; Sica et al., 2003; Zang et al., 2003). It has a similarly broad mRNA expression pattern to B7-H3 in both humans and mice, where it is expressed in lymphoid (spleen, and thymus) and nonlymphoid (lung, liver, small intestine, pancreas, placenta, ovary, testis, and skeletal muscle) tissues (Sica et al., 2003; Zang et al., 2003). Protein expression studies suggest that it is absent from freshly isolated human T and B cells, DCs, and monocytes but that it can be induced on these cells following stimulation. Immunohistochemical analyses demonstrate that it is not expressed on the majority of normal human tissues (Choi et al., 2003), although it has been reported to be expressed by some tissues, such as normal breast, Fallopian tubal epithelium, endometrial and endocervical glands, and pancreas (Tringler et al., 2005). It is, however, expressed on several tumor lines (prostate, lung, and colon) as demonstrated by quantitative real-time polymerase chain reaction analyses, and on human cancers (ovarian and lung) at higher levels than in the normal tissue counterparts as demonstrated by immunohistochemical analyses (Choi et al., 2003; Salceda et al., 2005; Tringler et al., 2005). Expression levels on lymphoid and antigen-presenting cells are currently controversial.

It is unclear whether the differences in mRNA expression patterns and immunohistochemistry relate to low-level protein expression, technical issues related to the antibodies employed, or translational regulation of protein levels. Administration of anti-B7x/B7-H4 antibodies to mice exacerbates EAE with concomitant increases in the numbers of $CD8^+$ and $CD4^+$ T cells infiltrating the brain (Prasad et al., 2003), and B7x/B7-H4Ig both reduces T-cell proliferation and cytotoxic T-cell activity, and extends survival in a murine model of graft-versus-host disease (Sica et al., 2003). The apparently inhibitory function, coupled to the demonstration of enhanced expression on human tumors, indicate that it is another potentially useful target in tumor immunotherapy.

Finally, BTLA is expressed on activated T and B cells, shows high expression by resting B cells, is induced on anergic $CD4^+$ T cells and has lower expression on macrophages, DCs, and NK cells (Han et al., 2004; Hurchla et al., 2005; Watanabe et al., 2003). It remains expressed on Th1 but not Th2 cells, suggesting that it may specifically downregulate Th1-mediated inflammatory responses. Its ligand has recently been identified as HVEM (Sedy et al., 2005). HVEM is constitutively expressed by naïve T cells, is downregulated after activation, and then reexpressed as the T cell returns toward a resting (memory) state. Lymphotoxins, inducible, competes with herpes simplex virus glycoprotein D for HVEM, expressed by T cells (LIGHT) can costimulate T cells through HVEM activation, but it remains unclear whether BTLA activates HVEM or what effects BTLA might exert on LIGHT or lymphotoxin (LT) α interactions with HVEM. BTLA binding does not occlude the TNF family binding site, which is on the opposite face of HVEM, suggesting that HVEM may form stable ternary complexes with BTLA and either LIGHT or LTα (Compaan et al., 2005). BTLA exerts inhibitory effects on both B and T cells (Watanabe et al., 2003). Both cell types show moderately enhanced responsiveness in BTLA$^{-/-}$ mice. The phenotype of these mice is more similar to that of PD-1 knockout than to that of CTLA-4 knockout mice (Han et al., 2004; Watanabe et al., 2003). They have an increased susceptibility to EAE suggesting that the function of BTLA is not entirely redundant, although no propensity to spontaneous autoimmunity with age has yet been documented. Thus, the negative regulation induced by BTLA ligation on B and T cells can potently regulate the strength of the immune response and alter the balance governing immune tolerance. The consequences of immunological blockade in tumor models await further study.

6. Conclusions

The potential for therapeutic immunological checkpoint blockade has been amply demonstrated in preclinical murine models of a variety of cancers and in combination with a variety of other therapeutic interventions. Clinical studies remain in their infancy but have demonstrated exciting initial responses in heavily pretreated patients with advanced stage disease. The association of clinical responses with immune related adverse events is perhaps not surprising given the mode of action of these therapies, but whether such adverse events are an inherent part of effective checkpoint blockade, or whether they can be dissociated remains an area for future study. These reactions have been organ-specific and no evidence of generalized systemic autoimmunity has been documented to date. Evidence for the antigen specificity of the clones causing toxicity is lacking but seems likely to differ from those of the clones mediating the therapeutic benefits. The majority resolves with systemic immune suppression without long-term sequelae, and antitumor responses do not appear to be compromised. This has led to current exploration of dose escalation as one potential way to improve response rates. While CTLA-4 blockade remains the archetypal example of these approaches, other immunological checkpoints offer further targets for intervention. Manipulation of any of these pathways will likely be most effective when combined with other therapeutic strategies, particularly as this may offer the best balance of benefits and toxicities. In addition, combined or sequential manipulation of multiple members of the costimulatory family may ultimately prove more effective in generation of sustained responses and immunological memory. It is anticipated that the results from preclinical studies of combinatorial approaches will help to inform the rational evolution of clinical strategies in the coming years.

References

Acuto, O., and Michel, F. (2003). CD28-mediated costimulation: A quantitative support for TCR signalling. *Nat. Rev. Immunol.* **3,** 939–951.

Annunziato, F., Cosmi, L., Liotta, F., Lazzero, E., Manetti, R., Vanini, V., Romagnani, P., Maggi, E., and Romagnani, S. (2002). Phenotype, localization, and mechanism of suppression of CD4(+) CD25(+) human thymocytes. *J. Exp. Med.* **196,** 379–387.

Aramaki, O., Shirasugi, N., Takayama, T., Shimazu, M., Kitajima, M., Ikeda, Y., Azuma, M., Okumura, K., Yagita, H., and Niimi, M. (2004). Programmed death-1-programmed death-L1 interaction is essential for induction of regulatory cells by intratracheal delivery of alloantigen. *Transplantation* **77,** 6–12.

Atkins, M. B., Lotze, M. T., Dutcher, J. P., Fisher, R. I., Weiss, G., Margolin, K., Abrams, J., Sznol, M., Parkinson, D., Hawkins, M., Paradise, C., Kunkel, L., and Rosenberg, S. A. (1999). High-dose recombinant interleukin 2 therapy for patients with metastatic melanoma: Analysis of 270 patients treated between 1985 and 1993. *J. Clin. Oncol.* **17,** 2105–2116.

Attia, P., Phan, G. Q., Maker, A. V., Robinson, M. R., Quezado, M. M., Yang, J. C., Sherry, R. M., Topalian, S. L., Kammula, U. S., Royal, R. E., Restifo, N. P., Haworth, L. R., *et al.* (2005). Autoimmunity correlates with tumor regression in patients with metastatic melanoma treated with anti-cytotoxic T-lymphocyte antigen-4. *J. Clin. Oncol.* **23,** 6043–6053.

Bachmann, M. F., Kohler, G., Ecabert, B., Mak, T. W., and Kopf, M. (1999). Cutting edge: Lymphoproliferative disease in the absence of CTLA-4 is not T cell autonomous. *J. Immunol.* **163,** 1128–1131.

Baecher-Allan, C., Brown, J. A., Freeman, G. J., and Hafler, D. A. (2001). CD4+CD25high regulatory cells in human peripheral blood. *J. Immunol.* **167,** 1245–1253.

Beck, K. E., Blansfield, J. A., Tran, K. Q., Hughes, S. M., Royal, R. E., Kammula, U. S., Topalian, S. L., Sherry, R. M., Rosenberg, S. A., and Yang, J. C. (2005). Enterocolitis in patients after antibody blockade of CTLA-4. *J. Immunother.* **28,** 647.

Blair, P. J., Riley, J. L., Levine, B. L., Lee, K. P., Craighead, N., Francomano, T., Perfetto, S. J., Gray, G. S., Carreno, B. M., and June, C. H. (1998). CTLA-4 ligation delivers a unique signal to resting human CD4 T cells that inhibits interleukin-2 secretion but allows Bcl-X(L) induction. *J. Immunol.* **160,** 12–15.

Blank, C., Brown, I., Peterson, A. C., Spiotto, M., Iwai, Y., Honjo, T., and Gajewski, T. F. (2004). PD-L1/B7H-1 inhibits the effector phase of tumor rejection by T cell receptor (TCR) transgenic CD8+ T cells. *Cancer Res.* **64,** 1140–1145.

Blansfield, J. A., Beck, K. E., Tran, K., Yang, J. C., Hughes, M. S., Kammula, U. S., Royal, R. E., Topalian, S. L., Haworth, L. R., Levy, C., Rosenberg, S. A., and Sherry, R. M. (2005). Cytotoxic T-lymphocyte-associated antigen-4 blockage can induce autoimmune hypophysitis in patients with metastatic melanoma and renal cancer. *J. Immunother.* **28,** 593–598.

Borriello, F., Sethna, M. P., Boyd, S. D., Schweitzer, A. N., Tivol, E. A., Jacoby, D., Strom, T. B., Simpson, E. M., Freeman, G. J., and Sharpe, A. H. (1997). B7-1 and B7-2 have overlapping, critical roles in immunoglobulin class switching and germinal center formation. *Immunity* **6,** 303–313.

Brown, J. A., Dorfman, D. M., Ma, F. R., Sullivan, E. L., Munoz, O., Wood, C. R., Greenfield, E. A., and Freeman, G. J. (2003). Blockade of programmed death-1 ligands on dendritic cells enhances T cell activation and cytokine production. *J. Immunol.* **170,** 1257–1266.

Brunner, M. C., Chambers, C. A., Chan, F. K., Hanke, J., Winoto, A., and Allison, J. P. (1999). CTLA-4-Mediated inhibition of early events of T cell proliferation. *J. Immunol.* **162,** 5813–5820.

Carreno, B. M., Bennett, F., Chau, T. A., Ling, V., Luxenberg, D., Jussif, J., Baroja, M. L., and Madrenas, J. (2000). CTLA-4 (CD152) can inhibit T cell activation by two different mechanisms depending on its level of cell surface expression. *J. Immunol.* **165,** 1352–1356.

Carter, L., Fouser, L. A., Jussif, J., Fitz, L., Deng, B., Wood, C. R., Collins, M., Honjo, T., Freeman, G. J., and Carreno, B. M. (2002). PD-1:PD-L inhibitory pathway affects both CD4 (+) and CD8(+) T cells and is overcome by IL-2. *Eur. J. Immunol.* **32,** 634–643.

Caton, A. J., Cozzo, C., Larkin, J., III, Lerman, M. A., Boesteanu, A., and Jordan, M. S. (2004). CD4+ CD25+ regulatory T cell selection. *Ann. NY Acad. Sci.* **1029,** 101–114.

Chai, J. G., Tsang, J. Y., Lechler, R., Simpson, E., Dyson, J., and Scott, D. (2002). CD4+CD25+ T cells as immunoregulatory T cells *in vitro*. *Eur. J. Immunol.* **32,** 2365–2375.

Chambers, C. A., Kuhns, M. S., and Allison, J. P. (1999). Cytotoxic T lymphocyte antigen-4 (CTLA-4) regulates primary and secondary peptide-specific CD4(+) T cell responses. *Proc. Natl. Acad. Sci. USA* **96,** 8603–8608.

Chambers, C. A., Kuhns, M. S., Egen, J. G., and Allison, J. P. (2001). CTLA-4-mediated inhibition in regulation of T cell responses: Mechanisms and manipulation in tumor immunotherapy. *Annu. Rev. Immunol.* **19,** 565–594.

Chambers, C. A., Sullivan, T. J., and Allison, J. P. (1997). Lymphoproliferation in CTLA-4-deficient mice is mediated by costimulation-dependent activation of CD4+ T cells. *Immunity* **7,** 885–895.

Chambers, C. A., Sullivan, T. J., Truong, T., and Allison, J. P. (1998). Secondary but not primary T cell responses are enhanced in CTLA-4-deficient CD8+ T cells. *Eur. J. Immunol.* **28,** 3137–3143.

Chen, L., Ashe, S., Brady, W. A., Hellstrom, I., Hellstrom, K. E., Ledbetter, J. A., McGowan, P., and Linsley, P. S. (1992). Costimulation of antitumor immunity by the B7 counterreceptor for the T lymphocyte molecules CD28 and CTLA-4. *Cell* **71,** 1093–1102.

Chen, L., McGowan, P., Ashe, S., Johnston, J., Li, Y., Hellstrom, I., and Hellstrom, K. E. (1994). Tumor immunogenicity determines the effect of B7 costimulation on T cell-mediated tumor immunity. *J. Exp. Med.* **179,** 523–532.

Chikuma, S., Abbas, A. K., and Bluestone, J. A. (2005). B7-independent inhibition of T cells by CTLA-4. *J. Immunol.* **175,** 177–181.

Choi, I. H., Zhu, G., Sica, G. L., Strome, S. E., Cheville, J. C., Lau, J. S., Zhu, Y., Flies, D. B., Tamada, K., and Chen, L. (2003). Genomic organization and expression analysis of B7-H4, an immune inhibitory molecule of the B7 family. *J. Immunol.* **171,** 4650–4654.

Chuang, E., Alegre, M. L., Duckett, C. S., Noel, P. J., Vander Heiden, M. G., and Thompson, C. B. (1997). Interaction of CTLA-4 with the clathrin-associated protein AP50 results in ligand-independent endocytosis that limits cell surface expression. *J. Immunol.* **159,** 144–151.

Collins, A. V., Brodie, D. W., Gilbert, R. J., Iaboni, A., Manso-Sancho, R., Walse, B., Stuart, D. I., van der Merwe, P. A., and Davis, S. J. (2002). The interaction properties of costimulatory molecules revisited. *Immunity* **17,** 201–210.

Compaan, D. M., Gonzalez, L. C., Tom, I., Loyet, K. M., Eaton, D., and Hymowitz, S. G. (2005). Attenuating lymphocyte activity: The crystal structure of the BTLA-HVEM complex. *J. Biol. Chem.* **280,** 39553–39561.

Curiel, T. J., Coukos, G., Zou, L., Alvarez, X., Cheng, P., Mottram, P., Evdemon-Hogan, M., Conejo-Garcia, J. R., Zhang, L., Burow, M., Zhu, Y., Wei, S., *et al.* (2004). Specific recruitment of regulatory T cells in ovarian carcinoma fosters immune privilege and predicts reduced survival. *Nat. Med.* **10,** 942–949.

Davila, E., Kennedy, R., and Celis, E. (2003). Generation of antitumor immunity by cytotoxic T lymphocyte epitope peptide vaccination, CpG-oligodeoxynucleotide adjuvant, and CTLA-4 blockade. *Cancer Res.* **63,** 3281–3288.

Davis, T. A., Tchekmedyian, S., Korman, A., Keler, T., Deo, Y., and Small, E. J. (2002). MDX-010 (human anti-CTLA4): A phase 1 trial in hormone refractory prostate carcinoma (HRPC). *ASCO Annual Meeting* (Abstract 74).

Demaria, S., Kawashima, N., Yang, A. M., Devitt, M. L., Babb, J. S., Allison, J. P., and Formenti, S. C. (2005). Immune-mediated inhibition of metastases after treatment with local radiation and CTLA-4 blockade in a mouse model of breast cancer. *Clin. Cancer Res.* **11,** 728–734.

Diehn, M., Alizadeh, A. A., Rando, O. J., Liu, C. L., Stankunas, K., Botstein, D., Crabtree, G. R., and Brown, P. O. (2002). Genomic expression programs and the integration of the CD28 costimulatory signal in T cell activation. *Proc. Natl. Acad. Sci. USA* **99,** 11796–11801.

Dong, H., Strome, S. E., Matteson, E. L., Moder, K. G., Flies, D. B., Zhu, G., Tamura, H., Driscoll, C. L., and Chen, L. (2003). Costimulating aberrant T cell responses by B7-H1 autoantibodies in rheumatoid arthritis. *J. Clin. Invest.* **111,** 363–370.

Dong, H., Strome, S. E., Salomao, D. R., Tamura, H., Hirano, F., Flies, D. B., Roche, P. C., Lu, J., Zhu, G., Tamada, K., Lennon, V. A., Celis, E., *et al.* (2002). Tumor-associated B7-H1 promotes T-cell apoptosis: A potential mechanism of immune evasion. *Nat. Med.* **8,** 793–800.

Dong, H., Zhu, G., Tamada, K., and Chen, L. (1999). B7-H1, a third member of the B7 family, co-stimulates T-cell proliferation and interleukin-10 secretion. *Nat. Med.* **5,** 1365–1369.

Dong, H., Zhu, G., Tamada, K., Flies, D. B., van Deursen, J. M., and Chen, L. (2004). B7-H1 determines accumulation and deletion of intrahepatic CD8(+) T lymphocytes. *Immunity* **20,** 327–336.

Doyle, A. M., Mullen, A. C., Villarino, A. V., Hutchins, A. S., High, F. A., Lee, H. W., Thompson, C. B., and Reiner, S. L. (2001). Induction of cytotoxic T lymphocyte antigen 4 (CTLA-4) restricts clonal expansion of helper T cells. *J. Exp. Med.* **194,** 893–902.

Egen, J. G., and Allison, J. P. (2002). Cytotoxic T lymphocyte antigen-4 accumulation in the immunological synapse is regulated by TCR signal strength. *Immunity* **16,** 23–35.

Fahlen, L., Read, S., Gorelik, L., Hurst, S. D., Coffman, R. L., Flavell, R. A., and Powrie, F. (2005). T cells that cannot respond to TGF-{beta} escape control by CD4+CD25+ regulatory T cells. *J. Exp. Med.* **201,** 737–746.

Fallarino, F., Grohmann, U., Hwang, K. W., Orabona, C., Vacca, C., Bianchi, R., Belladonna, M. L., Fioretti, M. C., Alegre, M. L., and Puccetti, P. (2003). Modulation of tryptophan catabolism by regulatory T cells. *Nat. Immunol.* **4,** 1206–1212.

Fischkoff, S. A., Hersh, E., Weber, J., Powderly, J., Khan, K., Pavlick, A., Samlowski, W., O'Day, S., Nichol, G., and Yellin, M. (2005). Durable responses and long-term progression-free survival observed in a Phase II study of MDX-010 alone or in combination with dacarbazine (DTIC) in metastatic melanoma. *ASCO Annual Meeting* (Abstract 7525).

Freeman, G. J., Long, A. J., Iwai, Y., Bourque, K., Chernova, T., Nishimura, H., Fitz, L. J., Malenkovich, N., Okazaki, T., Byrne, M. C., Horton, H. F., Fouser, L., *et al.* (2000). Engagement of the PD-1 immunoinhibitory receptor by a novel B7 family member leads to negative regulation of lymphocyte activation. *J. Exp. Med.* **192,** 1027–1034.

Gondek, D. C., Lu, L. F., Quezada, S. A., Sakaguchi, S., and Noelle, R. J. (2005). Cutting edge: Contact-mediated suppression by CD4+CD25+ regulatory cells involves a granzyme B-dependent, perforin-independent mechanism. *J. Immunol.* **174,** 1783–1786.

Greene, J. L., Leytze, G. M., Emswiler, J., Peach, R., Bajorath, J., Cosand, W., and Linsley, P. S. (1996). Covalent dimerization of CD28/CTLA-4 and oligomerization of CD80/CD86 regulate T cell costimulatory interactions. *J. Biol. Chem.* **271,** 26762–26771.

Greenwald, R. J., Boussiotis, V. A., Lorsbach, R. B., Abbas, A. K., and Sharpe, A. H. (2001). CTLA-4 regulates induction of anergy *in vivo*. *Immunity* **14,** 145–155.

Greenwald, R. J., Freeman, G. J., and Sharpe, A. H. (2005). The B7 family revisited. *Annu. Rev. Immunol.* **23,** 515–548.

Gregor, P. D., Wolchok, J. D., Ferrone, C. R., Buchinshky, H., Guevara-Patino, J. A., Perales, M. A., Mortazavi, F., Bacich, D., Heston, W., Latouche, J. B., Sadelain, M., Allison, J. P., Scher, H. I., and Houghton, A. N. (2004). CTLA-4 blockade in combination with xenogeneic DNA vaccines enhances T-cell responses, tumor immunity and autoimmunity to self antigens in animal and cellular model systems. *Vaccine* **22,** 1700–1708.

Groux, H., O'Garra, A., Bigler, M., Rouleau, M., Antonenko, S., de Vries, J. E., and Roncarolo, M. G. (1997). A CD4+ T-cell subset inhibits antigen-specific T-cell responses and prevents colitis. *Nature* **389,** 737–742.

Han, P., Goularte, O. D., Rufner, K., Wilkinson, B., and Kaye, J. (2004). An inhibitory Ig superfamily protein expressed by lymphocytes and APCs is also an early marker of thymocyte positive selection. *J. Immunol.* **172,** 5931–5939.

Harding, F. A., McArthur, J. G., Gross, J. A., Raulet, D. H., and Allison, J. P. (1992). CD28-mediated signalling co-stimulates murine T cells and prevents induction of anergy in T-cell clones. *Nature* **356,** 607–609.

Hathcock, K. S., Laszlo, G., Pucillo, C., Linsley, P., and Hodes, R. J. (1994). Comparative analysis of B7-1 and B7-2 costimulatory ligands: Expression and function. *J. Exp. Med.* **180,** 631–640.

Hinrichs, C. S., Palmer, D. C., Rosenberg, S. A., and Restifo, N. P. (2005). Glucocorticoids do not inhibit antitumor activity of activated CD8+ T cells. *J. Immunother.* **28,** 517.

Hirano, F., Kaneko, K., Tamura, H., Dong, H., Wang, S., Ichikawa, M., Rietz, C., Flies, D. B., Lau, J. S., Zhu, G., Tamada, K., and Chen, L. (2005). Blockade of B7-H1 and PD-1 by monoclonal antibodies potentiates cancer therapeutic immunity. *Cancer Res.* **65,** 1089–1096.

Hodi, F. S., Mihm, M. C., Soiffer, R. J., Haluska, F. G., Butler, M., Seiden, M. V., Davis, T., Henry-Spires, R., MacRae, S., Willman, A., Padera, R., Jaklitsch, M. T., *et al.* (2003). Biologic activity of cytotoxic T lymphocyte-associated antigen 4 antibody blockade in previously vaccinated metastatic melanoma and ovarian carcinoma patients. *Proc. Natl. Acad. Sci. USA* **100,** 4712–4717.

Huang, A. Y., Bruce, A. T., Pardoll, D. M., and Levitsky, H. I. (1996). Does B7–1 expression confer antigen-presenting cell capacity to tumors *in vivo? J. Exp. Med.* **183,** 769–776.

Hurchla, M. A., Sedy, J. R., Gavrielli, M., Drake, C. G., Murphy, T. L., and Murphy, K. M. (2005). B and T lymphocyte attenuator exhibits structural and expression polymorphisms and is highly Induced in anergic CD4+ T cells. *J. Immunol.* **174,** 3377–3385.

Hurwitz, A. A., Foster, B. A., Kwon, E. D., Truong, T., Choi, E. M., Greenberg, N. M., Burg, M. B., and Allison, J. P. (2000). Combination immunotherapy of primary prostate cancer in a transgenic mouse model using CTLA-4 blockade. *Cancer Res.* **60,** 2444–2448.

Hurwitz, A. A., Sullivan, T. J., Krummel, M. F., Sobel, R. A., and Allison, J. P. (1997). Specific blockade of CTLA-4/B7 interactions results in exacerbated clinical and histologic disease in an actively-induced model of experimental allergic encephalomyelitis. *J. Neuroimmunol.* **73,** 57–62.

Hurwitz, A. A., Yu, T. F., Leach, D. R., and Allison, J. P. (1998). CTLA-4 blockade synergizes with tumor-derived granulocyte-macrophage colony-stimulating factor for treatment of an experimental mammary carcinoma. *Proc. Natl. Acad. Sci. USA* **95,** 10067–10071.

Iwai, Y., Ishida, M., Tanaka, Y., Okazaki, T., Honjo, T., and Minato, N. (2002). Involvement of PD-L1 on tumor cells in the escape from host immune system and tumor immunotherapy by PD-L1 blockade. *Proc. Natl. Acad. Sci. USA* **99,** 12293–12297.

Iwai, Y., Terawaki, S., and Honjo, T. (2005). PD-1 blockade inhibits hematogenous spread of poorly immunogenic tumor cells by enhanced recruitment of effector T cells. *Int. Immunol.* **17,** 133–144.

Jordan, M. S., Boesteanu, A., Reed, A. J., Petrone, A. L., Holenbeck, A. E., Lerman, M. A., Naji, A., and Caton, A. J. (2001). Thymic selection of CD4+CD25+ regulatory T cells induced by an agonist self-peptide. *Nat. Immunol.* **2,** 301–306.

Karandikar, N. J., Vanderlugt, C. L., Walunas, T. L., Miller, S. D., and Bluestone, J. A. (1996). CTLA-4: A negative regulator of autoimmune disease. *J. Exp. Med.* **184,** 783–788.

Kataoka, H., Takahashi, S., Takase, K., Yamasaki, S., Yokosuka, T., Koike, T., and Saito, T. (2005). CD25+CD4+ regulatory T cells exert *in vitro* suppressive activity independent of CTLA-4. *Int. Immunol.* **17,** 421–427.

Keler, T., Halk, E., Vitale, L., O'Neill, T., Blanset, D., Lee, S., Srinivasan, M., Graziano, R. F., Davis, T., Lonberg, N., and Korman, A. (2003). Activity and safety of CTLA-4 blockade combined with vaccines in cynomolgus macaques. *J. Immunol.* **171,** 6251–6259.

Korman, A., Yellin, M., and Keler, T. (2005). Tumor immunotherapy: Preclinical and clinical activity of anti-CTLA4 antibodies. *Curr. Opin. Invest. Drugs* **6,** 582–591.

Krummel, M. F., and Allison, J. P. (1996). CTLA-4 engagement inhibits IL-2 accumulation and cell cycle progression upon activation of resting T cells. *J. Exp. Med.* **183,** 2533–2540.

Kundig, T. M., Shahinian, A., Kawai, K., Mittrucker, H. W., Sebzda, E., Bachmann, M. F., Mak, T. W., and Ohashi, P. S. (1996). Duration of TCR stimulation determines costimulatory requirement of T cells. *Immunity* **5,** 41–52.

Kwon, E. D., Hurwitz, A. A., Foster, B. A., Madias, C., Feldhaus, A. L., Greenberg, N. M., Burg, M. B., and Allison, J. P. (1997). Manipulation of T cell costimulatory and inhibitory signals for immunotherapy of prostate cancer. *Proc. Natl. Acad. Sci. USA* **94,** 8099–8103.

Latchman, Y., Wood, C. R., Chernova, T., Chaudhary, D., Borde, M., Chernova, I., Iwai, Y., Long, A. J., Brown, J. A., Nunes, R., Greenfield, E. A., Bourque, K., et al. (2001). PD-L2 is a second ligand for PD-1 and inhibits T cell activation. Nat. Immunol. 2, 261–268.

Leach, D. R., Krummel, M. F., and Allison, J. P. (1996). Enhancement of antitumor immunity by CTLA-4 blockade. Science 271, 1734–1736.

Lenschow, D. J., and Bluestone, J. A. (1993). T cell co-stimulation and in vivo tolerance. Curr. Opin. Immunol. 5, 747–752.

Levings, M. K., Sangregorio, R., Galbiati, F., Squadrone, S., de Waal, M. R., and Roncarolo, M. G. (2001a). IFN-alpha and IL-10 induce the differentiation of human type 1 T regulatory cells. J. Immunol. 166, 5530–5539.

Levings, M. K., Sangregorio, R., and Roncarolo, M. G. (2001b). Human cd25(+)cd4(+) T regulatory cells suppress naive and memory T cell proliferation and can be expanded in vitro without loss of function. J. Exp. Med. 193, 1295–1302.

Linsley, P. S., Brady, W., Grosmaire, L., Aruffo, A., Damle, N. K., and Ledbetter, J. A. (1991). Binding of the B cell activation antigen B7 to CD28 costimulates T cell proliferation and interleukin 2 mRNA accumulation. J. Exp. Med. 173, 721–730.

Liu, X., Gao, J. X., Wen, J., Yin, L., Li, O., Zuo, T., Gajewski, T. F., Fu, Y. X., Zheng, P., and Liu, Y. (2003). B7DC/PDL2 promotes tumor immunity by a PD-1-independent mechanism. J. Exp. Med. 197, 1721–1730.

Liyanage, U. K., Moore, T. T., Joo, H. G., Tanaka, Y., Herrmann, V., Doherty, G., Drebin, J. A., Strasberg, S. M., Eberlein, T. J., Goedegebuure, P. S., and Linehan, D. C. (2002). Prevalence of regulatory T cells is increased in peripheral blood and tumor microenvironment of patients with pancreas or breast adenocarcinoma. J. Immunol. 169, 2756–2761.

Luhder, F., Chambers, C., Allison, J. P., Benoist, C., and Mathis, D. (2000). Pinpointing when T cell costimulatory receptor CTLA-4 must be engaged to dampen diabetogenic T cells. Proc. Natl. Acad. Sci. USA 97, 12204–12209.

Luhder, F., Hoglund, P., Allison, J. P., Benoist, C., and Mathis, D. (1998). Cytotoxic T lymphocyte-associated antigen 4 (CTLA-4) regulates the unfolding of autoimmune diabetes. J. Exp. Med. 187, 427–432.

Luo, L., Chapoval, A. I., Flies, D. B., Zhu, G., Hirano, F., Wang, S., Lau, J. S., Dong, H., Tamada, K., Flies, A. S., Liu, Y., and Chen, L. (2004). B7-H3 enhances tumor immunity in vivo by costimulating rapid clonal expansion of antigen-specific CD8+ cytolytic T cells. J. Immunol. 173, 5445–5450.

Lurquin, C., Lethe, B., De Plaen, E., Corbiere, V., Theate, I., van Baren, N., Coulie, P. G., and Boon, T. (2005). Contrasting frequencies of antitumor and anti-vaccine T cells in metastases of a melanoma patient vaccinated with a MAGE tumor antigen. J. Exp. Med. 201, 249–257.

Maker, A. V., Attia, P., and Rosenberg, S. A. (2005a). Analysis of the cellular mechanism of antitumor responses and autoimmunity in patients treated with CTLA-4 blockade. J. Immunol. 175, 7746–7754.

Maker, A. V., Phan, G. Q., Attia, P., Yang, J. C., Sherry, R. M., Topalian, S. L., Kammula, U. S., Royal, R. E., Haworth, L. R., Levy, C., Kleiner, D., Mavroukakis, S. A., Yellin, M., and Rosenberg, S. A. (2005b). Tumor Regression and Autoimmunity in Patients Treated With Cytotoxic T Lymphocyte-Associated Antigen 4 Blockade and Interleukin 2: A Phase I/II Study. Ann. Surg. Oncol. 12, 1005–1016.

Mandelbrot, D. A., McAdam, A. J., and Sharpe, A. H. (1999). B7-1 or B7-2 is required to produce the lymphoproliferative phenotype in mice lacking cytotoxic T lymphocyte-associated antigen 4 (CTLA-4). J. Exp. Med. 189, 435–440.

Marrogi, A. J., Munshi, A., Merogi, A. J., Ohadike, Y., El Habashi, A., Marrogi, O. L., and Freeman, S. M. (1997). Study of tumor infiltrating lymphocytes and transforming growth factor-beta as prognostic factors in breast carcinoma. Int. J. Cancer 74, 492–501.

Masteller, E. L., Chuang, E., Mullen, A. C., Reiner, S. L., and Thompson, C. B. (2000). Structural analysis of CTLA-4 function *in vivo*. *J. Immunol.* **164,** 5319–5327.

Mokyr, M. B., Kalinichenko, T., Gorelik, L., and Bluestone, J. A. (1998). Realization of the therapeutic potential of CTLA-4 blockade in low-dose chemotherapy-treated tumor-bearing mice. *Cancer Res.* **58,** 5301–5304.

Naito, Y., Saito, K., Shiiba, K., Ohuchi, A., Saigenji, K., Nagura, H., and Ohtani, H. (1998). CD8+ T cells infiltrated within cancer cell nests as a prognostic factor in human colorectal cancer. *Cancer Res.* **58,** 3491–3494.

Nakano, O., Sato, M., Naito, Y., Suzuki, K., Orikasa, S., Aizawa, M., Suzuki, Y., Shintaku, I., Nagura, H., and Ohtani, H. (2001). Proliferative activity of intratumoral CD8(+) T-lymphocytes as a prognostic factor in human renal cell carcinoma: Clinicopathologic demonstration of antitumor immunity. *Cancer Res.* **61,** 5132–5136.

Nakaseko, C., Miyatake, S., Iida, T., Hara, S., Abe, R., Ohno, H., Saito, Y., and Saito, T. (1999). Cytotoxic T lymphocyte antigen 4 (CTLA-4) engagement delivers an inhibitory signal through the membrane-proximal region in the absence of the tyrosine motif in the cytoplasmic tail. *J. Exp. Med.* **190,** 765–774.

Nguyen, L. T., Radhakrishnan, S., Ciric, B., Tamada, K., Shin, T., Pardoll, D. M., Chen, L., Rodriguez, M., and Pease, L. R. (2002). Cross-linking the B7 family molecule B7-DC directly activates immune functions of dendritic cells. *J. Exp. Med.* **196,** 1393–1398.

Nishimura, H., Nose, M., Hiai, H., Minato, N., and Honjo, T. (1999). Development of lupus-like autoimmune diseases by disruption of the PD-1 gene encoding an ITIM motif-carrying immunoreceptor. *Immunity* **11,** 141–151.

Nishimura, H., Okazaki, T., Tanaka, Y., Nakatani, K., Hara, M., Matsumori, A., Sasayama, S., Mizoguchi, A., Hiai, H., Minato, N., and Honjo, T. (2001). Autoimmune dilated cardiomyopathy in PD-1 receptor-deficient mice. *Science* **291,** 319–322.

Ohigashi, Y., Sho, M., Yamada, Y., Tsurui, Y., Hamada, K., Ikeda, N., Mizuno, T., Yoriki, R., Kashizuka, H., Yane, K., Tsushima, F., Otsuki, N., *et al.* (2005). Clinical significance of programmed death-1 ligand-1 and programmed death-1 ligand-2 expression in human esophageal cancer. *Clin. Cancer Res.* **11,** 2947–2953.

Paust, S., Lu, L., McCarty, N., and Cantor, H. (2004). Engagement of B7 on effector T cells by regulatory T cells prevents autoimmune disease. *Proc. Natl. Acad. Sci. USA* **101,** 10398–10403.

Pentcheva-Hoang, T., Egen, J. G., Wojnoonski, K., and Allison, J. P. (2004). B7-1 and B7-2 selectively recruit CTLA-4 and CD28 to the immunological synapse. *Immunity* **21,** 401–413.

Perrin, P. J., Maldonado, J. H., Davis, T. A., June, C. H., and Racke, M. K. (1996). CTLA-4 blockade enhances clinical disease and cytokine production during experimental allergic encephalomyelitis. *J. Immunol.* **157,** 1333–1336.

Phan, G. Q., Touloukian, C. E., Yang, J. C., Restifo, N. P., Sherry, R. M., Hwu, P., Topalian, S. L., Schwartzentruber, D. J., Seipp, C. A., Freezer, L. J., Morton, K. E., Mavroukakis, S. A., *et al.* (2003a). Immunization of patients with metastatic melanoma using both class I- and class II-restricted peptides from melanoma-associated antigens. *J. Immunother.* **26,** 349–356.

Phan, G. Q., Yang, J. C., Sherry, R. M., Hwu, P., Topalian, S. L., Schwartzentruber, D. J., Restifo, N. P., Haworth, L. R., Seipp, C. A., Freezer, L. J., Morton, K. E., Mavroukakis, S. A., *et al.* (2003b). Cancer regression and autoimmunity induced by cytotoxic T lymphocyte-associated antigen 4 blockade in patients with metastatic melanoma. *Proc. Natl. Acad. Sci. USA* **100,** 8372–8377.

Prasad, D. V., Richards, S., Mai, X. M., and Dong, C. (2003). B7S1, a novel B7 family member that negatively regulates T cell activation. *Immunity* **18,** 863–873.

Radhakrishnan, S., Nguyen, L. T., Ciric, B., Flies, D., Van Keulen, V. P., Tamada, K., Chen, L., Rodriguez, M., and Pease, L. R. (2004). Immunotherapeutic potential of B7-DC (PD-L2) cross-linking antibody in conferring antitumor immunity. *Cancer Res.* **64,** 4965–4972.

Read, S., Malmstrom, V., and Powrie, F. (2000). Cytotoxic T lymphocyte-associated antigen 4 plays an essential role in the function of CD25(+)CD4(+) regulatory cells that control intestinal inflammation. *J. Exp. Med.* **192**, 295–302.

Reuben, J. M., Lee, B. N., Shen, D. Y., Gutierrez, C., Hernandez, I., Parker, C. A., Bozon, V. A., Gomez-Navarro, J., Lopez-Berestein, G., and Camacho, L. H. (2005). Therapy with human monoclonal anti-CTLA-4 antibody, CP-675, 206, reduces regulatory T cells and IL-10 production in patients with advanced malignant melanoma (MM). *ASCO Annual Meeting* (Abstract 7505).

Ribas, A., Glaspy, J. A., Lee, Y., Dissette, V. B., Seja, E., Vu, H. T., Tchekmedylan, N. S., Oseguera, D., Comin-Anduix, B., Wargo, J. A., Amornani, S. N., McBride, W. H., *et al.* (2004). Role of dendritic cell phenotype, determine spreading, and negative costimulatory blockade in dendritic cell-based melanoma immunotherapy. *J. Immunother.* **27**, 354–367.

Ribas, A., Bozon, V. A., Lopez-Berestein, G., Pavlov, D., Reuben, J. M., Parker, C. A., Seja, E., Glaspy, J. A., Gomez-Navarro, J., and Camacho, L. H. (2005b). Phase 1 Trial of Monthly Doses of the Human Anti-CTLA4 Monoclonal Antibody CP-675, 206 in Patients with Advanced Melanoma. *ASCO Annual Meeting* (Abstract 7524).

Ribas, A., Camacho, L. H., Lopez-Berestein, G., Pavlov, D., Bulanhagui, C. A., Millham, R., Comin-Anduix, B., Reuben, J. M., Seja, E., Parker, C. A., Sharma, A., Glaspy, J. A., *et al.* (2005a). Antitumor activity in melanoma and anti-self responses in a phase I trial with the anti-cytotoxic T lymphocyte-associated antigen 4 monoclonal antibody CP-675, 206. *J. Clin. Oncol.* **23**, 8968–8977.

Riley, J. L., Mao, M., Kobayashi, S., Biery, M., Burchard, J., Cavet, G., Gregson, B. P., June, C. H., and Linsley, P. S. (2002). Modulation of TCR-induced transcriptional profiles by ligation of CD28, ICOS, and CTLA-4 receptors. *Proc. Natl. Acad. Sci. USA* **99**, 11790–11795.

Robinson, M. R., Chan, C. C., Yang, J. C., Rubin, B. I., Gracia, G. J., Sen, H. N., Csaky, K. G., and Rosenberg, S. A. (2004). Cytotoxic T lymphocyte-associated antigen 4 blockade in patients with metastatic melanoma: A new cause of uveitis. *J. Immunother.* **27**, 478–479.

Rosenberg, S. A. (2000). Interleukin-2 and the development of immunotherapy for the treatment of patients with cancer. *Cancer J. Sci. Am.* **6**(Suppl. 1), S2–S7.

Rosenwald, A., Wright, G., Leroy, K., Yu, X., Gaulard, P., Gascoyne, R. D., Chan, W. C., Zhao, T., Haioun, C., Greiner, T. C., Weisenburger, D. D., Lynch, J. C., *et al.* (2003). Molecular diagnosis of primary mediastinal B cell lymphoma identifies a clinically favorable subgroup of diffuse large B cell lymphoma related to Hodgkin lymphoma. *J. Exp. Med.* **198**, 851–862.

Salceda, S., Tang, T., Kmet, M., Munteanu, A., Ghosh, M., Macina, R., Liu, W., Pilkington, G., and Papkoff, J. (2005). The immunomodulatory protein B7-H4 is overexpressed in breast and ovarian cancers and promotes epithelial cell transformation. *Exp. Cell Res.* **306**, 128–141.

Salomon, B., Lenschow, D. J., Rhee, L., Ashourian, N., Singh, B., Sharpe, A., and Bluestone, J. A. (2000). B7/CD28 costimulation is essential for the homeostasis of the CD4+CD25+ immunoregulatory T cells that control autoimmune diabetes. *Immunity* **12**, 431–440.

Sanderson, K., Scotland, R., Lee, P., Liu, D., Groshen, S., Snively, J., Sian, S., Nichol, G., Davis, T., Keler, T., Yellin, M., and Weber, J. (2005). Autoimmunity in a phase I trial of a fully human anti-cytotoxic T-lymphocyte antigen-4 monoclonal antibody with multiple melanoma peptides and Montanide ISA 51 for patients with resected stages III and IV melanoma. *J. Clin. Oncol.* **23**, 741–750.

Schwartz, J. C., Zhang, X., Fedorov, A. A., Nathenson, S. G., and Almo, S. C. (2001). Structural basis for co-stimulation by the human CTLA-4/B7-2 complex. *Nature* **410**, 604–608.

Sedy, J. R., Gavrieli, M., Potter, K. G., Hurchla, M. A., Lindsley, R. C., Hildner, K., Scheu, S., Pfeffer, K., Ware, C. F., Murphy, T. L., and Murphy, K. M. (2005). B and T lymphocyte attenuator regulates T cell activation through interaction with herpesvirus entry mediator. *Nat. Immunol.* **6**, 90–98.

Shahinian, A., Pfeffer, K., Lee, K. P., Kundig, T. M., Kishihara, K., Wakeham, A., Kawai, K., Ohashi, P. S., Thompson, C. B., and Mak, T. W. (1993). Differential T cell costimulatory requirements in CD28-deficient mice. *Science* **261**, 609–612.

Shin, T., Kennedy, G., Gorski, K., Tsuchiya, H., Koseki, H., Azuma, M., Yagita, H., Chen, L., Powell, J., Pardoll, D., and Housseau, F. (2003). Cooperative B7-1/2 (CD80/CD86) and B7-DC costimulation of CD4+ T cells independent of the PD-1 receptor. *J. Exp. Med.* **198**, 31–38.

Shiratori, T., Miyatake, S., Ohno, H., Nakaseko, C., Isono, K., Bonifacino, J. S., and Saito, T. (1997). Tyrosine phosphorylation controls internalization of CTLA-4 by regulating its interaction with clathrin-associated adaptor complex AP-2. *Immunity* **6**, 583–589.

Shrikant, P., Khoruts, A., and Mescher, M. F. (1999). CTLA-4 blockade reverses CD8+ T cell tolerance to tumor by a CD4+ T cell- and IL-2-dependent mechanism. *Immunity* **11**, 483–493.

Sica, G. L., Choi, I. H., Zhu, G., Tamada, K., Wang, S. D., Tamura, H., Chapoval, A. I., Flies, D. B., Bajorath, J., and Chen, L. (2003). B7-H4, a molecule of the B7 family, negatively regulates T cell immunity. *Immunity* **18**, 849–861.

Sotomayor, E. M., Borrello, I., Tubb, E., Allison, J. P., and Levitsky, H. I. (1999). *In vivo* blockade of CTLA-4 enhances the priming of responsive T cells but fails to prevent the induction of tumor antigen-specific tolerance. *Proc. Natl. Acad. Sci. USA* **96**, 11476–11481.

Stamper, C. C., Zhang, Y., Tobin, J. F., Erbe, D. V., Ikemizu, S., Davis, S. J., Stahl, M. L., Seehra, J., Somers, W. S., and Mosyak, L. (2001). Crystal structure of the B7-1/CTLA-4 complex that inhibits human immune responses. *Nature* **410**, 608–611.

Strome, S. E., Dong, H., Tamura, H., Voss, S. G., Flies, D. B., Tamada, K., Salomao, D., Cheville, J., Hirano, F., Lin, W., Kasperbauer, J. L., Ballman, K. V., and Chen, L. (2003). B7-H1 blockade augments adoptive T-cell immunotherapy for squamous cell carcinoma. *Cancer Res.* **63**, 6501–6505.

Suh, W. K., Gajewska, B. U., Okada, H., Gronski, M. A., Bertram, E. M., Dawicki, W., Duncan, G. S., Bukczynski, J., Plyte, S., Elia, A., Wakeham, A., Itie, A., *et al.* (2003). The B7 family member B7-H3 preferentially down-regulates T helper type 1-mediated immune responses. *Nat. Immunol.* **4**, 899–906.

Sun, M., Richards, S., Prasad, D. V., Mai, X. M., Rudensky, A., and Dong, C. (2002). Characterization of mouse and human B7-H3 genes. *J. Immunol.* **168**, 6294–6297.

Sutmuller, R. P., van Duivenvoorde, L. M., van Elsas, A., Schumacher, T. N., Wildenberg, M. E., Allison, J. P., Toes, R. E., Offringa, R., and Melief, C. J. (2001). Synergism of cytotoxic T lymphocyte-associated antigen 4 blockade and depletion of CD25(+) regulatory T cells in antitumor therapy reveals alternative pathways for suppression of autoreactive cytotoxic T lymphocyte responses. *J. Exp. Med.* **194**, 823–832.

Takahashi, S., Kataoka, H., Hara, S., Yokosuka, T., Takase, K., Yamasaki, S., Kobayashi, W., Saito, Y., and Saito, T. (2005). *In vivo* overexpression of CTLA-4 suppresses lymphoproliferative diseases and thymic negative selection. *Eur. J. Immunol.* **35**, 399–407.

Takahashi, T., Tagami, T., Yamazaki, S., Uede, T., Shimizu, J., Sakaguchi, N., Mak, T. W., and Sakaguchi, S. (2000). Immunologic self-tolerance maintained by CD25(+)CD4(+) regulatory T cells constitutively expressing cytotoxic T lymphocyte-associated antigen 4. *J. Exp. Med.* **192**, 303–310.

Tamura, H., Dong, H., Zhu, G., Sica, G. L., Flies, D. B., Tamada, K., and Chen, L. (2001). B7-H1 costimulation preferentially enhances CD28-independent T-helper cell function. *Blood* **97**, 1809–1816.

Tang, Q., Boden, E. K., Henriksen, K. J., Bour-Jordan, H., Bi, M., and Bluestone, J. A. (2004). Distinct roles of CTLA-4 and TGF-beta in CD4+CD25+ regulatory T cell function. *Eur. J. Immunol.* **34,** 2996–3005.

Taylor, P. A., Lees, C. J., Fournier, S., Allison, J. P., Sharpe, A. H., and Blazar, B. R. (2004). B7 expression on T cells down-regulates immune responses through CTLA-4 ligation via T-T interactions. *J. Immunol.* **172,** 34–39.

Thompson, R. H., Gillett, M. D., Cheville, J. C., Lohse, C. M., Dong, H., Webster, W. S., Krejci, K. G., Lobo, J. R., Sengupta, S., Chen, L., Zincke, H., Blute, et al. (2004). Costimulatory B7-H1 in renal cell carcinoma patients: Indicator of tumor aggressiveness and potential therapeutic target. *Proc. Natl. Acad. Sci. USA* **101,** 17174–17179.

Thornton, A. M., and Shevach, E. M. (1998). CD4+CD25+ immunoregulatory T cells suppress polyclonal T cell activation *in vitro* by inhibiting interleukin 2 production. *J. Exp. Med.* **188,** 287–296.

Thornton, A. M., and Shevach, E. M. (2000). Suppressor effector function of CD4+CD25+ immunoregulatory T cells is antigen nonspecific. *J. Immunol.* **164,** 183–190.

Tivol, E. A., Borriello, F., Schweitzer, A. N., Lynch, W. P., Bluestone, J. A., and Sharpe, A. H. (1995). Loss of CTLA-4 leads to massive lymphoproliferation and fatal multiorgan tissue destruction, revealing a critical negative regulatory role of CTLA-4. *Immunity* **3,** 541–547.

Townsend, S. E., and Allison, J. P. (1993). Tumor rejection after direct costimulation of CD8+ T cells by B7-transfected melanoma cells. *Science* **259,** 368–370.

Tringler, B., Zhuo, S., Pilkington, G., Torkko, K. C., Singh, M., Lucia, M. S., Heinz, D. E., Papkoff, J., and Shroyer, K. R. (2005). B7-h4 is highly expressed in ductal and lobular breast cancer. *Clin. Cancer Res.* **11,** 1842–1848.

Tseng, S. Y., Otsuji, M., Gorski, K., Huang, X., Slansky, J. E., Pai, S. I., Shalabi, A., Shin, T., Pardoll, D. M., and Tsuchiya, H. (2001). B7-DC, a new dendritic cell molecule with potent costimulatory properties for T cells. *J. Exp. Med.* **193,** 839–846.

van der Merwe, P. A., and Davis, S. J. (2003). Molecular interactions mediating T cell antigen recognition. *Annu. Rev. Immunol.* **21,** 659–684.

van Elsas, A., Hurwitz, A. A., and Allison, J. P. (1999). Combination immunotherapy of B16 melanoma using anti-cytotoxic T lymphocyte-associated antigen 4 (CTLA-4) and granulocyte/macrophage colony-stimulating factor (GM-CSF)-producing vaccines induces rejection of subcutaneous and metastatic tumors accompanied by autoimmune depigmentation. *J. Exp. Med.* **190,** 355–366.

Vanasek, T. L., Khoruts, A., Zell, T., and Mueller, D. L. (2001). Antagonistic roles for CTLA-4 and the mammalian target of rapamycin in the regulation of clonal anergy: Enhanced cell cycle progression promotes recall antigen responsiveness. *J. Immunol.* **167,** 5636–5644.

Vesalainen, S., Lipponen, P., Talja, M., and Syrjanen, K. (1994). Histological grade, perineural infiltration, tumour-infiltrating lymphocytes and apoptosis as determinants of long-term prognosis in prostatic adenocarcinoma. *Eur. J. Cancer* **30A,** 1797–1803.

Viguier, M., Lemaitre, F., Verola, O., Cho, M. S., Gorochov, G., Dubertret, L., Bachelez, H., Kourilsky, P., and Ferradini, L. (2004). Foxp3 expressing CD4+CD25(high) regulatory T cells are overrepresented in human metastatic melanoma lymph nodes and inhibit the function of infiltrating T cells. *J. Immunol.* **173,** 1444–1453.

Vijayakrishnan, L., Slavik, J. M., Illes, Z., Greenwald, R. J., Rainbow, D., Greve, B., Peterson, L. B., Hafler, D. A., Freeman, G. J., Sharpe, A. H., Wicker, L. S., and Kuchroo, V. K. (2004). An autoimmune disease-associated CTLA-4 splice variant lacking the B7 binding domain signals negatively in T cells. *Immunity* **20,** 563–575.

Viola, A., and Lanzavecchia, A. (1996). T cell activation determined by T cell receptor number and tunable thresholds. *Science* **273,** 104–106.

Wang, H. B., Shi, F. D., Li, H., Chambers, B. J., Link, H., and Ljunggren, H. G. (2001). Anti-CTLA-4 antibody treatment triggers determinant spreading and enhances murine myasthenia gravis. *J. Immunol.* **166,** 6430–6436.
Wang, S., Bajorath, J., Flies, D. B., Dong, H., Honjo, T., and Chen, L. (2003). Molecular modeling and functional mapping of B7-H1 and B7-DC uncouple costimulatory function from PD-1 interaction. *J. Exp. Med.* **197,** 1083–1091.
Watanabe, N., Gavrieli, M., Sedy, J. R., Yang, J., Fallarino, F., Loftin, S. K., Hurchla, M. A., Zimmerman, N., Sim, J., Zang, X., Murphy, T. L., Russell, J. H., et al. (2003). BTLA is a lymphocyte inhibitory receptor with similarities to CTLA-4 and PD-1. *Nat. Immunol.* **4,** 670–679.
Waterhouse, P., Penninger, J. M., Timms, E., Wakeham, A., Shahinian, A., Lee, K. P., Thompson, C. B., Griesser, H., and Mak, T. W. (1995). Lymphoproliferative disorders with early lethality in mice deficient in CTLA-4. *Science* **270,** 985–988.
Weiner, H. L. (2001). Induction and mechanism of action of transforming growth factor-beta-secreting Th3 regulatory cells. *Immunol. Rev.* **182,** 207–214.
Woo, E. Y., Chu, C. S., Goletz, T. J., Schlienger, K., Yeh, H., Coukos, G., Rubin, S. C., Kaiser, L. R., and June, C. H. (2001). Regulatory CD4(+)CD25(+) T cells in tumors from patients with early-stage non-small cell lung cancer and late-stage ovarian cancer. *Cancer Res.* **61,** 4766–4772.
Woo, E. Y., Yeh, H., Chu, C. S., Schlienger, K., Carroll, R. G., Riley, J. L., Kaiser, L. R., and June, C. H. (2002). Cutting edge: Regulatory T cells from lung cancer patients directly inhibit autologous T cell proliferation. *J. Immunol.* **168,** 4272–4276.
Yang, J. C., Beck, K. E., Blansfield, J. A., Tran, K., Lowy, I., and Rosenberg, S. A. (2005). Tumor regression in patients with metastatic renal cancer treated with a monoclonal antibody to CTLA4 (MDX-010). *ASCO Annual Meeting* (Abstract 2501).
Yang, Y. F., Zou, J. P., Mu, J., Wijesuriya, R., Ono, S., Walunas, T., Bluestone, J., Fujiwara, H., and Hamaoka, T. (1997). Enhanced induction of antitumor T-cell responses by cytotoxic T lymphocyte-associated molecule-4 blockade: The effect is manifested only at the restricted tumor-bearing stages. *Cancer Res.* **57,** 4036–4041.
Youngnak, P., Kozono, Y., Kozono, H., Iwai, H., Otsuki, N., Jin, H., Omura, K., Yagita, H., Pardoll, D. M., Chen, L., and Azuma, M. (2003). Differential binding properties of B7-H1 and B7-DC to programmed death-1. *Biochem. Biophys. Res. Commun.* **307,** 672–677.
Zang, X., Loke, P., Kim, J., Murphy, K., Waitz, R., and Allison, J. P. (2003). B7x: A widely expressed B7 family member that inhibits T cell activation. *Proc. Natl. Acad. Sci. USA* **100,** 10388–10392.
Zhang, L., Conejo-Garcia, J. R., Katsaros, D., Gimotty, P. A., Massobrio, M., Regnani, G., Makrigiannakis, A., Gray, H., Schlienger, K., Liebman, M. N., Rubin, S. C., and Coukos, G. (2003). Intratumoral T cells, recurrence, and survival in epithelial ovarian cancer. *N. Engl. J. Med.* **348,** 203–213.
Zhang, X., Schwartz, J. C., Almo, S. C., and Nathenson, S. G. (2003). Crystal structure of the receptor-binding domain of human B7-2: Insights into organization and signaling. *Proc. Natl. Acad. Sci. USA* **100,** 2586–2591.
Zhang, X., Schwartz, J. C., Guo, X., Bhatia, S., Cao, E., Lorenz, M., Cammer, M., Chen, L., Zhang, Z. Y., Edidin, M. A., Nathenson, S. G., and Almo, S. C. (2004). Structural and functional analysis of the costimulatory receptor programmed death-1. *Immunity* **20,** 337–347.
Zhang, Y., and Allison, J. P. (1997). Interaction of CTLA-4 with AP50, a clathrin-coated pit adaptor protein. *Proc. Natl. Acad. Sci. USA* **94,** 9273–9278.
Zhou, G., Drake, C. G., and Levitsky, H. I. (2005). Amplification of tumor-specific regulatory T cells following therapeutic cancer vaccines. *Blood* **107,** 628–636.

Combinatorial Cancer Immunotherapy

F. Stephen Hodi and Glenn Dranoff

*Department of Medical Oncology, Dana-Farber Cancer Institute,
Boston, Massachusetts*

Abstract	341
1. Introduction	341
2. Endogenous Host Responses	342
3. Enhancing Tumor Antigen Presentation	343
4. GM-CSF Secreting Tumor Cell Vaccines	344
5. Targets of Vaccine-Induced Tumor Destruction	347
6. Cytotoxic T Lymphocyte Antigen-4 Antibody Blockade	352
7. Combination Immunotherapy: The Next Paradigm?	358
References	358

Abstract

The formulation of therapeutic strategies to enhance immune-mediated tumor destruction is a central goal of cancer immunology. Substantive progress toward delineating the mechanisms involved in innate and adaptive tumor immunity has improved the prospects for crafting efficacious treatments. Schemes under active clinical evaluation include cancer vaccines, monoclonal antibodies, recombinant cytokines, and adoptive cellular infusions. While these manipulations increase tumor immunity in many patients, the majority still succumbs to progressive disease. Detailed analysis of subjects on experimental protocols together with informative studies of murine tumor models have begun to clarify the parameters that determine therapeutic activity and resistance. These investigations have highlighted efficient dendritic cell activation and inhibition of negative immune regulation as central pathways for intervention. This review discusses the development of genetically modified whole tumor cell vaccines and antibody-blockade of cytotoxic T lymphocyte associated antigen-4 (CTLA-4) as immunotherapies targeting these key control points. Early-stage clinical testing raises the possibility that combinatorial approaches that augment dendritic cell-mediated tumor antigen presentation and antagonize negative immune regulation may accomplish significant tumor destruction without the induction of serious autoimmune disease.

1. Introduction

The design of therapeutic strategies to stimulate potent, specific, and long-lasting antitumor immune responses is a central objective for cancer immunology. The crafting of genetic and biochemical techniques to characterize tumor antigens has led to the discovery that most cancer patients mount innate and adaptive reactions to developing neoplasms (Germeau et al., 2005). Stress-induced gene products in tumor cells, such as MHC class I chain-related protein A (MICA) and MHC class I chain-related protein B (MICB), frequently activate natural killer cells, phagocytes, and cytotoxic lymphocytes (Diefenbach and Raulet, 2002), whereas mutated or aberrantly expressed tumor-associated proteins often trigger T and B lymphocytes (Gilboa, 1999). Despite this broad immune recognition, however, the formation and progression of clinically evident disease implies that endogenous reactions are typically ineffectual (Gabrilovich, 2004). Analysis of the mechanisms underlying tumor escape from immune surveillance has underscored inefficient dendritic cell-mediated tumor antigen presentation and negative immune regulation as critical factors that restrain the potency of host responses (Dranoff, 2004). These insights in turn have guided the formulation of therapeutic strategies to overcome these defects, and early-stage clinical testing has established the ability of these schemes to effectuate substantive tumor destruction in some otherwise refractory patients.

2. Endogenous Host Responses

There is convincing evidence that multiple types of cancer can evoke specific cellular and humoral responses of prognostic importance (Old and Chen, 1998). $CD4^+$ and $CD8^+$ T cells that manifest major histocompatibility complex (MHC) restricted tumor cell reactivity can be detected in the blood, lymph nodes, and metastases of many patients (van der Bruggen et al., 1991). Dense intratumoral (but not peritumoral) T-cell infiltrates in the vertical growth phase of primary melanomas are strongly associated with a decreased incidence of recurrent disease and reduced mortality following complete resection (Clark et al., 1989). Intratumoral T-cell responses in follicular lymphomas and ovarian, colon, and renal cell carcinomas are similarly linked with improved patient outcomes after chemotherapy and surgery (Dave et al., 2004; Naito et al., 1998; Nakano et al., 2001; Zhang et al., 2003). Even brisk T-cell infiltrates in melanomas that have metastasized to regional lymph nodes are correlated with diminished mortality (Mihm et al., 1996). Furthermore, antibody reactions to mucin-1, transmembrane (MUC-1), a tandem-repeat containing glycoprotein that is overexpressed in carcinomas, are linked with prolonged survival in treated early-stage breast cancer patients (von Mensdorff-Pouilly et al., 2000). Together, these findings indicate that whereas endogenous host responses may alone be insufficient to prevent tumor formation, they can be associated with favorable clinical outcomes following standard cancer therapy. Future studies may clarify whether this spontaneous immunity plays a role in treatment efficacy and durability.

Significant work has been devoted to characterizing the molecular targets of these adaptive reactions (Old, 1981). T cell and antibody-based expression cloning techniques have unveiled a large repertoire of tumor-associated gene products that evoke immune recognition (Boon and van der Bruggen, 1996; Cox et al., 1994; Sahin et al., 1995). These include mutated or aberrantly expressed proteins, alternatively translated open reading frames and intronic sequences and overexpressed normal differentiation antigens (Rosenberg, 2001). This diversity of targets implies that some pathways of tumor antigen presentation are operative during carcinogenesis (Dunn et al., 2004), albeit insufficient to impede tumor progression.

Direct stimulation by tumor cells likely contributes to the abortive T-cell responses, since cancer cells typically lack the appropriate costimulatory molecules and cytokines necessary for effective immune priming (Greenwald et al., 2005). Dendritic cells, in contrast, might elicit stronger T-cell responses through cross-priming of tumor antigens (Paczesny et al., 2003). Dendritic cells are endowed with various surface receptors that facilitate the efficient capture of tumor cell debris (Albert et al., 1998). Subsequent dendritic cell maturation promotes tumor antigen processing for MHC class I and II molecule presentation to $CD8^+$ and $CD4^+$ T cells and CD1d molecule presentation to invariant natual killer T (NKT) cells (Munz et al., 2005). The coordinated display of costimulatory proteins, such as B7-1 and B7-2, and cytokines, such as IL-12 and IL-18, therein contributes to the activation of antigen-specific lymphocytes (Steinman and Mellman, 2004). While these many capabilities potentially confer an important role for dendritic cells in triggering adaptive antineoplastic responses, the tumor microenvironment impedes optimal dendritic cell activation (Bell et al., 1999), in part through the release of immunosuppressive cytokines such as vascular endothelial cell growth factor (VEGF) and interleukin-10 (IL-10) (Gabrilovich, 2004). Hence, the limited capacity of tumor cells to function directly as antigen presenting cells together with the impaired maturation of tumor-infiltrating dendritic cells culminates in inadequate adaptive immunity and successful tumor escape.

3. Enhancing Tumor Antigen Presentation

In light of this tumor-induced dendritic cell dysfunction, intense efforts have been directed toward devising therapeutic schemes that augment dendritic cell activation (Cerundolo et al., 2004). In one approach, large numbers of dendritic cells are generated *ex vivo* by culturing hematopoietic precursors in the presence of granulocyte-macrophage colony stimulating factor (GM-CSF) and other factors; these expanded cells are then charged with tumor antigen and inoculated into tumor-bearing hosts (Young and Inaba, 1996). Key variables under study include the source of hematopoietic progenitors, the mixtures of cytokines and other immunostimulatory molecules employed to promote dendritic cell maturation, method of antigen loading, and route of inoculation (Palucka *et al.*, 2005). In a second strategy, dendritic cells are triggered *in situ* through the provision of appropriate activating signals. These schemes include the administration of CpG oligonucleotides or imiquimod (which engage TLR9 and TLR7, respectively), α-galactosylceramide (which stimulates dendritic cell/NKT cell cross-talk), Flt3-ligand or GM-CSF protein, and chemical adjuvants such as ISCOMATRIX (Bendandi *et al.*, 1999; Chang *et al.*, 2005; Davis *et al.*, 2004; Fong *et al.*, 2001; Krieg, 2003; Slingluff *et al.*, 2003; Srivastava, 1993).

Both defined antigens and whole tumor cells have been incorporated into the *ex vivo* and *in vivo* dendritic cell targeting strategies (Finn, 2003). The application of molecularly characterized antigens provides advantages for precise immune monitoring, but may be limited by the intrinsic immunogenicity of specific gene products (Engelhard *et al.*, 2002; Van Der Bruggen *et al.*, 2002). The modification of peptide epitopes to increase MHC binding and T-cell receptor engagement may overcome this obstacle, particularly when coupled to a quantitative and functional assessment of the pool of potentially reactive T cells (Chen *et al.*, 2005). The use of whole tumor cells, in contrast, affords a large array of candidate antigens and exploits the hardwiring of the immune system to detect dominant targets (Pardoll, 2002). Nonetheless, there is limited understanding of the rules underlying the establishment of antigenic hierarchies, and the most immunogenic moieties remain to be delineated, shortcomings that present formidable challenges for immune monitoring. Overall, the definition of a battery of immunogenic gene products whose function is linked to tumor maintenance remains a critical goal for ongoing investigation (Gilboa, 2004).

4. GM-CSF Secreting Tumor Cell Vaccines

The mixture of cytokines produced in the tumor microenvironment plays a decisive role in dictating the outcome of the host response (Mach and Dranoff, 2000). Forni and colleagues established that the peritumoral injection of particular cytokines could provoke tumor destruction through a complex reaction consisting of macrophages, granulocytes, dendritic cells, natural killer cells, and T and B lymphocytes (Forni *et al.*, 1988). This response in some cases also engendered protective immunity against a subsequent live tumor challenge. These pioneering experiments uncovered the therapeutic potential of manipulating the cytokine balance in the tumor microenvironment.

A comparative analysis of the relative abilities of multiple immunostimulatory molecules to enhance host responses, following gene transfer into tumor cells, identified GM-CSF as the most potent of 33 products tested (Dranoff, 2002). The inoculation of irradiated tumor cells engineered to secrete GM-CSF elicited a dense local infiltrate composed of granulocytes, macrophages, and CD11b$^+$ dendritic cells (Dranoff et al., 1993). This coordinated reaction promoted dendritic cell maturation, as evidenced by high-level expression of B7-1, B7-2, MHC II, and CD1d, and resulted in improved tumor antigen presentation (Huang et al., 1994; Mach et al., 2000). Potent, specific, and long-lasting protection against subsequent wild-type tumor challenge required the activities of CD4$^+$ and CD8$^+$ T cells, CD1d-restricted NKT cells, and antibodies (Dranoff et al., 1993; Gillessen et al., 2003; Hung et al., 1998; Reilly et al., 2001).

To determine whether this cancer vaccination strategy might enhance tumor immunity in humans, we performed a phase I clinical trial of vaccination with irradiated, autologous melanoma cells engineered by retroviral mediated gene transfer to secrete GM-CSF in patients with metastatic melanoma (Soiffer et al., 1997, 1998). In the study, resected tumors were processed to single cell suspension by enzymatic and mechanical digestion and introduced into short-term culture. Replicating melanoma cells were infected with replication defective retroviruses expressing human GM-CSF, irradiated, and cryopreserved. Vaccines were produced for 29 of the 31 patients enrolled, and the GM-CSF secretion rates ranged from 84 to 965 ng/10^6 cells/24 h, values representing at least a two-log increase over endogenous levels. Patients were immunized intra-dermally and subcutaneously with 10^7 irradiated tumor cells (per treatment) administered at 28-, 14-, or 7-day intervals; no significant toxicities were observed.

Vaccination sites revealed brisk infiltrates of dendritic cells, macrophages, eosinophils, and lymphocytes in all 21 evaluable patients. While metastatic lesions resected prior to immunization revealed minimal host reactions, lesions resected following vaccination showed dense infiltrates of CD4$^+$ and CD8$^+$ T lymphocytes and plasma cells with extensive tumor destruction, fibrosis, and edema in 11 of 16 patients. Consistent with the pathologic evidence of tumor necrosis, T lymphocytes purified from infiltrated metastases manifested potent cytotoxicity and secreted a broad profile of cytokines in response to autologous tumor cells. High-titer antibodies recognizing melanoma-associated antigens were present in postvaccination sera, as revealed by flow cytometry and western analysis. An unexpected additional finding was the targeted destruction of the tumor vasculature by activated lymphocytes, eosinophils, and neutrophils. This accomplished zonal tumor necrosis, which extended the destruction mediated by direct lymphocyte-tumor cell engagement.

Whereas this initial study in melanoma established the biologic activity and safety of the vaccination strategy in patients, the use of retroviral vectors for vaccine production impeded further clinical development. In this context, retroviral vectors require replicating target cells for efficient gene transfer, necessitating the establishment of short-term cultures, and are potential carcinogens, thereby requiring extensive safety testing to ensure the absence of replication competent viruses (Mulligan, 1993). In contrast to these limitations, adenoviral vectors efficiently transduce many nonreplicating tumor cells and are associated with only minimal toxicities in *ex vivo* applications (Berkner, 1988; Shenk, 1996).

We thus conducted a second phase I trial in which autologous melanoma cells were engineered by adenoviral mediated gene transfer to secrete GM-CSF (Soiffer *et al.*, 2003). In this scheme, single cell suspensions of resected melanomas were transduced overnight with an E1, E3 replicative defective adenoviral vector encoding GM-CSF, washed and irradiated. The ability to manufacture vaccines for 34 of 35 enrolled patients validated the high efficiency of the production scheme. The average GM-CSF secretion achieved was 745 ng/10^6 cells/24 h, comparable to the level generated with retroviral vectors. Intra-dermal and subcutaneous injections of the transduced cells elicited no significant toxicity, and any adenoviral structural proteins retained in the tumor cell preparation did not measurably influence the generation of anti-melanoma immunity. Vaccination sites were characterized by dense dendritic cell, macrophage, granulocyte, and lymphocyte infiltrates in 17 of 26 evaluable patients. As a consequence of immunization, 17 of 25 patient developed delayed-type hypersensitivity (DTH) reactions to injections of unmodified, irradiated autologous cells. These reactions were composed of lymphocytes, macrophages and eosinophils. Moreover, metastatic lesions resected after vaccination showed dense T lymphocyte and plasma cell infiltrates effectuating tumor necrosis, fibrosis, and edema in 10 of 16 patients. While these reactions infrequently resulted in tumor regression, 10 of 26 evaluable patients with disseminated disease survived for at least 44 months, and 6 are currently alive and well at a minimum of 67 months from initiating vaccination. These encouraging survival data raise the possibility that regression may not be the most informative endpoint for this immunotherapy and have motivated the undertaking of a follow-up study to define survival more thoroughly in an additional cohort of 40 stage IV melanoma patients. Analysis of advanced melanoma patients immunized with irradiated, autologous tumor cells admixed with BCG similarly highlighted an association of tumor-infiltrating lymphocytes with prolonged survival (Haanen *et al.*, 2005).

To test whether vaccination with GM-CSF secreting tumor cells might augment immunity in other types of cancers, we conducted a phase I clinical trial using adenoviral mediated gene transfer in patients with stage IV nonsmall cell lung carcinoma (Salgia *et al.*, 2003). Vaccines were successfully prepared for

34 of 35 patients, achieving an average GM-CSF secretion rate of 513 ng/10^6 cells/24 h and no significant toxicities were observed. Immunization elicited local dendritic cell, macrophage, granulocyte, and lymphocyte infiltrates in 18 of 25 patients, and DTH reactions to irradiated, nontransduced tumor cells were evoked in 18 of 22 patients. Metastatic lesions resected after vaccination revealed T lymphocyte and plasma cell infiltrates with tumor necrosis in three of six patients. Seven patients achieved stable disease, and three remained alive and well for a minimum of 67 months since starting treatment. A subsequent multicenter national study confirmed the immunogenicity of this vaccination strategy in patients with advanced nonsmall cell lung carcinoma (Nemunaitis et al., 2004). In the absence of significant toxicity, 3 of 33 patients achieved durable complete responses to immunization.

Additional pilot trials testing autologous tumor cells engineered to secrete GM-CSF have been conducted in other diseases. Two studies in stage IV renal cell carcinoma patients revealed the induction of strong vaccine and DTH reactions associated with some clinical responses (Simons et al., 1997; Tani et al., 2004). A small trial in prostate carcinoma similarly disclosed robust vaccine and DTH reactions (Simons et al., 1999). Phase I investigations in ovarian cancer and acute myelogenous leukemia are currently underway. A potentially important simplification of autologous tumor vaccine manufacture involves the admixing of a generic cell line stably engineered to secrete GM-CSF with nontransduced autologous tumor cells (Borrello et al., 1999). This "bystander" approach is being explored for several hematologic and solid malignancies.

The relative complexity of autologous tumor cell vaccines together with the ability of dendritic cells to cross-present dying cells has motivated evaluation of allogeneic cancer cell lines stably engineered to secrete GM-CSF (Laheru and Jaffee, 2005). A phase I study of this approach in locally advanced pancreatic cancer patients treated in the adjuvant setting revealed increased DTH responses, and three subjects were disease-free for more than 25 months (Jaffee et al., 2001). Detailed immune analysis of the surviving patients identified mesothelin as a target antigen for vaccination, thereby validating the principle of cross-priming in patients (Thomas et al., 2004). GM-CSF secreting allogeneic prostate carcinoma cell lines demonstrated significant immunologic activity in initial testing, and large randomized phase III studies to determine impact on survival compared to standard care are underway in patients with metastatic disease (Assikis and Simons, 2004).

5. Targets of Vaccine-Induced Tumor Destruction

The clinical trials of vaccination with irradiated, autologous, GM-CSF secreting tumor cells established that this therapeutic manipulation consistently improves antitumor immunity in patients with advanced cancers. Nonetheless, the majority of treated subjects still succumb to progressive disease, indicating that defects in addition to impaired dendritic cell-mediated tumor antigen presentation remain to be addressed. To learn more about these pathways, we initiated efforts to identify the targets of vaccine responses, reasoning that a more detailed molecular analysis of the host reaction might provide insights into the basis for treatment sensitivity and resistance. Since the pathologic and laboratory investigations indicated that GM-CSF secreting tumor cell vaccines elicited a coordinated humoral and cellular antitumor response, we hypothesized that antibodies and T cells might, at least in some cases, recognize common antigens. Thus, the targets of vaccine-induced tumor destruction were characterized through screening cDNA expression libraries, prepared from densely infiltrated metastases, with postimmunization sera from long-term surviving patients.

5.1. ATP6S1

ATP6S1, a putative accessory subunit of the vacuolar H^+-ATPase complex, emerged from a library screen performed with sera from a vaccinated melanoma patient who remains disease-free 10 years after completion of therapy (Hodi et al., 2002). ATP6S1 is a broadly expressed protein that likely contributes to pH regulation in the secretory and endocytic pathways (Getlawi et al., 1996; Holthuis et al., 1995; Schoonderwoert et al., 2000; Supek et al., 1994). The Xenopus homolog is upregulated with pro-opiomelanocortin in response to dark adaptation (Holthuis et al., 1999), suggesting that ATP6S1 might play a role in melanocyte biology and/or melanoma pathogenesis. Indeed, diverse human cancers express high levels of ATP6S1 transcripts, consistent with a potential function in tumor maintenance. While expression in normal tissues and the absence of tumor-associated mutations render the immunogenicity of ATP6S1 unexpected, the Xenopus homolog can be detected at the cell membrane, following gene transfer in mammalian cells (Jansen et al., 1998), raising the possibility that antibodies might accomplish tumor destruction through cell surface interactions.

A longitudinal analysis of anti-ATP6S1 antibodies in the index melanoma patient revealed that vaccination increased titers at least 12-fold, in contrast to unaltered reactivity to Candida and mumps antigens (Fig. 1). The peak response to ATP6S1 was correlated with the development of erythema and hemorrhage in a subcutaneous metastasis, underscoring a potential link between immunity to this antigen and tumor destruction. Further investigations demonstrated that vaccine-induced increases in ATP6S1 specific antibodies were correlated, in several immunized metastatic melanoma and nonsmall cell lung carcinoma patients, with the induction of T- and B-cell infiltrates and

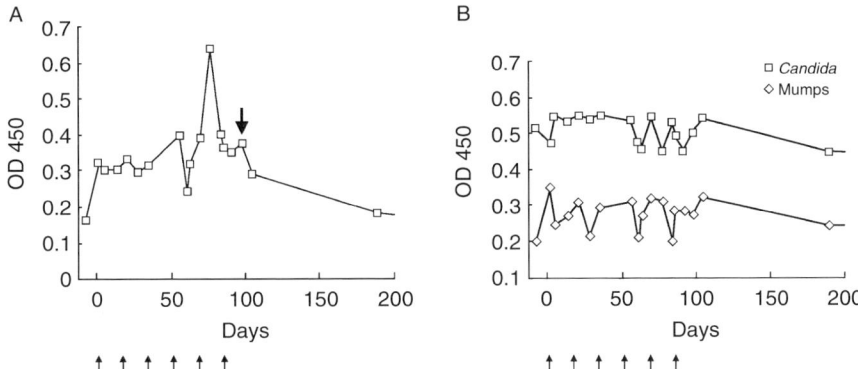

Figure 1 Vaccination stimulated humoral immunity to ATP6S1. (A) Longitudinal analysis of melanoma subject K08 reactivity to ATP6S1 by ELISA. The small arrows denote vaccinations and the large arrow indicates the appearance of erythema and hemorrhage in a subcutaneous metastasis. (B) Reactivity to mumps and *Candida* antigens. Patient sera were diluted 1:500 and ELISAs were developed with a labeled pan-IgG secondary antibody. Reprinted from Hodi *et al.* (2002).

tumor necrosis in distant metastases. Augmented immunity to ATP6S1 was also documented in a chronic myelogenous leukemia patient who experienced a complete remission following the infusion of $CD4^+$ donor lymphocytes after allogeneic bone marrow transplantation. Taken together, these results delineate an association between potent humoral responses to ATP6S1 and immune-mediated tumor destruction in diverse cancers.

5.2. Opioid Growth Factor Receptor

A putative opioid growth factor receptor (OGFr) (Zagon *et al.*, 2000), is a second gene product isolated in the library screen from the index melanoma patient (Mollick *et al.*, 2003). Noteworthy in the OGFr sequence are 20 amino acid tandem repeats in the carboxy-terminal domain, which manifest significant similarity (20% identity) to the tandem repeats found in the extracellular domain of MUC1, with positional conservation of 4 of the 5 prolines in each repeat (Gendler *et al.*, 1990; Siddiqui *et al.*, 1988). Unexpectedly, the patient sera also recognized a clone in the library in which OGFr was fused with the *LacZ* promoter in an alternative reading frame. This sequence encoded a putative second tandem repeat containing protein (which we designate as OGFr-ARF) that showed a higher overall identity to MUC1 (30%), with positional conservation of 2 of the 5 prolines per repeat.

ELISAs were performed, with bacterial-produced recombinant full-length wild-type OGFr protein and a synthetic peptide corresponding to the tandem repeat region of OGFr-ARF, to evaluate the immunogenicity of these gene products in more detail. Longitudinal study of the index melanoma patient disclosed increased reactivity to both targets as a function of vaccination, with kinetics that paralleled the humoral response to ATP6S1. Furthermore, high-titer IgG antibodies specific for OGFr and OGFr-ARF were frequently detected in other cancer patients. 11 of 45 (24%) and 5 of 45 (11%) metastatic melanoma patients generated antibodies to OGFr and OGFr-ARF, respectively, whereas 5 of 24 (21%) nonsmall cell lung carcinoma, 4 of 25 (16%) prostate carcinoma, and 5 of 6 breast or ovarian carcinoma patients developed reactions to OGFr, the alternative frame product, or both. OGFr was also a target for immune-mediated tumor destruction in a chronic myelogenous leukemia patient who achieved a complete remission as a consequence of donor lymphocyte infusions (Wu et al., 2000). Together, these findings establish that OGFr and OGFr-ARF are broadly immunogenic in cancer patients.

The repetitive epitopes in tandem repeat-containing proteins appear to stimulate immunoglobulin production efficiently, perhaps analogous to the T-cell independent B-cell responses directed to bacterial polysaccharides (Fehr et al., 1998). Antibody responses to the MUC1 tandem repeats are of prognostic importance in breast and ovarian cancer patients (von Mensdorff-Pouilly et al., 2000). CDR34, a protein with 34 inexact six amino acid tandem repeats, elicits antibody responses in a variety of solid tumors (Dropcho et al., 1987). Since this protein is normally expressed in the cerebellum, the spontaneous development of antitumor immunity may underlie the pathogenesis of paraneoplastic cerebellar degeneration in some cases. Additional work identified CT7, a protein with ten 35 amino acid repeats and some homology to MAGE 10 as a target for antibody responses in melanoma (Chen et al., 1998). Lastly, while previous investigations disclosed that alternatively translated reading frames of NY-ESO-1/LAGE-1, SART-1, tyrosinase related protein-1, and intestinal carboxyl esterase can trigger tumor-specific cytotoxic T cells (Rimoldi et al., 2000; Ronsin et al., 1999; Shichijo et al., 1998; Wang et al., 1996, 1998), OGFr represents the first example of a tumor antigen eliciting antibody responses to two alternatively translated gene products.

5.3. Melanoma Inhibitor of Apoptosis Protein

Library screening with sera from a second patient who achieved an objective tumor response and prolonged survival (4.5 years) as a consequence of vaccination yielded the melanoma inhibitor of apoptosis protein (ML-IAP) (Schmollinger et al., 2003). Melanoma inhibitor of apoptosis protein is a member of the inhibitor of apoptosis protein family and is characterized by a single baculoviral IAP repeat and a carboxy-terminal RING domain (Ashhab et al., 2001; Kasof and Gomes, 2000; Lin et al., 2000; Vucic et al., 2000). It antagonizes extrinsic and intrinsic apoptotic pathways through the inhibition of caspases 3, 7, and 9, the sequestration of SMAC/Diablo, and the participation of JNK1 (Sanna et al., 2002; Vucic et al., 2005). The gene is localized to chromosome 20q13.3, a locus commonly amplified in melanomas and other solid tumors (Barks et al., 1997; Korn et al., 1999), and immunohistochemistry reveals frequent expression in diverse malignancies. Increased ML-IAP levels likely contribute to carcinogenesis and tumor cell resistance to cytotoxic therapy and radiation (Crnkovic-Mertens et al., 2003; Nachmias et al., 2003).

Longitudinal analysis of the humoral response to ML-IAP indicated that vaccination increased overall specific titers and promoted isotype switching (Manis et al., 2002). Since the latter finding typically indicates the provision of T-cell help, $CD4^+$ lymphocytes were isolated from metastases that became densely infiltrated as a function of immunization. These purified T cells manifested strong proliferative responses to recombinant ML-IAP protein, but not irrelevant antigen (Fig. 2A). Bioinformatic tools were employed to identify candidate ML-IAP-derived class I epitopes that showed high-affinity binding to HLA-A2, one of the MHC class I alleles expressed by this patient (Parker et al., 1994). Soluble HLA-A2 tetramers folded with either JS34 or JS90 peptides detected ML-IAP specific $CD8^+$ T cells in necrotic metastases (Fig. 2B). These lymphocytes were functionally competent, mediating interferon-gamma production and cytolysis of ML-IAP expressing tumor cells (Fig. 2C and D). In this context, cytotoxic lymphocytes likely exploit the perforin-granzyme pathway to cleave critical cellular substrates through caspase-independent mechanisms (Andrade et al., 1998; Heibein et al., 2000; Sutton et al., 2000; Thomas et al., 2000; Zhang et al., 2001).

The influence of anti-ML-IAP immunity on disease progression was delineated through immunohistochemical analysis of serial metastases obtained during treatment (Fig. 3). Whereas nearly all melanoma cells evidenced strong ML-IAP expression in association with dense T- and B-lymphocyte infiltrates early during vaccination, recurrent tumors gradually revealed the accumulation of antigen-loss variants. Indeed, a metastasis resected shortly before the patient's demise revealed no ML-IAP staining and the absence of immune infiltrates. Taken together, these findings suggest that the vaccine-induced response exerted selective pressure on the melanoma cells, resulting in the emergence of antigen-loss escape variants. Subsequent investigations have confirmed the immunogenicity of ML-IAP in patients with melanoma, nonsmall cell lung carcinoma, gastrointestinal cancer, and breast carcinoma (Andersen et al., 2004a,b; Hariu et al., 2005; Yagihashi et al., 2003, 2005a,b).

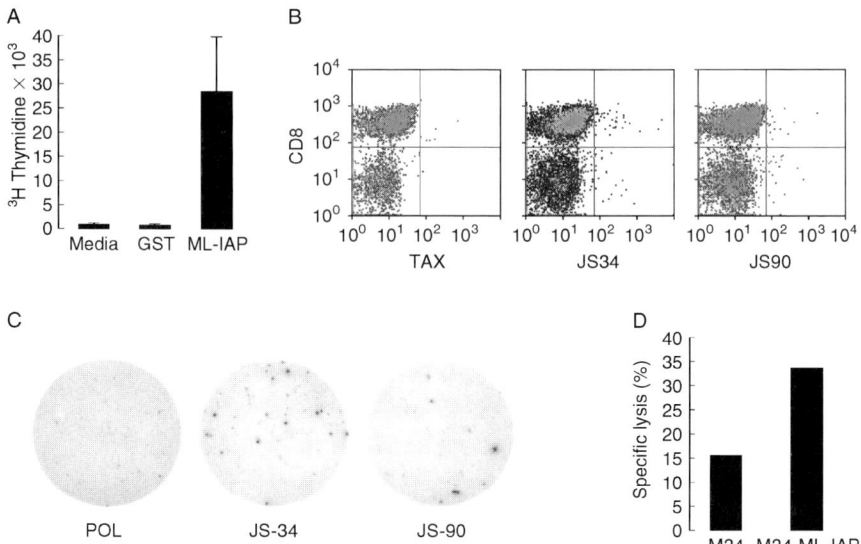

Figure 2 Tumor infiltrating lymphocytes manifest ML-IAP-specific reactivity. (A) Proliferative responses of CD4$^+$ T cells to bacterially produced recombinant ML-IAP or GST protein. (B) JS34- and JS90-tetramer-stained CD8$^+$ T cells. (C) JS34 and JS90 peptides stimulate CD8$^+$ T cell interferon-gamma production in an ELISPOT. (D) ML-IAP-specific cytotoxicity against autologous tumor cells engineered to express high levels of ML-IAP. Reprinted from Schmollinger et al. (2003). (**See Plate 12 in color insert at the end of the book.**)

Tumor escape through antigenic modulation highlights a defect in the breadth of the host response. A better understanding of the pathways that compensate for ML-IAP loss might suggest additional targets for therapy (Liston et al., 2003). In this context, antibody and T-cell responses to survivin, another IAP family member, were previously observed in some cancer patients (Andersen et al., 2001a,b; Hirohashi et al., 2002; Rohayem et al., 2000). While the vaccinated subject described here similarly mounted humoral reactions to survivin, resistant metastases devoid of this gene product eventually arose. The screening of cDNA expression libraries, derived from these resistant clones, with sera from other long-term responding patients might yield other antigens that complement the immunogenicity of inhibitor of apoptosis proteins (Schmollinger and Dranoff, 2004).

6. Cytotoxic T Lymphocyte Antigen-4 Antibody Blockade

An increasing number of immunotherapies have been reported to promote the emergence of antigen-loss escape variants (Dudley et al., 2005; Jäger et al.,

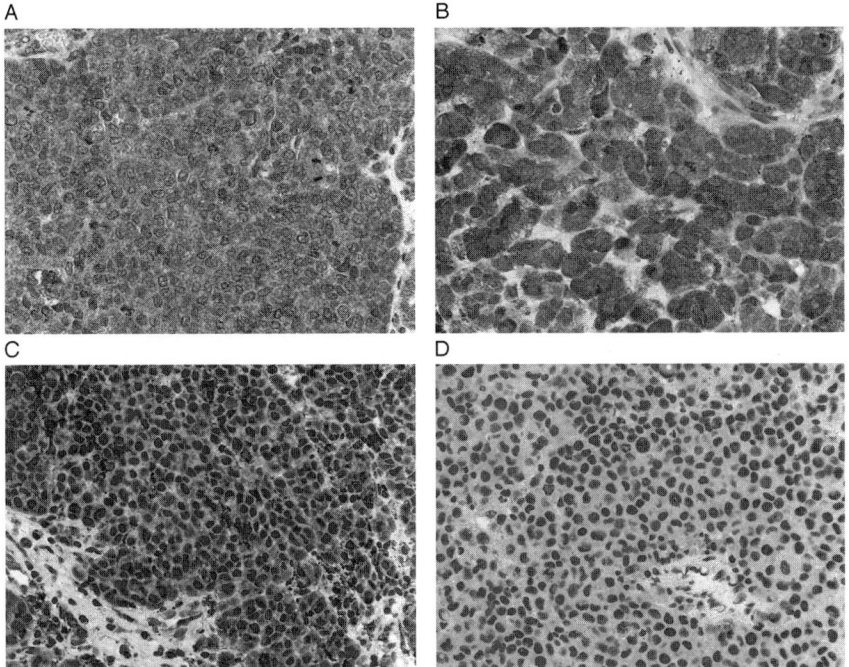

Figure 3 Vaccination promotes the emergence of antigen-loss escape variants. Tumor cells early during vaccination show strong ML-IAP expression (A, B). The evolution of ML-IAP negative tumor cells after prolonged immunization (C, D). Reprinted from Schmollinger et al. (2003). (**See Plate 13 in color insert at the end of the book.**)

1997; Khong et al., 2004; Riker et al., 1999; Yee et al., 2002). Although these results illustrate the ability of therapeutically induced immune responses to accomplish substantial tumor destruction, they also underscore the requirement for generating multivalent reactions. One mechanism that might limit the diversification of antitumor immunity involves regulatory circuits that normally function to maintain tolerance to self-antigens (Chambers et al., 2001). These pathways may increase the activation threshold for mounting responses toward less immunogenic tumor cell targets, particularly those that may also be expressed in some healthy tissues.

Cytotoxic T lymphocyte associated antigen-4 (CTLA-4) occupies a central position in this negative immune regulation (Thompson and Allison, 1997). Whereas CD28 engagement by B7-1 or B7-2 provides an important costimulatory signal for effector T cells, the subsequent triggering of CTLA-4 by these same ligands decreases cytokine production and restrains cellular proliferation

(Doyle et al., 2001; Salomon and Bluestone, 2001). Moreover, regulatory T cells, a distinct lineage that constrains potentially autoreactive T cells in the periphery, constitutively express CTLA-4 (Hori et al., 2003). The development of lethal autoimmune disease with multiorgan lymphocyte infiltrates in CTLA-4- and regulatory T-cell-deficient mice indicate that intact negative regulation is necessary for immune homeostasis (Fontenot and Rudensky, 2005; Tivol et al., 1995; Waterhouse et al., 1995).

In contrast to the severe consequences of abrogating regulation, the controlled attenuation of these pathways might enhance antitumor immunity with acceptable toxicities. Indeed, Allison and colleagues showed that the transient inhibition of CTLA-4 function with blocking antibodies increased the potency of tumor immunity (Leach et al., 1996). The administration of anti-CTLA-4 antibodies either as monotherapy or in conjunction with chemotherapy provoked tumor regression in a variety of immunogenic models (Kwon et al., 1997; Mokyr et al., 1998; Yang et al., 1997). Whereas the impact of CTLA-4 antibody blockade was less significant against poorly immunogenic tumors, combination therapy with vaccination evoked synergistic anticancer effects. Concurrent treatment with CTLA-4 blocking antibodies and GM-CSF secreting tumor cells proved highly efficacious against transplantable B16 melanomas and SM1 breast carcinomas or SV40 T antigen-induced prostate carcinomas in TRAMP mice (Hurwitz et al., 1998, 2000; van Elsas et al., 1999). Therapeutic immunity was mediated primarily through $CD8^+$ cytotoxic T cells, but could be associated with a partial loss of tolerance to normal tissues, including melanocytes and prostate epithelium (van Elsas et al., 2001).

Based on these provocative findings, we undertook a phase I clinical trial to obtain an initial assessment of the biologic activity of antagonizing CTLA-4 function in humans (Hodi et al., 2003). In light of the potential for autoreactivity with concurrent antibody/vaccine therapy in preclinical studies, a single infusion of the humanized CTLA-4 blocking monoclonal antibody MDX-CTLA-4 (3 mg/kg) was administered to nine previously immunized metastatic melanoma or ovarian carcinoma patients. To gain insights into whether specific characteristics of preexisting immunity might influence the response to subsequent CTLA-4 antibody blockade, we enrolled subjects that had earlier received vaccines composed of either GM-CSF secreting tumor cells or dendritic cells loaded with defined melanosomal antigens.

Infusion of MDX-CTLA-4 partially compromised tolerance to self, irrespective of prior therapy, as manifested by low titers of autoantibodies (antinuclear, antithyroglobulin, and rheumatoid factors) in four patients. All seven metastatic melanoma subjects developed erythematous cutaneous eruptions on the trunk and extremities; skin biopsies in five cases disclosed $CD4^+$ and $CD8^+$ T-cell infiltrates juxtaposed against normal melanocytes (Fig. 4). Despite this

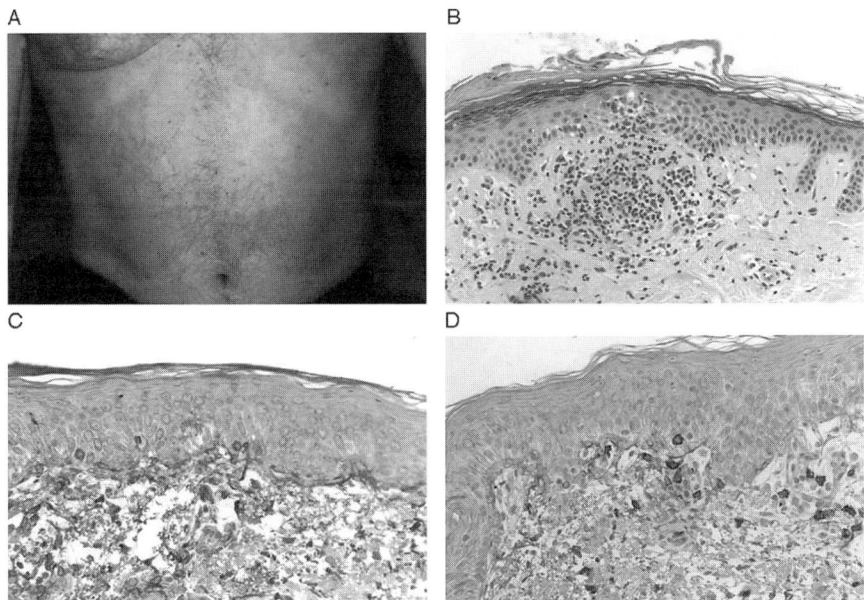

Figure 4 CTLA-4 antibody blockade partially compromises tolerance. (A) Erythematous cutaneous eruption. (B) Lymphocyte infiltrate extending into epidermis. (C) $CD4^+$ T cells apposed to dying melanocytes. (D) $CD8^+$ T cells apposed to dying melanocytes. Reprinted from Hodi *et al.* (2003). (**See Plate 14 in color insert at the end of the book.**)

autoreactivity, vitiligo was not observed, likely reflecting an incomplete destruction of melanocytes. While two ovarian carcinoma patients also developed rashes, these reflected T-cell reactions localized to superficial blood vessels in the dermis, without evidence for melanocyte targeting. Together, these findings suggest that CTLA-4 antibody blockade can overcome negative immune regulation involving some differentiation antigens that are expressed by tumor cells and normal tissues.

In addition to this autoreactivity, MDX-CTLA-4 infusion stimulated extensive tumor destruction in 3 of 3 metastatic melanoma patients and a reduction or stabilization of CA-125 levels in 2 of 2 metastatic ovarian carcinoma patients previously vaccinated with irradiated, autologous GM-CSF secreting tumor cells. In contrast, 4 of 4 metastatic melanoma patients previously immunized with defined melanosomal antigens failed to display tumor necrosis following CTLA-4 blockade. These preliminary findings raise the possibility that some vaccine-induced reactions might prove more sensitive to combination treatment with anti-CTLA-4 antibodies. Identifying those parameters most predictive of therapeutic activity is a key goal of ongoing investigation.

Pathologic examination of the necrotic lesions in responding patients revealed abundant $CD4^+$ and $CD8^+$ T cells, $CD20^+$ B cells producing immunoglobulin, and granulocytes (Fig. 5). A dense, circumferential lymphoid infiltrate was also found in disrupted tumor blood vessels, which resulted in zonal, ischemic necrosis. These histologic features imply the evolution of a coordinated innate and adaptive antitumor reaction. As similar infiltrates were engendered with GM-CSF secreting tumor vaccines, these results raise the possibility that MDX-CTLA-4 may amplify a long-lasting memory response in humans.

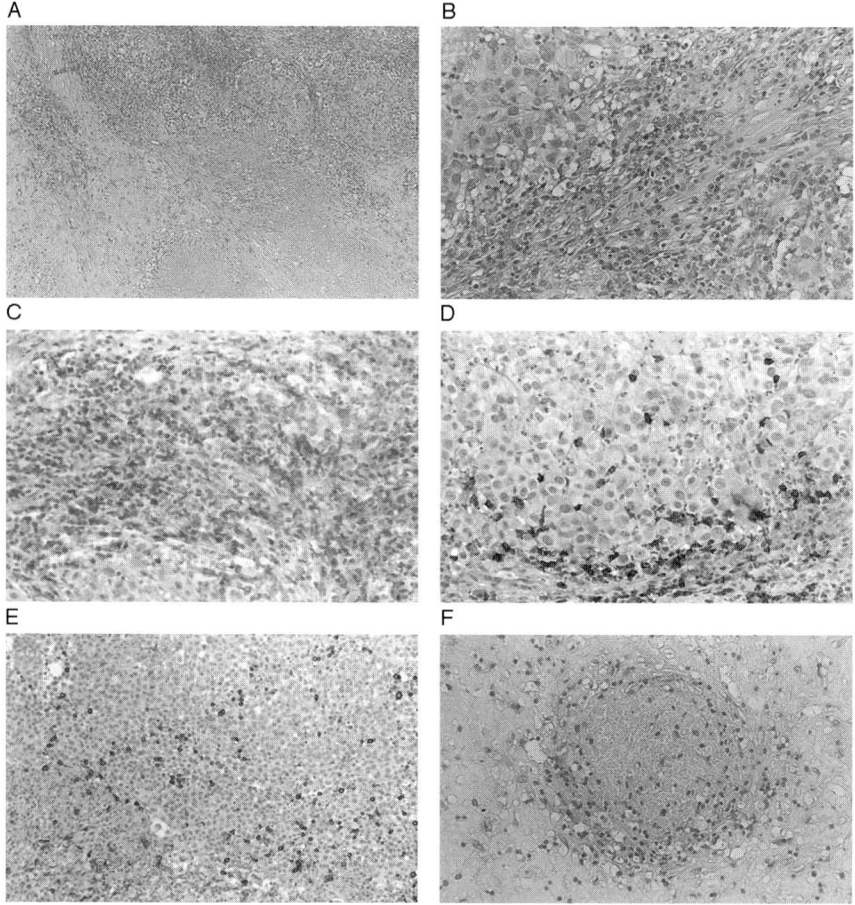

Figure 5 CTLA-4 antibody blockade stimulates extensive tumor necrosis. (A, B) Granulocyte and lymphocyte mediated tumor destruction of a mediastinal metastasis. (C) $CD4^+$ T cells. (D) $CD8^+$ T cells. (E) $CD20^+$ B cells. (F) Vasculopathy. Reprinted from Hodi et al. (2003). (**See Plate 15 in color insert at the end of the book.**)

Other early-stage clinical studies evaluated serial infusions of MDX-CTLA-4 administered concurrently with melanosomal antigen-derived peptide vaccines. Rosenberg and colleagues observed three tumor responses in a cohort of 14 metastatic melanoma patients, although 6 subjects (including those showing tumor destruction) developed serious autoimmune disorders (Phan et al., 2003). In addition to frank vitiligo, these severe toxicities included enterocolitis, hepatitis, dermatitis, pneumonitis, and hypophysitis. Interestingly, these pathologies are also found in patients harboring defects in regulatory T cells as a consequence of inherited mutations in the Foxp3 master transcription factor (Ochs et al., 2005).

Weber and associates administered repetitive doses of MDX-CTLA-4 and melanosomal-derived peptides to 19 patients with surgically resected stage III and IV metastatic melanoma (Sanderson et al., 2005). Eight patients developed dose-dependent serious autoimmune toxicities, including uveitis, enterocolitis, and vitiligo. A polymorphism in CTLA-4, which was previously linked to reduced T-cell surface expression and an increased risk of autoimmune diabetes (Ueda et al., 2003), may have been associated with a higher incidence of severe toxicity in this cohort. The risk of relapse also appeared to be reduced in patients who manifested autoimmune complications following MDX-CTLA-4.

Together, these three pilot trials illuminate the ability of CTLA-4 antibody blockade to elicit both substantial tumor destruction and serious autoimmunity. A major challenge for further study is to determine if these clinical outcomes can be consistently dissociated. Critical to this issue is whether the threshold for overcoming negative regulation of antitumor responses might be lower than that for unleashing autoreactive cells. In this context, the frequency, affinity, and functional status of tumor-specific effector cells that are present at the time of CTLA-4 blockade are all likely to be decisive. Further, targeting the immune reaction to antigens with selective, or at least increased, expression in cancer cells is likely to be advantageous.

As anti-CTLA-4 antibodies appear to amplify memory responses, it should be possible to activate preferentially preexisting antitumor effector cells, while minimizing the likelihood of breaching steady-state tolerance mechanisms. Toward this end, prior vaccination and/or an unusually strong endogenous host reaction might permit therapeutic activity without substantive toxicity. Indeed, our ongoing trials of CTLA-4 antibody blockade in patients previously immunized with autologous, GM-CSF secreting tumor cells continue to demonstrate the induction of tumor destruction with a low risk of serious autoimmunity (Hodi et al., in preparation). In many ways, this therapeutic challenge may be analogous to allogeneic bone marrow transplantation, where a therapeutic index between graft-versus-tumor effects and graft-versus-host disease does exist, albeit a narrow one (Antin, 1993). More detailed studies exploring the optimal dose, schedule, and integration of CTLA-4 antibody blockade with other treatments should clarify the extent to which tumor immunity and autoimmunity can be separated in the autologous setting.

7. Combination Immunotherapy: The Next Paradigm?

A deeper understanding of the mechanisms underlying the generation of tumor immunity has provided a framework for developing more potent immunotherapies. A major insight is that combinatorial approaches that address the multiplicity of defects in the host response are likely to be required for clinical efficacy. Treatment schemes that enhance tumor antigen presentation, inhibit negative immune regulation, and amplify T-cell effector functions should yield synergistic anticancer effects. The studies of dendritic cell-based vaccination and CTLA-4 blockade highlighted here are likely to be extended in the near future to include other manipulations that target negative regulation, including antibodies to PD-L1 (Iwai *et al.*, 2002), GITR (Watts, 2005), ICOS (Herman *et al.*, 2004), and CD25 (Shimizu *et al.*, 1999), and agents that override myeloid suppressor cells (Kusmartsev *et al.*, 2003). Moreover, NKT cell agonists, such as α-galactosylceramide (Chang *et al.*, 2005), activating antibodies to costimulatory molecules including 4-1BB (Kwon *et al.*, 2002), CD40 (Schultze *et al.*, 2004), CD28 (Vonderheide and June, 2003), and OX40 (Dannull *et al.*, 2005) and cytokines that enhance cytotoxic T-cell function, such as IL-15 (Klebanoff *et al.*, 2004) and IL-21 (Zeng *et al.*, 2005), represent exciting new opportunities to potentiate vaccine-induced effector responses. Whereas deciphering the optimal sequence and mixtures of these strategies poses an intriguing clinical challenge, the comprehensive evaluation of innate and adaptive tumor immunity coupled with the genetic profiling of cancer cells should help actualize the rich potential of active immunotherapy.

References

Albert, M., Pearce, S., Francisco, L., Sauter, B., Roy, P., Silverstein, R., and Bhardwaj, N. (1998). Immature dendritic cells phagocytose apoptotic cells via $\alpha_v\beta_5$ and CD36, and cross-present antigens to cytotoxic T lymphocytes. *J. Exp. Med.* **188,** 1359–1368.

Andersen, M. H., Becker, J. C., and Straten, P. (2004a). Identification of an HLA-A3-restricted cytotoxic T lymphocyte (CTL) epitope from ML-IAP. *J. Invest. Dermatol.* **122,** 1336–1337.

Andersen, M. H., Pedersen, L. O., Becker, J. C., and Straten, P. T. (2001a). Identification of a cytotoxic T lymphocyte response to the apoptosis inhibitor protein survivin in cancer patients. *Cancer Res.* **61,** 869–872.

Andersen, M. H., Pedersen, L. O., Capeller, B., Brocker, E. B., Becker, J. C., and thor Straten, P. (2001b). Spontaneous cytotoxic T-cell responses against survivin-derived MHC class I-restricted T-cell epitopes *in situ* as well as *ex vivo* in cancer patients. *Cancer Res.* **61,** 5964–5968.

Andersen, M. H., Reker, S., Becker, J. C., and thor Straten, P. (2004b). The melanoma inhibitor of apoptosis protein: A target for spontaneous cytotoxic T cell responses. *J. Invest. Dermatol.* **122,** 392–399.

Andrade, F., Roy, S., Nicholson, D., Thornberry, N., Rosen, A., and Casciola-Rosen, L. (1998). Granzyme B directly and efficiently cleaves several downstream caspase substrates: Implications for CTL-induced apoptosis. *Immunity* **8,** 451–460.

Antin, J. H. (1993). Graft-versus-leukemia: No longer an epiphenomenon. *Blood* **82,** 2273–2277.

Ashhab, Y., Alian, A., Polliack, A., Panet, A., and Yehuda, D. B. (2001). Two splicing variants of a new inhibitor of apoptosis gene with different biological properties and tissue distribution pattern. *FEBS Lett.* **495,** 56–60.

Assikis, V. J., and Simons, J. W. (2004). Novel therapeutic strategies for androgen-independent prostate cancer: An update. *Semin. Oncol.* **31,** 26–32.

Barks, J. H., Thompson, F. H., Taetle, R., Yang, J. M., Stone, J. F., Wymer, J. A., Khavari, R., Guan, X. Y., Trent, J. M., Pinkel, D., and Nelson, M. A. (1997). Increased chromosome 20 copy number detected by fluorescence *in situ* hybridization (FISH) in malignant melanoma. *Genes Chromosomes Cancer* **19,** 278–285.

Bell, D., Chomarat, P., Broyles, D., Netto, G., Harb, G., Lebecque, S., Valladeau, J., Davoust, J., Palucka, K., and Banchereau, J. (1999). In breast carcinoma tissue, immature dendritic cells reside within the tumor, whereas mature dendritic cells are located in peritumoral areas. *J. Exp. Med.* **190,** 1417–1425.

Bendandi, M., Gocke, C., Kobrin, C., Benko, F., Sternas, L., Pennington, R., Watson, T., Reynolds, C., Gause, B., Duffey, P., Jaffe, E., Creekmore, S., *et al.* (1999). Complete molecular remissions induced by patient-specific vaccination plus granulocyte-monocyte colony-stimulating factor against lymphoma. *Nature Med.* **5,** 1171–1177.

Berkner, K. L. (1988). Development of adenovirus vectors for the expression of heterologous genes. *Biotechniques* **6,** 616–629.

Boon, T., and van der Bruggen, P. (1996). Human tumor antigens recognized by T lymphocytes. *J. Exp. Med.* **183,** 725–729.

Borrello, I., Sotomayor, E., Cooke, S., and Levitsky, H. (1999). A universal granulocyte-macrophage colony-stimulating factor-producing bystander cell line for use in the formulation of autologous tumor cell-based vaccines. *Hum. Gene Ther.* **10,** 1983–1991.

Cerundolo, V., Hermans, I. F., and Salio, M. (2004). Dendritic cells: A journey from laboratory to clinic. *Nat. Immunol.* **5,** 7–10.

Chambers, C. A., Kuhns, M. S., Egen, J. G., and Allison, J. P. (2001). CTLA-4-mediated inhibition in regulation of T cell responses: Mechanisms and manipulation in tumor immunotherapy. *Annu. Rev. Immunol.* **19,** 565–594.

Chang, D. H., Osman, K., Connolly, J., Kukreja, A., Krasovsky, J., Pack, M., Hutchinson, A., Geller, M., Liu, N., Annable, R., Shay, J., Kirchhoff, K., *et al.* (2005). Sustained expansion of NKT cells and antigen-specific T cells after injection of alpha-galactosyl-ceramide loaded mature dendritic cells in cancer patients. *J. Exp. Med.* **201,** 1503–1517.

Chen, J. L., Stewart-Jones, G., Bossi, G., Lissin, N. M., Wooldridge, L., Choi, E. M., Held, G., Dunbar, P. R., Esnouf, R. M., Sami, M., Boulter, J. M., Rizkallah, P., *et al.* (2005). Structural and kinetic basis for heightened immunogenicity of T cell vaccines. *J. Exp. Med.* **201,** 1243–1255.

Chen, Y.-T., Gure, A., Tsang, S., Stockert, E., Jager, E., Knuth, A., and Old, L. (1998). Identification of multiple cancer/testis antigens by allogeneic antibody screening of a melanoma cell line library. *Proc. Natl. Acad. Sci. USA* **95,** 6919–6923.

Clark, W., Elder, D., Guerry, D., Braitman, L., Trock, B., Schultz, D., Synnestvedt, M., and Halpern, A. (1989). Model predicting survival in stage I melanoma based on tumor progression. *J. Natl. Cancer Inst.* **81,** 1893–1904.

Cox, A., Skipper, J., Chen, Y., Henderson, R., Darrow, T., Shabanowitz, J., Englehard, V., Hunt, D., and Slinghuff, C. (1994). Identification of a peptide recognized by five melanoma-specific human cytotoxic T cell lines. *Science* **264**, 716–719.

Crnkovic-Mertens, I., Hoppe-Seyler, F., and Butz, K. (2003). Induction of apoptosis in tumor cells by siRNA-mediated silencing of the livin/ML-IAP/KIAP gene. *Oncogene* **22**, 8330–8336.

Dannull, J., Nair, S., Su, Z., Boczkowski, D., DeBeck, C., Yang, B., Gilboa, E., and Vieweg, J. (2005). Enhancing the immunostimulatory function of dendritic cells by transfection with mRNA encoding OX40 ligand. *Blood* **105**, 3206–3213.

Dave, S. S., Wright, G., Tan, B., Rosenwald, A., Gascoyne, R. D., Chan, W. C., Fisher, R. I., Braziel, R. M., Rimsza, L. M., Grogan, T. M., Miller, T. P., LeBlanc, M., *et al.* (2004). Prediction of survival in follicular lymphoma based on molecular features of tumor-infiltrating immune cells. *N. Engl. J. Med.* **351**, 2159–2169.

Davis, I. D., Chen, W., Jackson, H., Parente, P., Shackleton, M., Hopkins, W., Chen, Q., Dimopoulos, N., Luke, T., Murphy, R., Scott, A. M., Maraskovsky, E., *et al.* (2004). Recombinant NY-ESO-1 protein with ISCOMATRIX adjuvant induces broad integrated antibody and CD4 (+) and CD8(+) T cell responses in humans. *Proc. Natl. Acad. Sci. USA* **101**, 10697–10702.

Diefenbach, A., and Raulet, D. (2002). The innate immune response to tumors and its role in the induction of T-cell immunity. *Immunol. Rev.* **188**, 9–21.

Doyle, A. M., Mullen, A. C., Villarino, A. V., Hutchins, A. S., High, F. A., Lee, H. W., Thompson, C. B., and Reiner, S. L. (2001). Induction of cytotoxic T lymphocyte antigen 4 (CTLA-4) restricts clonal expansion of helper T cells. *J. Exp. Med.* **194**, 893–902.

Dranoff, G. (2002). GM-CSF-based cancer vaccines. *Immunol. Rev.* **188**, 147–154.

Dranoff, G. (2004). Cytokines in cancer pathogenesis and cancer therapy. *Nat. Rev. Cancer* **4**, 11–22.

Dranoff, G., Jaffee, E., Lazenby, A., Golumbek, P., Levitsky, H., Brose, K., Jackson, V., Hamada, H., Pardoll, D., and Mulligan, R. C. (1993). Vaccination with irradiated tumor cells engineered to secrete murine granulocyte-macrophage colony-stimulating factor stimulates potent, specific, and long-lasting anti-tumor immunity. *Proc. Natl. Acad. Sci. USA* **90**, 3539–3543.

Dropcho, E., Chen, Y.-T., Posner, J., and Old, L. (1987). Cloning of a brain protein identified by autoantibodies from a patient with paraneoplastic cerebellar degeneration. *Proc. Natl. Acad. Sci. USA* **84**, 4552–4556.

Dudley, M. E., Wunderlich, J. R., Yang, J. C., Sherry, R. M., Topalian, S. L., Restifo, N. P., Royal, R. E., Kammula, U., White, D. E., Mavroukakis, S. A., Rogers, L. J., Gracia, G. J., *et al.* (2005). Adoptive cell transfer therapy following non-myeloablative but lymphodepleting chemotherapy for the treatment of patients with refractory metastatic melanoma. *J. Clin. Oncol.* **23**, 2346–2357.

Dunn, G. P., Old, L. J., and Schreiber, R. D. (2004). The immunobiology of cancer immunosurveillance and immunoediting. *Immunity* **21**, 137–148.

Engelhard, V. H., Bullock, T. N., Colella, T. A., Sheasley, S. L., and Mullins, D. W. (2002). Antigens derived from melanocyte differentiation proteins: Self-tolerance, autoimmunity, and use for cancer immunotherapy. *Immunol. Rev.* **188**, 136–146.

Fehr, T., Skrastina, D., Pumpens, P., and Zinkernagel, R. M. (1998). T cell-independent type I antibody response against B cell epitopes expressed repetitively on recombinant virus particles. *Proc. Natl. Acad. Sci. USA* **95**, 9477–9481.

Finn, O. J. (2003). Cancer vaccines: Between the idea and the reality. *Nat. Rev. Immunol.* **3**, 630–641.

Fong, L., Hou, Y., Rivas, A., Benike, C., Yuen, A., Fisher, G. A., Davis, M. M., and Engleman, E. G. (2001). Altered peptide ligand vaccination with Flt3 ligand expanded dendritic cells for tumor immunotherapy. *Proc. Natl. Acad. Sci. USA* **98**, 8809–8814.

Fontenot, J. D., and Rudensky, A. Y. (2005). A well adapted regulatory contrivance: Regulatory T cell development and the forkhead family transcription factor Foxp3. *Nat. Immunol.* **6**, 331–337.

Forni, G., Fujiwara, H., Martino, F., Hamaoka, T., Jemma, C., Caretto, P., and Giovarelli, M. (1988). Helper strategy in tumor immunology: Expansion of helper lymphocytes and utilization of helper lymphokines for experimental and clinical immunotherapy. *Cancer Metast. Rev.* **7**, 289–309.

Gabrilovich, D. (2004). Mechanisms and functional significance of tumour-induced dendritic-cell defects. *Nat. Rev. Immunol.* **4**, 941–952.

Gendler, S. J., Lancaster, C. A., Taylor-Papadimitriou, J., Duhig, T., Peat, N., Burchell, J., Pemberton, L., Lalani, E. N., and Wilson, D. (1990). Molecular cloning and expression of human tumor-associated polymorphic epithelial mucin. *J. Biol. Chem.* **265**, 15286–15293.

Germeau, C., Ma, W., Schiavetti, F., Lurquin, C., Henry, E., Vigneron, N., Brasseur, F., Lethe, B., De Plaen, E., Velu, T., Boon, T., and Coulie, P. G. (2005). High frequency of antitumor T cells in the blood of melanoma patients before and after vaccination with tumor antigens. *J. Exp. Med.* **201**, 241–248.

Getlawi, F., Laslop, A., Schagger, H., Ludwig, J., Haywood, J., and Apps, D. (1996). Chromaffin granule membrane glycoprotein IV is identical with Ac45, a membrane-integral subunit of the granule's H(+)-ATPase. *Neurosci. Lett.* **219**, 13–16.

Gilboa, E. (1999). The makings of a tumor rejection antigen. *Immunity* **11**, 263–270.

Gilboa, E. (2004). The promise of cancer vaccines. *Nat. Rev. Cancer* **4**, 401–411.

Gillessen, S., Naumov, Y. N., Nieuwenhuis, E. E., Exley, M. A., Lee, F. S., Mach, N., Luster, A. D., Blumberg, R. S., Taniguchi, M., Balk, S. P., Strominger, J. L., Dranoff, G., *et al.* (2003). CD1d-restricted T cells regulate dendritic cell function and antitumor immunity in a granulocyte-macrophage colony-stimulating factor-dependent fashion. *Proc. Natl. Acad. Sci. USA* **100**, 8874–8879.

Greenwald, R. J., Freeman, G. J., and Sharpe, A. H. (2005). The B7 family revisited. *Annu. Rev. Immunol.* **23**, 515–548.

Haanen, J. B., Baars, A., Gomez, R., Weder, P., Smits, M., de Gruijl, T. D., von Blomberg, B. M., Bloemena, E., Scheper, R. J., van Ham, S. M., Pinedo, H. M., and van den Eertwegh, A. J. (2005). Melanoma-specific tumor-infiltrating lymphocytes but not circulating melanoma-specific T cells may predict survival in resected advanced-stage melanoma patients. *Cancer Immunol. Immunother.* 1–8.

Hariu, H., Hirohashi, Y., Torigoe, T., Asanuma, H., Hariu, M., Tamura, Y., Aketa, K., Nabeta, C., Nakanishi, K., Kamiguchi, K., Mano, Y., Kitamura, H., *et al.* (2005). Aberrant expression and potency as a cancer immunotherapy target of inhibitor of apoptosis protein family, Livin/ML-IAP in lung cancer. *Clin. Cancer Res.* **11**, 1000–1009.

Heibein, J. A., Goping, I. S., Barry, M., Pinkoski, M. J., Shore, G. C., Green, D. R., and Bleackley, R. C. (2000). Granzyme B-mediated cytochrome c release is regulated by the Bcl-2 family members bid and Bax. *J. Exp. Med.* **192**, 1391–1402.

Herman, A. E., Freeman, G. J., Mathis, D., and Benoist, C. (2004). CD4+CD25+ T regulatory cells dependent on ICOS promote regulation of effector cells in the prediabetic lesion. *J. Exp. Med.* **199**, 1479–1489.

Hirohashi, Y., Torigoe, T., Maeda, A., Nabeta, Y., Kamiguchi, K., Sato, T., Yoda, J., Ikeda, H., Hirata, K., Yamanaka, N., and Sato, N. (2002). An HLA-A24-restricted cytotoxic T lymphocyte epitope of a tumor-associated protein, survivin. *Clin. Cancer Res.* **8**, 1731–1739.

Hodi, F. S., Mihm, M. C., Soiffer, R. J., Haluska, F. G., Butler, M., Seiden, M. V., Davis, T., Henry-Spires, R., MacRae, S., Willman, A., Padera, R., Jaklitsch, M. T., *et al.* (2003). Biologic activity of cytotoxic T lymphocyte-associated antigen 4 antibody blockade in previously vaccinated metastatic melanoma and ovarian carcinoma patients. *Proc. Natl. Acad. Sci. USA* **100**, 4712–4717.

Hodi, F. S., Schmollinger, J. C., Soiffer, R. J., Salgia, R., Lynch, T., Ritz, J., Alyea, E. P., Yang, J. C., Neuberg, D., Mihm, M., and Dranoff, G. (2002). ATP6S1 elicits potent humoral responses associated with immune mediated tumor destruction. *Proc. Natl. Acad. Sci. USA* **99**, 6919–6924.

Holthuis, J. C., Jansen, E. J., Schoonderwoert, V. T., Burbach, J. P., and Martens, G. J. (1999). Biosynthesis of the vacuolar H+-ATPase accessory subunit Ac45 in Xenopus pituitary. *Eur. J. Biochem.* **262**, 484–491.

Holthuis, J. C., Jansen, E. J., van Riel, M. C., and Martens, G. J. (1995). Molecular probing of the secretory pathway in peptide hormone-producing cells. *J. Cell Sci.* **108**, 3295–3305.

Hori, S., Takahashi, T., and Sakaguchi, S. (2003). Control of autoimmunity by naturally arising regulatory CD4+ T cells. *Adv. Immunol.* **81**, 331–371.

Huang, A. Y., Golumbek, P., Ahmadzadeh, M., Jaffee, E., Pardoll, D., and Levitsky, H. (1994). Role of bone marrow-derived cells in presenting MHC class I-restricted tumor antigens. *Science* **264**, 961–965.

Hung, K., Hayashi, R., Lafond-Walker, A., Lowenstein, C., Pardoll, H., and Levitsky, H. (1998). The central role of CD4$^+$ T cells in the antitumor immune response. *J. Exp. Med.* **188**, 2357–2368.

Hurwitz, A., Yu, T., Leach, D., and Allison, J. (1998). CTLA-4 blockade synergizes with tumor-derived granulocyte-macrophage colony-stimulating factor for treatment of an experimental mammary carcinoma. *Proc. Natl. Acad. Sci. USA* **95**, 10067–10071.

Hurwitz, A. A., Foster, B. A., Kwon, E. D., Truong, T., Choi, E. M., Greenberg, N. M., Burg, M. B., and Allison, J. P. (2000). Combination immunotherapy of primary prostate cancer in a transgenic mouse model using CTLA-4 blockade. *Cancer Res.* **60**, 2444–2448.

Iwai, Y., Ishida, M., Tanaka, Y., Okazaki, T., Honjo, T., and Minato, N. (2002). Involvement of PD-L1 on tumor cells in the escape from host immune system and tumor immunotherapy by PD-L1 blockade. *Proc. Natl. Acad. Sci. USA* **99**, 12293–12297.

Jaffee, E., Hruban, R., Biedrzycki, B., Laheru, D., Schepers, K., Sauter, P., Goemann, M., Coleman, J., Grochow, L., Donehower, R., Lillemoe, K., O'Reilly, S., *et al.* (2001). Novel allogeneic granulocyte-macrophage colony-stimulating factor-secreting tumor vaccine for pancreatic cancer: A phase I trial of safety and immune activation. *J. Clin. Oncol.* **19**, 145–156.

Jäger, E., Ringhoffer, M., Altmannsberger, M., Arand, M., Karbach, J., Jäger, D., Oesch, F., and Knuth, A. (1997). Immuno-selection *in vivo*: Independent loss of MHC class I and melanocyte differentiation antigen expression in metastatic melanoma. **71**, 142–147.

Jansen, E. J., Holthuis, J. C., McGrouther, C., Burbach, J. P., and Martens, G. J. (1998). Intracellular trafficking of the vacuolar H+-ATPase accessory subunit Ac45. *J. Cell Sci.* **111**, 2999–3006.

Kasof, G. M., and Gomes, B. C. (2000). Livin, a novel inhibitor-of-apoptosis (IAP) family member. *J. Biol. Chem.* **276**, 3238–3246.

Khong, H. T., Wang, Q. J., and Rosenberg, S. A. (2004). Identification of multiple antigens recognized by tumor-infiltrating lymphocytes from a single patient: Tumor escape by antigen loss and loss of MHC expression. *J. Immunother.* **27**, 184–190.

Klebanoff, C. A., Finkelstein, S. E., Surman, D. R., Lichtman, M. K., Gattinoni, L., Theoret, M. R., Grewal, N., Spiess, P. J., Antony, P. A., Palmer, D. C., Tagaya, Y., Rosenberg, S. A., *et al.* (2004). IL-15 enhances the *in vivo* antitumor activity of tumor-reactive CD8+ T cells. *Proc. Natl. Acad. Sci. USA* **101**, 1969–1974.

Korn, W. M., Yasutake, T., Kuo, W. L., Warren, R. S., Collins, C., Tomita, M., Gray, J., and Waldman, F. M. (1999). Chromosome arm 20q gains and other genomic alterations in colorectal cancer metastatic to liver, as analyzed by comparative genomic hybridization and fluorescence *in situ* hybridization. *Genes Chromosomes Cancer* **25**, 82–90.

Krieg, A. M. (2003). CpG motifs: The active ingredient in bacterial extracts? *Nat. Med.* **9**, 831–835.

Kusmartsev, S., Cheng, F., Yu, B., Nefedova, Y., Sotomayor, E., Lush, R., and Gabrilovich, D. (2003). All-trans-retinoic acid eliminates immature myeloid cells from tumor-bearing mice and improves the effect of vaccination. *Cancer Res.* **63**, 4441–4449.

Kwon, B., Lee, H. W., and Kwon, B. S. (2002). New insights into the role of 4-1BB in immune responses: Beyond CD8+ T cells. *Trends Immunol.* **23**, 378–380.

Kwon, E. D., Hurwitz, A. A., Foster, B. A., Madias, C., Feldhaus, A. L., Greenberg, N. M., Burg, M. B., and Allison, J. P. (1997). Manipulation of T cell costimulatory and inhibitory signals for immunotherapy of prostate cancer. *Proc. Natl. Acad. Sci. USA* **94**, 8099–8103.

Laheru, D., and Jaffee, E. M. (2005). Immunotherapy for pancreatic cancer – science driving clinical progress. *Nat. Rev. Cancer* **5**, 459–467.

Leach, D. R., Krummel, M. F., and Allison, J. P. (1996). Enhancement of antitumor immunity by CTLA-4 blockade. *Science* **271**, 1734–1736.

Lin, J.-H., Deng, G., Huang, Q., and Morser, J. (2000). KIAP, a novel member of the inhibitor of apoptosis protein family. *Biochem. Biophys. Res. Comm.* **279**, 820–831.

Liston, P., Fong, W. G., and Korneluk, R. G. (2003). The inhibitors of apoptosis: There is more to life than Bcl2. *Oncogene* **22**, 8568–8580.

Mach, N., and Dranoff, G. (2000). Cytokine-secreting tumor cell vaccines. *Curr. Opin. Immunol.* **12**, 571–575.

Mach, N., Gillessen, S., Wilson, S. B., Sheehan, C., Mihm, M., and Dranoff, G. (2000). Differences in dendritic cells stimulated *in vivo* by tumors engineered to secrete granulocyte-macrophage colony-stimulating factor or flt3-ligand. *Cancer Res.* **60**, 3239–3246.

Manis, J., Tian, M., and Alt, F. (2002). Mechanism and control of class-switch recombination. *Trends Immunol.* **23**, 31–39.

Mihm, M., Clemente, C., and Cascinelli, N. (1996). Tumor infiltrating lymphocytes in lymph node melanoma metastases—A histopathologic prognostic indicator and an expression of local immune response. *Lab. Invest.* **74**, 43–47.

Mokyr, M. B., Kalinichenko, T., Gorelik, L., and Bluestone, J. A. (1998). Realization of the therapeutic potential of CTLA-4 blockade in low-dose chemotherapy-treated tumor-bearing mice. *Cancer Res.* **58**, 5301–5304.

Mollick, J. A., Hodi, F. S., Soiffer, R. J., Nadler, L. M., and Dranoff, G. (2003). MUC1-like tandem repeat proteins are broadly immunogenic in cancer patients. *Cancer Immunity* **3**, 3–20.

Mulligan, R. C. (1993). The basic science of gene therapy. *Science* **260**, 926–932.

Munz, C., Steinman, R. M., and Fujii, S. (2005). Dendritic cell maturation by innate lymphocytes: Coordinated stimulation of innate and adaptive immunity. *J. Exp. Med.* **202**, 203–207.

Nachmias, B., Ashhab, Y., Bucholtz, V., Drize, O., Kadouri, L., Lotem, M., Peretz, T., Mandelboim, O., and Ben-Yehuda, D. (2003). Caspase-mediated cleavage converts Livin from an antiapoptotic to a proapoptotic factor: Implications for drug-resistant melanoma. *Cancer Res.* **63**, 6340–6349.

Naito, Y., Saito, K., Shiiba, K., Ohuchi, A., Saigenji, K., Nagura, H., and Ohtani, H. (1998). CD8+ T cells infiltrated within cancer cell nests as a prognostic factor in human colorectal cancer. *Cancer Res.* **58**, 3491–3494.

Nakano, O., Sato, M., Naito, Y., Suzuki, K., Orikasa, S., Aizawa, M., Suzuki, Y., Shintaku, I., Nagura, H., and Ohtani, H. (2001). Proliferative activity of intratumoral CD8(+) T-lymphocytes as a prognostic factor in human renal cell carcinoma: Clinicopathologic demonstration of antitumor immunity. *Cancer Res.* **61**, 5132–5136.

Nemunaitis, J., Sterman, D., Jablons, D., Smith, J. W., 2nd, Fox, B., Maples, P., Hamilton, S., Borellini, F., Lin, A., Morali, S., and Hege, K. (2004). Granulocyte-macrophage colony-stimulating factor gene-modified autologous tumor vaccines in non-small-cell lung cancer. *J. Natl. Cancer Inst.* **96**, 326–331.

Ochs, H. D., Ziegler, S. F., and Torgerson, T. R. (2005). FOXP3 acts as a rheostat of the immune response. *Immunol. Rev.* **203,** 156–164.

Old, L. (1981). Cancer immunology: The search for specificity-G.H.A. Clowes memorial lecture. *Cancer Res.* **41,** 361–375.

Old, L., and Chen, Y.-T. (1998). New paths in human cancer serology. *J. Exp. Med.* **187,** 1163–1167.

Paczesny, S., Ueno, H., Fay, J., Banchereau, J., and Palucka, A. K. (2003). Dendritic cells as vectors for immunotherapy of cancer. *Semin. Cancer Biol.* **13,** 439–447.

Palucka, A. K., Laupeze, B., Aspord, C., Saito, H., Jego, G., Fay, J., Paczesny, S., Pascual, V., and Banchereau, J. (2005). Immunotherapy via dendritic cells. *Adv. Exp. Med. Biol.* **560,** 105–114.

Pardoll, D. M. (2002). Spinning molecular immunology into successful immunotherapy. *Nat. Rev. Immunol.* **2,** 227–238.

Parker, K. C., Bednarek, M. A., and Coligan, J. E. (1994). Scheme for ranking potential HLA-A2 binding peptides based on independent binding of individual peptide side-chains. *J. Immunol.* **152,** 163–175.

Phan, G. Q., Yang, J. C., Sherry, R. M., Hwu, P., Topalian, S. L., Schwartzentruber, D. J., Restifo, N. P., Haworth, L. R., Seipp, C. A., Freezer, L. J., Morton, K. E., Mavroukakis, S. A., *et al.* (2003). Cancer regression and autoimmunity induced by cytotoxic T lymphocyte-associated antigen 4 blockade in patients with metastatic melanoma. *Proc. Natl. Acad. Sci. USA* **100,** 8372–8377.

Reilly, R., Machiels, J.-P., Emens, L., Ercolini, A., Okoye, F., Lei, R., Weintraub, D., and Jaffee, E. (2001). The collaboration of both humoral and cellular HER-2/neu-targeted immune responses is required for the complete eradication of HER-2/*neu*-expressing tumors. *Cancer Res.* **61,** 880–883.

Riker, A., Cormier, J., Panelli, M., Kammula, U., Wang, E., Abati, A., Fetsch, P., Lee, K. H., Steinberg, S., Rosenberg, S., and Marincola, F. (1999). Immune selection after antigen-specific immunotherapy of melanoma. *Surgery* **126,** 112–120.

Rimoldi, D., Rubio-Godoy, V., Dutoit, V., Lienard, D., Salvi, S., Guillaume, P., Speiser, D., Stockert, E., Spagnoli, G., Servis, C., Cerottini, J. C., Lejeune, F., *et al.* (2000). Efficient simultaneous presentation of NY-ESO-1/LAGE-1 primary and nonprimary open reading frame-derived CTL epitopes in melanoma. *J. Immunol.* **165,** 7253–7261.

Rohayem, J., Diestelkoetter, P., Weigle, B., Oehmichen, A., Schmitz, M., Melhorn, J., Conrad, K., and Rieber, E. (2000). Antibody response to the tumor-associated inhibitor of apoptosis protein survivin in cancer patients. *Cancer Res.* **60,** 1815–1817.

Ronsin, C., Chung-Scott, V., Poullion, I., Aknouche, N., Gaudin, C., and Triebel, F. (1999). A non-AUG-defined alternative open reading frame of the intestinal carboxyl esterase mRNA generates an epitope recognized by renal cell carcinoma-reactive tumor-infiltrating lymphocytes *in situ*. *J. Immunol.* **163,** 483–490.

Rosenberg, S. A. (2001). Progress in human tumour immunology and immunotherapy. *Nature* **411,** 380–384.

Sahin, U., Tureci, O., Schmitt, H., Cochlovius, B., Johannes, T., Schmits, R., Stenner, F., Luo, G. R., Schobert, I., and Pfreundschuh, M. (1995). Human neoplasms elicit multiple specific immune responses in the autologous host. *Proc. Natl. Acad. Sci. USA* **92,** 11810–11813.

Salgia, R., Lynch, T., Skarin, A., Lucca, J., Lynch, C., Jung, K., Hodi, F. S., Jaklitsch, M., Mentzer, S., Swanson, S., Lukanich, J., Bueno, R., *et al.* (2003). Vaccination with irradiated autologous tumor cells engineered to secrete granulocyte-macrophage colony-stimulating factor augments antitumor immunity in some patients with metastatic non-small-cell lung carcinoma. *J. Clin. Oncol.* **21,** 624–630.

Salomon, B., and Bluestone, J. A. (2001). Complexities of CD28/B7: CTLA-4 costimulatory pathways in autoimmunity and transplantation. *Annu. Rev. Immunol.* **19,** 225–252.

Sanderson, K., Scotland, R., Lee, P., Liu, D., Groshen, S., Snively, J., Sian, S., Nichol, G., Davis, T., Keler, T., Yellin, M., and Weber, J. (2005). Autoimmunity in a phase I trial of a fully human anticytotoxic T-lymphocyte antigen-4 monoclonal antibody with multiple melanoma peptides and Montanide ISA 51 for patients with resected stages III and IV melanoma. *J. Clin. Oncol.* **23,** 741–750.

Sanna, M. G., da Silva Correia, J., Ducrey, O., Lee, J., Nomoto, K., Schrantz, N., Deveraux, Q. L., and Ulevitch, R. J. (2002). IAP suppression of apoptosis involves distinct mechanisms: The TAK1/JNK1 signaling cascade and caspase inhibition. *Mol. Cell Biol.* **22,** 1754–1766.

Schmollinger, J. C., and Dranoff, G. (2004). Targeting melanoma inhibitor of apoptosis protein with cancer immunotherapy. *Apoptosis* **9,** 309–313.

Schmollinger, J. C., Vonderheide, R. H., Hoar, K. M., Maecker, B., Schultze, J. L., Hodi, F. S., Soiffer, R. J., Jung, K., Kuroda, M. J., Letvin, N. L., Greenfield, E. A., Mihm, M., *et al.* (2003). Melanoma inhibitor of apoptosis protein (ML-IAP) is a target for immune-mediated tumor destruction. *Proc. Natl. Acad. Sci. USA* **100,** 3398–3403.

Schoonderwoert, V. T., Holthuis, J. C., Tanaka, S., Tooze, S. A., and Martens, G. J. (2000). Inhibition of the vacuolar H+-ATPase perturbs the transport, sorting, processing and release of regulated secretory proteins. *Eur. J. Biochem.* **267,** 5646–5654.

Schultze, J. L., Grabbe, S., and von Bergwelt-Baildon, M. S. (2004). DCs and CD40-activated B cells: Current and future avenues to cellular cancer immunotherapy. *Trends Immunol.* **25,** 659–664.

Shenk, T. (1996). Adenoviridae: The viruses and their replication. *In* "Fields Virology" (B. N. Fields, D. M. Knipe, and P. M. Howley, Eds.), pp. 2111–2148. Lippincott-Raven Publishers, Philadelphia.

Shichijo, S., Nakao, M., Imai, Y., Takasu, H., Kawamoto, M., Niiya, F., Yang, D., Toh, Y., Yamana, H., and Itoh, K. (1998). A gene encoding antigenic peptides of human squamous cell carcinoma recognized by cytotoxic T lymphocytes. *J. Exp. Med.* **187,** 277–288.

Shimizu, J., Yamazaki, S., and Sakaguchi, S. (1999). Induction of tumor immunity by removing CD25+CD4+ T cells: A common basis between tumor immunity and autoimmunity. *J. Immunol.* **163,** 5211–5218.

Siddiqui, J., Abe, M., Hayes, D., Shani, E., Yunis, E., and Kufe, D. (1988). Isolation and sequencing of a cDNA coding for the human DF3 breast carcinoma-associated antigen. *Proc. Natl. Acad. Sci. USA* **85,** 2320–2325.

Simons, J., Mikhak, B., Chang, J.-F., DeMarzo, A., Carducci, M., Lim, M., Weber, C., Baccala, A., Goemann, M., Clift, S., Ando, D., Levitsky, H., *et al.* (1999). Induction of immunity to prostate cancer antigens: Results of a clinical trial of vaccination with irradiated autologous prostate tumor cells engineered to secrete granulocyte-macrophage colony-stimulating factor using *ex vivo* gene transfer. *Cancer Res.* **59,** 5160–5168.

Simons, J. W., Jaffee, E. M., Weber, C. E., Levitsky, H. I., Nelson, W. G., Carducci, M. A., Lazenby, A. J., Cohen, L. K., Finn, C. C., Clift, S. M., Hauda, K. M., Beck, L. A., *et al.* (1997). Bioactivity of autologous irradiated renal cell carcinoma vaccines generated by *ex vivo* granulocyte-macrophage colony-stimulating factor gene transfer. *Cancer Res.* **57,** 1537–1546.

Slingluff, C. L., Jr., Petroni, G. R., Yamshchikov, G. V., Barnd, D. L., Eastham, S., Galavotti, H., Patterson, J. W., Deacon, D. H., Hibbitts, S., Teates, D., Neese, P. Y., Grosh, W. W., *et al.* (2003). Clinical and immunologic results of a randomized phase II trial of vaccination using four melanoma peptides either administered in granulocyte-macrophage colony-stimulating factor in adjuvant or pulsed on dendritic cells. *J. Clin. Oncol.* **21,** 4016–4026.

Soiffer, R., Hodi, F. S., Haluska, F., Jung, K., Gillessen, S., Singer, S., Tanabe, K., Duda, R., Mentzer, S., Jaklitsch, M., Bueno, R., Clift, S., et al. (2003). Vaccination with irradiated, autologous melanoma cells engineered to secrete granulocyte-macrophage colony-stimulating factor by adenoviral-mediated gene transfer augments antitumor immunity in patients with metastatic melanoma. *J. Clin. Oncol.* **21,** 3343–3350.

Soiffer, R., Lynch, T., Mihm, M., Jung, K., Rhuda, C., Schmollinger, J., Hodi, F., Liebster, L., Lam, P., Mentzer, S., Singer, S., Tanabe, K., et al. (1998). Vaccination with irradiated, autologous melanoma cells engineered to secrete human granulocyte-macrophage colony stimulating factor generates potent anti-tumor immunity in patients with metastatic melanoma. *Proc. Natl. Acad. Sci. USA* **95,** 13141–13146.

Soiffer, R. T. L., Mihm, M., Jung, K., Kolesar, K., Liebster, L., Lam, P., Duda, R., Mentzer, S., Singer, S., Tanabe, K., Johnson, R., Sober, A., et al. (1997). A phase I study of vaccination with autologous, irradiated melanoma cells engineered to secrete human granulocyte-macrophage colony stimulating factor. *Hum. Gene Ther.* **8,** 111–123.

Srivastava, P. K. (1993). Peptide-binding heat shock proteins in the endoplasmic reticulum: Role in immune response to cancer and in antigen presentation. *Adv. Cancer Res.* **62,** 153–177.

Steinman, R. M., and Mellman, I. (2004). Immunotherapy: Bewitched, bothered, and bewildered no more. *Science* **305,** 197–200.

Supek, F., Supekova, L., Mandiyan, S., Pan, Y. C., Nelson, H., and Nelson, N. (1994). A novel accessory subunit for vacuolar H(+)-ATPase from chromaffin granules. *J. Biol. Chem.* **269,** 24102–24106.

Sutton, V. R., Davis, J. E., Cancilla, M., Johnstone, R. W., Ruefli, A. A., Sedelies, K., Browne, K. A., and Trapani, J. A. (2000). Initiation of apoptosis by granzyme B requires direct cleavage of bid, but not direct granzyme B-mediated caspase activation. *J. Exp. Med.* **192,** 1403–1414.

Tani, K., Azuma, M., Nakazaki, Y., Oyaizu, N., Hase, H., Ohata, J., Takahashi, K., OiwaMonna, M., Hanazawa, K., Wakumoto, Y., Kawai, K., Noguchi, M., et al. (2004). Phase I study of autologous tumor vaccines transduced with the GM-CSF gene in four patients with stage IV renal cell cancer in Japan: Clinical and immunological findings. *Mol. Ther.* **10,** 799–816.

Thomas, A. M., Santarsiero, L. M., Lutz, E. R., Armstrong, T. D., Chen, Y. C., Huang, L. Q., Laheru, D. A., Goggins, M., Hruban, R. H., and Jaffee, E. M. (2004). Mesothelin-specific CD8 (+) T cell responses provide evidence of *in vivo* cross-priming by antigen-presenting cells in vaccinated pancreatic cancer patients. *J. Exp. Med.* **200,** 297–306.

Thomas, D., Du, C., Xu, M., Wang, X., and Ley, T. (2000). DFF45/ICAD can be directly processed by granzyme B during the induction of apoptosis. *Immunity* **12,** 621–632.

Thompson, C. B., and Allison, J. P. (1997). The emerging role of CTLA-4 as an immune attenuator. *Immunity* **7,** 445–450.

Tivol, E. A., Borriello, F., Schweitzer, A. N., Lynch, W. P., Bluestone, J. A., and Sharpe, A. H. (1995). Loss of CTLA-4 leads to massive lymphoproliferation and fatal multiorgan tissue destruction, revealing a critical negative regulatory role of CTLA-4. *Immunity* **3,** 541–547.

Ueda, H., Howson, J. M., Esposito, L., Heward, J., Snook, H., Chamberlain, G., Rainbow, D. B., Hunter, K. M., Smith, A. N., Di Genova, G., Herr, M. H., Dahlman, I., et al. (2003). Association of the T-cell regulatory gene CTLA4 with susceptibility to autoimmune disease. *Nature* **423,** 506–511.

van der Bruggen, P., Traversari, C., Chomez, P., Lurquin, C., De Plaen, E., Van den Eynde, B., Knuth, A., and Boon, T. (1991). A gene encoding an antigen recognized by cytolytic T lymphocytes on a human melanoma. *Science* **254,** 1643–1647.

Van Der Bruggen, P., Zhang, Y., Chaux, P., Stroobant, V., Panichelli, C., Schultz, E. S., Chapiro, J., Van Den Eynde, B. J., Brasseur, F., and Boon, T. (2002). Tumor-specific shared antigenic peptides recognized by human T cells. *Immunol. Rev.* **188,** 51–64.

van Elsas, A., Hurwitz, A., and Allison, J. (1999). Combination immunotherapy of B16 melanoma using anti-cytotoxic T lymphocyte-associated antigen 4 (CTLA-4) and granulocyte/macrophage colony-stimulating factor (GM-CSF)-producing vaccines induces rejection of subcutaneous and metastatic tumors accompanied by autoimmune depigmentation. *J. Exp. Med.* **190,** 355–366.

van Elsas, A., Sutmuller, R. P., Hurwitz, A. A., Ziskin, J., Villasenor, J., Medema, J. P., Overwijk, W. W., Restifo, N. P., Melief, C. J., Offringa, R., and Allison, J. P. (2001). Elucidating the autoimmune and antitumor effector mechanisms of a treatment based on cytotoxic T lymphocyte antigen-4 blockade in combination with a B16 melanoma vaccine: Comparison of prophylaxis and therapy. *J. Exp. Med.* **194,** 481–489.

von Mensdorff-Pouilly, S., Verstraeten, A. A., Kenemans, P., Snijdewint, F. G., Kok, A., Van Kamp, G. J., Paul, M. A., Van Diest, P. J., Meijer, S., and Hilgers, J. (2000). Survival in early breast cancer patients is favorably influenced by a natural humoral immune response to polymorphic epithelial mucin. *J. Clin. Oncol.* **18,** 574–583.

Vonderheide, R. H., and June, C. H. (2003). A translational bridge to cancer immunotherapy: Exploiting costimulation and target antigens for active and passive T cell immunotherapy. *Immunol. Res.* **27,** 341–356.

Vucic, D., Franklin, M. C., Wallweber, H. J., Das, K., Eckelman, B. P., Shin, H., Elliott, L. O., Kadkhodayan, S., Deshayes, K., Salvesen, G. S., and Fairbrother, W. J. (2005). Engineering ML-IAP to produce an extraordinarily potent caspase 9 inhibitor: Implications for Smac-dependent anti-apoptotic activity of ML-IAP. *Biochem. J.* **385,** 11–20.

Vucic, D., Stennicke, H., Pisabarro, M., Salvesen, G., and Dixit, V. (2000). ML-IAP, a novel inhibitor of apoptosis that is preferentialy expressed in human melanomas. *Curr. Biol.* **10,** 1359–1366.

Wang, R., Parkhurst, M., Kawakami, Y., Robbins, P., and Rosenberg, S. (1996). Utilization of an alternative open reading frame of a normal gene in generating a novel human cancer antigen. *J. Exp. Med.* **183,** 1131–1140.

Wang, R.-F., Johnston, S., Zeng, G., Topalian, S. L., Schwartzentruber, D. J., and Rosenberg, S. (1998). A breast and melanoma-shared tumor antigen: T cell responses to antigenic peptides translated from different open reading frames. *J. Immunol.* **161,** 3596–3606.

Waterhouse, P., Penninger, J. M., Timms, E., Wakeham, A., Shahinian, A., Lee, K. P., Thompson, C. B., Griesser, H., and Mak, T. W. (1995). Lymphoproliferative disorders with early lethality in mice deficient in Ctla-4. *Science* **270,** 985–988.

Watts, T. H. (2005). TNF/TNFR family members in costimulation of T cell responses. *Annu. Rev. Immunol.* **23,** 23–68.

Wu, C., Yang, X.-F., McLaughlin, S., Neuberg, D., Canning, C., Stein, B., Alyea, E., Soiffer, R., Dranoff, G., and Ritz, J. (2000). Detection of a potent humoral response associated with immune-induced remission of chronic myelogenous leukemia. *J. Clin. Invest.* **106,** 705–714.

Yagihashi, A., Asanuma, K., Kobayashi, D., Tsuji, N., Shijubo, Y., Abe, S., Hirohashi, Y., Torigoe, T., Sato, N., and Watanabe, N. (2005a). Detection of autoantibodies to livin and survivin in sera from lung cancer patients. *Lung Cancer* **48,** 217–221.

Yagihashi, A., Asanuma, K., Tsuji, N., Torigoe, T., Sato, N., Hirata, K., and Watanabe, N. (2003). Detection of anti-livin antibody in gastrointestinal cancer patients. *Clin. Chem.* **49,** 1206–1208.

Yagihashi, A., Ohmura, T., Asanuma, K., Kobayashi, D., Tsuji, N., Torigoe, T., Sato, N., Hirata, K., and Watanabe, N. (2005b). Detection of autoantibodies to survivin and livin in sera from patients with breast cancer. *Clin. Chim. Acta* **362,** 125–130.

Yang, Y. F., Zou, J. P., Mu, J., Wijesuriya, R., Ono, S., Walunas, T., Bluestone, J., Fujiwara, H., and Hamaoka, T. (1997). Enhanced induction of antitumor T-cell responses by cytotoxic T lymphocyte-associated molecule-4 blockade: The effect is manifested only at the restricted tumor-bearing stages. *Cancer Res.* **57,** 4036–4041.

Yee, C., Thompson, J. A., Byrd, D., Riddell, S. R., Roche, P., Celis, E., and Greenberg, P. D. (2002). Adoptive T cell therapy using antigen-specific CD8+ T cell clones for the treatment of patients with metastatic melanoma: *In vivo* persistence, migration, and antitumor effect of transferred T cells. *Proc. Natl. Acad. Sci. USA* **99**, 16168–16173.

Young, J. W., and Inaba, K. (1996). Dendritic cells as adjuvants for class I major histocompatibility complex-restricted antitumor immunity. *J. Exp. Med.* **183**, 7–11.

Zagon, I. S., Verderame, M. F., Allen, S. S., and McLaughlin, P. J. (2000). Cloning, sequencing, chromosomal location, and function of cDNAs encoding an opioid growth factor receptor (OGFr) in humans. *Brain Res.* **856**, 75–83.

Zeng, R., Spolski, R., Finkelstein, S. E., Oh, S., Kovanen, P. E., Hinrichs, C. S., Pise-Masison, C. A., Radonovich, M. F., Brady, J. N., Restifo, N. P., Berzofsky, J. A., and Leonard, W. J. (2005). Synergy of IL-21 and IL-15 in regulating CD8+ T cell expansion and function. *J. Exp. Med.* **201**, 139–148.

Zhang, D., Beresford, P. J., Greenberg, A. H., and Lieberman, J. (2001). Granzymes A and B directly cleave lamins and disrupt the nuclear lamina during granule-mediated cytolysis. *Proc. Natl. Acad. Sci. USA* **98**, 5746–5751.

Zhang, L., Conejo-Garcia, J., Katsaros, D., Gimotty, P., Massobrio, M., Regnani, G., Makrigiannakis, A., Gray, H., Schlienger, K., Liebman, M., Rubin, S., and Coukos, G. (2003). Intratumoral T cells, recurrence, and survival in epithelial ovarian cancer. *N. Eng. J. Med.* **348**, 203–213.

INDEX

A

Activation-induced cell death (AICD), 107
Active immunization with differentiation antigens as altered self, 222
 with recombinant viruses expressing differentiation antigens, 225–226
 with syngeneic DNA linked to foreign sequences, 224–225
 with xenogeneic DNA, 223–224
Acute myeloid leukemia (AML), 110–111
Adalimumab, 94
ADCC. *See* Antibody, dependent cellular toxicity
Adenoviruses, 225
A20 (HA) tumors, 64
AICD. *See* Activation–induced cell death
Alemtuzumab, 101–103
Allogeneic hematopoietic stem cell transplantation (HSCT), 133
 approaches for characterizing donor T cells following, 144
 clinical evidence for GVL activity following, 139
 complexity of variables that influence outcome of, 135
 donor lymphocyte infusions induce GVL responses after, 141–143
 future directions, 158–160
 reconstitution of donor hematopoiesis following, 134–136
 sequence of immune reconstitution following, 136–138
 target antigens of donor T cells after, 146–150
Allogeneic stem cell graft, variables in, 135–136
Anoikis, 4, 5
Antibody(ies). *See also specific* antibody
 auto, 220

dependent cellular toxicity (ADCC), 84, 91
-directed enzyme prodrug therapy (ADEPT), 107–108
passive immunization with differentiation antigens against, 226–228
responses against tumor-associated antigens, 156
titers specific for 2 CML-associated tumor antigens, 157
toxin conjugates, 120
Anti-CTLA-4
 and chemotherapy, 321, 323
 and IL-2, 323
 mAb, 232
Antigenic targets, 85
Antigen(s), 52. *See also specific* antigens
 presenting cells (APC), 154, 178
Antitumor immune response, 9
ATP6S1, 348–349
Autoantibodies, 220
Autoimmune thyroiditis, 103
Autoimmunity, 217, 224
Autologous typing, 16
"Auto reactive" clones, 145
Avastin. *See* Bevacizumab

B

BALB-*Neu*T mice for mammary cancer study, 188–191
BAT antibody, 198
Bax/Bak proteins, 4
B-cell(s), 154–155
 tolerance to tumors, 56
Bevacizumab, 105–107
B7-H1, 185
Bimodal role of TGF-β in cancer, 61

Bispecific antibodies
    immunogenicity of, 96
B16 melanoma, 222
    cells, 229
Breast tumors, 101

C

CAMPATH series of anti-CD52
    antibodies, 101–102
CampathT. *See* Alemtuzumab
Cancer
    controlled by immune effector
        molecules
        cytokines, 20–22
        cytotoxic mediators: granule
            exocytosis, 25–26
        cytotoxictiy: TNF family death
            ligands, 26–28
        IFN-γ, 22–24
        Type I interferons, 24–25
    genetic instability in, 29
    immunoediting, 2, 7
        cellular and molecular model for, 9
        synopsis of tumor elimination phase
            of, 7–11
    Immunosurveillance Hypothesis, 5–7
    immunosurveillance/immunoediting in
        humans
        evidences to suggest, 32–35
    immunotherapy
        checkpoint blockade in, 298–299
        genetically engineered antibody fragments
            for, 95–96
        immunotoxins for treatment of,
            108–110
        gemtuzumab ozogamicin, 110–112
    recognition by immune cells, 16–20
    vaccine development, 265–266
CD25, 90
CD28, 301
    expression by mouse T cells
        B7.1, 302–303
        B7.2, 302–303
    T-cell responses, 301
CD33, 110
CD20 antigen, 96–97
Cd28:B7 immunoglobulin superfamily,
    extended, 300
Cd28/CTLA-4:B7.1/B7.2
    CD28, 301

CTLA-4 as a non cell-autonomous
    regulator: regulatory T cells and
    dendritic cells, 306, 308–310
CTLA-4 as a T cell intrinsic cell-
    autonomous negative
    regulator, 303–306
CD8+ CTL effector response, 178
CD8+ CTL tolerance, 178
CD4+ donor T cells, infusion of, 142–143
CD4+ melanoma-specific cytolytic CD4+ T
    cells, 182
CD94/NKG2, 150–151
CDR34, 350
CDT$^+$ CD25$^+$ Foxp3 expressing T regs, 89–90
CD8 T cell response evaluation, 250
CD4+ T cells, 224, 229
CD8 T cells, 69
CD8+ T cells, 136
CD8+ T cells, 10, 221
    adoptive transfer of, specific for
        differentiation antigens in adoptive
        immunotherapy, 228
    in immunization, role of, 224
CD4 T-cell tolerance, 63–64
Cell-contact mechanisms, 219
Cells. *See specific* cells
Centuximab
    effects on EGFR expressing cells, 103–105
Checkpoint blockade
    in cancer immunotherapy, 298–300
    in tumor immunotherapy
        adverse immune manifestations of CTLA-
            4 blockade, 316
        vaccination approaches, 310–311
        vaccination/CTLA-4 blockade
            model, 311–312
        other potential coinhibitory targets
            for, 323–328
Chemotherapeutic agents
    antibodies armed with, 107–108
Chemotherapy
    and anti-CTLA-4, 321, 323
    nonmyeloablative, 232
Chimeric antibodies, 85, 93
Chronic myelocytic leukemia (CML), 139
Coinhibition, 64–66
Cold antibody saturates CD20, 117
Coley's toxins, 5
Combination immunotherapy, 358
Complement-dependent cytotoxicity, 92

INDEX

Concomitant tumor immunity, 229–230
Costimulatory proteins, 343
C_pG deoxyoligonucleotide, benefits of, 180
CT7, 350
CTL. *See* Cytotoxic T-cell lymphocyte
CTLA-4, 219, 352–358
  anti-CTLA-4 mAb, 232
  blockade, 65–66, 311–312
  blockade in tumor immunotherapy, 312, 315–316
    adverse immune manifestations of, 316
  blockade of, 184, 228–229
  expression of, 88–89
  as a non cell-autonomous regulator: regulatory T cells and dendritic cells, 306
    blockade in cancer immunotherapy, 307
    regulatory mechanisms, 308–310
  and PD1 inhibitory receptors, blockade of, 88–89
  as a T cell intrinsic cell-autonomous negative regulator, 303
    engagement, effects of, 305–306
    expression of, 304–305
    interaction with B7.1, 304
CTLA-4 blockade, clinical trials of, 317
  adverse events, 318–319
  anti-CTLA- and chemotherapy, 321, 323
  anti-CTLA-4 and IL-2, 323
  specific trials
    monotherapy for malignant melanoma, 319–320
    monotherapy for renal cell carcinoma, 320
    and vaccines, 320–321
Cumulative incidence of chronic GVHD, 155
Cyclophosphamide, 185
  pretreatment, 265
Cytokine(s), 181
  antibodies armed with, 107
  release syndrome, 98
Cytotoxic agents, 91
Cytotoxicity: TNF family death ligands, 26–28
Cytotoxic mediators: granule exocytosis, 25–26
Cytotoxic T-cell lymphocyte (CTL)
  epitope vaccines, 177
  tolerization of, 178
Cytotoxic T-lymphocyte antigen-4. *See* CTLA-4
Cytotoxic T lymphocyte associated antigen-4. *See* CTLA-4

Cytotoxic T lymphocyte (CTL) antigen-4 antibody blockade, 352–358

D

Daclizumab, 85, 90
Death-inducing signaling complex (DISC), 3
Death receptors, 4
Dendritic cells (DC), 343
  activated Stat3 in, 62
  activation, independent pathways for, 179
  as adjuvants, 230
  dysfunction of, 58
  functional maturation of, 57–58
  immunotherapy, 233
  for tumor, 182–183
Differentiation antigens, 222
  active immunization with, 223–226
  passive immunization against, 226–228
Disabled antigen presenting cells, 62–63
DNA
  vaccination, 183
    factors effecting efficiency of, 193–196
    in HER2 mammary carcinogenesis, role of, 191–193
    limitations of, 196–199
  vaccines, 191–193, 223–224
Donor T cells, central role of, 143–146
Dormancy, 29. *See also* Immunoediting: when tumor cells survive

E

EC-TM plasmid
  electroporation, 195–196, 197, 199, 202–203
  immune reaction by, 204
  immunization, 201, 203
  injection, 191–193
Effector molecules mediating tumor suppression, 21
Electroporation, of EC-TM plasmid, 195–196
Endogenous host responses, 342–343
Enhanced green fluorescent protein (EGFP), 224–225
Enhancing tumor antigen presentation, 343–344
Epidermal growth factor (EGF), 104
  receptors (EGFR), 187
Exact MHC Class I binding peptide(s), 181
  vaccines, flaw in the design of, 177–178

F

FISH. *See* Fluorescence *in situ* hybridization
Fluorescence *in situ* hybridization (FISH), 100–101

G

Gemtuzumab ozogamicin, 110
  composition of, 111–112
  side effect of, 112
Genetic instability, 186
  in cancer, 29
Glucocorticoid-induced TNF receptor (GITR), 67
GM-CSF, 250
  secreting tumor cell vaccines, 344–347
Graft-*versus*-host disease (GVHD), 134, 146
Graft-*versus*-leukemia (GVL), 133, 140
  donor B cells as mediators of, 154–158
  donor natural killer cells as mediators of, 150–154
  effect, 138
Granulocyte-macrophage colony stimulating factor. *See* GM–CSF
Grave's disease. *See* Autoimmune thyroiditis
GVHD. *See* Graft-*versus*-host disease
GVL. *See* Graft-*versus*-leukemia

H

HA. *See* Hemagglutinin peptide
HAMA. *See* Human, -anti-mouse antibody
Heat-shock proteins (HSPs), 9
Hemagglutinin peptide (HA), 64
Hepatitis B virus (HBV), 183
Hepatitis C virus (HCV), 183
HER2
  lesions, cure *versus* control of, 204–205
  oncogene, 187–188, 191
  level of tumor, 99
HercepTest, 100
HerceptinT. *See* Trastuzumab
Heteroclitic peptides, 232
Heterodimeric receptor, 95
Histocompatibility antigens, 146–147
HLA. *See* Human, leukocyte antigen
Host immune system, mechanisms of, 30–31.
  See also Immunoediting: when cancer cells survive
Human
  -anti-mouse antibody (HAMA) responses, 93
    induction of, 118
  HER-2/*neu* (HER-2) protein, 98

leukocyte antigen (HLA), 136
minor histocompatibility antigens, 148
monoclonal antibody, 89
Humanized monoclonal antibody daclizumab (Zenapax), 94
Human papilloma virus (HPV) peptide, 178
HVEM, 328
Hypertension, risk of, 106–107
Hypopigmentation, 221

I

IFN-γ, 9, 10–11, 26
  -producing T cells, 183
IFN$_\alpha$, high-dose, 249
IgG, 95
IL-12, 23–24
IM-225, ErbituxT. *See* Centuximab
Immature myeloid cells (iMC), 59–60
Immune cells, cancer recognition by, 16–20
Immune effector molecules that control cancer
  cytokines, 20–22
  cytotoxicity: TNF family death ligands, 26–28
  cytotoxic mediators: granule exocytosis, 25–26
  IFN-γ, 22–24
  Type I interferons, 24–25
Immune evasion by tumors, categories of, 51
Immunization
  active, with differentiation antigens as altered self, 222
  with human DCT, 224
  human gp100 DNA, 224
  with recombinant adenoviruses, 225
  with recombinant viruses, 225–226
  with xenogeneic DNA, 223–224
  intramuscular, 226
  passive, with antibodies against differentiation antigens, 226
  with TA99 for tumor protection, 227
  with TA99-inducing vitiligo, 227–228
  smallpox, 224
  xenogeneic, 223–224
Immunoediting: when tumor cells survive
  equilibrium, 28
    possible outcomes for a tumor in, 29
  escape, 29–32
    activation of STAT3, 31
    basic categories, 30

INDEX

Immunogenecity
  comparison of, in vaccination with DC and vaccination with peptides in adjuvant, 250–251
  effect of vaccination with multipeptides and low-dose IL-2 on
    clinical results, 252
    immunologic results, 251–252
Immunoregulation, therapeutic interventions counteracting tumor-induced, 183–185
Immunosurveillance, 16
Immunotherapy
  adoptive, 228
  combination, 358
  with DCs, 233
Incomplete Freund's adjuvant (IFA), 177
Indolamine-2,3 dioxygenase (IDO), 60–61
Inhibitors of apoptosis (IAPs), 4
Innate and adaptive immunity, roles of
  NKT cells
    and other regulatory T cells, 12–13
    and $\gamma\delta^+$ T cells, 14–15
  other leukocytes, 15–16
  T cells, 11–12
Insulinoma, animal models of, 17–18
Interleukin (IL)
  -2 (IL-2), 231
  -12 (IL-12), 229
  therapy, 232
Intramuscular immunization, 226
"Intrinsic" tumorsuppressive mechanisms, 2
Iodine-131, 116
Irinotecan, fluorouracil, and leucovorin (IFL), 106–107

K

Keratinocytes of mouse, 222
Killer inhibitory receptors (KIR), 150
KIR ligand, 153

L

Lymphocyte(s)
  activation gene-3 (LAG-3), 192
  tumor infiltrating, 231–232
  vitiligo-infiltrating, 221
Lymphoproliferative autoimmunity, 64

M

Mammary cancer, 188–191
Mammary lesions, 204

in BALB-*neu* T mice, progression of rHER2, 188–189
Mass spectrometry, 246
MDP. *See* Melanocyte differentiation proteins
MDS. *See* Myelodysplasia
MDX-010, 320–321
Melanocyte differentiation proteins (MDP), 244
  -specific immune responses in tolerant mice enable control of tumor outgrowth
    immune responses to other MDP peptides and tumor control, 274–275
    tumor control in mTyr$_{369}$-tolerant mice after immunization with Tyr peptides, 273–274
Melanocytes, 219
  functions of, 220
Melanoma, 219
  antigens, 220
  associated peptides, 181
  -associated vitiligo, 221
    spontaneous, 230–231
  B16 melanoma, 222
  clinical trials in
    adoptive transfer of TILs, 231–232
    blockade of CTLA-4, 232
    vaccination with autologus DC, 233
  concurrent vitiligo and tumor immunity in, 221–222
  patients, 221
  peptides, 250
  regression, 244–245
Melanoma inhibitor
  of apoptosis protein, 350–352
  of apoptosis protein (ML-IAP), 350–352
MHC
  class I pathway, downregulation of, 52, 53
  expression, levels of, 54
Mice
  genetically modified, 185
  transgenic for the HER2 oncogene, 186–188
MIC proteins, 18–19
β2-Microglobulin, 53
Mitochondria, 3
mLAG-3Ig injection, 192
ML-IAP. *See* Melanoma inhibitor, of apoptosis protein
Monoclonal antibodies, 83–84
  approved for therapy of cancer, 86
  efficacy of, 93

Monoclonal antibodies (*continued*)
  mechanisms of action of, 91–92
  radionuclides cytokine armed with, 107
  systemic radioimmunotherapy with, 112–115
  targeting host immune cells, 87–88
  targeting nonneoplastic tissues, 85–87
  targeting of inhibitory cytokine
    TGF-β, 90–91
  targets of, in therapy of cancer, 85
Mouse autoimmune vitiligo, 222
MSC. *See* Myeloid suppressor cells
MT/*ret* transgenic mice, 230–231
Multipeptide vaccines
  effect of vaccination with, and low-dose IL-2 on immunogenecity
    clinical results, 252
    immunologic results, 251–252
  expanding the repertoire of melanoma reactivity using, 252–253
  improvement in breadth and magnitude of T-cell by twelve-peptide vaccines, 254–258
  long-term survivor of metastatic melanoma developed spontaneous shift of repertoire of CD8 T cell for melanoma antigens, 254
Murine
  anti-VEGF monoclonal antibody A6.4.1, 105
  models, 65, 143
  monoclonal antibodies
    ibritumomab tiuxetan, 115–116
    limitations of, 92
    ositumomab, 115–116
Murine Model to evaluate immunity to the MDP-derived peptide Ag From tyrosinase, 266–267
Muromonab-CD3 (Orthoclone OKT-3), 92
Myelodysplasia (MDS), 135
Myeloid suppressor cells (MSC), 59–60
MYLOTARGT; CMA-676. *See* Gemtuzumab ozogamicin

N

Natural killer (NK) cells, 136, 224, 227
  inhibition of, 151
Neonatal Fc receptor (FcRn), 94–95
Neoplastic stem cells, 204
Neo-vascularization bevacizumab (Avastin™), 85
NFκB signaling, 55

NK cell lytic function, 151–152
NKT cells, 9, 14
Non-Hodgkin's lymphoma (NHL), 83, 92
Nonmyeloablative chemotherapy, 232

O

OGFr. *See* Opioid growth factor receptor
Oncogenes, 4
Opioid growth factor receptor (OGFr), 349–350

P

P53, 41
Paraneoplastic neurologic disorders/degenerations (PNDs), 33–34
Passive immunization with antibodies against differentiation antigens, 226
  cellular and molecular requirements for TA99-induced tumor-protection, 227
  cellular and molecular requirements for TA99-induced vitiligo, 227–228
Peptide-pulsed exogenous DC
  influence on T-cell avidity, response magnitude, and tumor control, 279–282
  overcoming the limited antitumor immune response in individual LN, 277–279
  route of immunization for determining location of T-cell activation and antitumor efficacy, 275–277
Peptide(s)
  ELISPOT assays, 144
  heteroclitic, 232
  vaccines; *See also* Multipeptide vaccines; Twelve-peptide vaccine
    for cancer, 181–182
    long, 180
    not previously tested in humans, 255–257
    synthetic MHC-associated, 246–248; *See also* Multipeptide vaccines
Perforin (pfp), 25
p185^{neu}, 187–188, 201
Preneoplastic lesion, 202
Preventive vaccination, 177
Primary cell death, 2–4
Proapoptotic effectors, 4
Programmed cell death-1, 89
Programmed death 1 (PD1), 65
Proinflammatory chemokine genes, 58
Proinflammatory cytokines/chemokines, 55

INDEX 375

Propagation-incompetent alphavirus vectors. *See* Virus–like replicon particles
Prophylaxis, 103
Proteins, melanocyte differentiation, 244

R

Radioimmunotherapy, targets for systemic, 113
Radiolabeled monoclonal antibodies, 113
Radiolabeled tositumomab, 116
Radionuclides emitting alpha particles, 115
RAG-2, 11–12, 23
Recombinant viruses for immunization, 225–226
Regulatory T cells, 63, 67
r-HER2 lesions in mammary gland of BALB-*neu* T mice, progression of, 188–189
Rheumatoid arthritis, 103
Rituxan, MabTheraT. *See* Rituximab
Rituximab, 96
   efficacy of, 97–98

S

Scurfin, 90
Self-antigens, 216
   overcome ignorance or tolerance to, 217–219
   strategies to overcome ignorance or tolerance to, 218
Self-major histocompatability complex (MHC), 299
Self-proteins, 299
Self-tolerance to $m\text{Tyr}_{369}$ and its effect on tumor control, nature of
   controlled entry of activated Tyr-specific CD8 T cells into skin, 271–272
   deletion of $m\text{Tyr}_{369}$-specific CD8 cells by Ag encounter in peripheral LN, 267–268
   endogenous Tyr presentation by radioresistant antigen presenting cells, 268–271
   residual repertoire of Tyr-specific T cells in Tyr^+ mice, 271
   self-tolerance to Tyr impairs control of B16-AAD tumor outgrowth, 273
Sentinel-immunized node (SIN), evaluation of immune responses in, 250
Serological expression cloning technique (SEREX), 17

Sf9 insect cells, 222
SIN. *See* Sentinel-immunized node
Single nucleotide polymorphisms (SNP), 147
Smallpox immunization, 224
Spectrum of target antigens, 150
Spontaneous melanoma-associated vitiligo, 230–231
Spontaneous regression/complete remission (SR/CR) phenotype, 15
Sporadic tumors, 183
Stat3 pathway, 56–58
Steroid, 318
Surface receptors, 223
SV40 large T viral oncoprotein, 183
Synthetic MHC-associated peptide vaccines, 246–248
Synthetic peptide-based cancer vaccines, clinical trials with, 181–182

T

TA99, 226
   immunization with, for tumor protection, 227
TAM. *See* Tumor, -associated macrophages
TAP genes, downmodulation of, 53
Targets of vaccine-induced tumor destruction, 347
   ATP6S1, 348–349
   melanoma inhibitor of apoptosis protein, 350–352
   opioid growth factor receptor, 349–350
T-cell regulatory function, modulation of, 260–265
T-cell responses by combination of CD4 and CD8 T-cell vaccination, modulation of, 260
   immunogenicity and clinical benefit of vaccination with a mixture of 6 melanoma helper peptides, 261
   preliminary clinical outcomes, 264
   preliminary immunologic findings, 262–264
   trial design for evaluation of MHP in combination vaccines for patients with advanced melanoma (E1602), 264
   trial design for evaluation of MHP in combination with cyclophosphamide for melanoma patients in the adjuvant setting (Mel44), 264

T-cell responses by combination of CD4 and
    CD8 T-cell vaccination, modulation of
    (*continued*)
  effects of cyclophosphamide
    pretreatment, 265
  vaccination with helper peptide
    mixtures, 265
T cell(s), 9, 51–52, 198, 218–219
  CD4+ T cells, 224, 229
  CD8+ T cells, 221
  overcoming effects of suppressor
    populations of, 229–230
  receptor (TCR), 137–138, 217
  response to class I MHC restricted peptides,
    ex vivo analysis of, 259–260
TGF-β, 90–91
Thymic T cells, analysis of, 63
TIL. *See* Tumor, infiltrating lymphocytes
Tissue disruption, 55
TLR ligands, 181
Toxins
  antibodies armed with, 107
  conjugates, 112
Transforming growth factor beta (TGF-β), 61–62
Trastuzumab, 99–101
  and breast cancer, 98
Trastuzumab therapy, 100
Treg, 13
  cells, *See* T cells
  markers, 67
T regs. *See* T regulatory cells
T regulatory cells (T regs), 89–90
Tumor(s). *See also specific* Tumors
  antigen(s), 245–246
    categories of, 17
  load, 70
  antigen presentation
    downmodulation of, 52–55
    enhancing, 343–344
  -associated antigens (TAA), 54, 134, 145
  -associated macrophages (TAM), 60
  B-cell tolerance to, 56
  cells, 91
    malignant phenotype of, 299–300
  elimination, 55
  immune effector molecules that control
    cancer, 20–28
  phase, synopsis of, 7–11
  recognition of cancer by immune
    cells, 16–20

  roles of innate and adaptive
    immunity, 11–16
  immune recognition of, 52
  immunity, 224
    from autoimmunity, mechanisms of
      uncoupling, 233
  immunosurveillance, 22
  -induced immunoregulation, therapeutic
    interventions counteracting, 183–185
  infiltrating lymphocytes (TIL), 231–232
  microenvironment
    immunologic barriers within, 55–62
    multiple immunologic checkpoints in, 57
  model, effect of cyclophosphamide in, 68
  necrosis factor apoptosisinducing ligand
    (TRAIL), 26–27
  necrosis factor 2 (TNF2), 91
  protection, coordinated low-avidity
    mechanisms for, 199–203
  -specific antigens, 150
  suppression, effector molecules
    mediating, 21
  suppressors, 2–5
  tolerance, 51–52
Twelve-peptide vaccine (12 MP vaccine), 254
  competition for binding to class I MHC
    molecules does not diminish CD8
    T–cell responses to lower affinity
    peptides, 257–258
  immunogenic peptides not previously tested
    in humans, 255–257
  result of vaccination with mixtures of, 255
Type I interferons, 24–25
Tyrosine kinases, 187
TYRP1 DNA, 224

U

Unique antigens, 216
Unmodified monoclonal antibodies
  alemtuzumab, 101–103
  bevacizumab, 105–107
  centuximab, 103–105
  rituximab, 96–98
  trastuzumab, 98–101

V

Vaccination
  with autologus DCs, 233
  comparison of immunogenecity between DC
    and peptides in adjuvant, 250–251

with cytotoxic T-cell lymphocytes
    (CTL), 177
DNA, 183
    factors effecting efficiency of,
        193–196
    in HER2 mammary carcinogenesis, role
        of, 191–193
    limitations of, 196–199
    with exact MHC class I binding
        peptides, 177–178
    with heteroclitic peptides, 232
    with long peptides, 178–179
        with overlapping 32–35 amino acid long
            peptides, 180
    with single melanoma peptide and
        nonspecific helper peptide in
        adjuvant, 248
        immunization gp100$_{280-288}$ and
            tetanus peptides induces CD8
            and CD4 immune responses
            in the blood,
            248–249
        survival results of, 249

Vaccines
    cytotoxic T-cell lymphocytes (CTL)
        epitope, 177
    DNA, 191–193
    exact MHC Class I binding
        peptide, 177–178, 181
    synthetic peptide-based cancer, 181–182
Vaccinia virus, 224
Vascular endothelial growth factor
    (VEGF), 105–106
Virus-induced malignancies, 32
Virus–induced tumors. *See* Sporadic tumors
Virus-like replicon particles (VRP), 226
Vitiligo, 219–220
    -infiltrating lymphocytes, 221
    mouse autoimmune, 222
VRP. *See* Virus-like replicon particles

X

Xenogeneic immunization, 223–224

Y

Yttrium-90 ibritumomab tiuxetan, 116

Contents of Recent Volumes

Volume 80

Protein Degradation and the
  Generation of MHC Class
  I-Presented Peptides
  Kenneth L. Rock, Ian A. York,
  Tomo Saric, and Alfred L. Goldberg

Proteoanalysis and Antigen
  Presentation by MHC Class
  II Molecules
  Paula Wolf Bryant,
  Ana-Maria Lennon-Duménil,
  Edda Fiebiger, Cécile Lagaudriére-Gesbert,
  and Hidde L. Ploegh

Cytokine Memory of T Helper Lymphocytes
  Max Löhning, Anne Richter, and
  Andreas Radbruch

Ig Gene Hypermutation:
  A Mechanism Is Due
  Jean-Claude Weill, Barbara Bertocci,
  Ahmad Faili, Said Aoufouchi,
  Stéphane Frey, Annie De Smet,
  Sébastian Storck, Auriel Dahan,
  Frédéric Delbos, Sandra Weller,
  Eric Flatter, and Claude-Agnés Reynaud

Generalization of Single
  Immunological Experiences
  by Idiotypically Mediated
  Clonal Connections
  Hilmar Lemke and Hans Lange

The Aging of the Immune System
  B. Grubeck-Loebenstein and
  G. Wick

Index

Volume 81

Regulation of the Immune Response by
  the Interaction of Chemokines and
  Proteases
  Jo Van Damme and Sofie Struyf

Molecular Mechanisms of
  Host-Pathogen Interaction: Entry
  and Survival of Mycobacteria in
  Macrophages
  Jean Pieters and John Gatfield

B Lymphoid Neoplasms of Mice:
  Characteristics of Naturally Occurring and
  Engineered Diseasse and Relationships to
  Human disorders
  Herbert Morse et al.

Prions and the Immune System:
  A Journey Through Gut Spleen,
  and Nerves
  Adriano Aguzzi

Roles of the Semaphorin Family in
  Immune Regulation
  H. Kikutani and A. Kumanogoh

HLA-G Molecules: from Maternal-Fetal
  Tolerance to Tissue Acceptance
  Edgardo Carosella et al.

The Zebrafish as a Model Organism to Study
  Development of the Immune System
  Nick Trede et al.

Control of Autoimmunity by
  Naturally Arising Regulatory
  CD4+ T Cells
  S. Sakaguchi

Index

Human Models of Inherited Immunoglobulin
  Class Switch Recombination and Somatic
  Hypermutation Defects (Hyper-IgM
  Syndromes)
  Anne Durandy, Patrick Revy, and
  Alain Fischer

The Biological Role of the C1 Inhibitor
  in Regulation of Vascular Permeability
  and Modulation of Inflammation
  Alvin E. Davis, III, Shenghe Cai,
  and Dongxu Liu

Index

Volume 82

Transcriptional Regulation in Neutrophils:
  Teaching Old Cells New Tricks
  Patrick P. McDonald

Tumor Vaccines
  Freda K. Stevenson, Jason Rice, and
  Delin Zhu

Immunotherapy of Allergic Disease
  R. Valenta, T. Ball, M. Focke,
  B. Linhart, N. Mothes,
  V. Niederberger, S. Spitzauer,
  I. Swoboda, S.Vrtala, K. Westritschnic, and
  D. Kraft

Interactions of Immunoglobulins Outside the
  Antigen-Combining Site
  Roald Nezlin and Victor Ghetie

The Roles of Antibodies in Mouse Models of
  Rheumatoid Arthritis, and Relevance to
  Human Disease
  Paul A. Monach, Christophe Benoist, and
  Diane Mathis

MUC1 Immunology: From Discovery to
  Clinical Applications
  Anda M. Vlad, Jessica C. Kettel,
  Nehad M. Alajez, Casey A. Carlos, and
  Olivera J. Finn

Volume 83

Lineage Commitment and Developmental
  Plasticity in Early Lymphoid
  Progenitor Subsets
  David Traver and Koichi Akashi

The CD4/CD8 Lineage Choice: New Insights
  into Epigenetic Regulation during T Cell
  Development
  Ichiro Taniuchi, Wilfried Ellmeier, and
  Dan R. Littman

CD4/CD8 Coreceptors in Thymocyte
  Development, Selection, and Lineage
  Commitment: Analysis of the CD4/CD8
  Lineage Decision
  Alfred Singer and Remy Bosselut

Development and Function of T Helper 1 Cells
  Anne O'Garra and Douglas Robinson

Th2 Cells: Orchestrating Barrier Immunity
  Daniel B. Stetson, David Voehringer,
  Jane L. Grogan, Min Xu, R. Lee Reinhardt,
  Stefanie Scheu, Ben L. Kelly, and
  Richard M. Locksley

Generation, Maintenance, and Function of
  Memory T Cells
  Patrick R. Burkett, Rima Koka,
  Marcia Chien, David L. Boone, and
  Averil Ma

CD8⁺ Effector Cells
  Pierre A. Henkart and Marta Catalfamo

An Integrated Model of Immunoregulation Mediated by Regulatory T Cell Subsets
  Hong Jiang and Leonard Chess

Index

Volume 84

Interactions Between NK Cells and B Lymphocytes
  Dorothy Yuan

Multitasking of Helix-Loop-Helix Proteins in Lymphopoiesis
  Xiao-Hong Sun

Customized Antigens for Desensitizing Allergic Patients
  Fátima Ferreira,
  Michael Wallner, and
  Josef Thalhamer

Immune Response Against Dying Tumor Cells
  Laurence Zitvogel, Noelia Casares,
  Marie O. Pëquignot,
  Nathalie Chaput,
  Mathew L. Albert,
  and Guido Kroemer

HMGB1 in the Immunology of Sepsis (Not Septic Shock) and Arthritis
  Christopher J. Czura,
  Huan Yang,
  Carol Ann Amella, and
  Kevin J. Tracey

Selection of the T-Cell Repertoire: Receptor-Controlled Checkpoints in T-Cell Development
  Harald Von Boehmer

The Pathogenesis of Diabetes in the NOD Mouse
  Michelle Solomon and
  Nora Sarvetnick

Index

Volume 85

Cumulative Subject Index
Volumes 66–82

Volume 86

Adenosine Deaminase Deficiency: Metabolic Basis of Immune Deficiency and Pulmonary Inflammation
  Michael R. Blackburn and
  Rodney E. Kellems

Mechanism and Control of V(D)J Recombination Versus Class Switch Recombination: Similarities and Differences
  Darryll D. Dudley, Jayanta Chaudhuri, Craig H. Bassing, and Frederick W. Alt

Isoforms of Terminal Deoxynucleotidyltransferase: Developmental Aspects and Function
  To-Ha Thai and John F. Kearney

Innate Autoimmunity
  Michael C. Carroll and V. Michael Holers

Formation of Bradykinin: A Major Contributor to the Innate Inflammatory Response
  Kusumam Joseph and Allen P. Kaplan

Interleukin-2, Interleukin-15, and Their Roles in Human Natural Killer Cells
  Brian Becknell and Michael A. Caligiuri

Regulation of Antigen Presentation and Cross-Presentation in the Dendritic Cell Network: Facts, Hypothesis, and Immunological Implications
Nicholas S. Wilson and Jose A. Villadangos

Index

Volume 87

Role of the LAT Adaptor in T-Cell Development and T_h2 Differentiation
Bernard Malissen, Enrique Aguado, and Marie Malissen

The Integration of Conventional and Unconventional T Cells that Characterizes Cell-Mediated Responses
Daniel J. Pennington, David Vermijlen, Emma L. Wise, Sarah L. Clarke, Robert E. Tigelaar, and Adrian C. Hayday

Negative Regulation of Cytokine and TLR Signalings by SOCS and Others
Tetsuji Naka, Minoru Fujimoto, Hiroko Tsutsui, and Akihiko Yoshimura

Pathogenic T-Cell Clones in Autoimmune Diabetes: More Lessons from the NOD Mouse
Kathryn Haskins

The Biology of Human Lymphoid Malignancies Revealed by Gene Expression Profiling
Louis M. Staudt and Sandeep Dave

New Insights into Alternative Mechanisms of Immune Receptor Diversification
Gary W. Litman, John P. Cannon, and Jonathan P. Rast

The Repair of DNA Damages/Modifications During the Maturation of the Immune System: Lessons from Human Primary Immunodeficiency Disorders and Animal Models

Patrick Revy, Dietke Buck, Françoise le Deist, and Jean-Pierre de Villartay

Antibody Class Switch Recombination: Roles for Switch Sequences and Mismatch Repair Proteins
Irene M. Min and Erik Selsing

Index

Volume 88

CD22: A Multifunctional Receptor That Regulates B Lymphocyte Survival and Signal Transduction
Thomas F. Tedder, Jonathan C. Poe, and Karen M. Haas

Tetramer Analysis of Human Autoreactive CD4-Positive T Cells
Gerald T. Nepom

Regulation of Phospholipase C-γ2 Networks in B Lymphocytes
Masaki Hikida and Tomohiro Kurosaki

Role of Human Mast Cells and Basophils in Bronchial Asthma
Gianni Marone, Massimo Triggiani, Arturo Genovese, and Amato De Paulis

A Novel Recognition System for MHC Class I Molecules Constituted by PIR
Toshiyuki Takai

Dendritic Cell Biology
Francesca Granucci, Maria Foti, and Paola Ricciardi-Castagnoli

The Murine Diabetogenic Class II Histocompatibility Molecule I-A^{g7}: Structural and Functional Properties and Specificity of Peptide Selection
Anish Suri and Emil R. Unanue

RNAi and RNA-Based Regulation of Immune
  System Function
  Dipanjan Chowdhury and
  Carl D. Novina

Index

Volume 89

Posttranscriptional Mechanisms Regulating
  the Inflammatory Response
  Georg Stoecklin Paul Anderson

Negative Signaling in Fc Receptor Complexes
  Marc Daëron and Renaud Lesourne

The Surprising Diversity of Lipid Antigens for
  CD1-Restricted T Cells
  D. Branch Moody

Lysophospholipids as Mediators of Immunity
  Debby A. Lin and Joshua A. Boyce

Systemic Mastocytosis
  Jamie Robyn and Dean D. Metcalfe

Regulation of Fibrosis by the Immune System
  Mark L. Lupher, Jr. and W. Michael Gallatin

Immunity and Acquired Alterations in
  Cognition and Emotion: Lessons from SLE
  Betty Diamond, Czeslawa Kowal,
  Patricio T. Huerta, Cynthia Aranow,
  Meggan Mackay, Lorraine A. DeGiorgio,
  Ji Lee, Antigone Triantafyllopoulou,
  Joel Cohen-Solal Bruce, and T. Volpe

Immunodeficiencies with Autoimmune
  Consequences
  Luigi D. Notarangelo, Eleonora Gambineri,
  and Raffaele Badolato

Index

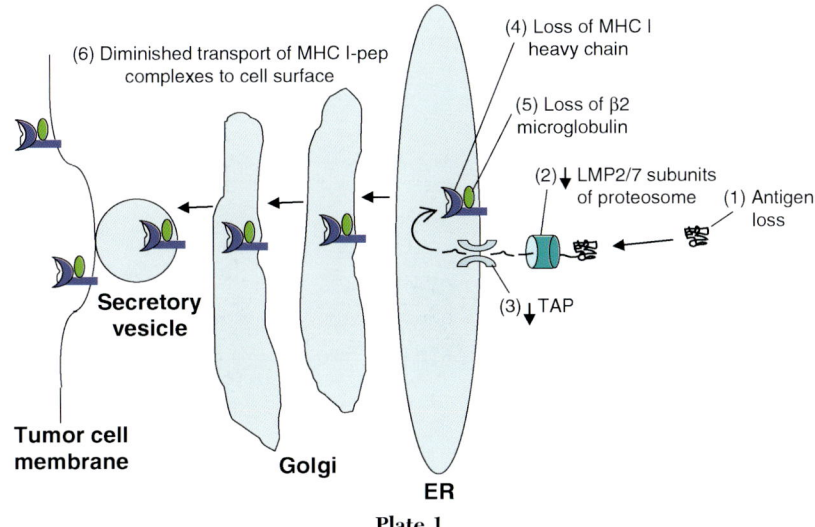

Plate 1

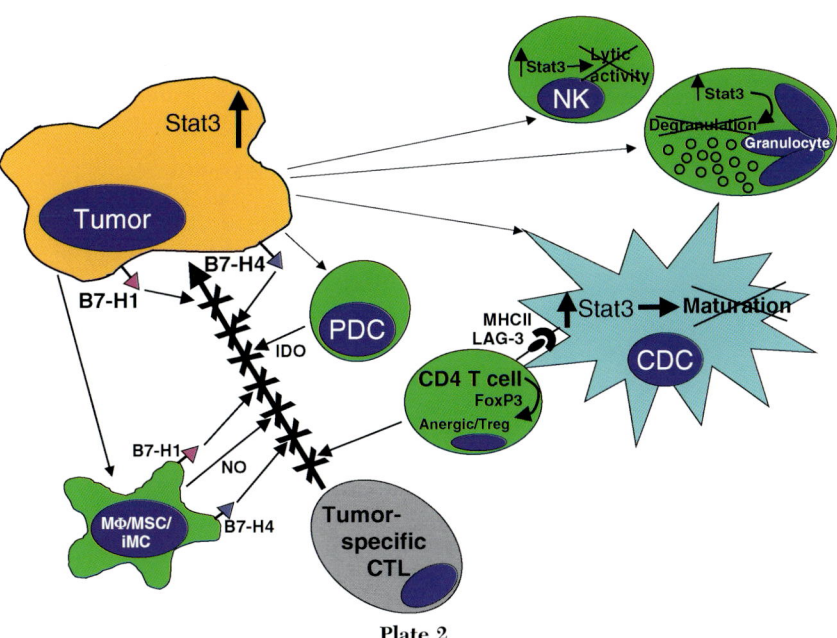

Plate 2

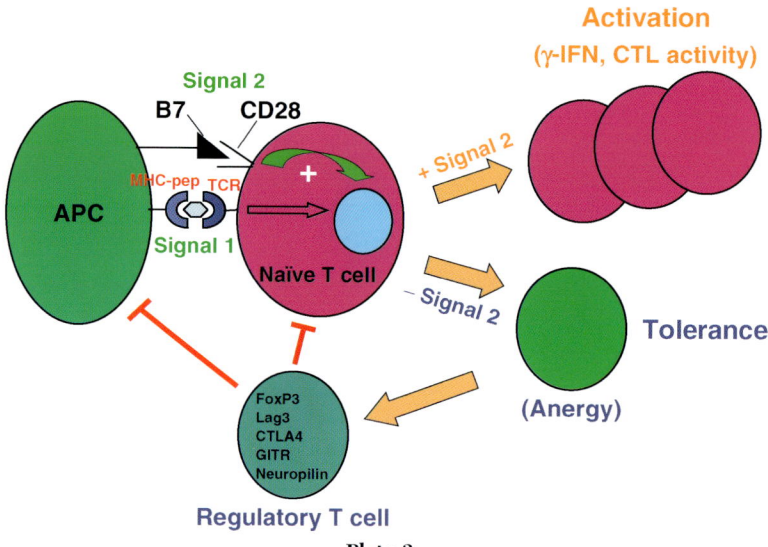

Plate 3

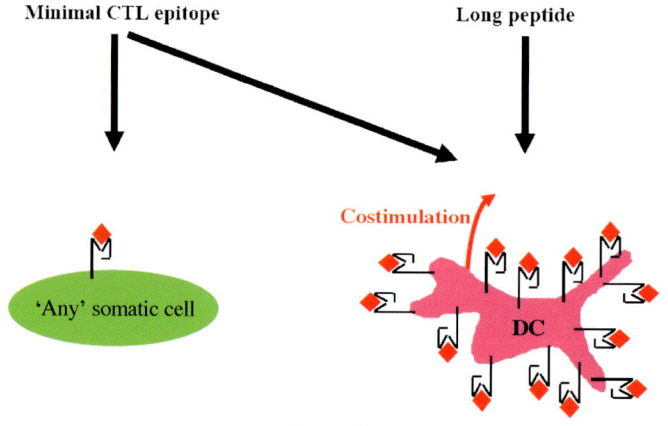

Plate 4

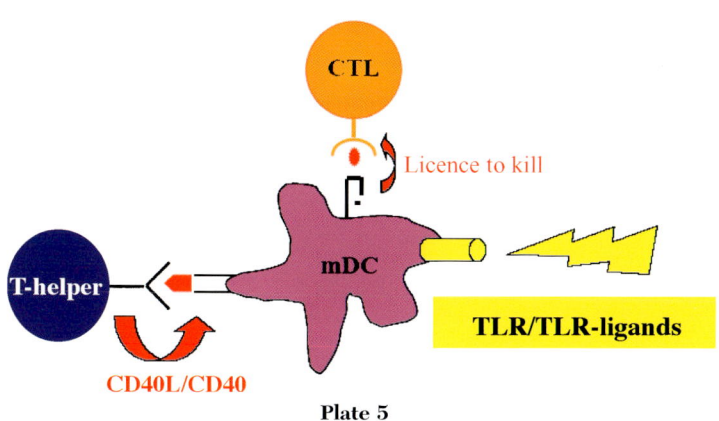

Plate 5

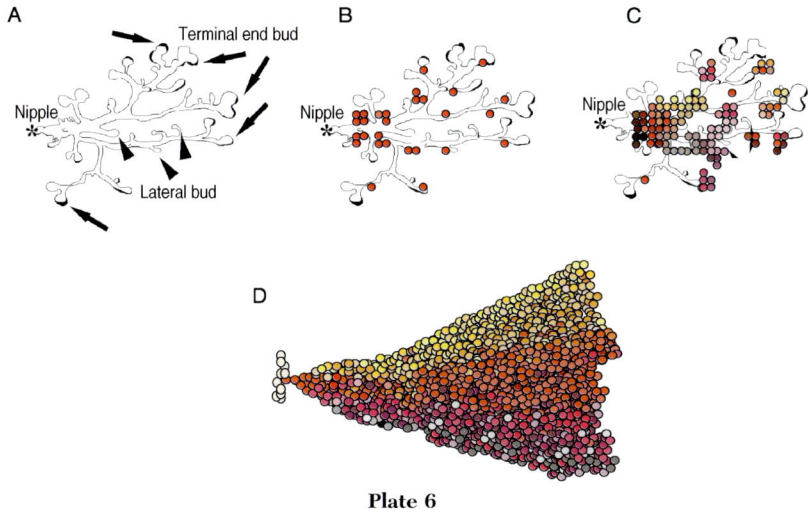

Plate 6

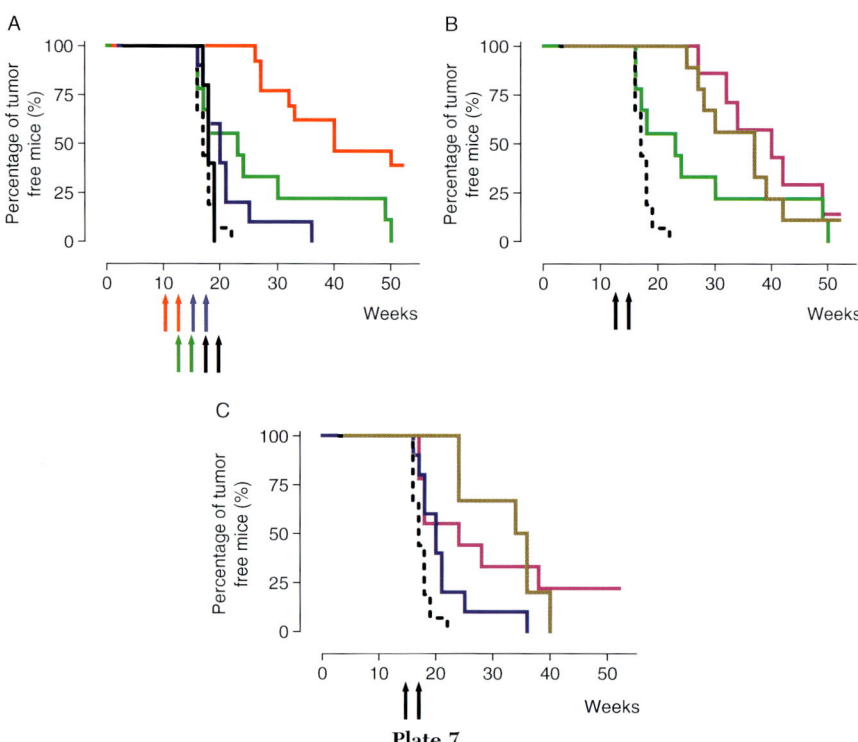

Plate 7

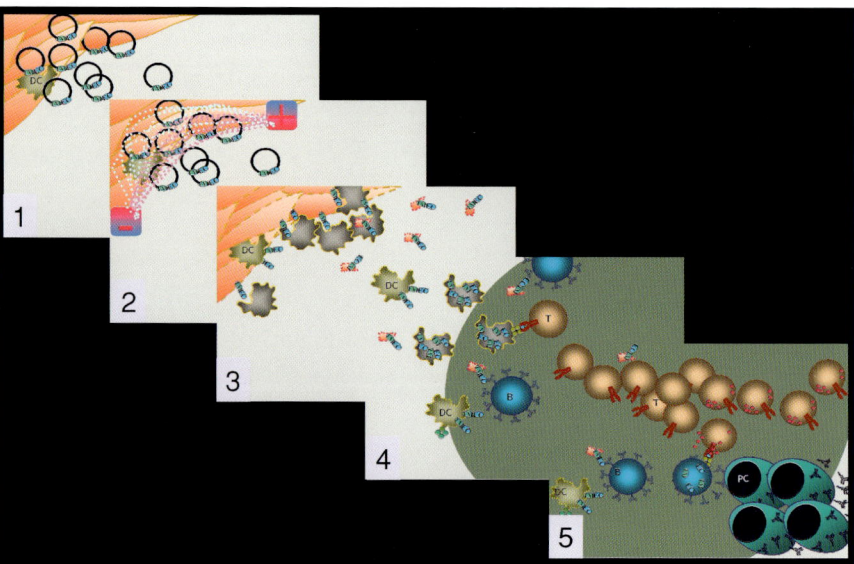

Plate 8

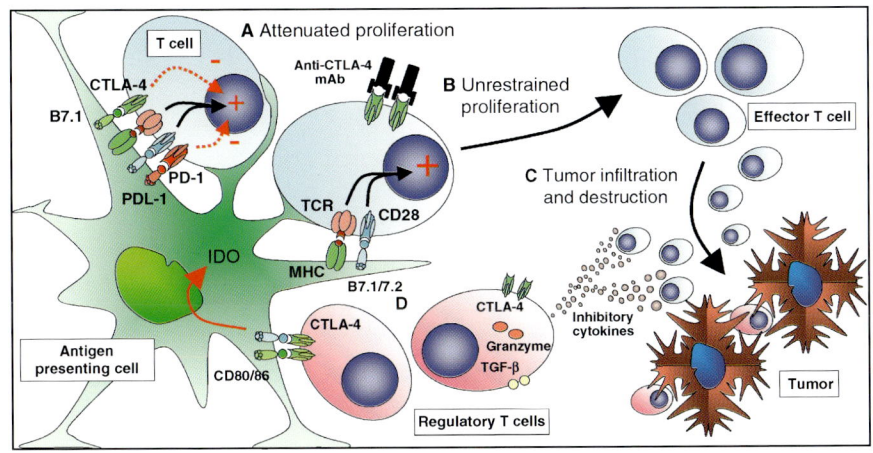

Plate 9

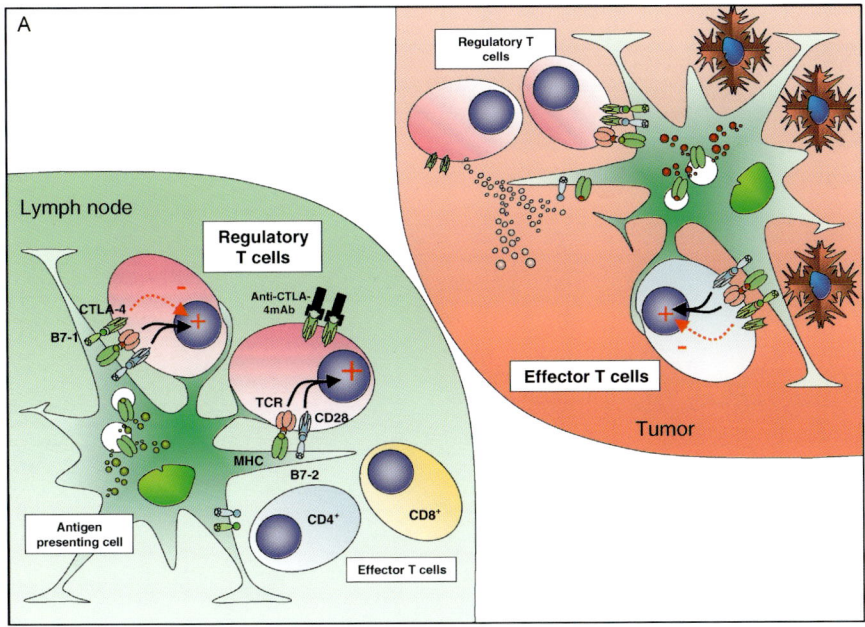

Plate 10 (Continued)

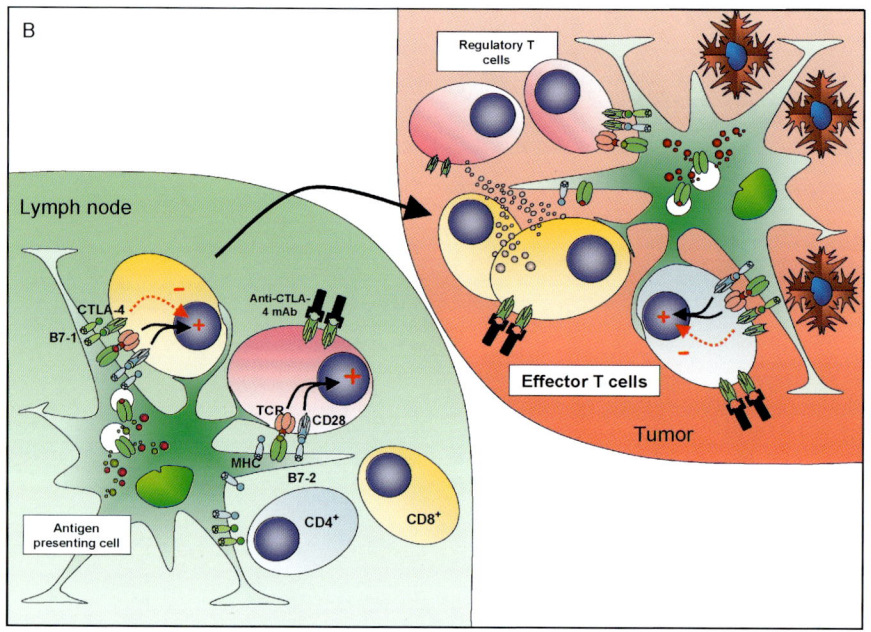

Plate 10

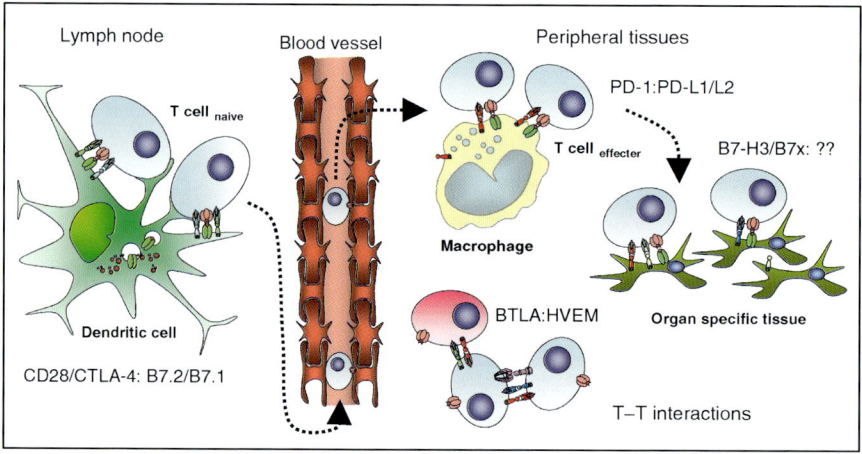

Plate 11

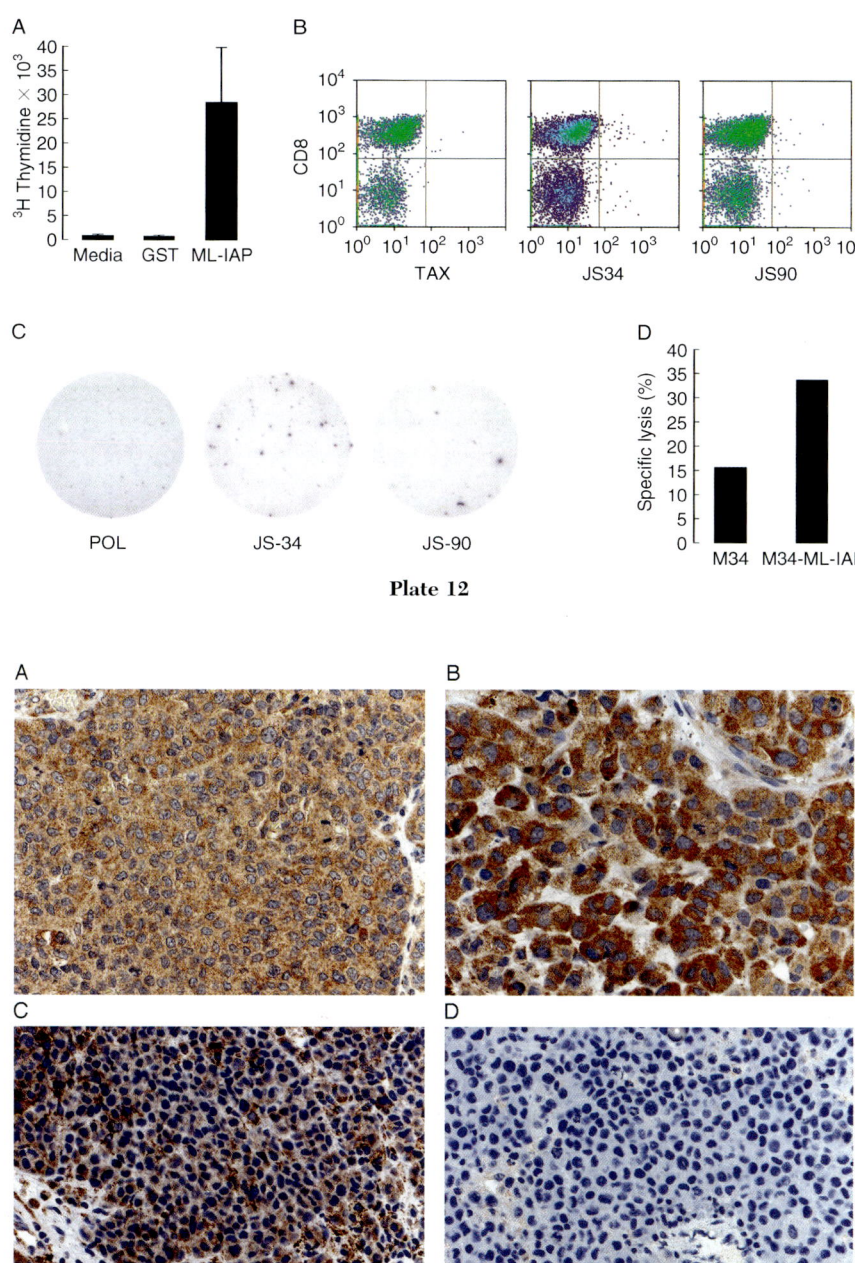

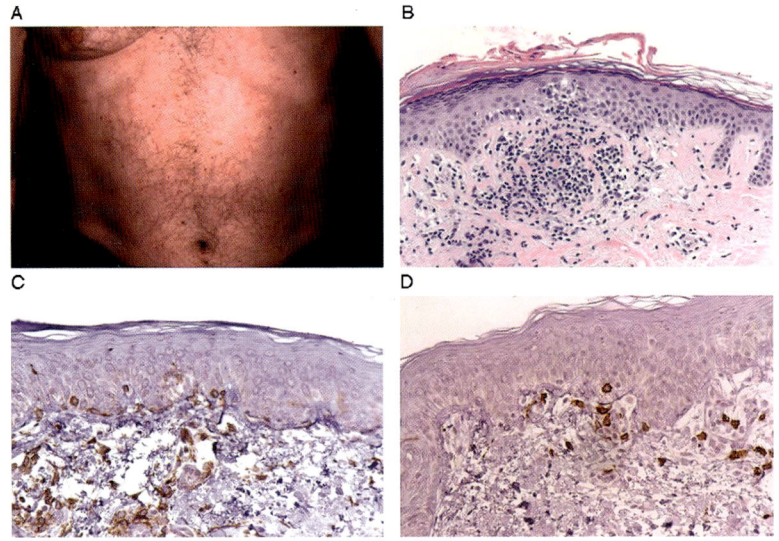

Plate 14

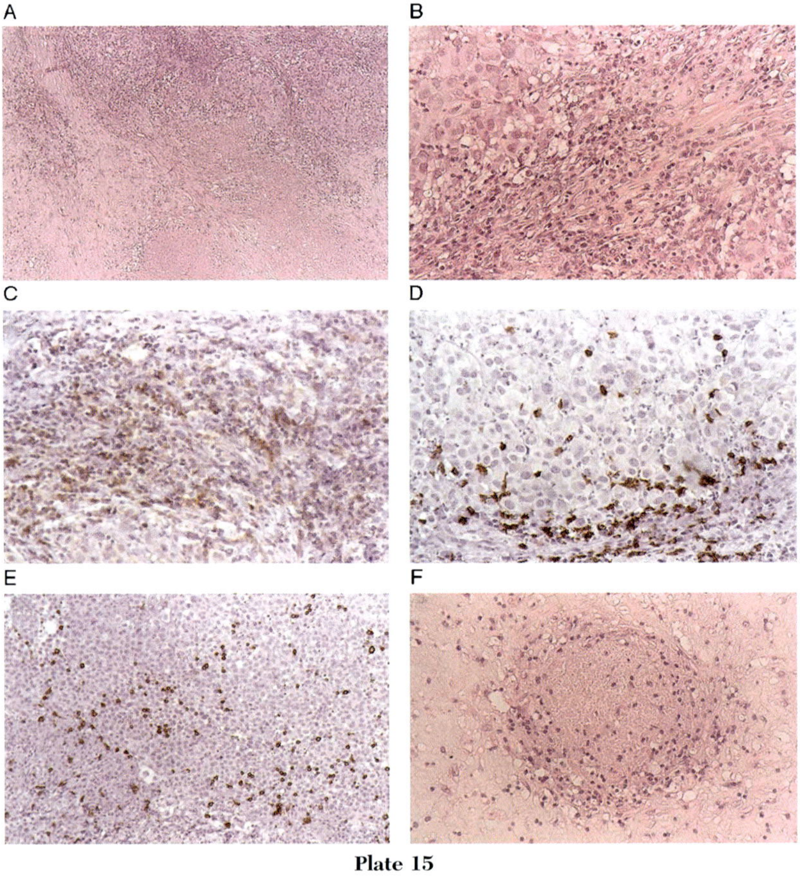

Plate 15